Cutting-Edge Therapies for *Autism*

2011–2012

Ken Siri and Tony Lyons

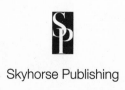

Skyhorse Publishing

This book is for Lina, Alex, and all the kids suffering from autism, and for their parents struggling to give them the best possible life.

ACKNOWLEDGEMENTS

Ken and Tony are deeply indebted to in-house Skyhorse Publishing editor Joey Sverchek, without whom we could not possibly have completed this project. We are also indebted to Teri Arranga of AutismOne who spent countless hours going over the manuscript, the jacket, and the press release and gave us excellent editorial advice.

Tony would like to thank his ex-wife Helena who has worked with Lina to the brink of insanity, utilizing many of the therapies described in this book, staying up with her when she can't sleep, calming her down when she is disregulated, holding, comforting, and carrying her, joining and engaging with her and giving her as much love as any human being has ever received from another human being. She is pulling Lina with both hands out of the abyss of autism.

Ken would like to thank his parents, Ken and Carole, for standing by him and Alex and for all their support and guidance.

CONTENTS

Foreword *by Rita Shreffler* ix

Preface *by Ken Siri and Tony Lyons* xi

Introduction Navigating the Autism SuperHighway: How To Determine If a Therapy Is Right for Your Child and Family xix

THERAPIES

1. Allergy Desensitization: An Effective Alternative Treatment for Autism
   by Dr. Darin Ingels 2

2. Allergy-Like Symptoms, Blood-Brain Barrier Disruption, and Brain Inflammation *by Dr. Theoharis Theoharides* 6

3. Animals in the Lives of Persons with Autism Spectrum Disorder(ASD): Companions to Co-Therapists *by Dr. Aubrey Fine* 12

4. Antiepileptic Treatments *by Dr. Richard E. Frye* 23

5. Antifungal Treatment *by Dr. Lewis Mehl-Madrona* 28

6. Applied Behavior Analysis: What Makes a Great ABA Program? Sorting Through the Science, the Brands, and the Acronyms *by Dr. Jonathan Tarbox and Dr. Doreen Granpeesheh* 35

7. Aquatic Therapy *by Andrea Salzman* 42

8. Architecture and Autism: Providing Supports for the Autistic Child or Adult Through the Built Environment *by Cathy Purple Cherry* 48

9. Art Therapy Approaches to Treating Autism *by Nicole Martin and Dr. Donna Betts* 56

10. Berard Auditory Integration Training *by Sally Brockett* 61

11. Biofilm Protocol *by Ken Siri* 66

12. Breaking Through Behavior *by Alison Berkley and Amanda Friedman* 72

13. The Camphill Communities Anthroposophical Approach to Autism *by Dr. Marga Hogenboom and Paula Moraine* 76

14. CARD eLearning and Skills: Web-Based Training, Assessment, Curriculum and Progress Tracking for Children with Autism
by Dr. Doreen Granpeesheh and Dr. Adel C. Najdowski 86

15. Center for Autism Spectrum Disorders, Munroe-Meyer Institute
by Dr. Tiffany Kodak and Dr. Alison Betz 92

16. Chelation: Removal of Toxic Metals *by Dr. James B. Adams* 97

17. Craniosacral and Chiropractic Therapy: A New Biomedical Approach to ASD *by Dr. Charles Chapple* 101

18. Dance/Movement Therapy *by Mariah Meyer LeFeber* 109

19. Dietary Interventions for Autism: Different Approaches
by Karyn Seroussi and Lisa Lewis, Ph.D. 114

20. Dietary Interventions for Autism: Specific Carbohydrate Diet
by Judith Chinitz 121

21. Drama Therapy *by Sally Bailey* 129

22. Early Start Denver Model
by Dr. Sally Rogers, Dr. Laurie Vismara, and Dr. Geraldine Dawson 133

23. Elevated Male Hormones: Their Role and Treatment in Autism Spectrum Disorders *by David A. Geier, Lisa Sykes, and Dr. Mark R. Geier* 139

24. Enzymes for Digestive Support in Autism *by Dr. Devin Houston* 146

25. How Enzymes Complement Therapeutic Diets *by Kristin Selby Gonzalez* 149

26. The Floortime Center *by Jake Greenspan and Tim Bleecker* 152

27. Food Selectivity and Other Feeding Disorders in Autism
by Dr. Petula Vaz and Dr. Cathleen Piazza 158

28. Gastrointestinal Disease: Emerging Consensus *by Dr. Arthur Krigsman* 163

29. Helminthic Therapy and Immune Abnormalities *by Judith Chinitz* 171

30. The Holistic Approach to NeuroDevelopment and Learning Efficiency (HANDLE) *by Carolyn Nuyens and Marlene Suliteanu* 178

31. Homeopathy—The Houston Homeopathy Method
by Cindy Griffin and Lindyl Lanham 184

32. Homotoxicology and Beyond *by Mary Coyle* 191

33. Integrated Play Groups Model *by Dr. Pamela Wolfberg* 198

34. Integrative Educational Care *by Dr. Mary Joann Lang* 202

35. Intestine, Leaky Gut, and Autism: Is it Real and How to Fix it (including with Probiotics)? *by Dr. Alessio Fasano* 210

36. Intravenous Immunoglobulin (IVIG) *by Dr. Michael Elice*   217

37. Low Dose Naltrexone (LDN) *by Dr. Jaquelyn McCandless*   224

38. Medicinal Marijuana: A Novel Approach to the Symptomatic
    Treatment of Autism *by Dr. Lester Grinspoon*   228

39. Melatonin Therapy for Sleep Disorders *by Dr. James Jan*   235

40. MERIT: Integrating ABA with Developmental Models *by Jenifer Clark*   241

41. Methyl-B$_{12}$: Myth or Masterpiece *by Dr. James Neubrander*   248

42. Mitochondrial Dysfunction and its Treatment *by Dr. Richard E. Frye*   253

43. Music Therapy *by Leah Kmetz*   257

44. Neurofeedback for the Autism Spectrum *by Dr. Siegfried and
    Susan F. Othmer*   262

45. Neuroimmune Dysfunction and the Rationale and
    Use of Antiviral Therapy *by Dr. Michael Goldberg*   268

46. Nutrigenomics and Optimizing Supplement Choices *by Dr. Amy Yasko*   273

47. Nutritional Supplementation for Autism *by Larry Newman*   279

48. Occupational Therapy and Sensory Integration *by Markus Jarrow*   291

49. Parent Support *by Dr. Lauren Tobing-Puente*   300

50. Physical Therapy *by Meghan Collins*   305

51. Psychotropic Medications and Their Cautious Discontinuation
    by Dr. Georgia A. Davis   308

52. Relationship Development Intervention *by Laura Hynes*   315

53. Sensory-Based Antecedent Interventions
    by Dr. Ginny Van Rie and Dr. L. Juane Heflin   323

54. Sensory Gyms, Academics, and Growing Minds
    by Amanda Friedman and Alison Berkley   327

55. The Sensory Learning Program *by Mary Bolles*   335

56. Sound-Based Therapies—Davis Model of Sound Intervention
    by Dorinne Davis   339

57. Speech-Language Therapy *by Lavinia Pereira and Michelle Solomon*   348

58. The Struggle to Speak: Implementation of the Kaufman
    Speech to Language Protocol (K-SLP) *by Nancy R. Kaufman*   359

59. Technological-Based Interventions for Autism—There's an App for That!   363

   A. Computer-Based Intervention—What's It All About? *by Valerie Herskowitz*   364

   B. AAC: Augmentative and Alternative Communication *by Patti Murphy*   369

   C. HandHold Adaptive *by Robert Tedesco*   379

   D. Introducing Proloquo2Go *by Rachel Coppin*   383

60. Traditional and Indigenous Healing *by Dr. Lewis Mehl-Madrona*   387

61. Transcranial Direct Current Stimulation, Implicit Teaching, and Syntax Acquisition in Minimally Verbal Children with Autism: Getting Kids to Speak *by Dr. Harry Schneider*   394

62. Transcranial Magnetic Stimulation *by Dr. Joshua M. Baruth, Dr. Estate Sokhadze, Dr. Ayman El-Baz, Dr. Grace Mathai, Dr. Lonnie Sears, and Dr. Manuel F. Casanova*   402

THERAPIES OF THE FUTURE

63. Vision Therapy *by Dr. Jeffrey Becker*   412

64. The Role of the Microbiome/Biome and Cysteine Deficiency in Autism Spectrum Disorder: the Implications for Glutathione and Defensins in the Gut-Brain Connection *by Dr. Jeff Bradstreet*   417

65. Research at the University of Louisville Autism Center *by Dr. Manuel Casanova, Dr. Estate Sokhadze, Dr. Ayman El-Baz, Dr. Joshua M. Baruth, Dr. Grace Mathai, and Dr. Lonnie Sears*   425

66. Three Drugs that Could Change Autism *by Meghan Thompson*   430

Afterword *by Teri Arranga*   435

References   437

Autism Organizations   472

Schools for Persons with Autism Spectrum Disorders   486

Recommended Reading   504

Index   507

FOREWORD

The word "autism" first became a part of my family's vocabulary when our son was two years old back in 1994. While it did not become an official diagnosis until several years later, the therapist who first mentioned this as a possible explanation for our son's alarming regressions and personality changes believed we should seek further evaluation. And that we did, seeking answers from every source we could think of and securing every service available to us in our quest to regain what had so mysteriously been taken away.

By the time our son was entering kindergarten, the therapies he'd undergone—occupational, speech, and behavioral—seemed to have really paid off. All involved with his care believed that he was ready to attend public school with no special services required. Our joy at witnessing his remarkable gains was short-lived, as we saw a re-regression in the months after he received the recommended kindergarten booster shots. His regression the first time around had been too gradual to connect with the vaccines he'd received, but now we watched in despair as the terrifying tantrums returned with a vengeance, obsessive and compulsive tendencies ruling each hour of our lives. Often we were afraid to send him to school, not knowing what horrors lay ahead on any given day, fearing the school's number would show up on the caller ID display and once again we would pick him up and bring him home for whatever period of time the school deemed appropriate.

Although not everyone affected by autism is part of the "second-hit phenomenon," the term was one I was to hear increasingly in the ensuing years—another strange-sounding phrase entering into our personal vernacular. A host of other terms had now become all too familiar: vaccine injury, self-injurious behavior, oppositional defiant disorder, and intermittent explosive disorder to name a few. My husband and I were now well-versed in the terminology and becoming increasingly frustrated that these completely subjective labels were being thrown at our child and so many others without the benefit of clinical investigation to determine what underlying, undiagnosed medical conditions might be manifesting in behavioral symptoms. Realizing that these underlying pathologies and abnormalities were being ignored by most in mainstream medicine, we joined the rapidly growing number of parents seeking biomedical treatments for their children from professionals who recognized the importance of clinical involvement.

I once heard someone say that "if you've seen one person with autism, you've seen one person with autism." Just as the symptoms of autism vary widely, so does the degree of success with available treatments and therapies among the individuals affected. Ken Siri and Tony Lyons have done a remarkably thorough job in pulling together both traditional and emerging treatments for autism and related disorders. Whether you've been on the autism journey for a long time, or have a newly-diagnosed child, *Cutting-Edge Therapies for Autism* is an invaluable resource, each topic addressed by the most renowned experts in the field.

At the time of this writing, nearly 1 percent of children in this country are diagnosed with autism, and one in six has a learning or behavior disorder. While those are overwhelming numbers, the good news is that there is much real hope for all families dealing with autism. What was once thought to be a mysterious genetic disorder is increasingly being recognized as a medical condition that can and does respond to medical treatments, often in conjunction with more traditional therapies. I hear from parents every day who report significant gains in their children, and some are also seeing a complete loss of the diagnosis through the interventions presented in this book. With gratitude to the medical professionals brave enough to look for real answers, I stand firmly with the parents who refuse to give up hope in restoring their children's health.

—**Rita Shreffler**
Executive Director
National Autism Association

PREFACE

EDITOR'S NOTE: Ken and I both have children on the autism spectrum. We don't have any financial connection to any organization, doctor, or therapist included in this book. We conceived of the book as a way to learn more ourselves in order to help our children. We are happy to be able to present what we have learned regarding the resources and treatments currently available and those which are emerging. Our team of contributors is impressive. It includes leading doctors, therapists, teachers, scientists, educators, social workers, and parents. —**Tony Lyons**

What's New in the Second Edition, 2011–2012

Time flies. It has been one year since our inaugural edition of Cutting Edge Therapies For Autism—what has changed you ask? More than we expected is the answer. Our kids, Lina and Alex, are a year older and making progress in their respective therapies, providing inspiration and hope that our research efforts will find the right combination of approaches for each to realize their potential.

In this second edition we present more than seventy therapies over the course sixty-seven chapters. Twenty-five of the chapters are brand new for this edition, including two special sections—one on technology-based interventions (chapter 60) and another ASD drugs in the clinical pipeline (chapter 67) that could change autism by treating not just its symptoms but its underlying causes. Of the remaining chapters, a number include significant updates and the rest are chapters we include again this year to complement our new offerings or serve to broaden coverage.

Teri Arranga, of AutismOne and *Autism Science Digest*, returns to provide us with our Afterword and Rita Shreffler, National Autism Association Executive Director, joins the team, contributing a Foreword.

We have also added to our resource lists at the back of the book and are happy to take suggestions for other therapies or resources for future editions. Email us at autism@skyhorsepublishing.com with suggestions.

The central purpose of this book is to provide people interested in autism therapies—including parents, grandparents, teachers, therapists, doctors and researchers—with articles about the cutting-edge work being done in the field. This field changes rapidly and we plan to update the book annually. *Cutting-Edge Therapies for Autism* is for people who want to learn as much as they possibly can about the therapies available, and about how to do everything in their power to help the growing number of children who are suffering.

Autism is the country's fastest-growing medical emergency, affecting more children than cancer, diabetes, Down syndrome and AIDS combined. Approximately 1 million people in the United States currently suffer from some form of autism.

Autism is difficult to define. No two kids have the same exact set of symptoms or respond to the same combination of therapies. Each child's treatment plan needs to be unique, taking into consideration the specific symptoms the child exhibits, the results of tests administered, and the observations of the child's doctors, therapists, teachers and, just as importantly, parents.

Case study #1: Lina

My daughter Lina was a bright, happy, talkative, social little girl. She had some ongoing problems with eczema but, other than that, was very healthy. Just before she turned three, she was given a regimen of antibiotics for bronchitis. Shortly thereafter, she received her measles mumps and rubella (MMR) booster shot. About two weeks later, she started to drool uncontrollably. It looked like her lips and jaw muscles had gone totally numb. The pediatrician took some tests and found that she had been exposed to the Epstein-Barr Virus, but couldn't tell us anything more. The drooling episode lasted a couple of weeks, during which time her speech became garbled and she began to stutter. It took an incredible effort for her to push words out of her mouth. She was like a toy running low on batteries, losing steam, losing control. As things inside of her began to disconnect, she was becoming disconnected from the world around her. A friend came over with her daughter for a play date and, after a few minutes with Lina, she asked, with real fear in her eyes: "What's going on with Lina? She seems like a different person." Lina seemed to improve after that, but then gradually deteriorated. She was first diagnosed with Sensory Processing Disorder, then Pervasive Development Disorder (PDD), and then, finally, autism. For some kids autism means screaming, biting, throwing things out the window, breaking everything in sight, even head banging. Life with them and for them can be harsh. When I look at Lina I see a peaceful, loving, gentle girl struggling to get out of a body that isn't functioning correctly. She's the victim—not me, not her mother, not her teachers, not society. The other day after slamming doors, screaming uncontrollably, and throwing things, she was able to calm down and walked over to me. I was sitting in my home office and, exhausted, she put her cheek on my arm, pulled my fingers to her back and said: "Can I please have a tickle, scratch, scratch." Lina clearly has attention deficit hyperactivity disorder (ADHD), she's obsessive compulsive (OCD), she has sensory processing disorder (SPD), is often manic, has gut and sleep issues, and her language is a constant struggle. But her mother, Helena, and I are fighting these symptoms and Lina is fighting them and we'll keep fighting them together and, God willing, we'll continue to see progress.

Case study #2: Alex

My son Alex was born in June of 1998 and developed normally, meeting or exceeding all his milestones until just after the age of 3. He attended day-care early (from age 4 months old) and was a popular and happy kid. While at daycare, Alex was able to pick up some Spanish in addition to his native English and could count to 10 in English, Spanish and Japanese by his second birthday. Medically, Alex was healthy as an infant and toddler, although he did have frequent sinus and ear infections that were treated with inhaled albuterol. He had all his vaccinations on time, the last of which followed his third birthday. By late summer folks at daycare began to comment that Alex was uncharacteristically spending more time on his own, sometimes staring out the window. A visit to his pediatrician produced an all too common "Don't worry, it's just a stage." Then Alex began to lose some speech, though he was still able to say, "Turn that off, that's scary," in response to TV coverage of 9/11. By Christmas 2001, Alex had lost a significant amount of speech, frequently stimmed by clapping his hands loudly (you never heard such a clap) and clearly had ADHD. At a holiday party that season, a person who owned a daycare center told me she thought Alex was autistic. This began our year-long journey into the autism abyss. By the end of 2002 Alex was non-verbal and a fully diagnosed member of the autism epidemic.

There is no general consensus on what causes autism—either classic Kanner's autism or the regressive kind. Some people think it's entirely genetic, while others think it's caused by Pitocin, fluoride in tap water or tooth paste, GAMT (guanidinoacetate methyltransferase) deficiency, chemicals in foods or household products, parental age, stress, treatments for asthma given to pregnant women, vaccines and/or the preservative thimerosal in some vaccines, viruses in the stomach or perhaps a specific retrovirus known as XMRV (which is under investigation by the CDC), gastrointestinal (GI) tract problems, immune problems, impaired intestinal functioning, environmental toxins, vitamin D deficiency, seizures, mobile phone radiation, encephalitis, hypoglycemia, antibiotics, and the list goes on and on. In compiling this book we have noticed a consensus beginning to emerge that the symptoms of autism result from a perfect storm of factors that come together to create a kind of system overload, a tipping point, in a genetically predisposed child's developing immune system. Recent studies point toward this overload causing problems at the cellular level, impairing the ability of nerve cells to transmit information properly through the synapses of the brain. Furthermore, the dramatic increase in the incidence of autism spectrum disorders points toward environmental factors playing a significant role. Further supporting this is the fact that scientists have found that by introducing environmental toxins or antibiotics they can create autistic symptoms in rats.

So what happened to Lina and Alex? We believe that they were genetically predisposed to contract autism, but required a big push and that the push came from a virus and a high fever, followed by antibiotics and a barrage of vaccines, all of which occurred at a fragile developmental stage. The antibiotics disregulated the immune system and the vaccines, thrown in as an additional stressor at the worst possible time, were the final straw. We also believe that the disregulated, hyper-active immune system created an autoimmune response whereby the immune system couldn't tell the difference between healthy tissue and the antigens that it normally fights and then probably attacked the healthy tissue of both the stomach lining and the brain. We believe that this combination of factors created a gut malfunction, a kind of climate change in the stomach that made it difficult for our kids to digest certain proteins that are necessary for healthy blood-cell development and healthy nerve cell activation. The proteins in the blood cells are necessary for the healthy development of the cognitive centers of the brain and in the nerve cells they help the neurotransmitters fire up correctly, send proper messages (like pain, hot and cold, sound etc.) and connect the right and left lobes of the brain. We think that the human body can normally withstand severe complications and stressors but, for the young, predisposed child, this chain of events is just too much. While we're not scientists, like everyone reading this book, we're doing our very best to try to solve the puzzle.

As far as treatments for autism, most doctors still tell parents with absolute certainty that it is an incurable lifelong condition and that treatments simply don't work. Kim Stagliano, author of the book *All I Can Handle: I'm No Mother Teresa* about life with three autistic daughters writes:

> An autism diagnosis can erase a person's ability to get solid medical care. If you brought your 6-year-old to a hospital in the throes of a seizure, the neurologists would run tests and look for the cause. When I brought my 6-year-old in, I was told, "She has autism. She has different circuitry." And then when I requested tests, I was told, "We're just not that aggressive with autism." My child has a brain and a gut and immune system just like any other child. Why does her autism negate that?

In looking at a more than 50 percent increase in the incidence of autism between 2002 to 2006, Dr. Thomas Insel director of the National Institute of Mental Health (NIMH) and chair of the Interagency Autism Coordinating Committee (IACC) the nation's top autism research coordinator, had this to say in an interview with David Kirby for the *Huffington Post*:

> This tells you that you really have to take this very seriously. From every-thing they are looking at, this is not something that can be explained away by methodology, by diagnosis.

He goes on to say that we should not be looking at autism as a single thing, with one cause, one treatment, one explanation. There may, in fact, be 10 or 20 or more distinct variations.

> I think this is a collection of many, many different disorders…It's quite believable to me that there are many children who develop autism in the context of having severe gut pathology, or having autoimmune problems, or having lots of other problems. And some of these kids really do recover. And this is quite different from the autism that was originally described in the 1940s and 1950s—where it looks like you have it and you are going to have it for the rest of your life.

If autism is caused by the comorbidity of the underlying medical conditions, and if there are really endless variations of autism, then why on earth wouldn't we treat these conditions, mandate that insurance companies pay for these treatments, and get on to the business of trying to heal the underlying conditions. Dr. Insel agrees and says: "We've got to be able to break apart this spectrum disorder into its component parts and identify who's going to respond to which interventions." He advocates for genetic mapping as a way to pinpoint the underlying medical conditions so that we can figure out whether an individual had been "exposed to organophosphates, or perhaps to some infection, or some autoimmune process" that interferes with the way the brain develops. Others are beginning to express similar sentiment. Dr. Christo-pher Walsh, Ballard Professor of Neurology and Chief of the Division of Genetics at Children's Hospital in Boston says: "I would like every kid on the spectrum to have not 'autism' but a more specific disorder. By isolating the genes involved and understanding their functions, researchers can begin to develop particular treat-ments aimed at particular disorders." Dr. James Gusella, Ballard Professor of Neu-rogenetics and director of the Center for Human Genetic Research at Massachusetts General Hospital (MGH) says: "Autism is a problem that no one person or discipline can figure out alone."

Throughout the book, we use the word "treatment" in the broadest possible sense. Nevertheless, the therapies included by no means constitute an exhaustive list. Most of the practitioners included can tell you about cases where their therapy helped decrease the symptoms of a specific child, helped the child relate better, speak better, helped minimize gut problems, or helped control behavioral problems. And they have parents to support their claims. On the other hand, most of these therapies have not undergone rigorous trials, the kind of trials that cost substantial amounts of money and often take years to complete and evaluate. As a result, there are some people who contest the claims of the practitioners or parents. In any case, by including a specific treatment, we are not endorsing that treatment or telling you that it will work for your child or patient. Nor are the more than seventy doctors, teachers, therapists, parents, and other experts who have contributed to this book endorsing any treatment other than the one that they are writing about. Furthermore, practically none of these therapies are endorsed by any state or the federal government or covered by health insurance.

We certainly believe that the government should mandate insurance coverage for extensive genetic, blood and spinal fluid testing before any definitive diagnosis can be given. We have heard of cases where children showed the symptoms of autism or other disorders such as cerebral palsy, multiple sclerosis, or schizophrenia, but in fact had easily treatable disorders and were fully rehabilitated. We believe these kids, like any other kids, deserve the best medical care available, including full coverage for any treatment that is recommended by a specialist in any specific underlying medical condition. Some states have already started heading in this direction. For now, the only FDA approved drugs are Abilify and Risperdal and the only therapy approved by most states is applied behavior analysis (ABA), based on the teachings of B. F. Skinner. Recently, however, practitioners and researchers have begun advocating for approaches that combine the various therapies and scientists are trying to develop ways to measure how particular therapies improve brain connections in a specific individual.

Autism costs families an incredible amount of money. Estimates range from $60,000 to $100,000 per year and that assumes that you can either find an adequate public school in your district or, more likely, a private school that your city will agree to pay for. If you can't get the school paid for, then the cost could be as high as $200,000 per year. Whoever pays, autism is a growing problem and states and the federal government need to address it. Right now, autism costs the United States an estimated 35 billion dollars per year, but that could well be the trickle that turns into a flood. We believe that by funding more research and by agreeing either to pay for a broader range of therapies or to require insurance companies to do that, states and the federal government will save money in the long run.

Dr. Insel admits that when he was in training as a psychiatrist he "never saw a child with autism." He says that he wanted to see kids with autism, but he simply couldn't find any. Now, Insel says, "I wouldn't have to go any further than the block where I live to see kids with autism." This is an epidemic. We've come from a time when 1 in 10,000 babies born in the United States exhibited symptoms of autism to a time when the statistics are roughly 1 in 100. Think about that for a moment, 1% of kids born in this country become autistic. And those statistics, which come from the Centers for Disease Control (CDC), are based on data collected four years ago, so that the current rate is estimated to be 1 in 91.

If you were to take the 57% increase in the incidence of autism between 2002 and 2006, as calculated by the CDC (which the CDC itself says cannot be explained away by a shift in diagnostic criteria) and extrapolate forward, then at least half of all children born in the United States will be autistic by 2046. And these statistics fail to differentiate between classic autism, which is characterized by a child sitting in a corner rocking back and forth with little interest in social interaction, and regressive autism, where a normally developing child suddenly loses speech, interest in social interaction with peers and develops various biomedical symptoms. Ten years ago no one talked or wrote about regressive autism and now this is the fastest growing segment of the autistic population. What if this is just a different disorder? What if it's a disorder that has gone from 1 in 200 million to 1 in 200 in a 10 year period? Then, certainly, we're looking at a medical disaster of unprecedented proportions that is here, now and warrants a response at least as dramatic as the CDCs response to swine flu or the AIDS epidemic. We could well be at the tipping point of a crisis that will soon consume our future.

We are not doctors or scientists or government officials, but dads who love our kids and want to do the very best we can for them. We don't know for sure what caused our kids' autism and maybe we never will. If it was an immune system overload, we think that in most cases the cure is going to come not from a one-off drug, but from a coun-terassault, an all-out systemic approach, from DIR, from ABA, from dietary interventions, from GI tract treatments, from nutritional supplements, from anti-virals, from physical therapy, from sensory integration therapy, from brain therapy, from whatever fits the individual child. The current unwillingness of insurance companies, states and the federal government to pay for therapies is typical short-term thinking. Costs will only escalate, as untreated children become adults who need to be cared for by the state. A long-term approach will ultimately save money and will undoubtedly lead to at least some children being cured. This is war and if we want these children back, if we want to stop the progress of this disorder, we are going to have to fight. There will be people, lots of people, who will keep pointing out that there is no known cure, that they believe the struggle is hopeless. They will tell you that the best thing to do is to try to protect your own sanity and save your money. Our mission is to give our children, everyone's autistic children, their lives back to the fullest extent possible. We want to be involved in finding a remedy or a series of therapies that act together to bring these kids back to themselves and to their families and to the world.

Lina and Alex may never be typical kids. But perhaps they can be in a position to make informed decisions about their own lives, to communicate with people, to experience friendship and love and passion and hope. And who knows, perhaps if we help cure them, they will be the ones who develop a cure for cancer! Whatever the outcome, until there is a cure, we will do our very best to look for promising therapies for the symptoms of autism and continue to publish *Cutting-Edge Therapies for Autism* in April of every year.

—**Ken Siri and Tony Lyons**

INTRODUCTION

NAVIGATING THE AUTISM SUPERHIGHWAY: HOW TO DETERMINE IF A THERAPY IS RIGHT FOR YOUR CHILD AND FAMILY

If you are intently reading or just skimming through the chapters of this book, the assumption is that your child or a child you know was recently or at some time in the past diagnosed with an autism spectrum disorder.

At this point you have hopefully, to one degree or another, started to come to terms with the diagnosis and what it means for your child, for you, and for your family. You are now ready to enter the Autism Superhighway, inch by inch, or at full speed.

In either case, it is now time to gather your team of co-navigators who will assist you in putting together a GPS system with the appropriate approaches, methods, and interventions. These should all be based on your child's unique and individual profile. This profile is essential in guiding the course of treatment.

For any child with autism, determining a course of treatment using only information you have read in a book or researched on the Internet is ill-advised. One needs a qualified team of specialists to properly evaluate, diagnose, prescribe, and monitor your child's strengths and areas of need.

This book is intended to provide an overview of a variety of approaches, methods, and interventions that alone or in combination may help place a child on the road to recovery from autism. It needs to be said that at this time there is no cure for autism. There are many children, however, who have received timely and comprehensive interventions and no longer meet the diagnostic criteria for an autism spectrum diagnosis. No matter the severity of manifestations, significant benefit can be gained by the child, the family, or both, with early and intensive interventions. However, if any clinician, specialist, or intervention approach promises a cure, be very leery and scrutinize carefully the validity of these claims.

Your primary pediatric care provider should be knowledgeable about the various medical, developmental, and behavioral issues that children with autism spectrum disorders may encounter. They should be aware of the available treatment options and the specialists in your area to whom you need to be referred. They need to be open minded to ALL treatments, whether they are based on a Western medicine approach or an alternative/complementary medical philosophy. Most importantly, there needs to be close collaboration and communication between your family, your specialists/therapists, and your child's primary care pediatric physician.

Unfortunately a common etiology for autism has not been discovered. Each child may broadly share common general manifestations but the triggers and causes for these manifestations may vary greatly from one child to another. It appears that the way parents and professionals view autism today is in transition. Although many continue to view it as strictly a psychiatric or a neurologic disorder, newer viewpoints are being embraced. Autism is increasingly being viewed as a disorder with multifactorial etiologies defined by its behavioral manifestations. These include impairments in communication and social interactions, repetitive behaviors, and sensory processing and regulatory issues. Therefore, autism needs to be considered a "spectrum" disorder that not only is impacted by issues in the brain and nervous system but one that is impacted by dysfunction in the immune, gastrointestinal, and metabolic systems. Since the etiology as well as the manifestations of autism are influenced by a variety of multiple factors, a cookie-cutter or a one-size-fits-all approach to treatment and intervention programming is steering you onto the wrong road. Creating an individual profile is therefore essential to navigating the Autism Superhighway. This profile must include an assessment of the child's present developmental level. It needs to analyze the child's individual medical, genetic, behavioral, sensory processing, and regulatory profile. Consideration of parenting skills, cultural beliefs, and expectations need to be factored in.

The child's profile should and will change over time. The key to successful outcomes is establishing a cohesive team approach, with ongoing monitoring of progress to ensure treatments remain relevant and goals are always current and realistic.

One cannot promise that the Autism Superhighway your child and your family will be travelling on will offer a smooth or detour-free trip. There will be bumps, curves, and forks in the road. Remember, this is a long journey, not a short road trip. There will be many moments when you think "are we there yet?" but there will also be many scenic road stops and enjoyable attractions. Be sure to take the time to enjoy the major highlights along the way.

—**MARK FREILICH, M.D.**

THERAPIES

ALLERGY DESENSITIZATION: AN EFFECTIVE ALTERNATIVE TREATMENT FOR AUTISM

BY DR. DARIN INGELS

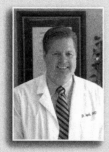

Darin Ingels, ND

2425 Post Road, Suite 100
Southport, CT 06890
Ph. 203-254-9957
NEFHA.com
nefha@nefha.com

Darin Ingels, ND, is a respected leader in natural medicine with numerous publications, international lectures, and more than 20 years experience in the healthcare field. He received his bachelor of science degree in medical technology from Purdue University and his doctorate of naturopathic medicine from Bastyr University in Seattle, Washington. Dr. Ingels completed a residency program at the Bastyr Center for Natural Health. He is a licensed naturopathic physician in the State of Connecticut and State of California, where he maintains practices in both states. Dr. Ingels is a member of the American Association of Naturopathic Physicians, the Connecticut Naturopathic Physicians Association, the New York Association of Naturopathic Physicians, the American Academy of Environmental Medicine, the American College for Advancement in Medicine, and the Holistic Pediatric Association. He has served on the board of directors for the Naturopathic Physicians Licensing Exam (NPLEX) as the chair of microbiology and immunology. Dr. Ingels' practice focuses on autism spectrum disorders with special emphasis on chronic immune dysfunction, including allergies, asthma, recurrent or persistent infections, and other genetic or acquired immune problems. He uses diet, nutrients, herbs, homeopathy, and immunotherapy to help his children achieve better health.

Allergies and asthma affect more than 50 million people living in the United States and comprise the sixth leading cause of physician office visits. Children with autism often have impaired immune function and may be predisposed to allergy symptoms.[1,2] Studies also show that children with autism have multiple defects in immune function and that the severity of immune dysfunction is proportional to the severity of autism.[3] Unfortunately, allergies are often underdiagnosed and undertreated due to lack of verbal skills of the child or the lack of understanding by parents of what symptoms may be caused by allergy. The immune system produces five different antibodies (also known as immunoglobulins) in response to substances that are recognized as being foreign (e.g., bacteria, viruses, allergens, etc.). Immunologists refer to them as IgG, IgM, IgA, IgD and IgE. Each immunoglobulin serves a primary role in our normal immune function, and IgE is the one most associated with allergies. Common symptoms of allergy, including runny nose, itchy eyes, sneezing, and asthma, are often precipitated by IgE, which triggers the cascade of events leading to allergic symptoms. However, there is good evidence that many allergic reactions do not involve IgE at all and can be mediated by different immune mechanisms. Non-IgE reactions have been identified as causing neuropsychiatric symptoms such as irritability, hyperactivity, mood disorders, or cognitive deficits; gastrointestinal or motility problems; skin rashes; and sleep disturbances.[4] Conventional allergy testing specifically looks mostly at IgE reactions (whether by blood test, intradermal, or scratch testing), so it is not uncommon for a child with autism to get allergy testing and be told they do not have any allergies. However, IgE testing excludes most non-IgE reactions and, therefore, has limited value in diagnosing these types of allergies.

Treatment of allergies usually consists of over-the-counter or prescription oral antihistamines (e.g., Benadryl®, Zyrtec®, or Claritin®), leukotriene inhibitors (Singulair®), or steroids. Nasal and inhaled steroids may also be prescribed to prevent inhaled allergy reactions. While medications may be used to suppress symptoms, they do not treat the underlying cause of allergies. Subcutaneous immunotherapy (SCIT), commonly referred to as "allergy shots" may be used to help desensitize the immune system to specific allergens, such as pollen, mold, or house dust mites. It is rarely used in the United States to treat food allergy due to its risk of triggering life-threatening (anaphylactic) reactions. However, children with autism who suffer from allergies and asthma now have a viable alternative to conventional injection immunotherapy in treating their symptoms. Although injection immunotherapy has been the gold standard for allergy desensitization for almost 100 years, over 300 published studies show that sublingual immunotherapy (SLIT) is equally or more effective than allergy shots in reducing allergy and asthma symptoms.[5,6,7,8] The allergy extracts used in SLIT are identical to those used in injection immunotherapy, but rather than receiving a shot on a weekly or monthly basis, oral drops are administered under the tongue, often on a daily basis.

Recent research shows that during SLIT, the allergen is absorbed into the oral mucosa. The underlying dendritic cells, which are part of the immune system, produce a series of chemicals that ultimately result in a decrease in IgE and other molecules that produce allergy symptoms as well as decreasing inflammation in target tissues.[9,10] This mechanism of action is similar to that observed in conventional immunotherapy.

Although SLIT seems relatively new in the United States, it has been used clinically for more than three decades. Its use has increased steadily in the past 15 years but mostly in other countries, especially those in Europe. There are many advantages to SLIT over injection immunotherapy. SLIT may be used in children who are not eligible to receive conventional allergy injections or who may have sensory issues that would prohibit using injections. There are no reports of SLIT causing anaphylaxis, making it a safer alternative to injections. SLIT is more convenient than injection immunotherapy, since the drops are administered at home by the parent, meaning fewer office visits and no needles. There are no significant medical disadvantages of SLIT treatment; however, many insurance companies in the United States do not reimburse for SLIT, which may be financially limiting for some individuals.

The practical application and successful use of SLIT is dependent on accurate assessment of a child's allergies and sensitivities. Since conventional allergy tests only pick up on the serious types of allergic reactions, other assessment tools may be helpful in identifying more subtle allergic triggers. Environmental medicine physicians have specialized training in some of these alternative methods. Provocation/neutralization is a technique where a small amount of a food substance is injected just under the skin. If a child is allergic or sensitive to the food, then an area of redness will appear on the skin and the child may start to exhibit physical signs of reaction, including red ears, irritability, screaming, head banging, etc. When the neutralizing dose is subsequently injected, the area of redness goes away and the physical symptoms stop. It can be a very powerful tool for the parent to observe how specific foods affect their child. A similar technique is used to test for inhalant allergies, such as mold, pollen, or dust mites.

However, testing most children with autism with a needle technique is difficult and time consuming. Other noninvasive methods may be more suitable for these children. Electrodermal screening (EDS) is an effective method of determining a child's sensitivities. Although there has been little research comparing EDS to conventional allergy testing, many practitioners have found it to be an invaluable tool in identifying hidden sensitivities. EDS is a noninvasive technology that allows the practitioner to measure energy patterns in the body. Dr. Alfred Gilman and Dr. Martin Rodbell won the Nobel Prize in Physiology and Medicine in 1994 by discovering that cells communicate electrically before they communicate chemically. This means we have a way of measuring how the energy of different allergens affects the energy of our own bodies.

EDS has the capacity to assess for sensitivities to foods, molds, pollen, animal dander, and even more subtle triggers, such as chemicals, hormones, and neurotransmitters. While conventional allergy testing looks specifically at IgE or IgG antibodies,

EDS looks at the broader scope of immune reactions, particularly delayed reactions. It is not uncommon for a child with autism to go through allergy testing and be told that they do not have any allergies. Since the term "allergy" has a strict definition of IgE reaction, this may very well be true. However, this does not necessarily mean that the child does not react to various allergens. EDS is an effective means to measure delayed or subtle sensitivities that are often missed through conventional allergy testing.

The author of this article and other physicians have successfully treated thousands of children with autism with SLIT and have not observed any significant side effects or severe reactions to the treatment. Some children do get hyperactive or agitated during their initial course of treatment, but this usually resolves after a couple of weeks. Sometimes the dose has to be adjusted down for very sensitive children. Although injection immunotherapy can take a year or longer to begin controlling allergies or asthma, SLIT will often diminish symptoms within weeks. The combination of EDS and SLIT has enabled our practice to successfully treat children with autism for their various allergies and sensitivities. SLIT is a safe, effective treatment that should be considered as a first line therapy for the treatment of allergies and asthma in children with autism.

ALLERGY-LIKE SYMPTOMS, BLOOD-BRAIN BARRIER DISRUPTION, AND BRAIN INFLAMMATION

BY DR. THEOHARIS THEOHARIDES

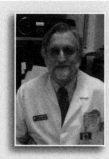

Theoharis C. Theoharides. MS, PhD, MD, FAAAAI

Professor of Pharmacology, Internal Medicine and Biochemistry
Director, Molecular Immunopharmacology and Drug Discovery Laboratory
Tufts University School of Medicine, Boston, MA
Clinical Pharmacologist, Massachusetts Drug Formulary Commission (1986–2011)

Department of Pharmacology and Experimental Therapeutics
Tufts University School of Medicine
136 Harrison Avenue
Boston, MA 02111
(617) 636-6866
Fax: 617-636-2456
www.mastcellmaster.com

Dr. Theoharis Theoharides is the Director of the Molecular Immunopharmacology and Drug Discovery Laboratory, as well as a Professor of Pharmacology, Biochemistry and Internal Medicine at Tufts University, in Boston, Massachusetts. He received all his degrees from Yale University, is a member of seventeen scientific societies and four Academies. He has published over three hundred research papers and three textbooks. Dr. Theoharides is much more that just an eminent physician and pharmacologist; he goes a step further in posing new theories and defining the cutting edge of allergy and inflammation research. He was the first to show that mast cells can be stimulated by non-allergic triggers, such as stress hormones, to secrete inflammatory mediators selectively leading to disruption of the gut-blood-brain barriers. Based on his discoveries, Dr. Theoharides proposed the novel concept that mast cells play a critical role in brain inflammation and autism. Dr. Theoharides extends his expertise beyond theory into practical options and offers hope for patients with diseases such as autism which, to date, have defied treatment.

Autism treatment has been elusive. In the majority of cases, the cause of autism is unknown. Although some possible autism susceptibility genes have been identified, no single or group of genes can explain the disturbing rise in the incidence of autism from 2 children out of every 100,000 only twenty years ago to 1 out of every 100 children presently. To date, most research has focused on the behavioral and neurologic manifestations of autistic spectrum disorders instead of what led to them.[1]

Gut-Blood-Brain Barrier Disruption, Mast Cells and Brain Inflammation

Many autism patients have evidence of "allergic symptomatology," but most test negative to various allergens on allergy tests such as skin prick or serum RAST tests, indicating the involvement of environmental and other triggers.[2] Moreover, "allergic" symptoms are asociated with different diagnoses, some of which are listed below.[3] It is, therefore, important for parents and their children's caregivers to understand that many of these subcategories are NOT treatable with antihistamines or immunotherapy.

Diseases involving mast cell activation
- Auto-inflammatory diseases
- Allergic rhinitis
- Angioneurotic edema
- Asthma
- Atopic dermatitis
- Eczema
- Food allergy
- Food intolerance
- Idiopathic urticaria
- Idiopathic mast cell activation disorder
- Mastocytosis
- Non-clonal mast cell activation syndrome
- Non-IgE food allergy
- Urticaria pigmentosa

Allergic Symptomatology and Autism

The observation that most children with autism have either a family or personal history of immune or allergic disorders prompted the proposal that autism may be a "neuroimmune" disorder.[4] There have been numerous studies that support this proposal (for review see [2,3]). One study investigated infants born in California between 1995–1999 and reported that maternal asthma and allergies during the second trimester of pregnancy were correlated with a greater than two-fold elevated risk of autism in their children. In another study, 30 percent of autistic children had a family history of allergies as compared to 2.5 percent in age-matched "neurologic controls." A more recent study reported that immune allergic response, represented by the frequency of atopic dermatitis, asthma and rhinitis was increased in 70 percent of Asperger patients compared to 7 percent in age-matched healthy controls. In a National Survey of Children's Health, parents of autistic children reported symptoms of allergies more often than those of other children, with food allergies being the most prevalent complaint. Another study reported an increased prevalence of non-IgE mediated food allergy in the autism group compared to normal controls. It is also interesting that a recent study conducted in Germany reported an independent association between atopic eczema and Attention-Deficit Hyperactivity Disorder (ADHD), which has considerable phenotypic overlap with autism.

The link between allergic symptomatology and autism is also supported by the observation that in many cases, autistic symptoms worsen when a patient's "allergic" symptoms flare-up. However, even in these symptomatic cases "allergy" tests, such as skin prick or RAST, are often negative. These circumstances suggest a non-allergic trigger of mast cells.[2]

Mast Cells and Autism

The possible association between autism and mast cells was first investigated because many symptoms that characterize patients with autism are also present in patients with mastocytosis, a spectrum of disorders that involve proliferation and activation of mast cells in the skin (urticaria pigmentosa, UP) and other organs. The *Mastocytosis Society, Inc.* (www.tmsforacure.org) together with the American Academy of Allergy, Asthma and Immunology recently produced a video, entitled *Mast Cell Activation Symptomatology* (available to physicians and patients), which highlights the fact that allergies may be only one aspect of mast cell activation. Preliminary research results indicate that the prevalence of autism spectrum disorders, including pervasive developmental disorder-not otherwise specified (PDD-NOS) in mastocytosis patients is ten-fold higher (1/10 children) than the general population.[5]

We hypothesized that autism starts when the protective *gut-blood and blood-brain barriers* break down either during pregnancy or early in life.[1] Such a barrier disruption allows neurotoxic molecules to reach the brain ultimately resulting in inflammation and defective nerve processing.[6] This premise is supported by the fact that many autistic patients have antibodies against brain proteins, which implies that immune cells reached the brain through a leaky blood-brain-barrier.[7]

Recent research has also shown that mast cells, immune cells typically known for causing allergic reactions,[8] are located close to the blood vessels making up the gut-blood-brain barriers, and can be activated by environmental, infectious, and stress triggers leading to disruption of these protective barriers.[9-11] One such mast cell trigger, neurotensin, a neuropeptide found in the brain and gut, was recently reported to be increased in the serum of young children with autism.[12] Other molecules, such as mercury, have been shown to have a synergistic action with neurotensin.[13] Mast cell activation could be particularly critical during gestation, since mast cell-derived mediators might act epigenetically to alter the expression of autism susceptibility genes.[14]

Environmental and Stress Mast Cell Triggers

Mast cells are critical for allergic reactions, but are also important in regulating immunity and inflammation.[8] Mast cells are located close to blood vessels both in the gut and in the brain. Functional mast cell-neuron interactions occur in these locations increasing both intestinal and brain permeability. This may help to explain the intestinal and neurologic complaints of autistic patients. Many substances originating in the environment, intestine or brain can trigger mast cell secretion of pro-inflammatory and vasoactive molecules.[15] These triggers include: bacterial and viral antigens; environmental toxins such as polychlorinated biphenyl (PCB) and mercury;[13] and neuropeptides such as neurotensin and corticotropin-releasing hormone (CRH). CRH is typically secreted under stress, which stimulates selective release of vascular endothelial growth factor (VEGF).

The ability of viruses to trigger mast cell activation is an important consideration in their contribution to autism pathogenesis. A number of rotaviruses have been isolated from asymptomatic neonates and could activate mast cells at that age. Once activated, mast cells secrete numerous vasoactive, neurosensitizing and proinflammatory substances that are relevant to autism including IL-6. IL-6 can disrupt the gut-blood-brain barriers as well as promote the development of Th17 cells, which are critical for the development of autoimmune diseases.

Available Therapies

There are no true anti-allergic drugs available. Cortisone, a steroid, would come close to it by suppressing the immune system response, but it cannot be given for long periods of time to children because of its numerous side effects, especially the associated potential for growth inhibition, and making the patients susceptible to infections.

Recent developments have led to a new formulation that could help reduce allergic type symptoms/inflammation both in the gut and the brain.

Non-Drug

NeuroProtek® is unique dietary formulation, which may help a patient's body to reduce gut and brain inflammation, and gut-blood-brain barrier disruption. NeuroProtek uses a unique combination of three natural molecules, called flavonoids, selected from about thirty thousand such molecules found in nature. It contains luteolin obtained from chamomile or chrysanthemum (>95 percent pure), quercetin and the quercetin glycoside rutin obtained from saphora (>95 percent pure) mixed in unrefined olive kernel oil imported from Greece to increase their absorption by forming micropsheres (liposomes). NeuroProtek is formulated in small softgel capsules that must be taken two per 44 lb weight per day with some food for 6-12 months before any noticeable benefits

Why Use Select Flavonoids?

Flavonoids are naturally occurring compounds with antioxidant and anti-inflammatory properties.[16] It is easy for many impure flavonoids to be sold under such names as "bioflavonoids," "citrus flavonoids," "soy flavonoids," or "Pycnogenol." Whether taken as pills, tablets, or hard capsules, all flavonoids are difficult to absorb (less than 10 percent) in powder form and are extensively metabolized to inactive ingredients in the liver. In addition, very few flavonoids are beneficial; instead, many such as morin have no anti-inflammatory activity, while pycnogenol is weakly active (as compared to luteolin or quercetin), but could cause liver toxicity. Unfortunately, such preparations DO NOT specify either the source or the purity of the flavonoids. This problem is even worse given that many autistic patients could have reactions to the impurities, fillers, or dyes. As an additional consideration, the most common source of the flavonoid quercetin is fava beans, which can induce hemolytic anemia (destruction of all the blood cells) in those 15 percent of people of Mediterranean origin (such as Greeks, Italians, Jews, and North Africans) who lack the enzyme glucose-phosphate dehydrogenase (G_6PD).

The selection of the specific flavonoids, as well as their source (chamomile, chrysanthemum, saphora), purity (>95 percent) and absorption (about 25 percent in olive seed oil) were taken into consideration in developing the dietary supplement NeuroProtek.

Luteolin, and its closely structurally related flavonoids quercetin and rutin, have potent antioxidant and anti-inflammatory actions and mast cell blocking actions.[17, 18] Luteolin and quercetin can also inhibit the release of histamine and prostaglandin D_2 (PGD_2), as well as the pro-inflammatory molecules IL-6, IL-8, and TNF from human cultured mast cells. Moreover, quercetin inhibits mast cell-dependent stimulation of activated T cells involved in autoimmune diseases.[19] Luteolin also inhibits IL-6 release from microglia cells, as well as IL-1- mediated release of IL-6 and IL-8 from astrocytes, Luteolin also inhibited autistic-like behavior in mice.[20]

NeuroProtek should best be taken with food starting with one capsule first per day, and increasing to two capsules per 44 lbs weight per day. For best results, capsules should be spread out throughout the day. The total number should not exceed 6–8 capsules per day regardless of the age or weight of the patient.

Risks and Side Effects

There are no side effects known. However, this formulation (as well as any flavonoids) must be used with caution with drugs that are heavily metabolized by the liver as it may affect the resulting blood levels of such compounds.

Potentially Useful Drugs

The following is a list of drugs that may be useful in addressing some symptoms, especially for the subgroup of autistic patients with allergic symptoms. Please note, they are not approved for autism and they should be discussed with a healthcare professional.

Cyproheptadine (Periactin) is a combined histamine-1 and serotonin receptor (5-HT$_2$) antagonist. It produced significant improvement over that of the antipsychotic haloperidol in a double-blind trial of forty children with autism, randomized to either haloperidol and cyproheptadine versus haloperidol and placebo. The apparent benefit of cyproheptadine may be related to the higher platelet serotonin levels reported in over 40 percent of patients with autism. Although high platelet serotonin may not reflect availability in the brain, it could affect the neuroenteric plexus in the gut that utilizes serotonin.

Disodium cromoglycate (cromolyn, sodium, Gastrocrom) is an inhibitor of *rodent* mast cell histamine secretion, but weak inhibitor of human mast cells.[21] Nevertheless, it is often used (100 mg orally 2-3 times/day) to treat GI symptoms in mastocytosis patients.

Ketotifen (Zaditen), is a histamine-1 receptor antagonist not available in the USA.[22] It has been reported to also partially inhibit mast cell activation and is often used (1 mg orally once per day) for treating symptoms associated with mast cell activation, but also for eosinophilic esophagitis and gastroenteritis.

Hydroxyzine (Atarax) is a potent histamine-1 receptor antagonist, which also partially inhibits mast cell activation and has mild anti-anxiety actions.[23] It is often used (5–25 mg orally once per day usually at night) for treating symptoms associated with allergies and mast cell activation, but also ADHS.

Rupatadine (Rupafin) is a newer histamine-1 receptor antagonist, available in Europe and Latin America, but not yet in the USA. It also inhibits mast cell release of inflammatory mediators and blocks platelet activating factor (PAF).[24] It can be used (10–20 mg orally per day) for eosinophilic esophagitis and gastroenteritis.

ANIMALS IN THE LIVES OF PERSONS WITH AUTISM SPECTRUM DISORDER(ASD): COMPANIONS TO CO-THERAPISTS

BY DR. AUBREY FINE

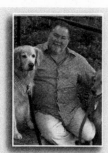

Aubrey H. Fine, Ed.D.

Professor
Department of Education
CA Poly University
3801 W. Temple Ave.
Pomona, CA 91768
ahfine@csupomona.edu

Psychologist Dr. Aubrey Fine has been in the field of Animal-Assisted Therapy (AAT) for over twenty-five years. He is the editor of the most widely accepted book on the subject, *The Handbook on Animal-Assisted Therapy*, has had a featured monthly column in *Dog Fancy* magazine on the human-animal bond entitled "The Loving Bond." He has also been a guest on numerous national TV and radio shows including on programs on ABC, Animal Planet, KTLA, and CNN. His newest book, *Afternoons with Puppy*, released by Purdue University in December 2007, is a heartwarming account about the evolving relationships and outcomes among a therapist, his therapy animals, and his patients over the course of over two decades. Over this period, he has applied AAT with a variety of children with diverse forms of etiology and has witnessed many moving outcomes as a result of incorporating animals as therapeutic agents. An active faculty member at California State Polytechnic University since 1981, he was awarded the prestigious Wang Award in 2001 for exceptional commitment, dedication, and exemplary contributions within the areas of education and applied sciences.

A special thanks is given to Karina Grasso who helped in the research for this chapter. Your efforts are greatly appreciated.

*H*is mother always wanted him to have a dog, but she wasn't quite sure how he would react. That is when I got the call. I decided that Magic would be his best match. Magic is a very gentle, calm and attentive four-year-old golden retriever, who seems very comfortable working with all children. She always approaches very slowly, giving all those she interacts with ample time to get acclimated.

When they first met, Bob was apprehensive and used poor eye contact. He also mumbled his speech and spoke with a pedantic flair. That didn't seem to be an obstacle for Magic. She moved closely next to Bob, waiting for him to pet her. Their relationship was just beginning. Over the following weeks not only did he become more comfortable with her presence, he also began to speak up and with more clarity. Puppy love and companionship may have been the initial goal, but Bob's family would quickly learn, that animal-assisted interventions could have much more to offer.

Introduction

The unique bond between humans and animals and its powerful impact on human well-being has been documented over hundreds of years (Wells, 2009). It is apparent that in most cases, pets fill a void in most owners' lives. Instead of coming home to an empty house, people come home to the greetings of happy loving animals such as dogs or cats. Our pets provide companionship and unconditional love as well as providing friendship to those who may lack social contact. Within this chapter, attention will be given to explain the value of the human-animal bond and describe how animal-assisted interventions including equine-assisted therapy and pet companionship can be a viable alternative to persons with any autism spectrum disorder (ASD). Before specifically discussing the roles that animals can have with people who have ASD, attention will begin with explaining the value of the human-animal bond and the field of animal-assisted interventions (AAI).

Understanding the Human-Animal Bond

The sense of being needed and having a purpose in life has been researched by numerous scholars as one of the number of reasons why the bond between animals and people is established. Some also believe that our relationships with animals provide social supports in vulnerable times as well as opportunities for healthy interaction. For example, I think of one young man with autism whose best friend was a Labrador that he got on his tenth birthday. Alex always loved dogs. His parents recognized this when he was much younger. They noticed how much he enjoyed being around animals and his connection with them. The animals didn't appear to be as judgmental of his developmental differences and seemed to be accepting of his kindness and attention. It seemed logical for the family to get him a dog of his own. At first, there were challenges, especially when introducing any puppy in a family. Nevertheless the early hardship of training and cementing a bond between the two was outweighed by their evolving friendship. His beloved Dreamer, his dog, was always eager to see him, especially when he came home from school. At school, he was shunned by peers and at times was the brunt of their jokes and avoidance. When he returned home, that wasn't the case. He and Dreamer would frolic and play with each other for hours. Most of the time, Dreamer just sat by him vigilantly, waiting for their next adventure together. Alan (fictional name) seemed to cherish his friendship with Dreamer and through touch and in times in total silence they seemed to communicate well. The presence of his pet acted as a safe refuge and provided him with what we all would have considered unconditional love.

McNicholas and Colis (2000 and 2006) suggest that animals may be more forgiving than their human counterparts and are more accepting than fellow humans of those who may have awkward social and communication skills. This would seem to be the case with Alan and Dreamer. She seemed to respond differently to Alan and seemed more patient with his developmental differences.

Numerous research studies and papers have also been written over the past few decades that illustrate the unique physiological benefits that animals' foster. The roots of these findings go back to the pioneer works of Friedmann, Katcher, and Lynch (Friedmann et al, 1990) who have demonstrated the value of caressing an animal on cardiovascular health and decreased anxiety because of the physical contact of the pet. Since that time, there have been other researchers who have unearthed other specific physiological outcomes that have been enhanced due to the bond such as an increase in oxytocin and other healthy neurotransmitters as a consequence of gently stoking and petting dogs (Odenthal and Meintjes, 2003; and Dayton, 2010). The researchers have also found that petting and interacting with the dogs also caused a decrease in the cortisol (stress hormones) levels. In essence, the research (Wells, 2009, has an outstanding review of the literature) leaves us with an understanding that interacting with animals may be similar to a welcoming spa treatment that promotes a relaxed state. In fact, two researchers named Headey and Grabka (cited in Dayton, 2010) attempted to quantify the health correlates of pet ownership using national survey data in Australia, Germany and China. Their results suggested that compared with people who didn't have pets, those who live with other species seem to benefit from better overall health, get more exercise, sleep better, take fewer days off work, and see their doctor less. Although these finding are interesting, little is still known on how interactions with animals impact some of these variables with persons with ASD. Attention to some of the findings and practical solutions will be given later in the chapter.

Defining Animal-Assisted Interventions

The reputation of AAI has blossomed in the past several decades ever since Boris Levinson coined the term pet therapy (Levinson, 1969). As a clinician, Levinson suggested that animals could provide a calming effect in therapy. Ever since that time, numerous terms have been used to explain the therapeutic use of animals. Terms such as "pet therapy," "animal-facilitated counseling," "animal-assisted therapy and activities," "pet-mediated therapy," and "pet psychotherapy" have been commonly used interchangeably as descriptive terms. Nevertheless, the two most widely utilized terms are "animal-assisted therapy" and "animal-assisted activities". Both of these alternatives could be classified under the rubric of animal-assisted interventions.

The Delta Society's *Standards of Practice for Animal-Assisted Therapy* (1996) defines animal assisted therapy (AAT) as an intervention with specified goals and objectives delivered by a health or human service professional with specialized expertise in using an animal as an integral part of treatment. On the other hand, but equally valuable, animal-assisted activities (AAA) occur when specially trained professionals, paraprofessionals or volunteers accompanied by animals interact with people in a variety of environments (Delta Society, 1996). In AAA, the same activity can be repeated for many different people or groups of people, the interventions are not part of a specific treatment plan and are not designed to address a specific emotional or medical condition, and detailed documentation does not occur.

On the other hand, equine-assisted therapy has also had a long history in supporting diverse groups of people including persons with autism. Although not a household pet, horses have been found to be extremely helpful to children with autism, especially because of the added benefit of being in the outdoors. Horses also appear to be quite capable of perceiving human emotions. This ability is an asset to their interactions with people. Children eventually learn that calmer behavior usually gets the horses to feel more comfortable around them. Rupert Isaacson, the author of *Horseboy*, and father of a child with autism has had positive experiences with horse riding with many children with ASD. In a recent interview on January 19, 2011, Isaacson pointed out that he believed the best horses to utilize in therapy seemed to be alpha mares. He believes that these horses often are more confident and are not afraid of new challenges. They also seem to take on more caring and giving roles in their herds. For example, it is not uncommon in the wild to see alpha mares take on the maternal responsibilities of juveniles who have been abandoned or separated from their mothers. We will discuss this point a bit more, later in this chapter.

Therapeutic horseback riding has been used to help people with their balance and posture while taking advantage of the bond between the horse and the individual. Some believe that the effectiveness of horse riding stems from the kinesthetic stimulation that occurs during riding. Originally, therapeutic riding was given attention by some Germans who in the early 1960s believed that riding horses could be a viable treatment for people with compromised motor control and neurological disorders (Frewin & Gardiner, 2005). They called the process Hippotherapy, utilizing the Greek word Hippos, which means horse. The term hippotherapy actually means providing treatment with the help of a horse. The primary focus of the intervention pertains to the movement of the horse.

In the United States, The North American Riding for the Handicapped Association (NARHA) was formed in 1969 with the mission of promoting equine assisted therapies and activities for people with special needs. It was at this time that hippotherapy began to attract more attention in this country. As years progressed, the use of horses within therapy has grown beyond its use for physiological benefits and attention is now given to the psychological benefits that include our interacting with the horses and taking care of their needs (husbandry). Responsibility for another or someone else may be an important factor in the bonding process. Equine psychotherapy was formally started in the late 1990s. In 1999, the Equine Assisted Growth and Learning Association (EAGALA) was established. EAGALA is also devoted to the development of high standards and professionalism in the field of EFT. Both organizations offer training programs, which include conferences, continuing education, and support groups.

Understanding the Underlying Mechanisms of Animal-Assisted Interventions

The author, in previous articles (most recently in 2010) has identified several tenets that he believes are some of the major purposes of incorporating animals as an aspect of therapy. Briefly two of the tenets are as follows:

Tenet 1: Animals Acting as a Social Lubricant

As stated earlier, this tenet has been the primary force behind AAI including equine-assisted therapy. The animals act as a social lubricant and ease the stress of therapy by being comforting. The animals also act as a link in conversation between clinician and client, and help establish trust and rapport between patient and clinician. The mere presence of an animal can also give clients a sense of comfort, which further promotes rapport in the therapeutic relationship. In regards to persons with ASD, the literature does suggest a similar outcome. For example, Martin and Farnum (2002) noted several improvements in children with ASD when they interacted with therapy dogs. It appears that the animals in therapy promoted more playful moods and better attentiveness in the youngsters who participated in the project. Martin and Farnum concluded that these changes in their behavior were a direct consequence of being around the dogs. They also explained that "animals are believed to act as transitional objects, allowing children to first establish bonds with them and then extend these bonds to humans" (Martin and Farnum, 2002).

Tenet 2: Animals as Teachers

Perhaps one of the strongest outlets for applying AAI is how clinicians have often utilized animals for teaching as well as role models. This is one of the greatest advantages of incorporating animals into therapy. Teaching animals and supporting their growth can also have therapeutic benefits for the clients. There have been many clinicians who have used the bonding relationship with the animal as a method to enhance developmental skills. For example, in a study with a child with autism, Barol (2006) used the relaxed atmosphere that the dog promoted to teach skills that were normally avoided by the young boy. Prior to the onset of her study, Barol met with the therapeutic team to discuss what sorts of activities they would offer the child using the therapy dog as a motivational tool. For example, traditionally when asked to cut things in occupational therapy, the boy would often be uncooperative, squeal and whine. However, when asked to do a similar task when cutting up bacon-like dog treats, he seemed more willing to cooperate. In addition, the speech and language therapist worked with the child to say "Here Henry" when he gave the dog the treat. In essence, the responsibility of taking care of the animal seemed to be the impetus for his actions.

Pet Companionship and AAI: Suggestions for Applications

It is clear that there has been a recent interest in the roles that animals have in the lives of persons with ASD. Before I actually cover the therapeutic benefits of animals, I want to stress that companion animals can be wonderful in the lives of all children including children with ASD. Depending on the needs of the child, adjustments will be needed in selecting the best pet for a specific child. For example, some children will enjoy the companionship of more slow moving animals while others may need pets that are more engaging and will seek out more interaction.

There also have been a handful of studies in the last decade that have demonstrated that AAI could be useful in supporting persons with ASD with many of their developmental needs. Ming-Lee Yeh (2008) suggested several interesting outcomes from her three years of research on evaluating a canine animal-assisted therapy (AAT) treatment for children with ASD in Taiwan. She reported significant improvements for the children on the social skills subscale and total score on the VABS (The Vineland Adaptive Behavior Scale, VABS, Chinese version). She also reported that after interacting with dogs, children revealed significant improvements in various dimensions of communication and language as well as increasing their on-task behavior.

Grandin, Fine, and Bowers (2010) have suggested several reasons why AAI may be more appropriate for some people with ASD, while others may react indifferently. One argument that was made pertains to the fact the some people may respond negatively to their interactions due to their sensory oversensitivity. For example, a person with ASD may not be able to tolerate the smell of a dog. Another may have auditory oversensitivity and may not be able to tolerate the sound of a dog barking. The impact of sensory oversensitivity is extremely variable and can have a very strong effect on an interaction. For instance, when Bob first met Magic, he seemed very conscious of how she smelled. Attention was given to bathe her right before his visits with a very neutral smelling shampoo. On the other hand, a barking dog or a squawking bird may not bother some, while others will find it extremely aversive and offensive. Simply put, some people with various levels of ASD may avoid animals because they have extreme sensitivity to either sound or smell (it may not have anything to do with the animal specifically). One needs to carefully consider this point prior to introducing an animal.

Some believe that persons with ASD may respond differently to animals due to their differences in cognitive problem solving. For example, Grandin and Johnson (2005) hypothesize that one of the reasons why some children and adults with ASD relate really well to animals is due to sensory based thinking. They suggest that there may be some similarities in the way that both people with ASD and perhaps companion animals process information. In essence, animals do not think in words. They believe that dogs' cognitions are filled with detailed sensory information and their world is filled with pictures, smells, sounds, and physical sensations. Grandin et al (2010) summarized their impressions about some of the safeguards to consider when utilizing animals in therapy with the following conclusions. Table 1 summarizes these perceptions.

Table 1

Guidelines to consider when applying AAI with persons with ASD	
1.	Children and adults with ASD may relate better with companion animals because they both use sensory-based thinking.
2.	Sensory oversensitivity may have a tremendous impact on the outcome and is extremely variable. This means that some people may not be able to tolerate smells or sudden sounds from an animal. On the other hand, some will have no sensory problems with animals and will be attracted to them.
3.	Animals, specifically dogs, may communicate their behavioral intentions more easily to persons with ASD especially because their relationships are simpler.

Additionally, AAI can also be applied with individuals who have a milder version of ASD. Perhaps one of the greatest benefits has been how the animals have supported companionship and friendship in the lives of people who have felt very isolated and lonely. Fine and Eisen (2008) in *Afternoons with Puppy*, discussed several cases of youth with Asperger's syndrome and autism and the roles that animals had in their lives. One case that clearly stands out was about a teenage boy diagnosed with high functioning autism who had tremendous social skill difficulties. Unfortunately, the boy led a very isolated life until he developed an interest in the birds in my office. Eventually he adopted a bird and it provided him with compassion and joy. He often would sit next to the bird when he was anxious and upset. The bird seemed to provide him with a blanket of warmth that helped him regulate his anxiety. He also realized the importance of handling the bird gently. They seemed to become protective of each other and enjoyed each other's company. Grandin (2011) agrees with this point of view and believes that one of the strongest benefits of having a pet for a person with ASD is for companionship. The animal can also act as a social lubricant and help the individual feel wanted.

How Horses Can Help

"Because she listens to me." Five words said it all! This simple phrase was volunteered by an eight-year -old boy with autism named Stan when describing his love for his new equine friend named Lady and his perceptions of therapeutic horseback riding.

Stan's story with horses starts about three years earlier when his parents decided to look for another option to help him in his development. He was diagnosed when he was three and continues to be vey uncommunicative and distractible. When Stan started at the Queen of Hearts Therapeutic Riding Center program, his progress was somewhat uneventful with a 27-year-old horse named Buddy. His sessions primarily consisted of being lead on a horse by three instructors—one on each side of him and an instructor leading. Although Stan seemed to enjoy the interaction, the gains hoped for didn't materialize. It was after about a year, that Robin Kilcoyne, the executive director, decided to alter his program. That's when the lights turned on for Sam and things began to change. Stan was introduced to a new horse named Lady and there was an immediate connection. The activities were altered and Stan was taught to western ride so more creative activities could be implemented while he was riding. For example, he went on letter searches around the ring or had the opportunity to direct Lady to various spots around the ring where he was able to drop a ball in a basket. Stan also was taught to use simple words to get Lady to respond to him, such as whoa, walk on and trot. To Sam's initial amazement, Lady followed his lead. Ultimately, it was the friendship between the two that cemented their bond. Stan often found himself coming early and staying later to interact and talk with his new four-legged friend. Lady often responds with a bowed head and a wiggling nose nudging his cheek. Stan doesn't even bribe her to come his way. She seems attuned to his presence.

Although Stan continues to have his challenges, his friendship with Lady is still flourishing. He now rides her more independently and is often seen trotting around the ring. His early comment about his friend was accurate. Lady does listen and follow his direction. More importantly, she is his beloved friend!

It seems that the greatest benefit derived in therapeutic riding comes from the movement of the horse (because of the multisensory benefits derived from the interaction). However, therapeutic riding may also assist in enhancing communication and social behavior (Foxall, 2002; and Mason, 2004). For example, Rupert Isaacson, (personal communication, January 19, 2011) agrees that one advantage of using horses is that a child can teach a horse to do tricks using very limited words and vocabulary. Children can use one-word phrases to possibly get the horse to bow, smile, or even lay down (very similar to what was done with Stan). This can be very empowering and reinforcing to a child especially when the horse responds. The interaction between them seems to act as a social catalyst similar to the other animals discussed earlier. In our discussion, Isaacson also noted an approach he called "Back Riding" which is when an adult and child riding together. He believes that this technique is extremely useful for promoting communication. He believes that the combination of deep pressure (holding the child), speaking into the child's ear (not face-to-face speaking, which may agitate the child), and the movement of the horse all combine to create an optimum opportunity for the child to receive and retain information. Perhaps it is the movement of the horse that causes a neurological awakening, and makes the child more capable of interacting with the external world.

However, just like any animal assisted intervention, a child needs to be receptive to the interaction. He or she needs to be ready for the process and sometimes that means one has to be patient and adjust. Over the years I have experienced this dilemma and I have learned that sometimes just giving the process time to simmer, actually can be extremely effective. This principle reminds me of the old proverb that should be seriously taken into consideration. In essence we have to appreciate that "when the mind is ready the teacher comes." In the case of equines and therapeutic riding, it sometimes may mean that you must bring the horse into the child's orbit and be patient with the outcomes. It sometimes may mean that a lesson may not even include riding for the day, but just being in the environment and nearby the horse.

In regards to therapeutic riding, trainers including Isaacson, believe that training a horse in the skill of collection is extremely valuable in supporting children with ASD. In essence, collection is when a horse carries more weight on his/her hind legs than the front legs. The movement makes it easier for the horses to change direction quickly.

When horses are capable of moving with collection it enhances their power and causes more of a rocking motion. It is this rocking motion that seems to cause a euphoric response in children with autism.

Therapeutic riding requires that the person with ASD work on his/her balance. Some believe that the horse's gait simulates the pace at which a human walks, making the pelvic position and swaying while riding a horse very similar to the sway one experiences when walking (Reide, 1988). Even though the horse has a smooth gait at the walk, the horse's stride is quite long, which requires one to work on balance and posture while riding. OTs often use horses to deliver controlled sensory input to an individual. For example, this occurs while one manipulates the movement of the horse, its speed and gait. The process can also be altered by using different horses, whose physical size and make-up may cause a different response for an individual. For example one may select a horse with increased movements for a person who is in need of more sensory seeking (hypotonicity) while one may want to select a horse with more rhythmical movement for an individual who is more sensory avoidant or has hypertonicity.

According to Isaacson, smaller children relish periods of time where they lay full length on the horse's back. Some children seem to get great comfort from this, and he has observed that their self-stimming is often curbed during these opportunities. He feels that back riding is helpful because it is similar to laying on a big couch.

Finally, the research points out that the most effective sessions last for twenty-minute intervals and that the riding arena should have limited distraction so that a child will not be over stimulated. Once the twenty-minute ride is completed, one could have the person engage in another activity. Grandin, Fine, and Bowers (2010) note that depending on the functional skills of the person with ASD, the individual may also be encouraged to engage in many other chores including grooming the horse, leading it to and from its stall, perhaps help in feeding or giving the horse treats, or even saddling the horse before they ride. This additional contact with the horse may provide many of the same therapeutic benefits offered through interaction with more traditional therapy animals such as dogs. After the break, the child could get back on the horse for another twenty-minute session of riding (Grandin, et al, 2010).

Concluding Remarks

George Eliot (1857) in his book *Mr. Gilfil's Love Story, Scenes of Clerical Life*, once stated that *"animals are such agreeable friends—they ask no questions, they pass no criticisms"*. His comments seem very après pros in our concluding remarks for this paper. The love and unconditional regard received from a pet or a therapy animal may represent a catalyst for emotional and psychological growth. A well-trained therapy animal working alongside a seasoned therapist may be a viable team used to promote various developmental and functional skills. On the other hand, families may want to consider adopting an animal for companionship. However, one must realize the importance of selecting a compatible pet, and the need for effective training. Provisions need to be thought through to support not only the welfare of the person but also the animal. Although AAI shouldn't be unrealistically viewed as a panacea, one should not overlook the power of our connection to animals. We may find some significant benefits derived from this relationship.

ANTIEPILEPTIC TREATMENTS

BY DR. RICHARD E. FRYE

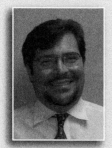

Richard E. Frye, M.D., Ph.D.

Department of Pediatrics, Division of Child and Adolescent Neurology
and The Children's Learning Institute
7000 Fannin—UCT 2478, Houston, TX 77030
Richard.E.Frye@uth.tmc.edu

Dr. Richard E. Frye received his M.D. and Ph.D. in physiology and
biophysics from Georgetown University. He completed his residency
in pediatrics at University of Miami and residency in child neurology at
Children's Hospital Boston. Following residency Dr. Frye completed a
clinical fellowship in behavioral neurology and learning disabilities at
Children's Hospital Boston and a research fellowship in psychology at Boston University. Dr.
Frye also completed a M.S. in biomedical science and biostatistics at Drexel University. Dr.
Frye is board certified in General Pediatrics and in Neurology with Special Competency in
Child Neurology. Dr. Frye has been funded to study brain structure function in individuals
with neurodevelopmental disorders, mitochondrial dysfunction in autism and clinical trials for
novel autism treatments. Dr. Frye is the medical-director of the University of Texas medically
based autism clinic. The purpose of this unique clinic is to diagnose and treat medical disorders
associated with autism, such as mitochondrial disorders and subclinical electrical discharges, in
order to optimize remediation and recovery.

Seizures, epilepsy, and subclinical electrical discharges are common in individuals
with Autism Spectrum Disorder (ASD). Seizures are most commonly treated with
antiepileptic medication but non-antiepileptic medication and treatments are used to
treat seizures when seizures are difficult to control. Antiepileptic medication have a
special role in ASD as some individuals with ASD have epileptic encephalopathies
as a result of uncommon epilepsy syndromes such as Landau-Kleffner syndrome and
electrical status epilepticus during slow-wave sleep. In addition, individuals with ASD
have been found to have a high rate of seizure-like electrical discharges on electroencephalogram (EEG) despite not having any clear clinical symptoms of seizures. Such
abnormalities are referred to as subclinical electrical discharges. While a wide range

of antiepileptic treatments have been developed to treat epilepsy in general, few treatments have been studied on children with ASD specifically.

Success Rates

Success in variable and depends on the indication for treatment. In some cases, dramatic results occur with antiepileptic treatment. It is best to select the most likely treatment that will produce minimal side effects based on the profile of the patient. Poor results with a particularly treatment should lead to consideration of alternative therapies or to prompt the investigation of underlying medical disorders that have not been investigated. Seizure-like events that do not respond to antiepileptic treatments should be reviewed carefully. If a video electroencephalograph has confirmed an electrographic correlate to the clinical behavior, more extensive metabolic or neuroimaging investigations might be indicated.

Adverse Effects

Most antiepileptic treatments can have adverse effects. Adverse effects of antiepileptic drugs are highly dependent on the medication. In general, newer antiepileptic drugs, such as lamotrigine, oxcarbazepine, topiramate, levetiracetam, have few serious adverse effects than older antiepileptic drugs, such as phenobarbital, phenytoin, primidone, and carbamazepine. The exception to this is valproate, which is an older antiepileptic medication that appears to have good efficacy for many individuals with ASD. However, the toxicity of valproic acid on the liver, pancreas, and blood cells must be carefully monitored and valproic acid must be avoided in individuals with mitochondrial disorders. The adverse effect profiles have not been studied in ASD specifically, so it is not known whether individuals with ASD have a higher incidence of adverse effects than other populations of individuals with epilepsy. However, it is best to avoid older antiepileptic drugs (phenobarbital, phenytoin, primidone) that have a high incidence of cognitive and neurological side-effects as adverse effects may exacerbate existing behavioral and cognitive abnormalities. In general, almost all antiepileptic drugs can cause neurological side effects (ataxia, tremor, nystagmus), behavioral side effects (hyperactivity, agitation, aggressiveness), gastrointestinal side-effects (abdominal pain, nausea) and an allergic reaction which can be severe in some cases. Serious side effects can often be avoided with careful monitoring. It is best to have a practitioner with experience in these medications prescribe an antiepileptic drug and monitor the patient. Care should especially taken when using multiple antiepileptic drugs as adverse effects can be additive. Since almost all antiepileptic drugs elevate the rate to birth defects, it is important to carefully consider the choice of antiepileptic drugs in potentially sexually active females.

There are specific adverse effects that ever practitioner should be aware of and should communicate to the patient when prescribing antiepileptic drugs:

Valproate: Valproate can result in serious adverse effects. The most serious adverse effects are hepatotoxicity (liver toxicity), hyperammonemia (high ammonia), and pancreatitis (inflammation of the pancreas). Precautions can be taken to prevent these adverse effects from occurring. In general, complete blood count, liver function tests and amylase and lipase should be monitored during the initially period of starting the medication and if the patient experiences gastrointestinal symptoms. Once a stable dose has been selected, the patient can be monitored approximately every three months. Hepatotoxicity is believed to be more prevalence in children under two years of age, so it is best to avoid prescribing valproate to very young children. In children with Alperts' syndrome, a syndrome causes by depletion of mitochondrial DNA, valproic acid can be fatal. In general, L-carnitine may mitigate liver damage resulting from valproic acid and, thus, cotreatment with carnitine is recommended. Common adverse effects of valproate include, weight gain and thinning of the hair. The latter is believed to respond to selenium (10–20 mcg per day) and zinc (25–50 mg per day). Long-term use of valproate has been linked to bone loss, irregular menstruation and polycystic ovary syndrome.

Lamotrigine: Lamotrigine has a low incidence of serious adverse effects and is generally well-tolerated. The most serious adverse effect of lamotrigine is a life threatening whole body rash known as a Steven-Johnson's reaction. Increasing the lamotrigine dose slowly towards the target dose can reduce the risk of this reaction occurring.

Oxcarbazepine: Hyponatremia (low blood sodium) can develop in some individuals.

Topiramate: Common adverse effects include weight loss and cognitive and psychomotor slowing. Topiramate is minimally metabolized by the liver and is excreted mostly unchanged by the kidney. Topiramate can cause a metabolic acidosis (high blood acid), nephrolithiasis (kidney stones) and oligohidrosis (decreased sweating). This medicine should be avoided in individuals with kidney disorders and extra care during hot weather is necessary. Glaucoma (increased eye pressure) has occurred in rare cases, so any vision symptoms should be considered evaluated.

Levetiracetam: Levetiracetam has a low incidence of serious adverse effects and is probably one of the safest antiepileptic drugs. The most prevalent adverse effects are behavioral, including agitation, aggressive behavior and mood instability. Levetiracetam has been linked to suicide in a few individuals without ASD. Preliminary reports suggest that cotreatment with pyridoxine (vitamin B6) helps reduce adverse behavioral effects.

Vigabatrin: Vigabatrin is associated with a progressive and permanent visual loss. Thus, its used is usually restricted to control of seizures in Tuberous Sclerosis.

Children With ASD have a High Incidence of Medical Disorders That May Guide The Practitioner To Choose a Particular Antiepileptic Drug.

ASD Symptoms	Avoid	Possible Alternative
Gastrointestinal Disorders	Valproate	Lamotrigine
Mitochondrial Disorders	Valproate	Levetiracetam, Lamotrigine
Poor growth	Topiramate	Lamotrigine
Overweight	Valproate	Topiramate, Lamotrigine, Levetiracetam
Behavioral problems	Levetiracetam	Lamotrigine, Valproate, Topiramate

Other Medications That Have Not Been Specifically Development as Antiepileptic Drugs Can Be Useful in Epilepsy That Is Not Well Controlled with Antiepileptic Medications.

Steroids: One-time treatment or regular scheduled treatments of high-dose steroids may help in refractory epilepsy, particularly epileptic encephalopathy syndromes. Daily steroids may also be effective but are difficult to maintain because of the high risk of adverse effects. Common adverse effects include weight gain, edema, mood instability and insomnia. Serious adverse effects include hypertension, immunosuppression, gastrointestinal ulceration, glucose instability and osteoporosis. Anyone on steroids for an extended period should be closely monitored for serious adverse effects.

Intravenous Immunoglobulin: Regularly scheduled infusion of intravenous immunoglobulin may help in refractory epilepsy, particularly epileptic encephalopathy syndromes. Common adverse effects include rash, headache and fever and require prophylactic pretreatment. This treatment is contraindicated in individuals with kidney or heart problems and should be administered by a practitioner familiar with the treatment. May individuals develop increasingly severe allergic reactions to intravenous immunoglobulin treatment. In such cases, changing the brand may reduce adverse effects.

Dietary Treatment Can Be Useful in Epilepsy That Is Not Well Controlled with Medications.

Low Carbohydrate Diets: Low carbohydrate diets, such as the ketogenic diet, have been very effective at controlling seizures in some children with refractory epilepsy. The ketogenic diet is a very restrictive diet, so some have tried the modified Atkins diet and found it to be effective. Any dietary treatment should be conducted under the guidance of a trained professional. The ketogenic diet can cause acidosis (high blood acid) anyone on this diet needs to be carefully monitored.

Elimination Diets: Isolated cases of improvement in seizures with elimination of certain foods or preservatives have been reported but no large studies have confirmed this practice as effective. Any dietary changes should be monitored by a trained professional.

Surgery Can Be Useful In Epilepsy That Is Not Well Controlled with Other Treatments or Diets.

Vagus Nerve Stimulator: The vagus nerve stimulator is a small device that is implanted under the skin that has a wire that wraps around the vagus nerve. The device stimulates the vagus nerve which has neural inputs into the brain. It is believed that stimulation of the brain results in changes in several levels of neurotransmitters, particularly gamma-aminobutyric acid, which can help control seizures. This device can cause alternations in vocalization, coughing, throat pain and hoarseness. More serious side effects include spasms of the vocal cords, obstruction of the airway and sleep apnea.

Corticetomy: If seizures are found to arise from one small area of the brain, it is possible for a neurosurgeon to remove the dysfunctional part of the brain. In order to determine if one portion of the brain is generating seizures, a patient must typically go through several extended hospitalization. Brain surgery can have serious adverse effects, so this option is typically reserved for the most refractory patients.

Multiple Subpial Transection: If a dysfunctional portion of the brain is found but cannot be removed, it is possible for a neurosurgeon to make cuts small cuts in the brain areas surrounding the dysfunctional areas. Like corticetomy, this requires brain surgery which can have serious adverse effects and requires an extended in hospital workup.

Individuals with Epilepsy, Especially Those with Frequent or Prolonged Seizures, Should Have an Emergency Medication Readily Available to Stop Any Generalized Seizure That Is Sustained for Over 5 Minutes.

Diazepam: The most common emergency medication is rectal diazepam. The most common adverse reaction is drowsiness. Respiratory depression can occur if given at high doses. If it is necessary to use this medication, medical personnel should be called to evaluate the patient.

For More Information:

The Epilepsy Foundation of America
www.epilepsyfoundation.org

American Epilepsy Outreach Foundation
www.epilepsyoutreach.org

ANTIFUNGAL TREATMENT

BY DR. LEWIS MEHL-MADRONA

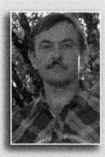

Lewis Mehl-Madrona, MD, Ph.D., MPhil

Education and Training Director
Coyote Institute for Studies of Change and Transformation
Burlington, VT and Honolulu, HI
Department of Family Medicine
University of Hawaii School of Medicine
Honolulu, HI
PO Box 9309
South Burlington, VT 05407
mehlmadrona@gmail.com
(808) 772-1099

Dr. Lewis Mehl-Madrona graduated from Stanford University School of Medicine and completed his family medicine and his psychiatry training at the University of Vermont College of Medicine. He earned a Ph.D. in clinical psychology at the Psychological Studies Institute in Palo Alto and also became a licensed psychologist in California. He took a Master's in Philosophy degree from Massey University in New Zealand in Narrative Studies in Psychology. He is American Board certified in family medicine, geriatric medicine, and psychiatry. He is the author of *Coyote Medicine, Coyote Healing, Coyote Wisdom, Narrative Medicine,* and, most recently, *Healing the Mind through the Power of Story: The Promise of Narrative Psychiatry.* He is the Education and Training Director for Coyote Institute for Studies of Change and Transformation, based in Burlington, Vermont and in Honolulu, Hawaii and is Clinical Assistant Professor of Family Medicine at the University of Hawaii in Honolulu.

Overview. The reduction in amount of fungi in the digestive tract is part of a larger group of interventions commonly called biological therapies. In this review, we will focus on the evidence for fungal involvement in the symptoms of autistic children, discuss the ways in which the amount of fungi in the gut can be reduced, and review the evidence that exists to support these practices.

Autism and Digestive Difficulties

Children diagnosed with autism do have considerable digestive difficulties. In 2003, Rosseneu studied eighty children diagnosed with autism who also had digestive symptoms, finding that 61 percent had abnormal gram negative endotoxin-producing bacteria, 55 percent had overgrowth of *Staphylococcus aureus* and 95 percent had an overgrowth of *Escherichia coli*. He did not find abnormal amounts of fungus.

Candida Overgrowth

The main fungal culprit implicated in autism is *Candida albicans* (Edelson, 2006). Generally this fungus is kept under control by the bacteria that live within the gut. However, exposure to antibiotics can kill these bacteria resulting in a proliferation of *Candida*. It lives on the moist dark mucous membranes which line the mouth, vagina, and intestinal tract. Ordinarily it exists only in small colonies, prevented from growing too rapidly by the human host's immune system, and by competition from other microorganisms in and on the body's mucous membranes. When something happens to upset this delicate natural balance, *Candida* can grow rapidly and aggressively, causing many unpleasant symptoms to the host. Vaginal yeast infections present the most common case in point.

High levels of *Candida* are thought to release toxins which are absorbed into the bloodstream through the blood, thereby causing difficulties. Edelson links an overgrowth of *Candida* to confusion, hyperactivity, short attention span, lethargy, irritability, and aggression. He further cites headaches, abdominal pain, constipation, excess gas, fatigue, and depression as linked to *Candida* overgrowth. Support for the *Candida* overgrowth theory is often sought in the observation that people treated for *Candida* become worse for two to three days before becoming better. This worsening is supposed to relate to "die-off" of the yeast. As the fungi die, their cell walls open, releasing the intracellular contents into the gut. Some components of this intracellular material are thought to be cause symptoms in humans. Further proof is offered in the form of organic acid analysis of the urine. When organic acids are found in the urine that are only produced by yeast, presumably the yeast are releasing these acids into the gut to pass through the gut wall into the bloodstream to be removed by the kidneys. Popular books on *Candida* include William Crook's *The Yeast Connection Handbook*. Organic acid urine testing is performed at The Great Plains Laboratory in Overland Park, Kansas.

Many children afflicted with autism have had frequent ear infections as young children and have taken large amounts of antibiotics. These are thought to exaggerate the yeast problem. Other possible contributors to *Candida* overgrowth are hormonal treatments; immunosuppressant drug therapy; exposure to herpes, chicken pox, or other "chronic" viruses; or exposure to chemicals that might upset the immune system.

Another reported reason for fungal overgrowth is a faulty immune system. A relationship between autism and immunity was proposed over forty years ago based on the detection of autoimmune conditions in family members of children diagnosed with autism (Money et al., 1971; Ashwood et al., 2004. Pardo and Eberhart, 2007). Numerous scientific reports of immune abnormalities in people with autism have been published (Ashwood and Van de Water, 2004, Hornig and Lipkin, 2001). These include defects in antibody production, imbalances between the different parts of the immune system, and higher rates of infections in children diagnosed with autism. The production of lymphocytes has been found to be decreased (Stubbs & Crawford, 1976).

A year later, Stubbs (1977) supported an altered immune response among "five of thirteen autistic children who had undetectable titers despite previous rubella vaccine, while all control children had detectable titers. This finding of undetectable titers in autistic children suggests these children may have an altered immune response." Children diagnosed with autism do not always respond to vaccination, having no evidence of being immunized a year after a rubella vaccine was given.

In one study, 46 percent of families of children diagnosed with autism have two or more members with autoimmune disorders such as type I diabetes, rheumatoid arthritis, hypothyroidism, and lupus (Pardo & Eberhart, 2007). Antibodies have been found in children diagnosed with autism against their own nerves and their myelin covering, nerve receptors, and even brain parts (Jepson, 2007). The commonly recognized clumsiness of many autistic children has been linked to antibodies attacking the Purkinje cells in the cerebellum (Rout and Dhossche, 2008) which are the cells that control coordinated movements. Inflammation has been found in the brains of children with autism (Vargas et al, 2005).

Oxalic Acid and Yeast

Oxalate and its acid form oxalic acid are organic acids that are primarily from three sources: the diet, from fungus such as *Aspergillus* and *Penicillium* and *Candida* (Fomina et al, 2005, Ruijter et al, 1999; Takeuchi et al, 1987), and from human metabolism (Ghio et al, 2000).

Researcher Susan Owens discovered that the use of a diet low in oxalates markedly reduced symptoms in children with autism and PDD. For example, a mother with a son with autism reported that he became more focused and calm, that he played better, that he walked better, and had a reduction in leg and feet pain after being on a low-oxalate diet. Prior to the low-oxalate diet, her child could hardly walk up the stairs. After the diet, he walked up the stairs easier (Great Plains, 2008).

Oxalates in the urine are much higher in individuals with autism than in normal children. In one study, 36 percent of the children with a diagnosis of autism had values higher than 90 mmol/mol creatinine, the value consistent with a diagnosis of genetic hyperoxalurias, while none of the normal children had values this high.

Supplements can also reduce oxalates. Calcium citrate can be used to reduce oxalate absorption from the intestine. Citrate is the preferred calcium form to reduce oxalate because citrate also inhibits oxalate absorption from the intestinal tract. Children over the age of 2 need about 1000 mg of calcium per day (Great Plains, 2008). N-Acetyl-glucosamine is used to stimulate the production of the intercellular cement hyaluronic acid to reduce pain caused by oxalates (Vulvar Pain Foundation, 2008). Chondroitin sulfate is used to prevent the formation of calcium oxalate crystals (Shirane et al, 1988). Vitamin B6 is a cofactor for one of the enzymes that degrades oxalate in the body and has been shown to reduce oxalate production (Chetyrkin et al, 2005). Increased water intake also helps to eliminate oxalates (Great Plains, 2008). Probiotics may be very helpful in degrading oxalates in the intestine. Individuals with low amounts of oxalate-degrading bacteria are much more susceptible to kidney stones (Kumar et al, 2002). Both *Lactobacillus acidophilus* and *Bifidobacterium lactis* have enzymes that degrade oxalates (Azcarate-Pearil et al, 2006). Increased intake of essential omega-3 fatty acids, commonly found in fish oil and cod liver oil, reduces oxalate (Baggio et al, 1996).

Non-pharmacological Therapies

The most common means of restoring *Candida* populations to desirable levels is through ingesting healthy bacteria, generally species of *Lactobacillus*. These potions of bacteria are generally called probiotics, and are safe and effective. Reduction of dietary sugar and carbohydrates is also advocated, along with a yeast-free diet.

Saturated Fatty Acids

Undecylenic and caprylic acids are common medium-chain saturated fatty acids used to treat fungal infections. Common sources of caprylic acid are palm and coconut oils, whereas undecylenic acid is extracted from castor bean oil. Palm and coconut oil and castor bean oil are also used. Both have been shown to be comparable to a number of common antifungal drugs. A typical dosage for caprylic acid would be up to 3600 mg per day in divided doses with meals. Undecylenic acid is commonly taken in dosages of up to 1000 mg per day in divided doses.

Useful herbs include berberine, an alkaloid found in an herb called barberry *(Berberis vulgaris)* and related plants as well as in goldenseal, Oregon grape root and Chinese goldthread. This herb is commonly used in Chinese and ayurvedic medicines for its antifungal. *Oregano vulgare* is an effective antifungal. Carvacrol, one of its components, was found to inhibit *Candida* growth. Garlic *(Allium sativum)* contains a large number of sulphur containing compounds with antifungal properties. Because of the many different compounds with anti-fungal properties in garlic, yeast and fungi are less likely to become resistant. Fresh garlic was significantly more potent against *Candida albicans* than other preparations. Colloidal silver is a suspension of silver particles in water. Colloidal silver is said to be effective against yeast and fungi species including *Candida*. It works by targeting the enzyme involved with supplying the fungus with oxygen. Cellulase is the enzyme that breaks down cellulose, the main component of the yeast cell wall. When it comes into contact with yeast cells, the cell wall is damaged and the organism dies. Plant tannins are natural substances found in black walnut and other plants. They are found in red wines and redwood trees. They have an antifungal effect.

Antifungal medications.

Antifungal medications include fluconazole, ketoconazole, itraconazole, or terbinafine and are used, sometimes for as long as one to two months. Antifungals are usually monitored with liver function tests every one to three months, since these drugs can cause liver damage. Sometimes Amphotericin B is used as an oral liquid because it is not absorbed by the intestines into the blood stream but will still kill intestinal yeast. Nystatin is another oral medication that is not absorbed by the intestines and is relatively safe to use over long periods of time.

Outcomes

No systematic studies have been conducted of antifungal regiments for children diagnosed with autism. Difficulties exist in making such studies. Autism is most likely what is called a polymorphic condition. Many pathways lead to the same symptoms. Some of these pathways could involve *Candida*; others, not. Finding the children who would respond could be a challenge. Many case reports exist of children who have improved with antifungal treatment. Case reports, however, cannot rule out the possibility of the treatment working because of what I call the "Pygmalion effect"—that people become what we expect them to become. It's a kind of social placebo effect. When we believe in a treatment, we can make it powerfully effective, even though it may have no intrinsic biological efficacy

In general, candidal overgrowth in the intestines of children diagnosed with autism has not been documented (Wakefield et al., 2000) by endoscopy. In 1995, two brothers were reported whose symptoms were associated with *Candida* overgrowth. Both improved following *Candida* elimination (Shaw, 1995).

One example of a common kind of story comes from the book, *Feast Without Yeast: 4 Stages to Better Health*: The authors' 4½-year-old son was writhing on the floor screaming. "He had been behaving this way on and off for six months. . . . At age two he had been fine. From two-and-a-half to age four, his development had slowed down, but had not stopped. Starting a few days after his fourth birthday, he began to lose his speech . . .

"He lost his toilet training, stopped eating and lost . . . weight. . . . [He] could not use his hands. He sat in a swing spinning much of the day. He had lost all emotional contact except with his mother, and that was fleeting . . .

"We took away chocolate, peanut butter, orange juice, aged cheeses, and some other foods. The improvement was immediate. Avi looked and acted as if a weight had been lifted from his head. Only then could we see the onset of separate headaches, when we would make a mistake and give him foods we weren't supposed to, or when he would eat something that we learned later caused problems. We saw the headaches set in about three times a week instead of being chronic.

His symptoms . . . began to diminish. He no longer screamed all the time. His behavior improved. He seemed more with us, more engageable. If he accidentally ate the wrong foods, the screaming began again . . . "

"We got our next break about eight weeks later with the Jewish holiday of Passover. For this holiday, all foods containing yeast, leavening and fermented foods are eliminated. This holiday lasts eight days. Three days into Passover, our son was clearly improving again. He appeared much more comfortable. . . . His behavior had improved to the point that he was accepted into a special education speech and language summer program.

"After that first Passover holiday, one of the many health care professionals we were seeing suggested we look at an outstanding book called *The Yeast Connection* by Dr. William Crook. Dr. Crook compiled treatment histories of people who have problems with something called *Candida albicans*, a type of fungus which at times resembles yeast. We found that Dr. Crook recommended eliminating many of the foods we had found to be problematic for Avi, although there were some very significant differences at that time. . . . Within a few days of starting on the nystatin, Avi made a year's growth in playground development. He got off the swings, where he usually spent his hours of playground time. He began climbing jungle gyms, sliding down slides, and beginning to look like a four year old kid again. Avi still did not get his speech back, but he was beginning to be able to function.

Once we eliminated barley malt and all other malted products (maltodextrin, malted barley flour, and so on), vinegar, and yeast, the improvement was dramatic. We began to see the light at the end of the tunnel, but little did we know how long that tunnel was. Reaching the end of the tunnel is still a goal, although after more than eight years, we are much closer. Eight years ago, simply decreasing Avi's headaches to once a week or once every two weeks, and seeing his behavior improve and his autistic symptoms decrease, were major victories. We had turned the tide before we lost Avi altogether. He was coming back to us, very, very slowly. It took two more years, and much more experimentation, to completely eliminate Avi's debilitating headaches. Another two years of experimentation eliminated Avi's eczema and itching.

"Many people ask us whether this treatment has been a cure; for our son. We cannot say that it has been, but we cannot say that it has not been. Avi still does not talk fluently, but he has words, and can communicate. He types independently, too.

"Talking is not the only important part of life. Avi now is able to relate to people emotionally. He is out of pain.

Avi has now started his fourth year of high school, and is doing great.

"Before we began treating Avi with dietary intervention, Avi could not tolerate the presence of other children before starting on this diet. He could not tolerate being touched. Now Avi loves tickles, hugs, and touches, even from strangers."

Another famous case occurred in 1981, when Duffy, the 3½-year-old son of Gianna and Gus Mayo of San Francisco began to developmentally regress. The Mayos were lucky enough to take Duffy to allergist Alan Levin who found that Duffy's immune system was severely impaired. Duffy had been given a number of treatments with antibiotics, which were intended to control his ear infections. Levin tried Nystatin, an antifungal drug which is toxic to *Candida* but not to humans. Duffy at first got worse (a common reaction, caused by the toxins released by the dying *Candida* cells). Then he began to improve. Since Duffy was sensitive to molds, the Mayos moved inland to a dryer climate. Since *Candida* thrives on certain foods (especially sugars and refined carbohydrates) Duffy's diet required extensive modification. Duffy became active, greatly improved child with few remaining signs of autism. The Los Angeles Times published a long, syndicated article about Duffy in 1983, which resulted in letters and phone calls from parents of autistic children throughout the country. There were many autistic children whose problems started soon after long-term antibiotic therapy, or whose mothers had chronic yeast infections, which they had passed along to the infants.

I have similar cases to report. I can say that the process of eradicating *Candida* has benefited many children in my practice. What I cannot say is that the problems were caused by the *Candida*. Healing is a process. When we believe in a process, then healing happens. David Peat in *Blackfoot Physics,* discusses the embeddedness of the English language in nouns and in a linear, mechanical, "thing" view of the world. We want things to work. Instead, it is more common that processes work. The process of eliminating *Candida* has helped many children, which is different from saying that eliminating *Candida* helped them. I don't know how many "things" are interchangeable in a process of healing. I don't know how much any individual "thing" matters. Double-blind, randomized, controlled trials are ideal for comparing to things. They are poor for determining if a process of healing can help a particular condition. Within a process of healing, these trials help us to compare two "things". We have yet to accomplish a clinical trial on eliminating yeast, but, for now, I continue to enthusiastically pursue the process of healing through eliminating yeast. This process I know to work.

APPLIED BEHAVIOR ANALYSIS: WHAT MAKES A GREAT ABA PROGRAM? SORTING THROUGH THE SCIENCE, THE BRANDS, AND THE ACRONYMS

BY DR. JONATHAN TARBOX AND DR. DOREEN GRANPEESHEH

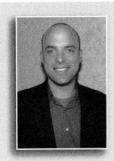

Jonathan Tarbox, Ph.D., BCBA-D

Center for Autism and Related Disorders
19019 Ventura Blvd, 3rd Floor
Tarzana, CA 91356
j.tarbox@centerforautism.com

Dr. Jonathan Tarbox is the Director of Research and Development at the Center for Autism and Related Disorders. Dr. Tarbox has worked in a variety of positions in the fields of behavior analysis and autism, including basic research, applied research, and practical work; with individuals with and without autism and other developmental disabilities, of all ages, and their families and care providers. His early career involved positions at both the New England Center for Children and the Kennedy Krieger Institute. Dr. Tarbox is a Board Certified Behavior Analyst-Doctoral and has a PhD in Behavior Analysis from the University of Nevada, Reno. Dr. Tarbox has over 40 publications in peer-reviewed journals, book chapters in scientific texts, and articles in popular media, and serves on the editorial board of several scientific journals. Dr. Tarbox's primary research interests include verbal behavior, rule-governed behavior, private events, and recovery from autism.

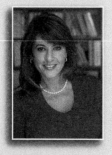

Doreen Granpeesheh, Ph.D., BCBA-D

Dr. Doreen Granpeesheh has dedicated over thirty years to helping individuals with autism lead healthy, productive lives. While completing her PhD in Psychology under Ivar Lovaas, she worked on the world-renowned 1987 study that showed a recovery rate of nearly 50%. Dr. Granpeesheh is a licensed psychologist in four states and is a Board Certified Behavior Analyst-Doctoral (BCBA-D). In 1990 Dr. Granpeesheh founded the Center for Autism & Related Disorders (CARD). CARD achieves success with every child through world-class treatment, staff training, curricula, and research. CARD provides services at 18 clinics in six U.S. states, as well as sites in Australia, New Zealand and partnerships in Dubai and Johannesburg. CARD employs over 800 staff and is a leading employer of BCBAs. Dr. Granpeesheh is on numerous Scientific and Advisory Boards for governmental and advocacy groups, and is the recipient of frequent honors, including the 2011 American Academy of Clinical Psychiatrists Winokur Award.

Treatment programs for children with autism that are based on Applied Behavior Analysis (ABA) have exploded over the last two decades and the result may appear to be a dizzying array of terminology, acronyms, and brands. Many parents of children with ASD may find it confusing and frustrating to navigate all of this information. This chapter will attempt to help by providing a brief overview of the core defining features of ABA programs, as well as describing the major models, brands, and acronyms.

Core Defining Features of Top-Quality ABA Programs

Applied Behavior Analysis, as a scientific discipline, involves applying scientifically validated principles of learning and motivation, and procedures derived from them, to solving problems of social significance. Autism is probably the best known problem to which ABA has been applied.

PRINCIPLES

The basic learning principles that form the foundation of any good ABA program are: 1) reinforcement, 2) extinction, 3) establishing or motivating operations, 4) stimulus control, and 5) generalization. The principle of reinforcement refers to the fact that people continue to do behaviors that produce desirable outcomes—it's what motivates us all to do what we do. Extinction simply refers to the discontinuation of reinforcement—when reinforcement stops, behavior decreases. Establishing operations are situations that help make reinforcement powerful, for example, being hungry makes food a strong reinforcer. Stimulus control is the process of how behavior becomes cued or signaled by the environment (e.g., the behavior of stopping at a red light). Generalization refers to how people apply learning to all relevant aspects of their lives. Good quality treatment programs have supervisors with advanced training and knowledge of behavioral principles and how they can be applied to teaching children with autism.

PROCEDURES

There are many intervention procedures derived from behavioral learning principles, but the basic ones common to all good ABA programs for children with autism include: 1) prompting, 2) preference assessment, 3) discrimination training, 4) shaping, 5) chaining, 6) explicit programming for maintenance and generalization, and 7) the provision of thousands of learning opportunities per day. All good ABA programs should have at least these seven features explicitly built into their daily operations.

DISCRETE TRIAL TRAINING AND NATURAL ENVIRONMENT TRAINING

The vast majority of comprehensive ABA treatment programs for autism include a large amount of time dedicated to discrete trial training (DTT), a teaching procedure that involves repeated practice of skills, gradually increasing in difficulty and gradually decreasing in structure and contrivance. DTT is still, by far, the most scientifically supported teaching procedure for children with autism. All good ABA programs today also incorporate a significant amount of naturalistic ABA teaching procedures, referred to as Natural Environment Training (NET). There are many different varieties of NET, including incidental teaching, milieu teaching, and Pivotal Response Training. Each has unique features, but all contain these basic elements: 1) teaching is done in the natural environment (e.g., during play, while getting dressed, while making a sandwich, etc.), 2) teaching interactions are initiated by the child, 3) prompting is used when necessary, and 4) the natural consequence of the behavior is used as a reinforcer, whenever possible. Good quality comprehensive ABA programs do not choose between NET and DTT, they include both. Both NET and DTT are generally considered necessary to ensure sufficient learning opportunities and effective generalization of skills.

A FUNCTIONAL APPROACH TO CHALLENGING BEHAVIOR

All good ABA programs are proficient at decreasing the challenging behaviors of children with autism and replacing them with other more adaptive behaviors. The best approach to decreasing challenging behavior is to first understand the function of the behavior, i.e., what the child is getting by engaging in the behavior. The most common functions of challenging behavior that have been identified in research are: 1) getting attention from others, 2) getting out of doing something the child does not want to do (e.g., school work), 3) getting access to a preferred item or activity, and 4) automatic reinforcement (aka, "self-stimulation"). That same source of reinforcement can then be used to teach appropriate alternative behaviors, such as asking for what one wants. Teaching a child to ask for what he wants instead of engaging in challenging behavior to get it is called Functional Communication Training (FCT) and has been proven effective by a large amount of research. Positive Behavioral Supports (PBS) is a model of ABA treatment for challenging behavior that emphasizes arranging the individual's environment to avoid challenging behavior, as well as establishing other preventive measures, such as systems and family supports.

GENERALIZATION AND MAINTENANCE

All good ABA programs place a heavy emphasis on generalization and maintenance of skills. This means that when a child learns new skills and/or his challenging behaviors decrease, these same improvements should also be seen in other settings, with other people (not just the therapists), and they should maintain across time. Good programs take explicit steps to encourage these outcomes, they do not merely hope for them.

DATA

All good ABA programs rely on regular data collection to ensure child progress and to make decisions regarding when to implement, change, or terminate particular treatment procedures. All good ABA programs assume that the teaching procedure is what causes learning, so if a child is not learning, it is unacceptable to blame the child or the diagnosis. The data must be used to evaluate procedures and the procedures must be changed until something effective is found.

TRAINING AND SUPERVISION

All good ABA programs place a heavy emphasis on training and continued professional development for staff. A single brief seminar or "in-service" training for new therapists or teacher's aids is never sufficient to establish excellent staff performance. Frequent supervision must be done by a supervisor who is an expert in designing ABA programs for children with autism, ideally a Board Certified Behavior Analyst with several years experience in top-quality ABA programs for children with autism.

RELATIONSHIP-BUILDING

All good ABA programs focus on building a positive relationship with the child by relying on positive reinforcement and rapport-building, and by providing the child sufficient help to ensure success. All good ABA programs begin with the assumption that every child with autism is capable of learning and that every child deserves a chance at learning the maximum number of skills possible, in a positive and fun environment.

INTENSITY

ABA treatment requires hard work. The research has clearly shown that the best gains are achieved when children receive at least 30 hours per week of one-to-one therapy, for two or more years. Many children require three or four years to reach their maximum potential. No research has yet been published that provides a shortcut around this level of intensity. ABA treatment implemented at this level of intensity, starting before the age of 4, and addressing all areas of deficit, is often referred to as Early Intensive Behavioral Intervention (EIBI) and sometimes as Intensive Behavioral Treatment (IBT).

CURRICULUM

Good ABA programs must use a comprehensive curriculum that addresses all areas of human functioning, since every child with autism is different, and some require learning in every area of development.

PARENT INVOLVEMENT

All good ABA programs require parent involvement. At a minimum, parents should attend regular supervision meetings, at least every two weeks. Parents must be taught the basics of ABA and are reminded that their child has an opportunity to learn, any time he is awake, 7 days per week. However, parent training is *not* a substitute for professional-quality therapy and supervision. No research has yet shown that professional therapy and supervision can be replaced with parent training. No one would even suggest such a thing for surgery, and ABA therapy is no less complex or difficult to supervise.

Models and Brands of ABA for Children with Autism

LOVAAS THERAPY

In 1987, Ivar Lovaas published the first controlled outcome study showing that ABA can produce robust treatment effects for children with autism, including recovery in a subset of cases. Virtually all contemporary ABA programs contain some elements of the original Lovaas approach. However, most contemporary programs have made changes to the original Lovaas approach, most notably including a heavier emphasis on NET. It should be noted that therapy based on the Lovaas approach is still the most scientifically supported treatment for autism in the world.

PIVOTAL RESPONSE TRAINING

Pivotal Response Training (PRT) is a form of NET. It is not something different from ABA, it is one set of procedures *within* ABA. It is distinguished from some other forms of NET by the fact that it explicitly involves reinforcing child *attempts* to respond, even if the response is incorrect. A large amount of research has shown that PRT is an effective teaching tool, but it is not a comprehensive intervention. It is one critical piece of comprehensive EIBI programs. No controlled outcome studies have yet been published on the effects of treatment programs include only PRT and exclude other ABA teaching procedures, such as DTT.

VERBAL BEHAVIOR

There is a currently a lot of confusion about what verbal behavior is and how or whether it should be part of ABA treatment for children with autism. In the last decade or so, some groups (perhaps unintentionally) have spoken and acted as though verbal behavior is something different from ABA. This idea is highly uninformed. The term "verbal behavior" comes from B. F. Skinner's analysis of language in terms of behavioral principles, which yielded the concepts of the "verbal operants": mand, tact, echoic, intraverbal, and so on. All good ABA programs should be thinking about and teaching language from the standpoint of behavioral principles and this is all that the term "verbal behavior" properly refers to. Skinner's verbal operants are useful tools for analyzing a child's language development and more basic verbal operants should be taught before more advanced ones (e.g., teach mands before intraverbals). The terms "Verbal Behavior Analysis" (VBA) and "Applied Verbal Behavior" (AVB) are not something different from ABA, they refer to ABA programs that place a heavy emphasis on incorporating Skinner's verbal operants into their programs. No research has been published that has compared these programs to other comprehensive EIBI programs that place less of an emphasis on verbal operants.

PICTURE COMMUNICATION AND SIGN LANGUAGE

All good ABA programs should include some provision for establishing language in children who have particular difficulty in learning to speak vocally and/or learning to respond to vocal speech. In these cases, most programs will either teach basic sign language or some form of picture communication system. The most researched form of picture communication is the Picture Exchange Communication System (PECS). PECS involves teaching children to exchange symbolic pictures in order to communicate. Research shows that both PECS and sign language are effective for children with autism, when implemented by clinicians who are experts in ABA.

CARD

The Center for Autism and Related Disorders (CARD) model of ABA intervention for children with ASD is a comprehensive approach to EIBI. The CARD model includes all major ABA principles and procedures described above, and customizes the proportion of each procedure for each child, based on his/her individual strengths, deficits, and preferences. The CARD curriculum is the most comprehensive curriculum available for children with autism and the CARD model is known for placing significant emphasis on higher order skills, such as perspective-taking, executive functions, and derived relational responding. The entire CARD system has also recently been made available online (see description of SKILLS in the CARD chapter in this book).

CABAS

Comprehensive Application of Behavior Analysis to Schooling (CABAS) is a comprehensive model of ABA instruction, based largely on Skinner's analysis of verbal behavior. The model focuses heavily on establishing concept formation ("generalized operants") and has a well-developed, but not publicly available, curriculum.

What's Coming Next

It is always difficult to predict the future but a few areas of development are worthy of special mention. First, it is likely that in the next several years, an additional certification will be created for ABA practitioners in autism. The BCBA certification assures foundational knowledge in ABA but not with respect to autism, in particular. Many parents of children on the spectrum have been demanding an additional guarantee of expertise in ABA treatment for autism and it is likely that such a certification will come about in the near future. Finally, the global demand for ABA services and the severe shortage of expert clinicians has created a need for faster training and dissemination of ABA expertise. It seems likely that information technology will play a part in meeting this demand, with university training systems moving increasingly to online education, as well as organizational communication systems moving toward Web-based meetings and teleconferencing. The coming decade is likely to be a critical period for designing systems for training and dissemination that will increase efficiency without sacrificing quality, in order to meet the ever-increasing demand for ABA services around the world.

AQUATIC THERAPY

BY ANDREA SALZMAN

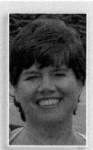

Andrea L. Salzman, MS, PT

Aquatic Therapy University
3500 Vicksburg Lane #250
Plymouth, MN 55447
(800) 680-8624
info@aquatic-university.com
www.aquatic-university.com (Aquatic Therapy University)
www.aquatic-sensory-integration.com (Aquatic Sensory Integration)

Ms. Salzman is the Director of Practice for Aquatic Therapy University
(ATU) which provides curriculum-based studies in aquatic therapy. Salzman has served as:
• Editor-in-Chief, Journal of Aquatic Physical Therapy;
• Seminar Instructor, two hundred-plus aquatic therapy seminars;
• Founder, Aquatic Resources Network, clearinghouse of information on aquatic therapy and
related topics;
• Creator, Aquatic Health Research Database (AHRD);
• Author, five textbooks and over three hundred magazine articles;
• Manager, Regions Hospital Therapy Pool;
• Adjunct Faculty, College of St. Catherine's PT program.
In 2010, Salzman was honored with the highest award given to aquatic physical therapists, the
Judy Cirullo Leadership Award, from the American Physical Therapy Association. Salzman has
also received the Aquatic Therapy Professional of the Year and Tsunami Aquatic Awards from
the Aquatic Therapy and Rehabilitation Institute (ATRI).
Special thanks to Jennifer Tvrdy, OTDR/L for her assistance in making Aquatic Sensory
Integration techniques accessible to parents and therapists everywhere.

Parents have a powerful weapon in their fight against autism: water. The bathtub,
shower, or public pool can offer countless opportunities to tame transitional
stresses, promote social encounters, correct out-of-kilter motor systems, and promote
sensory integration.

In water, parents have the power to harness buoyancy, viscosity, turbulence, surface tension, refraction, and thermal shifts.[1] Aquatic therapy offers so much promise
for this population that entire therapy pools have been designed with these children in

mind. [2-3] Additionally, training seminars, textbooks, and DVDs have been developed to teach therapists and parents to perform sensory integration in water.[4-5] Even Internet-based social networking sites have gotten into the act by devoting entire discussion groups to aquatic therapy for the sensory-challenged child.[6]

As always in the field of physical medicine, research lags behind anecdotal evidence. Intuitively, many pediatric clinicians believe in the power of the pool. In the literature, clinicians have reported a substantial increase in swim skills, attention, muscle strength, balance, tolerating touch, initiating/maintaining eye contact, and water safety during their sessions with young children with autism.[7-10] Parents who require assistance creating aquatic treatment ideas and skill-specific challenges can benefit from reading their findings.

To date, there are no gold-standard clinical trials which support aquatic therapy for the treatment of autism. This is interpreted—in all probability, prematurely—by some as a reason to deny aquatic therapy for this diagnosis.

As one example, Aetna Insurance has made a special notation of the fact that they will not reimburse for aquatic therapy services for autism or asthma (strangely specific rulings), while they will reimburse for water-based treatment of the musculoskeletal patient.[11] In this author's opinion, this represents a fundamental misunderstanding of what aquatic therapy is.

Insurers who deny aquatic therapy, yet readily approve of their land-based counterparts, do not understand that the pool is just another tool. Much like a therapeutic ball, a bolster, a mat or a swing, the pool is a means to an end, not a treatment in and of itself.

Truly, there is no such procedure as aquatic therapy. Instead, there is neuromuscular re-education, trained in the water. Or therapeutic exercise performed in a space dominated by buoyancy. Or sensory training practiced in a room overloaded with warm, viscous molecules. Insurers who would never consider denying therapists the right to use a splash-table or bucket in the clinic have little leg to stand on when denying those same clinicians the right to a *really big* pail.[12]

So what special opportunities can the pool provide? In addition to the normal therapy pursuits of strengthening, balance training, and range of motion (ROM), the pool is an excellent location to work on:

- Transitional stress
- Social interactions
- Body awareness and kinesthesia
- Tactile processing
- Vestibular processing
- Visual processing

Transitional Stress

According to Laurie Jake, CTRS, CEDS, children with autism have difficulty with change because they are unable to distinguish relevant from irrelevant information, resulting in huge difficulties with decision-making. Such kids often cannot "make up their minds" or make a simple A-versus-B choice.

These kids have a need for sameness and have a strong need for rituals and routine. Free time is very difficult for them to manage. Additionally, children with autism have organizational and sequencing problems. These children don't know where to start, what comes next, or when a task is finished. The child's life can become one long series of tragic interruptions.[13]

Water activities can provide autistic children with the opportunity to embrace change. Even the act of entering the pool from the deck is a massive leap into uncertainty, and parents looking for ways to promote acceptance of change can use the pool for this end.

For instance, parents who are greeted with unceasing crying jags every evening at bath time can try this trick for co-bathing. Take a towel, swaddle the child, offer the child the bottle, and then lower the child into a warm bath cradled in your arms. This works best if the child can be handed to an already-positioned parent ready in the tub. The transition is smoothed by the act of swaddling, immersion in skin-temperature water, and positioning in the cradling/nursing position. Yet, the child is successfully making a transition. Over time, the props can be removed and the transition can become more dramatic.

Even more than the bathtub, a therapy or community pool can be a daunting place for children with sensory integration issues. As a shield, children often seek out a comfort place in the pool—a place where they feel the safest. Parents or therapists who choose to work in the water should work from the child's chosen safe spot, leave for a little bit, and return again and again.

In addition to aiding with transitional skills, water activities can also provide autistic children with the opportunity to socialize and form attachments. It helps that pool-time seems less like therapy and more like fun. For many children on the spectrum, abnormal or absent social interactions are the painful realities of life with a disability.[13]

Social Interactions

Children with autism often choose to work in solitude even when surrounded by others. In water, parents can encourage their children to work with others. A parent could divide a pair of water crutches between two children and then challenge both to work together for a common goal, such as picking up a ball, lifting it out of the water, and carrying it to a target site, suggests Kari Valentine, OTR/L. Since neither child can achieve this with only one crutch, they will have to work together.

Some therapists who work in water have found role-playing scenes from books or a beloved movie a natural way to encourage interaction. As an example, it is possible to tap into the Harry Potter phenomenon by acting out the "best Potter moments" in the pool. Use a large dumbbell as a pogo stick and have races to outrun dragons and Death Eaters and the like. The rewards? Enhanced body awareness, balance, and the ability to adapt to changes in the plot of a verbal story—as well as to engage in creative play.

Once childhood morphs into adolescence, friendships, friendly competition, and a healthy interest in the opposite sex can become powerful motivators. The pool is a natural environment for these normal social interactions to take place. Oftentimes the pool is such a natural place for play, that children can exceed their parents' socialization expectations.[14]

Body Awareness and Kinesthesia

Many children with autism are afraid of movement, afraid of water splashing their face, and unable to use equilibrium reactions in an effective way. And while the pool may be the perfect place to work on these deficits, there is also a potential risk that the weightlessness which occurs in water will disrupt already atypical feedback loops. Additionally, the refraction of light on the water's surface can limit a child's ability to self-monitor limb placement, and visual cues are untrustworthy. So, does it even make sense to work on body awareness and kinesthesia in the pool?

Although it is true that quiet, full-body immersion can dampen proprioceptive input, the wise therapist or parent knows how to harness the effects of turbulence and momentum for enhancing body awareness and kinesthesia. Simple childhood games like whirlpool (running in one direction in a circle and then quickly reversing direction to move against the "current") can create opportunities for feedback loops which are unachievable on land.

Shay Vanderloo, COTA suggests that parents get creative to help facilitate a child's interest in water. Vanderloo believes in the power of role-playing. For instance, the parent can create a make-believe Egyptian adventure. Wrap the child in different textured wet towels and then challenge him to break through the towels to get free to save the "ruby"—a toy jewel floating on a mat—by jumping into the pool. The goal? To increase kinesthetic input, and diminish hypersensitivity.[15]

Kary Valentine, OTR/L suggests positioning flotation mats shaped like animals so the child can crawl, walk, or slide on his belly with weight on his back. After navigating the animal train, send the child to the water gun area where his hands, feet, legs, and arms re squirted with water to help with desensitization and body awareness.

Therapists or parents who want to jack up the mental intensity during water-gun time can have their patients call out the names of the body part hit by the stream of water. Or, better yet, both parent and child can take turns. The parent begins the game by "hitting" the child's right hand with a stream of water. The child then tries to replicate this effort by using his gun to return the favor.[15]

If a child is having difficulty with weightlessness, it is possible to achieve proprioceptive input by having him scrunch his body into a ball while hanging onto the wall and then push backwards, shooting into the middle of the pool.

The game "Simon says" can be used to both assess and encourage proprioceptive awareness. Make use of this kid's game to teach better body control. Or make use of wet, clingy items such as towels, fabric shower curtains, and even discarded clothing to morph a dress-up game into a therapeutic session designed to enhance proprioception.[15]

Tactile Processing

The water in a pool provides a singular opportunity to alter tactile input. During water activities, the hairs on the body "catch" water molecules as the molecules whisk by, creating a mild shearing effect on the limb. Additionally, the deeper the limb is immersed beneath the surface, the greater the hydrostatic pressure. Initially, this pressure can cause the tactile receptors to fire, but over time, the constant pressure can result in a shut-down effect.

Thus, it is possible to increase—or decrease—the amount of tactile input the child receives by putting him into the pool. But what if the child is so averse to noxious stimulation that he won't even place his face near the water's surface? Stock up a therapeutic toolbox with everyday items easily purchased such as car wash mitts, sponges, and window clings. In the water, it becomes possible to stroke cheeks with cheap paint rollers and drape soaking-wet bath towels over heads to increase tolerance for abrasive touch and pressure.[16]

Vestibular Processing

In the water, the therapist or parent has the ability to challenge the vestibular system in ways unachievable on land. In fact, in some ways, the water offers the perfect environment to enhance vestibular input

An inexpensive way to convert your therapy pool into a vestibular challenge is to perform hammock swings. Purchase a child's parachute or a net hammock. Spread out the parachute or hammock and have the child climb aboard. Swing the fabric through the water: up, down, side to side, tilted, and rotated. Move the child rapidly, then slowly, then rapidly again. The child can sit, kneel, lie supine, or even stand in the hammock during this task. To make this task more interactive, ask the child to sing in time to movements and to anticipate movements before they happen.[17]

Another option? The floatation mat. Rolling is always a strong vestibular task, and one of the best ways to perform this in the pool is on a floatation mat.

Visual Processing

In the pool, the therapist or parent has the ability to challenge the visual system in ways unachievable on land. Because light refracts when traveling from air to water (making it difficult to track what the body is doing underneath the surface), the pool can create a nice training ground for children who rely too heavily on visual cues.

Additionally, there are certain elements intrinsic to a swimming pool (turbulence, airborne splashing, flowing current from jets) which create a visual, tactile, and proprioceptive feast. This makes it possible for children to "feel" what they see. Sight becomes palpable. And this amplifies the therapeutic possibilities.[18]

Parents and therapists who choose to take their children to the water's edge will find a host of opportunity within. It becomes immediately possible to challenge or protect, to stimulate or soothe—all with little effort and much satisfaction. In the water, parents will find a weapon in their arsenal, and a companion for their journey along the spectrum.

For More Information

Aquatic Sensory Integration. Training opportunities for parents and therapists of children with sensory issues. Books, DVDs and hands-on educational seminars. Aquatic Therapy University. Plymouth, MN. Ph: (800) 680-8624. Web: www.aquatic-sensory-integration.com.

AquaticNet Social. Networking Site for Aquatic Therapists & Parents. Aquatic Resources Network. Plymouth, MN. Web: www.aquatictherapist.ning.com.

Aquatic Health Research Database. Over eight thousand aquatic therapy-related research abstracts, including research on the benefits of aquatic therapy for children. Aquatic Resources Network. Plymouth, MN. Ph: (800) 680-8624. Web: www.aquaticnet.com.

ARCHITECTURE AND AUTISM: PROVIDING SUPPORTS FOR THE AUTISTIC CHILD OR ADULT THROUGH THE BUILT ENVIRONMENT

BY CATHY PURPLE CHERRY

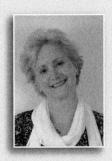

Cathy Purple Cherry, AIA, LEED AP

Purple Cherry Architects
One Melvin Ave.
Annapolis, MD 21401
410-990-1700
info@purplecherry.com
www.purplecherry.com

Cathy Purple Cherry, AIA, began her architectural studio in 1995, which thrives in Annapolis, Maryland with a passionate focus on the design of facilities for individuals with special needs combined with sensitivity to sustainable design. Cathy is personally connected to the special needs community by her life experiences with her autistic son and disabled brother and strives to connect these experiences with the incredible design skills of her firm. Ms. Cherry currently works as a Special Needs Design Architectural consultant on many projects nationally being designed and constructed to better serve our special needs population. She sits on the Boards of Directors for The Summit School in Edgewater, MD, which serves students with learning differences; Opportunity Builders, Inc. in Millersville, MD, which provides vocational training and other services to adults with developmental disabilities and Echoing Hope Ranch Oversight/Advisory Board, which provides programs and other services for children on the spectrum and their families. Ms. Cherry has presented to the National Association of Private Special Education Centers (NAPSEC) members at previous conferences and continues to support NAPSEC and its members. Ms. Cherry also has presented at NAPSEC's member conference, ASAH New Jersey, Association of parents, which have appeared in *School Planning and Management*, *Parenting Special Needs*, *Autism Advocate*, *The Autism File*, and *Autism & Aspergers Digest*.

Along with behavioral and educational strategies used to teach and assist children and adults with autism, there are also ways to impact their success through alteration and treatment of their physical environments. To understand what areas of the built environment could change to support them, you must first understand some of the challenges of children and adults on the spectrum, and how the physical environment can support successful behaviors. There are some simple and some more complex alterations that can be made to the living, academic and work environments for the ASD spectrum. Each of the challenge areas identified below also identifies some of the physical changes that can be made to help further support these individuals to success.

Difficulty with Social Skills

An individual with autism often has difficulty understanding personal space—the zone around each of us that we require to be comfortable in conversation. In not having a typical "zone", an autistic individual does not experience any discomfort in violating another person's personal space. When that other person is uncomfortable with anyone near them, this can lead to verbal or physical conflict. It can also just simply lead to a lot of frustration. The autistic person may also not have an inner voice—the silent voice in our mind that helps tell what is appropriate/ a stream of consciousness. The lack of these two neurotypically inherent skills makes it challenging for autistic individuals to develop proper social skills. To help reinforce proper standing distances, a series of touching circles can be placed on the floor with center marks in each circle. Continuous practicing with several individuals standing or sitting on the circle centers may help reinforce proper distances. These circles could be a permanent floor pattern contained within a social skills room. Seating should also be individual with separate single chairs in a living environment to help aid appropriate seating distances. If necessary, the child or adult may be assigned a "special" chair which belongs only to him or her. In home settings, halls and spaces between kitchen counters should be made wider to permit ample room for passage without violation of this space. In tightly contained areas such as in cars, it may be necessary to buffer two children with a neurotypical adult seated between them or to separate by row and side. See also Easily Distracted—*Waiting* below to understand how personal space and the exercise of waiting link together.

Challenges with Redirection and Change

Individuals on the spectrum often have great difficulty transitioning from one place to another or from one task to another. To support success for transition, in addition to clearly posted schedules, soft warning lights or sounds can be integrated into a building. In using light and/or sound, the designer must proceed cautiously to understand the best way to change the lighting (possibly from standard to dim or like a traffic light with different color warnings) or sound (from silence to a gentle instrument sound or soft song). Integrating these warning signals into the lighting or annunciation system of an environment will help provide a repetitive warning for change to the ASD individual. At home, a parent could utilize the alarm system of their phone as long as the alarm is set on a soft muted tone. Colored cards could also be used.

Repetitive and Compulsive Behaviors/Perseveration/ Hoarding Trash

Children and adults on the spectrum often tend to be fascinated with specific objects, and therefore, have a tendency to obsess repeatedly about these items. These fascinations can be different for each ASD person. Many can be distracted by running water or fascinated by fire. In school environments, hand sinks should be tucked behind partial walls to block any line of sight during learning. Also, no appliances that use gas and create a flame such as gas fireplaces or gas cooktops should be used. Personal items should be concealed and small items should not be left on counters. One simple solution to help reduce distraction and hoarding is to always provide ample storage in all settings by integrating locked closets or cabinets in every space to allow clutter and obsessive items to be out-of-sight and reinforce out-of-the–mind. To allow each child a collection of "special things", designate a specific drawer or provide a dedicated colored bin in his or her bedroom. However, be prepared as redirecting these perseverating thoughts is easier said than done and will take continuous effort.

Easily Distracted

Many children with ASD struggle with attention issues. The following environmental design solutions to specific challenges can help to reduce distractibility.

Clutter–Clutter in a space is too often the greatest source of distraction even for a neurotypical child or adult. The best strategy is to provide ample enclosed storage space for objects, not open shelves. In educational settings, these cabinets should be lockable to prevent students from trying to get any item they desire. Message boards that have a "curtain" or doors to control when the board can be viewed are also an option. Designing into the physical environment the organizational needs of a space is the key to reducing clutter. This also applies to hallways of schools as well. Ideally, all adaptive equipment can be stored in closets to remove these objects from sight.

Room Door and Window Placement–In a school or work environment, class or work rooms across a corridor from each other should have their exit doors staggered. This eliminates a visual connection between the opposite rooms and further helps prevent noise transfer from one room to the other room. Consideration should also be given to the placement of windows within each classroom. If windows are held higher such that when students are sitting down and learning they cannot see individuals and movement outside, this will help reduce distraction while still allowing for natural light to enter the room. Further, the amount of glass within the entry door to each classroom should be minimized to reduce the opportunity to see movement outside of the learning environment.

Waiting–If you expect a child or adult with autism to wait in a particular area to exit the classroom, line up to wait their turn or wait for a bus, you should provide a clearly marked area for this "waiting" function. The ability to understand waiting or taking turns is difficult for ASD children. This is often a skill that needs to be reinforced continuously. To reinforce waiting and staying in place, you can create a pattern in the finished flooring, purchase a special chair in a special color to be easily defined as different from others or simply tape on the floor for "x" marks the spot. This strategy also applies to making a line of children waiting to exit the classroom or to take a turn.

Unusual Responses to Sensory Stimuli

Lighting–Appropriate lighting should be selected to eliminate glare and flickering movement from the lamping. The flickering in fluorescent lights seen by some neurotypical children is intensified for the autistic child. The lower frequency (60-cycle) of fluorescent bulbs seems to be the issue though more studies need to done. So, if fluorescent bulbs must be used, use the newer ones and eliminate all old bulbs. Natural lighting is the best. Providing natural light inside a building of similar light quality to the outside for the same day seems to allow these children to transition well. Therefore, the ability to be able to control the lighting in each space is very important.

Sound–Sensory bombardment and inappropriate noises can trigger inappropriate actions, cause frustration, impede learning and affect the ability to focus. General sound levels (decibels of sound systems and acoustical reverberation within a space) as well as white noise (produced by sounds of different frequencies coming together) can further cause learning problems for ASD individuals with auditory issues. White noise from mechanical and electrical systems can also interfere with an autistic child's ability to properly process sound. Architectural applications that can assist in managing some levels of sound include installation of sound absorption materials as wall or ceiling panels, providing carpet in selected areas, placing rubber balls on the bottom of furniture legs, hanging baffles and banners within a classroom or work area, utilizing fabrics on furniture and installing airflow silencers in the ductwork. In addition, use of technology with high-frequency sounds like in CRT monitors and TV sets should be minimized. Chalk boards can be disturbing to some children so white boards should be used if possible. Lastly, no mechanical equipment should be located near a classroom or bedroom whether inside or outside so that the motor noise cannot be heard.

Off-Gassing–While strong odors can be annoying to neurotypical individuals, many autistic children and adults are particularly sensitive to odors from materials. Major indoor triggers include irritants such as commercial products (paints, cleaning agents, pesticides and perfumes), building components (sealants, plastics, adhesives and insulation materials), animal and insect allergens, environmental tobacco smoke, and molds. In an effort to design tighter, more energy conscious buildings, indoor pollution levels have generally increased. "Volatile organic compound" or VOC is the name given to a substance that contains carbon and that evaporates (becomes a vapor) or "off-gases" at room temperature. VOCs are often referred to as the "new car smell" in a building recently completed or renovated. VOCs are commonly found in carpet, paint, composite wood products (i.e. casework), adhesives, floor wax, cleaning products/chemicals, and air freshener sprays. The possible immediate effects of VOC exposure for some individuals (whether on the spectrum or neurotypical) include eye, nose, and throat irritation; headaches; allergic skin reaction like a rash; difficulty breathing; nausea and/or vomiting; nosebleeds; fatigue; dizziness; loss of coordination; and confusion. The possible long-term effects after repeated exposure may include damage to the heart, liver, kidneys, or the central nervous system and cancer. Our children overall and, even more specifically, our children with special needs, are affected by the quality of the air they breathe in any setting. Eliminating the odors and exposures is the goal for the ASD environment.

Temperature–Some individuals on the spectrum can have sensitivities to cold and heat. Thus, the heating and cooling system should be designed so that the temperature in each classroom, workspace or bedroom can be controlled separately by the supervisor. This will allow the staff to create the most comfortable environment for the ASD occupants. Desks and beds should be placed such that they are not close to the window glass which emits the cooler temperatures during the cold nights.

Color–Individuals with ASD can respond differently than neurotypical peers to colors and patterns. Those with visual sensitivities must be considered when selecting finish applications in the built environment. Intense colors, complex patterns and bold contrast can create problems with sustained attention for the autistic individual. At times, minimizing the offending stimuli can help improve the individual's ability to perform in other areas. For others with ASD, however, bright colors can offer successful simulation and help draw focus. The saturation of the color should be watched. Color has historically been used in various cultures for therapeutic treatment for neurotypical individuals for many years. The affect of certain colors on ASD children can vary so you may have to try multiple colors to determine the one that is right for your child. Research has shown that some ASD children see colors more intensely. However, this is not true for all. Generally, the following is often understood of the impact of color on neurotypical individuals: Red is believed to stimulate the mind and increase circulation and appetite. Blue is believed to be calming and to reduce blood pressure. Bright yellow reflects light and can over stimulate. Pale yellow can be soothing. Green is believed to soothe and is associated with nature and creativity. Orange can over stimulate and agitate. Light pink/rose is believed to be soothing and is often used in detention settings. Color can certainly set a mood. The effect of color, however, can also wear off after a person is in the space over time. It is commonly believed that soft, muted colors are more calming than bright, vibrant colors. Thus, if a child is incredibly active, one might try using calm colors in the sleeping or teaching areas. On the other hand, intense colors that initially stimulate may have a positive effect on some children who might be prone to complacency.

When changing colors of a room, one change at a time should occur in order to understand the impact of any change. Do not use stimulating colors in a sleeping area. Start by painting one wall to see the effect on the child. Ideally, there would be two clearly separate spaces for every ASD child in their bedroom. One would be for daytime play with possibly more stimulating colors and one would be for sleeping with calming colors.

Communication Challenges

Some individuals on the spectrum may be non-verbal or be challenged with written language. Colors can be used to communicate simple expectations such as "do not touch", "do not enter" and "stand here for waiting". Simple patterns and colors integrated as wayfinding elements can be used to help guide individuals with autism through learning or work spaces by clearly defining circulation paths. These visual cues are helpful reminders to ASD individuals and work as daily prompts in the home, school and work environment.

Fight or Flight

A defense mechanism often used by individuals with autism is the "fight or flight" response. The "fight" reaction can present itself as self-mutilation, physical harm to the environment or physical harm to others. The "flight" might display itself by the individual fleeing or running away. These reactions can be supported by some of the environmental applications listed below.

Durability of Materials–The durability of selected materials should be considered for environments that support the ASD population. Within the spectrum, explosive issues, such as intermittent explosive disorder or bipolar, can also co-habitat with ASD. Further, when the autistic child experiences puberty, their physical strength can be used in ways not expected even by them. When the child or adult experiences the "fight or flight" mode, the need, exists to use durable materials. The following materials can be selected for increased durability–color-thru floor linoleum tile and stained concrete floors; wall protection panels, linoleum wall panels, spray-on durable paints and corner guards; impact resistant drywall, plywood sheathing under drywall, and concrete block. The implication is that durable materials are hard and institutional in appearance. This impression is incorrect. Today's materials include creative colors, patterns, and textures and can be combined to create a warm, colorful and inviting environment.

Secure Boundaries–It is important for autistic children and adults to have their boundaries more clearly defined than their neurotypical peers. ASD children do not always assimilate boundaries in one setting to other areas that they visit. Restrictions must be clearly indicated. Boundaries must be clearly marked. There are also two types of physical boundaries–the boundary of not violating a siblings or roommates personal space and the perimeter boundary to keep the individuals within a safe area such as a school yard. See Impulsivity below for more regarding personal space boundaries. For the fight or flight mode, the perimeter of yards should be defined either by secure fencing or with landscaping. Landscape will not prevent fleeing children from leaving the area but it will help some individuals with understanding their perimeter play area. All doors of homes, schools and work environments supporting these individuals should have warning alarms so that all responsible adults can be aware of any escapes.

Time–Out Rooms–Individuals with autism may require time-out rooms to allow the child or adult to regain self-control during periods of outburst. These time-out rooms must be durable and, ideally, sound isolated. Most importantly, these spaces should be separated from the public gathering areas of the school so as to provide the isolated individual with greater dignity. The solution to this is to locate the room for privacy. This further removes the audience from the individual that, at times, can be stimulating and removes the disruption from others in adjacent spaces. These spaces, however, should not be scary but rather should try to promote calmness through the use of pale colors, soft music and possible graphics on the unreachable ceiling.

Struggles with Independence/Constant Prompting/Life Skills

All parents of ASD children usually come to a place where developing independence skills becomes the most significant thing they want for their child. So, in knowing this early, there are many ways to structure your child's environment to reinforce these skills in preparation for adulthood. Making available learning environments within our school settings such as "apartment" rooms, cafés, school stores, social group rooms and mail rooms all create opportunities for ASD students to develop skills necessary for adulthood—laundering, bed making, food preparation, turn-taking, money management and organizing. Further, providing opportunity for these responsibilities is the key to imparting a feeling of importance for the autistic child. Understanding that the ASD child requires constant prompting and reinforcement, the learning and home environments should make modifications to provide the necessary reminders such as color or image coded lockers, color or image coded doors, color or image coded shelves, etc. Using appropriate surfaces on counters such as stones and quartz solid surfaces permits the child to not have to worry for multiple issues when preparing meals on these surfaces or doing art projects, and laundry counters should be larger than normal to allow the child to lay out entire garments versus managing folds against the body like neurotypical individuals fold.

Impulsivity

Out-of-Sight, Out-of-Mind—The goal with this motto is to remove all harmful objects from view and potential reach depending upon the ASD individual. As well, other possessions of any value should be hidden from view. An individual with autism may be very impulsive and, thus, will take anything he or she desires and hoard in hidden areas of their room. The goal is to reduce if not prevent this from happening by "hiding" any objects that could cause harm (scissors, cutting knives, matches, etc.) or that have value or ownership. "Keep Out" signs should be posted on rooms that should not be entered by the ASD individual to help reinforce rules. If necessary, items should be locked away. Thus, in designing a classroom, home or work environment, strategies to store objects in different ways should be discussed. Locked closets and cabinets, high out-of-reach spaces and "hidden" rooms can all be used. To further reinforce boundaries for which these individuals cannot cross, doors to private areas should either be locked, of a different color or of a different style to reinforce the edge of the boundary.

Conclusion

There are many aspects that can be altered to create more successful opportunities for our kids with autism. Medical interventions and academic opportunities have obviously been in the forefront of the strategies. What should now be hopefully apparent is that you can alter the built environment as well so that it becomes a contributing factor to your child's success in life.

ART THERAPY APPROACHES TO TREATING AUTISM

BY NICOLE MARTIN AND DR. DONNA BETTS

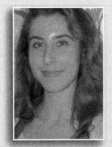

Nicole Martin, MAAT, LPC, ATR

Sky's The Limit Studio, LLC
Lawrence, KS 66044
(785) 424-0739
arttherapyandautism@yahoo.com
arttherapyandautism.com

Sky's The Limit was founded in 2007 by Nicole Martin, a registered art therapist, licensed professional counselor, and artist living in Lawrence, Kansas. As the big sister of a brother with autism, she is dedicated to improving public access to creative arts therapy services tailored specifically to the needs of people on the spectrum. STL's treatment model is a synthesis of her many years of experience working in developmental/behavioral art therapy, applied behavior analysis, and recreational arts and disabilities programs. She is the author of *Art as an Early Intervention Tool for Children with Autism* (2009) and various articles, and received her training at the School of the Art Institute of Chicago.

Donna Betts, Ph.D., ATR-BC

Art Therapy Program
The George Washington University
1925 Ballenger Avenue, Suite 250
Alexandria, VA 22314
dbetts@gwu.edu
www.art-therapy.us
www.gwu.edu/~artx/

Dr. Betts is a registered and board-certified art therapist and assistant professor in the George Washington University graduate art therapy program. Dr. Betts serves on GW's Autism Initiative Committee, which is working toward the establishment of the GW Autism Research, Treatment & Policy Institute. Her own research addresses the clinical utility of art therapy approaches with individuals on the autism spectrum. Dr. Betts is also the author of the Face Stimulus Assessment (FSA), (Betts, 2003, 2009) a performance-based, nonverbal drawing instrument used primarily to identify strengths of people with autism and related disabilities, establish treatment goals, and determine progress in therapy. Ongoing research related to the reliability and validity of the FSA is another focus of Dr. Betts's work.

Art therapy is a mental health profession that uses the creative process of art-making to improve and enhance the physical, mental, and emotional well-being of individuals of all ages (AATA, 2009a). Art therapy is based on the belief that the creative process involved in artistic self-expression helps people to increase self-esteem and self-awareness, achieve insight, develop interpersonal skills, resolve conflicts and problems, manage behavior, and reduce stress.

Creative expression has been used for healing throughout history (AATA, 2009b). In the early 20th century, psychiatrists became interested in the artwork created by their patients with mental illness. Educators simultaneously discovered that children's art expressions reflected emotional, developmental, and cognitive growth. By midcentury, hospitals, clinics, and rehabilitation centers increasingly incorporated art therapy programs along with traditional therapies.

Today, art therapy integrates the fields of human development, visual art (drawing, painting, sculpture, and other art forms), and the creative process with models of counseling and psychotherapy (AATA, 2009a). Art therapy is used in a number of settings with individuals of all ages, and with a variety of mental and emotional problems and disorders, and physical, cognitive, and neurological problems.

Art therapy is an effective approach when working with individuals with autism spectrum disorder (ASD). Art therapy involves the application of techniques specifically designed to reduce the symptoms of autism and promote healthy self-expression. A number of clinical reports support the use of art therapy with ASD, as well as with individuals with developmental disabilities in general (Gilroy, 2006).

The art therapist is adept at facilitating therapeutic processes with the use of visual art media and modalities such as painting and drawing, sculpture, cartooning, clay modeling, animation, and puppetry. The sensory appeal of the art materials makes them desirable tools for self-regulation and self-soothing. Projects designed to tackle specific treatment goals are limitless and may include group murals (to work on collaboration, reciprocity, and flexibility skills), portrait drawing (to work on face processing and relationship skills), friendship boxes (to work on memory and relationship skills), and many more (Martin, 2009a).

Art therapy differs from art education due to the therapist's expertise in the psychological application of art techniques, master's-level training in child development, knowledge of autism spectrum disorders, and how to tailor projects accordingly. An art therapist working in this specialty should be fluent in developmental/behavioral art therapy approaches, have a solid understanding of early childhood artistic development, have experience in the use of current best practices in behavioral and communication supports for individuals with autism, and be a patient and enthusiastic coach. Improving artistic skills and striving for aesthetic beauty are desirable qualities and will help maintain the client's enthusiasm, but remain secondary to the focus on personal growth and reduction of symptoms.

No possible risks or side effects from art therapy with this population have been published to date; however, the risks that can arise from poorly selected art materials and their poorly supervised use must be carefully considered. Art therapists should know the toxicity level and ingredients of all their art supplies as well as the allergies, diet restrictions, and behavioral patterns of their clients, and pair them wisely. For example, a child on a gluten-free diet should avoid traditional playdough since it contains wheat flour, and a child who tends to throw objects should not use sharp tools without close supervision. Art therapists can start by offering a sensible variety of nontoxic materials and then increasing the variety, number, and quality as the child matures. Art materials should also be carefully matched to the child's symptoms and energy level; a poor match can aggravate or encourage symptomatic behavior, while a good match can soothe and create an appropriate outlet for symptoms (Martin, 2009a).

The wide range of symptoms experienced by people with ASD makes them very unique in presentation, so treatments must be tailored to a range of varying needs (Evans & Dubowski, 2001). It is especially important to offer a safe, predictable, and stable environment by providing therapy at the same time every week and setting up materials in an orderly fashion. By doing so, the art therapist establishes psychological continuity and a stable environment for the client (Stack, 1998). Treatment takes place within the professional therapeutic relationship between the art therapist and the client, in either private sessions or a group setting. Additionally, an art therapist can train the client's caregivers and teachers in the use of art therapy techniques in order to help generalize progress to the client's natural environment, such as home or school.

To begin, the art therapist assesses the individual's skills and interests in order to formulate individualized treatment goals. Using a combination of formal and informal assessment, the art therapist determines the client's capacity for imagination and socialization, artistic developmental level, the impact of different art materials on the client's senses and behavior, and the client's initial interests and personality, before developing appropriate treatment goals. Assessment tools such as the Face Stimulus Assessment (Betts, 2003, 2009) and the Portrait Drawing Assessment (Martin, 2008) can provide insight into the skills of clients with autism.

Art therapy helps clients with autism on many different levels. Major treatment goal areas include socialization, communication, and sensory regulation (Martin, 2009b). Martin (2009a) highlights six treatment goal areas that distinguish art therapy from other therapies used to treat autism: imagination/abstract thinking skills, sensory regulation and integration, emotional understanding and self-expression, artistic developmental growth, visual-spatial skills, and appropriate recreation/leisure skills.

Early intervention is crucial. Goals that a child with ASD might accomplish in art therapy include age-appropriate drawing or modeling skills, improved self-expression and reduced anxiety or frustration, independent or semi-independent use of art making as a coping skill or self-soothing tool, improved social skills such as project collaboration and flexibility, and age-appropriate imagination and ideation skills.

The art therapist's ability to troubleshoot possible hindrances to the client's interest in art—such as sensory discomfort, perfectionism, anxiety, difficulty translating or generating ideas, compulsive/impulsive behaviors, lack of personal relevancy, or past punitive experiences associated with art materials—and take corrective action, means that art therapy has the potential to benefit the majority of individuals with autism, not just those who demonstrate a precocious talent.

To illustrate with a case example, an individual with autism who is withdrawn may be approached through the objects and activities that he or she prefers (Kramer, 1979). By beginning with the familiar and progressively introducing the new, clients with ASD are more willing to accept the unfamiliar. For instance, Dr. Betts once worked with a student who was obsessed with his own wet saliva. The boy was fascinated with the patterns of movement he created with his spit, and this is what kept him engaged in the kinesthetic activity. Thus, Dr. Betts came up with a way to divert the boy away from his excessive interest in saliva by introducing a dry substance—sand. In his art therapy sessions, the boy was encouraged to play with sand and its containers in a tabletop box. As he learned about how to manipulate his environment through sand play, his obsession with the spit eventually disappeared. With Dr. Betts's continuous encouragement and praise for using the sand, contained within the boundaries of a box, the client progressed toward a more flexible and mature ego functioning. He therefore made gains that addressed his Individualized Education Program (IEP) goals related to cognitive, behavioral, and emotional growth.

Including art therapy as a component of early intervention treatment helps individuals with autism form good habits for a lifetime of using art as a vital means of expression. Appropriate art therapy goals and projects can be created for a person with ASD at any age, level of functioning, or initial interest level. All individuals with autism can benefit from learning how to express their thoughts, feelings, and interests in a creative, hands-on way, whether to ease and enhance communication, externalize feelings of anxiety, or simply realize their potential as imaginative, productive human beings.

Ongoing Research

Dr. Betts is currently engaged as a co-investigator in a George Washington University Medical Faculty Associates funded research project entitled "Assessing Medication

Responsiveness in Persons with Autism Spectrum Disorders (ASD)." Led by Principal Investigator Dr. Valerie Hu of GW's Department of Biochemistry and Molecular Biology, the primary purpose of this project is to gather and use validated responses to psychotropic medication in the autistic population in order to assess the range of responses to specific medications in the ASD population. This information will be used to reduce the heterogeneity of potential subjects for genetic and biological profiling studies. Successful identification of clearly positive responders to a specific type of medication will lead to submission of an NIH proposal to study this subgroup of individuals vs. non-responders using genotype, gene expression, and metabolomics analyses to identify genetic variants and biological pathways associated with the positive response. Indicators of medication responsiveness will be measured by a patient/parents/caregivers questionnaire, a clinician questionnaire and an art-based assessment designed and evaluated by Dr. Betts.

10

BERARD AUDITORY INTEGRATION TRAINING

BY SALLY BROCKETT

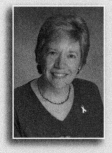

Sally Brockett, MS

Mrs. Brockett is the Director of the IDEA Training and Consultation Center in North Haven, Connecticut. She founded the center in 1992 to focus on interventions for developmental disabilities after 12 years as a special education teacher with all categories of disabilities. After training in France with Dr. Guy Berard, the Berard method of auditory integration training (AIT) and consultation became a special focus of her work. Mrs. Brockett has completed advanced training in AIT with Dr. Guy Berard and is approved by him as a certified International Professional Instructor in the Berard method. Mrs. Brockett founded the Berard AIT International Society and has served on the Board of Directors since its beginning. She and Dr. Berard have coauthored *Hearing Equals Behavior: Updated and Expanded*, the newest edition of Dr. Berard's book about his method of auditory integration training.

Introduction

Dr. Guy Berard, a French ENT physician, developed a listening program that was used primarily to assist in certain cases of hearing impairment. However, he quickly discovered that learning-related skills and abilities, such as attentive listening, concentration, auditory discrimination and memory skills often improved following the training program. Berard's auditory integration training (AIT) program requires that individuals passively listen to processed music through headphones for a total of 10 hours (half hour sessions usually over 10-12 days). The Berard program is now noted for its use as an educationally related intervention.

Interest in Berard's Program Expands

Dr. Berard meticulously describes his understanding of the auditory imbalances that interfere with efficient listening and learning in his book, *Audition Égale Comporte-ment* published in French in 1982, followed by the English translation in 1993, Hearing

Equals Behavior. English speaking professionals and parents were then introduced to the concept that *how* we hear plays a very significant role in *how* we behave and learn. Unfortunately, even today, there are professionals who are not aware that many individuals who are struggling with academics and behavioral problems have inefficient auditory skills that interfere with effective listening and processing which puts them at a great disadvantage in the classroom and workplace.

In 1991, the publication of Annabel Stehli's book, *"The Sound of a Miracle"*, quickly grabbed public attention and created a lot of interest in Berard AIT. The program began to receive recognition as an intervention for behavior and learning difficulties, in addition to its use for auditory hypersensitivity. This book chronicles the story of Annabel Stehli's daughter, Georgianna, who had severe autism and was institutionalized. She progressed dramatically after receiving Berard AIT at the age of eleven. She was able to be integrated into mainstream education following Berard AIT and intensive teaching provided initially by her mother. Parents, especially those with children on the autism spectrum, began seeking this intervention for their own children after learning about Mrs. Stehli's experience with her own daughter.

Research on the Berard Method of AIT

Dr. Bernard Rimland, and his assistant Dr. Stephen M. Edelson, from the Autism Research Institute, organized research studies to document the effectiveness of the method. They had heard many anecdotal reports from parents about the success of this intervention and wanted to document its efficacy. These studies focused on the autism population, but later studies by other researchers included subjects with attention deficit disorder (ADD), central auditory processing disorder (CAPD), and other disabilities. By 1998 there were 28 studies completed and 82% demonstrated positive effects from AIT.

Dr. Rimland recommended the term "auditory integration training" be used to refer to the Berard method of training. This term was agreed upon because it took into account the "integration" of the senses and processing that occurs with Berard AIT. Unfortunately, "auditory integration training" or AIT was not trademarked and new types of listening programs have also used the term AIT. In order to help distinguish Dr. Berard's method from these others, Berard Practitioners now use "Berard AIT" instead of just AIT. However, it is still confusing for parents who may not realize that all AIT is not the same, and the research that applies to the Berard method does not apply to other methods.

Berard AIT in the 21st Century

Berard AIT has expanded to more than 30 countries around the world and continues to spread to new regions. Currently, there are Berard AIT Instructors in 7 countries and seminars for professionals are provided in several different languages. New research continues to document the benefits derived from this method, which currently is available for those as young as 3 years of age. There is no upper age limit since the brain is capable of reorganizing through neural plasticity until death.

Jeffrey Lewine, PhD., neuroscience researcher at the MIND Research Network in Albuquerque, New Mexico, is directing a major new research project to explore auditory hypersensitivity and auditory processing problems experienced by those on the autism spectrum. Berard AIT is one of the programs being evaluated as an intervention for these issues.

As new understanding of the brain emerges, and new technologies develop, there may be changes in the Berard AIT protocol. New equipment may become available and adjustments may be made in the program. However, any changes must first undergo high quality, scientific study to measure whether the suggested change actually provides equal or greater benefit in terms of functional performance of the clients.

The Berard AIT Procedure

The Berard AIT program requires ten hours of listening. Each day consists of two 30-minute sessions separated by a minimum of a three hour break (go to the park, relax at a hotel or other activities of interest). Preferably the ten days are consecutive, running through weekends, although many practitioners may provide the training with a weekend break in the middle, which is acceptable.

Participants listen with headphones to music specially modulated through an instrument approved for Berard AIT called an Earducator™ (or the Audiokinetron) during the training sessions. The Berard AIT device modulates the music during all sessions which provides random dampening and amplification of high and low frequencies. The process is non-intrusive with the volume adjusted to be comfortably loud, below an average of 85 dB.

An audio test according to the Berard protocol is obtained with participants who are able to cooperate with this evaluation. This shows how the participant hears across all the frequencies and helps to identify conditions that may cause disruption in the auditory system. This information is used to determine if any narrow-band filters will be used during the training sessions. When the audio tests can be obtained, this evaluation is repeated after 5 days of training, and again at the end of the 10 day training period to see how the listening pattern is responding.

There are many young children and those with disabilities who cannot cooperate with the audio test protocol due to inability to focus on the tones and spontaneously communicate when they do hear the tones. Research with subjects with autism spectrum disorder in the 1990's showed that even when the audio test cannot be obtained, the training can still be done and significant benefits achieved.

How Does Berard AIT Compare with Other Similar Approaches?

The Berard method is provided under direct supervision by trained professionals and requires only 10 hours of listening while most sound-based intervention programs require 40 or more hours. Due to the nature of the stimulation provided by the Berard AIT device, the changes usually occur more quickly and include a broad area of response. Parent observations of improvements in language, social skills, cognition, fine motor skills and reduction of challenging behaviors and sound sensitivity are supported by data obtained through research studies and clinical observations. It is easier to monitor results from Berard AIT since there is a definitive ending of the training after 10 days. Typically, the majority of change occurs within the first 3 months after the program is completed, and the benefit is usually permanent. The Berard method is also well-researched and statistically significant results are documented. Professionally trained practitioners achieve similar results around the world when using the approved equipment and following the protocol. Berard AIT is not offered as a home program through the use of CDs.

Results Achieved with Berard AIT

There are results from research studies and anecdotal reports of success with Berard AIT that document behavioral and learning improvements following the 10 hours of training. The largest study to date was completed by the Autism Research Institute and included 445 subjects on the autism spectrum with an age range from 4 to 41 years. A significant reduction of sound sensitivity and a sharp reduction in problem behaviors occurred and was maintained through 9 months of post-AIT evaluations. A pilot study of the effect of Berard AIT on sensory processing problems was conducted by IDEA Training Center by Sally Brockett, Director. The median change was a 79% reduction of sensory problems 6 months after AIT. A long-term study with students in Sweden by Lars Persson, Director of the Berard's Method Center, documents that at 21 months after AIT, 38% of those students who received AIT were returned to regular education classes, while only 5.6% of students in the control group were returned to regular education classes. A summary of studies on AIT is posted at http://www.berardaitwebsite.com/sait/aitsummary.html. There are also pre and post AIT results at http://www.ideatrainingcenter.com/ait-results.shtml and http://www.ideatrainingcenter.com/stories.shtml which show the types of responses participants may achieve with Berard AIT.

Berard AIT balances the hearing and eliminates sound sensitivity and distortions for most participants. The changes in the auditory system also impact on the vestibular system which regulates many aspects of sensory processing. As the sensory problems diminish, the individual may feel more relaxed, less hypervigilant and defensive. There is typically a reduction in challenging behaviors and they can then focus their attention on other things, such as communication, socialization, and learning. Many participants seem to progress from the "bottom up". As the hearing distortions and misperceptions, and sensitivity if it is present, are reduced or eliminated, they show progress with other areas of development and behavior. This may include receptive and expressive communication, self-confidence, social and emotional relatedness, faster and higher level cognitive processing. Many also show progress with gross and fine motor skills due to the changes in the vestibular system and most likely, the cerebellum, which regulates many aspects of motor function.

When participants experience the changes that result from Berard AIT, they may have a transition period of irritability, hyperactivity, fatigue or other challenging behaviors before things stabilize and they adjust to the new perceptions, differences in their processing, and changes in sensory experiences. Behaviors may fluctuate during the 10 days of training and even for a short time afterwards while the body is still integrating the changes. These types of "positive-negative" behaviors are frequently seen when individuals receive various types of interventions such as vision therapy, hyperbaric oxygen therapy, sensory integration therapy, etc., due to the changes that occur and the need to re-organize and then stabilize.

To learn more about this intervention, visit the official Berard AIT website at www.berardaitwebsite.com. An international list of Berard Practitioners is available on the website as well as many articles that explain more details about the program. Professionals interested in becoming a practitioner will find a list of approved Berard Instructors. Dr. Berard's book, Hearing Equals Behavior, has been out of print during the recent years. A new edition, Hearing Equals Behavior: Expanded and Updated Material, will be published soon, if it is not already available. Look for an announcement of publication on this website.

11

BIOFILM PROTOCOL

BY KEN SIRI

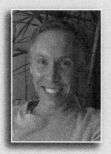

Kenneth J. Siri

Ken Siri, a former Wall Street analyst who covered the healthcare industry, is the single father of an autistic boy. Now a freelance writer, he is also the author of *1001 Tips for the Parents of Autistic Boys*. Ken has become active in the autism community in New York City where he and his son reside.

Introduction

Doctors now know that autism is not only a neurological condition but also an immune inflammatory condition, impacting the gut along with the brain. In fact, many of the symptoms associated with autism (stimming, hyperactivity, self-injurious behaviors, aggression) are related to the gut. Doctors on the cutting edge of autism research, such as Dr. Anju Usman, have had success treating autistic children by addressing persistent gut dysbiosis. A highly promising cutting-edge therapy in this realm is known as the biofilm protocol.

What is a Biofilm?

- A biofilm is a collection of microbes growing as a community, forming a matrix of extracellular polymeric substance (EPS) separated by a network of open water channels.
- The architecture is an optimal environment for cell-cell interactions, including the intercellular exchange of genetic material, communication signals, and metabolites, which enables diffusion of necessary nutrients to the biofilm community.

- The matrix is composed of a negatively charged polysaccharide substance, held together with positively charged metal ions (calcium, magnesium, and iron).
- The matrix in which the microbes are embedded protects them from UV exposure, metal toxicity, acid exposure, dehydration salinity, phagocytosis, antibiotics, antimicrobial agents and the immune system. *(Usman DAN! Presentation, October 9, 2009)*

Treatment Development

The gastrointestinal (GI) tract or gut contains the largest collection of microorganisms in the body (over a trillion bugs) and is the first line of defense in the body's immune system (the gut accounts for about 70 percent of the body's immune system). A healthy gut contains "good" bacteria; symbiotic flora growing in the GI tract, known as microbiota. These good bugs fight off pathogens and allergens.

This complex ecosystem of organisms needs to be in balance; stresses including a history of excessive antibiotics can unbalance the gut, killing off healthy flora and microbes (good bugs), allowing clostridia and yeast (bad bugs) to overgrow.

When the balance of good and bad bugs is disrupted, the immune system becomes weakened, leading to chronic infections, inflammation, and autoimmunity. This condition, of gut bugs out of balance, is known as dysbiosis.

Once bad bugs take over the GI tract, they are notoriously difficult to eliminate. Frontline treatment typically involves changing the diet and adding probiotics. If the patient has a serious dysbiosis problem (yeast), then antifungals (typically nystatin and Diflucan) are used. For many of our autistic kids the results from this standard therapy are fleeting or nonexistent, as they have had undiagnosed or improperly diagnosed GI issues for significant periods of time (often years). When these typical treatments do not work, it may be that the bad bugs have become protected by a pathogenic biofilm, which was produced over time by the dysbiosis.

Pathogenic Biofilm Indicators—a stool test ordered by a doctor can help confirm

- History of frequent antibiotics usage, and or usage at a young age (typically for ear infections) while the immune system was developing
- Dairy intolerance

- Poorly formed stools (color, consistency, undigested food)
- Chronic constipation and or diarrhea
- Aggression, self-injurious behavior, irritability, mood swings
- Poor sleeping behaviors
- Colic or reflux
- Thrush and history of diaper rash—skin problems, eczema, acne, rash
- Abdominal distention, bloating
- Initial response to antifungals, but relapse after discontinuation

How does this happen? Well, in order to hide from the body's immune system, bad bugs (when untreated) cause a chronic infection in the child, generating the pathogenic biofilm, which acts as a protective matrix, cloaking the same bad bugs from the immune system. This allows the bad bugs to thrive and produce toxic byproducts, leading to food sensitivities, GI dysfunction, and autoimmunity. This protective matrix makes pathogenic biofilm difficult to diagnose and treat.

GI (Gastrointestinal) Dysfunction

- Maldigestion—Food sensitivities (dairy, gluten, soy, etc), poor weight gain, low essential amino acids, low stomach acid/bloating
- Malabsorption—vitamin deficiencies, fatty acid deficiencies, dry skin, irregular stool
- Immune Dysregulation/Inflammation—stims, sleep disorders, aggression, and self-injurious behaviors.

Treatment of pathogenic biofilm can help the immune system restore normal gut flora and improve symptoms associated with autism. Unfortunately, pathogenic biofilms are resistant to many antimicrobials and antibiotics in standalone therapy.

Note: There are two types of biofilm communities, symbiotic, and pathogenic. Symbiotic are produced by good gut bugs and protect the gut lining. Symbiotic biofilms occur normally in the body around mouth, teeth, lungs, sinuses, and other areas. Pathogenic biofilm are those that can cause a disease.

Practitioners use a biofilm protocol to deal with the most persistent GI issues. The goal of the protocol is to sterilize the organisms in the gut which are creating the pathogenic biofilm and leading to abdominal illness and digestive problems as evidenced by poor stool quality (infrequent, discolored, poor consistency). The following is the latest iteration of the protocol.

The Protocol

A biofilm approach follows four steps:

1. Lysis/Detachment
   a. Oral Na (sodium) EDTA, ethylenediaminetetraacetic acid (an iron chelating compound), and enzymes (nattokinase, lumbrokinase, chitosan) are given on an empty stomach.

   Note: EDTA works as an antifungal enhancing agent, lactoferrin acts to block further biofilm development, and the enzymes help to break down or degrade the biofilm.

       i. Patients with dairy allergies should not take lactoferrin
       ii. Patients with shellfish allergy should not take chitosan
       iii. If severe GI issues are present, enzymes should not be give on an empty stomach
       iv. Avoid iron, calcium, or magnesium supplements within two hours of administration.

2. Microbial killing
   a. Natural antimicrobials or pharmaceutical agents given one hour after lysis/detachment. Agents will depend upon testing
   b. Start with natural antimicrobials; pharmaceuticals later, if organisms remain
   c. Killing bugs is secondary to creating a hostile environment for them

3. Cleanup
   a. Activated charcoal to help prevent symptoms of die-off and aid in removal of toxins, such as ammonia
       i. Remember to give activated charcoal space, at least two hours from step two and any other supplements/meds (they get absorbed by the charcoal).

4. Rebuild/Nourish the gut lining
   a. An hour plus outside microbial killing
   b. Utilize probiotics, prebiotics
   c. Probiotic- and prebiotic-rich foods
   d. Nutritious, nontoxic foods; think organic, hormone-free, antibiotic-free. Consider Specific Carbohydrate Diet (SCD). Use digestive enzymes with meals
   e. Supportive nutrients
       i. Probiotics are live organisms which confer a health benefit. You want a good quantity and quality of organisms

ii. Prebiotics are nondigestible food ingredients that benefit the patient, stimulating the growth of beneficial bacteria. Can be given as supplement and/or in foods—legumes, peas, soybeans, fruit, garlic, onions, leeks, and chives. Act as a food source for good bacteria. Also act to inhibit pathogens and reduce clostridia toxins

iii. Give away from microbial killing phase (two plus hours)

Layman translation is as follows:

Step 1 Lysis/Detachment

Break open the biofilm protecting the bad gut bugs utilizing the combination of Na EDTA and the enzymes mentioned above. To make life easier, there are now multiple products on the market that combine these. InterFase by Klaire Labs and Biofilm Defense by Kirkman Labs are examples. Either, or the combination above, are given on an empty stomach.

Step 2 Antimicrobial killing

An hour after completing the lysis/detachment step is the optimal time to give the antimicrobials. Your doctor can suggest a cocktail, but they typically include Diflucan, neomycin, and other antifungals/antimicrobials. Your doctor will also devise the dosage of each drug given the patient's size and specific gut issues.

Note: The antifungals will require a prescription, and the enzymes are typically only available to physicians, so working closely with a doctor trained in biofilm will be necessary. Easiest formulation is capsules/pills, some are available in suspension but it is worth it to transition a child to capsules if they are not already familiar. We have had success using applesauce on a spoon with a single pill/capsule each time, working from the smallest to largest each session.

Step 3 Cleanup

The body, properly fortified with nutritious food, will perform this task on its own in most cases. If experiencing a die-off reaction (increased negative behaviors) use of activated charcoal (from you local health food store) will assist in the cleanup. It may also be useful to give the activated charcoal anyway, during the initial week or so, to capture the ammonia and other byproducts generated from the lysis/detachment step. Remember, with activated charcoal, give two hours outside any supplement or medication, as the charcoal will not discriminate what is absorbs.

Step 4 Rebuild the gut

Here, probiotics are given following a meal (dinner works best) to help grow the good gut bug colonies. Again, this should be at least two hours after or before activated charcoal is given. After a meal is ideal, as a full stomach is occupied and less likely to have digestive juices available to destroy the probiotics (i.e., acid in the stomach is occupied). Note that if enzymes are given to help the patient digest certain proteins, notably dipeptidyl peptidase-IV (DPP-IV) or other proteases to help digest gluten and casein, their use may need to be suspended during the biofilm treatment, as these enzymes could inflame a seriously stressed GI tract.

Ideally this treatment is continued until stools normalize and the gut returns to normal. Enzymes may then be reintroduced.

Results

Parents should expect a die-off reaction with increased gas and loose, broken-up stools, and potentially increased negative behaviors (stimming, upset, aggression) for a short period of time. The duration of treatment is based on how quickly stools and bloating normalize, typically reported to be weeks to months. Do not get discouraged—the treatment takes time, as pathogenic biofilm has taken time to be created, and will likewise require time to be removed. As stools and bloating normalize, expect to see improved overall behaviors, better sleep, disappearing rash, and markedly improved mood, allowing for increased regulation and attention and focus.

Potential side effects include irritability, aggression, stimming, hyperactivity, sleep disturbances, and rash. These could be the due to yeast or bacteria flare-up, detox reaction (too rapid a removal of heavy metals leading to vitamin and mineral deficiency), and stress on liver or kidney. Die-offs usually create an excess release of toxins, including ammonia, which is why activated charcoal should be used at the start of the treatment.

12

BREAKING THROUGH BEHAVIOR

BY ALISON BERKLEY AND AMANDA FRIEDMAN

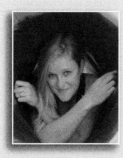

Alison Berkley
Alison@emergeandsee.net

Amanda Friedman
Amanda@emergeandsee.net

Emerge and See
www.emergeandsee.net
Twitter: EmergeandSeeEdu
Facebook: Emerge and See Education Center
and Social Groups
(917) 312-6600
(914) 494-9888
361 E 19th Street @ 1st Avenue, New York, NY

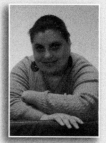

Emerge & See is excited to again be included in *Cutting-Edge Therapies for Autism*. Journeying into their 2nd year of operation at Watch Me Grow (a sensory gym providing OT, PT, speech & counseling services) E&S has begun preparing to reach beyond their education center, social groups, and workshops by applying to open a school. Amidst running programs, hosting community workshops on Medicaid, Embedded Educational Skills in Play, and events including Mommy Makeovers and Family Photo Shoots, Emerge & See owners, Amanda Friedman and Alison Berkley have submitted the initial application for NYC and Albany to open a non-for-profit private school for children and young adults with Autism and other developmental differences. The Atlas School intends to serve students between 7 and 21 years old and utilize a unique method of individualized components of TEACHH, ABA, and DIR/Floortime as well as a self-created FunQual (Functional Quality of Life) Curriculum to address activities of daily living (ADLs) and social/emotional skill sets. The Atlas School will carry on Emerge & See's philosophy of supporting the whole child with regards to academic growth (following NYS Standards), social awareness, and sensory integration. Emerge & See Education Center and Social Groups will continue to service children ages 3.5–21 in 1:1 tutoring sessions, after-school and holiday social groups, academic assessments and by hosting community workshops. Beginning January 2011 Emerge & See will be available to do trainings for families, schools, and community programs eager to understand Autism and how to support the ASD population. The company name serves to reflect our most highly valued philosophy: that we aim for our students to fully emerge into the world around them, but to also have the world see them for who they are. Hence, the name Emerge & See.

"Non-functional behavior" is a term often used within the special education field and Emerge & See is eager to see it eradicated from general use. We believe that, despite our inability to always understand, *all* behavior has a purpose and communicative intent. We deny so much from students in order to make them meet social "norms", of which many are a façade in the first place, and must allow children to capitalize on their multiple learning styles. In order to bring students "into our world" we must not hold them captive by our words, desks, and concepts when they crave to touch and explore. Even for neuro-typical learners scientists and psychologists are realizing the importance of utilizing all of the senses in education. "The connection between touch and understanding is deeply instinctual, beginning in infancy and continuing, in varying forms, throughout our lives. Experiments have found that touch is as important as vision for learning and retaining information. Studies also show that tactile activities such as playing with blocks help children improve everything from their math abilities to their thinking skills. We are knowledge architects, building edifices through physical experiences. Yet many school curricula are based on the old paradigm that knowledge flows from an expert instructor to a passive student. This mode of teaching is especially evident after children leave kindergarten for the long trek through elementary, middle and high school, where instruction relies less on hands-on exploration and more on rote memorization designed to improve test results. In contrast, haptics, the study of how the sense of touch affects the way people interact with the world-suggests that if educators engaged all of their students' senses, the children would not only learn better, they would *think* better too." (Cabrera, Derek and Colosi, Laura, Scientific American, September/October 2010).

All too often, when students are overwhelmed by their immediate environment, due to heightened auditory sensitivity, or processing delays, anxiety, or bouts of confusion, they are punished for their reactions. If we only could place ourselves in their shoes, maybe then we would gain a greater empathy and desire to understand before we try to change. When students with Autism or other delays, who have lower developmental capabilities than their chronological age, bite or act out in a "rage" they are immediately labeled and often deemed uneducable. Parents of other children complain and ask for these children to be isolated and segregation and harsh judgment ensues. Emerge & See puts a call to arms out to the public to realize that all people have the ability to progress and deserve to have someone observe, analyze, and attempt to shape a new avenue for their behavior. The fight or flight response is long established and respected when spoken of as instinctual yet is ignored when in the context of explaining children's behavior to a perceived threat. "It's not loud in here!" "What is there to be scared of?" "That's just absurd!" are all comments which belittle the experience of those functioning with a brain that is designed uniquely and a sensory system in desperate need of organization. Instead of placing judgment, we need to understand a child's /young adult's perception of the environment and demands being placed on them. We must then find an avenue on which to build a relationship and trust so that we may come into their awareness and help them to better and more safely navigate the "real world" so they may safely access their loved ones, their education, and the path to their independence and future.

Now that it has been established that all behavior serves some function, it is important to consider that some behaviors that we adults deem inappropriate (and thus try to extinguish) are merely age-appropriate expressions of child development. Parents and teachers are all too quick to attribute an unwanted or aversive behavior to the "Autism". They fail to first identify certain behaviors as part and parcel of natural child development. When a neuro-typical child is learning to write, for instance, they may form their letters backwards (so-called mirror writing). Yet, we don't automatically assume that the child is dyslexic. We *first* look at the child's age and writing skill profile to see if they are simply passing a naturally occurring developmental milestone. Likewise, we should never *assume* a child with autism is behaving a certain way simply because they are "autistic". There is always a neurological or environmental cause to be found. We simply have to remind ourselves to first identify behavior, and then attribute causality.

So many of us question self-stimulatory behaviors and try to deny its potency without first stopping to understand the fascination or sensation it brings to the child. Parents and educators often try to eliminate stimulatory objects and behaviors without offering a reasonable substitute. Although those same adults have their own quirks, hobbies, and obsessions, they unlike have been given tools to handle their eccentricities; why not offer the same resources to our students with autism? "A productive obsession provokes all sorts of mental states – euphoria when something goes brilliantly, irritation when you feel thwarted, fatigue after hours of mental struggle, excitement as one idea leads to another. You can prepare for these states and decide before hand how you will handle them. Have you grown a little too agitated? (A hot shower works wonders.) Keep inventing strategies and remember the ones that have proven effective in the past." (Maisel, Eric and Ann, Psychology Today, May/June 2010). Emerge & See fosters students' access to such coping mechanisms, thus recognizing the full intentions behind their stimulatory behavior, but also helping shape that behavior so that it does not impede social interactions or functioning in the "real world".

For so many of our students, especially the non-verbal and less-verbal, independence is thwarted when so much is assumed for them. Emerge & See aims to find their voice, choice, and specialty skills so as to empower and enable progress. There is passion and curiosity on every developmental level; perhaps not all students will go the academic route but they all are entitled to learn about the world around them, about what they may enjoy, and about having the right to either try and fail, or try and succeed... to give no tries is to oppress. We do not believe in cementing children and young adults into one category nor assuming a ceiling of ability based on standards that do not address the creativity and heart of a person. Therein we continue to observe and assess every glance, utterance, and movement our students make! This includes "scripting" which is when students repeat (echolalia) and quote (often repetitively) from familiar movies, television shows, computer games, etc. Often times, the timing of these scripts has purpose. Emerge & See is aware that it is often a hiccup of the brain, a safety default of the child/young adult, however does not deny that in the midst of all dialogue it can occur with great intentionality and poignancy.

Behavior is shaped by our own desires to succeed. This is no different for students of multiple abilities... The desire to please others often creates an anxiety level that negates true knowledge and leads to the assumption that because someone does not perform well on an assessment or a first play date they are unable to be successful. What Emerge & See aims to do is find the most natural connections to expand upon avoiding added stressors but working through those that clearly exist. "Once we feel stressed, we often try to control what we're doing in order to ensure success. So if we're doing a task that normally operates largely outside of conscious awareness, such as an easy golf swing, what screws us up is the impulse to think about and control our actions. Suddenly we're too attentive to what we're doing, and all the training that has improved our motor skills is for naught, since our conscious attention is essentially hijacking motor memory (Flora, Carlin, The Brain, Fall 2010). Therefore, it is essential to respect the student's internal coping of their immediate environment, transitions and understanding of the demands and expectations we are asking of them. All behavior comes from either an internal or external trigger. It is up to us to empower our students and loved ones to command those triggers and evolve as individuals in control. As Dr. Stanley Greenspan once said, "There is no greater feeling than that of being understood." Emerge & See advocates that self-understanding transforms a community as well as an individual.

13

THE CAMPHILL COMMUNITIES ANTHROPOSOPHICAL APPROACH TO AUTISM

BY DR. MARGA HOGENBOOM AND PAULA MORAINE

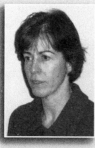

Marga G.E. Hogenboom, artsexamen Utrecht, MRCGP

Camphill Medical Practice
Murtle Estate
Bieldside
Scotland
AB15 9EP
00441224868935
marga@hogenboom.co.uk
www.camphillschools.org.uk

Dr. Marga Hogenboom has worked for seventeen years as a general practitioner and school medical officer in The Camphill Medical Practice in Scotland. She specialises in Anthroposophic medicine. The Camphill School Aberdeen has ninety pupils and is accredited by the Autistic Society in the U.K. She is co-author of the books *Autism: A Holistic Approach* and *Living with Genetic Syndromes Associated with Intellectual Disability.*

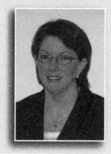

Paula Moraine, M.Ed.

pmoraine@gmail.com

Paula Moraine has been an educator for thirty-five years, working with children and adults in classrooms, residential homes, and universities. She is currently the Director of the Community Outreach Center for Literacy and Tutoring Program in Bel Air, Maryland.

The Camphill communities are therapeutic life-sharing communities, residential and day schools, and training centres for individuals with a wide range of special needs. Camphill communities are initiatives for social change, recognizing that every individual has special gifts and every individual can learn. The social change in Camphill communities might be characterized as moving from a life organized around more norm-based social hierarchies to social structures based on symbiotic collaboration. For the person with autistic spectrum disorder (ASD), who is socially challenged through the very nature of ASD, simply living in a Camphill community can be therapeutic and palliative. The information in this chapter will refer primarily to children with ASD, but the principles are applicable to adults as well.

The Camphill community was founded in 1940 by Dr. Karl Koenig, an Austrian educator, pediatrician, and social innovator. With a small group of colleagues, the first Camphill community was formed, and from the beginning the work was based on the principles and ideals of Rudolf Steiner and Anthroposophy. The work of Curative Education began with children in Aberdeen, Scotland, and gradually grew into the realm of Social Therapy to include teenagers and adults with special needs.

Camphill communities combine daily life with the arts, conventional and alternative medicine, therapy, nutritional insights, and education. Camphill centres strive to combine the wisdom of Anthroposophy with current medical research, social change, and educational innovation. Camphill's comprehensive approach to daily therapy, Waldorf education in the classroom, meaningful work, and a rhythmic, ordered home life form a foundational support for individuals with ASD.

So what is cutting edge about the Anthroposophical approach to autism that has been in existence since 1940? Why is so little known about this unique approach for children and adults with ASD? The Camphill schools and adult communities have always included people with a wide range of abilities and needs that include ASD, genetic syndromes, and cognitive and developmental delays or disabilities. There has never been a time when the Camphill communities catered specifically to the needs of the ASD individual, but the balance of daily life and therapeutic activity has always been core to the mission of Camphill. Part of why this unique approach has not gained notoriety is due to the important fact that the therapeutic value lies deeply ingrained in the daily life of the community. Gradually, though, the Camphill communities are becoming more actively involved in academic, educational, and medical research and training which will likely lead to more and more being known about this community-based, therapeutic approach to daily life.

Autism and the Senses

Autism/ASD remains a riddle in the 21st century with no known definitive cause, though a consensus is slowly forming that individuals with ASD are burdened by very fragmented and distorted sensory perceptions. This fragmentation occurs on all levels of sensory input from proprioception (sensing orientation and movement in the body), to the sense of smell, vision, hearing, taste, and touch.

Sensory information that is disjointed causes a person with ASD to live in a different consciousness and have altered and mostly confusing perceptions of their environment and the people around them. This causes a high level of anxiety and does seem to extend to the inner experience of the individual causing a fragmentation in self perception. Most people experience their thoughts, feelings and actions as having a level of cohesion. This is not necessarily so in people with autism. Thoughts can become isolated, break off from any unity with other thoughts, and can often become obsessions. The emotional life might not be mature, but there is an immediate reaction of distress in response to the world around them which can express itself in shouting, jumping up and down, physical mannerisms, repetitive actions, and acting out behaviours which can be perceived as aggression. This leads to the real question: "What is the deep, underlying cause of the inability to integrate sensory perceptions for a harmonious balance in the realms of thinking, feeling, and action?" The holistic view of Anthroposophy suggests that a human being has a physical, soul/emotional, and spiritual make-up. Even though we don't know the deep, underlying cause of ASD, the reality is that a daily, therapeutic life encourages the individual with ASD to more fully connect the physical and soul/emotional experiences with the spiritual, and that anything we do to balance or harmonize sensory experience will lead to a better integration of thoughts, feelings, and actions.

The Senses

We are all familiar with the senses of sight, hearing, taste, touch, and smell, but Rudolf Steiner spoke about twelve senses, giving us a comprehensive description and insight into their interrelationships. Steiner organized them into three groups of Lower Senses (Touch, Life Sense, Self-Movement, and Balance); Middle Senses (Smell, Taste, Vision, and Warmth); Higher Senses (Hearing, Sense of the Word, Thought, and Sense of the other). Through Anthroposophy we understand that the lower senses connect us to our physical body, the middle senses give us insight into our soul/emotional experiences, and the higher senses connect us to the more spiritual aspect of our human nature.

The Lower Senses

TOUCH

We gradually learn about the boundary between self and the world through touch. We combine touch with other sensory input to establish a knowledge-base about the world around us. Without a sense of touch, our information about the world is altered and incomplete.

LIFE SENSE

With the sense of life, we experience our body at the level of being well / unwell, or rested / tired, knowing when we need to sleep, rest, be active, etc. If the sense of life is out of balance, the child might not be able to experience or communicate pain effectively, will be distressed or upset, but will not always be able to communicate what is needed.

SENSE OF SELF-MOVEMENT

Movement gives us information about our body and a sense of where we are in the world. A child with ASD often exhibits repetitive, compulsive movements, demonstrating little control over the decision to move.

SENSE OF BALANCE OR EQUILIBRIUM

Equilibrium comes about through a balance of all three directionalities in space: left / right; above / below; front / behind. Physiologically equilibrium can be found in the semi-circular canals of the ear. The sense of balance comes about through finding our balance in relationship to the world around us

The Middle Senses

SENSE OF SMELL

There is no outer, physical boundary to smell. We have to take it fully inside ourselves, and smells can therefore be overwhelming and cause a strong reaction of either attraction or revulsion. The child with ASD can be overpowered by the sense of smell, which can result in reactive behaviours that are not within the child's realm of self-control to adjust.

SENSE OF TASTE

The experience of taste is an intimate experience. Most frequently, taste is connected to eating and the four common 'tastes' of sweet, salt, sour, and bitter. What is a pleasant taste experience for one person might be unpleasant and offensive to another. For such an intimate and personalized experience, it is not surprising that children with ASD often have strong likes and dislikes in food, and strong reactions to anything that doesn't taste good to them. The taste, texture, and temperature come together and if any of these are not in balance, the food is unacceptable.

VISION

Through our eyes we take in color, light, movement, and form. In order to identify an object, we most frequently will look at it to determine what it is. Our eyes use other sensibilities in that we use our eyes to regain our balance, to determine if something is level, to establish how close or how far away it is, to ascertain the movement of the object – and all these in addition to color and light. Color and form provide sensory input that can be overwhelming or soothing, painful or relaxing.

SENSE OF WARMTH

This can be referred to as the temperature sense, but it is a physical experience of the contraction and expansion caused by warmth or cold. When it is cold, we contract and withdraw. When it is warm, we generally expand and reach out. The child with ASD may appear "cold" but they have a real need for human warmth and connectedness.

The Higher Senses

HEARING

Hearing comes about through tonal frequencies that are a vibrating movement. Sounds are heard continuously, although we generally choose which sounds might be meaningful enough to process. The child with ASD might have strong reactions to actual sounds, including actual pain, so it is important to be sensitive to both the sound levels and the amount of sound a child with ASD is exposed to.

SENSE OF WORD

This is the sense that enables us to understand what others say, allowing us to decipher the sounds in speech. If a child is unable to engage in this way, then communication is compromised and an alternate communication options must be used.

SENSE OF THOUGHT

The sense of thought enables us to perceive and understand the thoughts of others. Through our sense of thought we understand the meaning behind the words. The very young child thinks in quite concrete terms, and is not able to understand nuance and innuendo. The child with ASD may understand the explicit meaning, and miss any implicit intention or meaning.

SENSE OF EGO OR SENSE OF SELF

This is possibly the most interesting sense that Steiner included in the twelve senses. The sense of 'I' is often referred to as the sense of 'self' and the sense of 'other'. What is it that makes it possible for us to experience the 'I' in ourselves? What makes it possible to experience the 'I' of others? Very young children don't refer to themselves with 'I' initially when they learn to speak. First they refer to themselves with their own name, or simply 'me'. It is quite a moment when it becomes clear to the child that they are an 'I' and you are a 'you'. What does the child with ASD experience as either a sense of 'I' or a sense of 'other'?

Assessment

When a child enters the Camphill school community, a process of assessment begins with a differentiated diagnosis that includes detailed insight into the sensory functions of the child. Although this is done for every child, for the child with ASD this sensory assessment is particularly essential. The children all have special needs in some area, and it is often wise to look at the lower senses, specifically the sense of life or wellbeing as this is frequently the source of many disturbances experienced by the child. They may have poor sleep patterns, challenging eating habits, emotional disturbances, obsession behaviours, self-harming behaviours, and physiological challenges that might include digestive disturbances. The therapeutic way of life in Camphill often produces the quickest positive changes in these areas. The rhythmic and predictable life style is comforting to the child and they begin to sleep easier, eat with fewer irritations, and begin to relax into the daily routine. The feeling of safety that is a direct result of the rhythmical routines, gradually allows the child to release his or her need for the parent to be present at all times. The symbiotic relationship that the child with ASD has with the parents can be gradually transformed so the child can enter into a new kind of therapeutic relationship with the care giver or teacher. This transfer has the specific benefits of demonstrating that the child can establish social interaction, and it creates in the care giver, teacher, or therapist a sense of awe at the emerging individual. The therapeutic relationship between the staff and the student can be an intensely healing opportunity for the child.

The next level of change comes about when the child begins to experience improved integration with his or her physical body, or when the physical body becomes a more 'friendly place' to spend inhabit. This happens when the child feels more integration between thinking, feeling, and action. The compulsions ease somewhat, and the child can undertake an activity with guidance. Gradually, the third level is achieved, and the child can engage in an independent activity, which naturally makes the child more confident and willing to further engage in learning. This kind of progress is rarely a straight line from effort to success. The ASD child might have many stops and starts, as well as successes and failures, but they are guided, supported, and cared for throughout the entire learning process.

The Camphill community teaches these approaches in university courses and training seminars around the world. The courses encompass meditative, self-reflective, diagnostic training that uses current research and comparative literature to enhance the knowledge base of the students in Curative Education. New approaches and insights into ASD are continuously assessed for their compatibility with the Camphill ideals of respecting the spiritual essence of the child, supporting the need for healing the fragmented sensory experience, and educating the cognitive, emotional, and will-based needs of the child. Many of the modern tools are incorporated into daily life and the classroom learning such as visual diaries, protective headphones, sensory integration supports, dietary supports, and medical interventions.

Case study—'Peter'

Peter as reported in Jackson, R. (Ed). *Holistic Special Education—Camphill Principles and Practice*. Edinburgh, Scotland: Floris Press, 2006.

Life at home with Peter as a toddler was not easy. The parents got very little sleep and became more and more reclusive in order to avoid bizarre situations when out in public with their son. He would run up to people in the store and feel their bare legs, play obsessively with water and flood the bathroom, or cause damage to items he touched. At the age of three, he climbed through the back yard fence and managed to escape, almost running in front of a car. He did not speak and life became exhausting for the parents. The parents and Peter's sibling were not able to spend time together and the older sibling increasingly retreated into his own room. Peter came to Camphill at age seven as a weekly boarder, meaning he stayed at Camphill during the week and spent the weekends at home with his family. This was initially very difficult for his parents and caused them a great deal of soul searching. Peter began to settle into his routine, and began responding very well to the structured environment. He participated in school, made his first drawing, and began speaking his first words at the age of nine. Now, Peter is nineteen, and his parents jokingly complain that he never stops speaking. Peter benefitted not only from the general daily rhythms and routines, but also from the specific therapies he was given. For Peter, his speech and language therapy was pivotal in his successful growth and learning, contributing to his progress and maturity. He is an outgoing, observant adult, who can even give you a hug! His language and reasoning is still improving, and he still has ASD, but his engages with appropriate and interesting conversation. Although he will still touch the light switch when entering a room, he acknowledges and orientates to the people in the room. He is now living in a Camphill community for adults and is able to contribute to the entire community through his work.

Case Study—'John'

John has ASD. He also has high arousal levels and anxiety. He is restless, avoids interaction with others, and has a low stress threshold. John does not respond well to transitions, is over-responsive to sounds, and subsequently finds large settings noisy and upsetting. John does not like to be touched – he doesn't like to have his hair washed, his nails trimmed, and he reacts to certain types of clothing. He prefers crispy food textures and sticky spreads on his bread. When he is anxious, he will hide under his covers and withdraw into his own space. If he stress level is high, he might kick or hit himself. He will try self-calming strategies such as crouching with a large beanbag over his head, or self-distracting movements like waving his hands. When he is in a good mood, he enjoys the vestibular self-stimulation of rocking, swinging, and bouncing. John's therapeutic plan includes addressing his anxiety through providing safe options for withdrawal when sensory stressors are too strong. A predictable, calm environment eases his overload of sensory experiences. He receives massage therapy with measured touch and pressure, and movement therapy to address his needs for proprioception, touch, and vestibular balance.

Therapeutic Approaches in Daily Life

Therapy in Camphill can take place in a therapeutic environment specifically prepared to provide the therapeutic experience. Some examples are art therapy, play therapy, massage therapy, equine or horse riding therapy, movement or eurythmy therapy, therapeutic speech, color and light therapy, and therapeutic music. These therapeutic interventions are provided by a trained therapist, and repeated over a longer period of time. Specific therapies are combined with medical support, natural medicines, and healthy nutrition to form a medical triad of interventions. Therapies are conducted in an exquisitely prepared environment, by a fully trained practitioner. The details of each therapy won't be discussed here, but time, care, and attention are paid to the individual child, implementing the child's care plan through each designated therapy.

Camphill intentionally establishes a rhythmical, predictable, structured life style as a therapeutic element. The daily rhythm encourages healthy sleep patterns through regular sleeping/waking times, daily events such as mealtime are ordered and predictable. The mealtime is a learning opportunity on many levels. The house community members gather before the meal for a time of relaxation and quiet, meals begin and end with a simple grace, and the activity of eating is guided for maximum comfort and ease of digestion. Children have to eat every day, so a therapeutic attitude surrounds each meal. There are many positive effects gained through dietary intervention. If a child has any difficulty living in the physical body, it will often manifest in digestive disturbances. The child might not be able to fully digest the food, leading to the discomfort of undigested foods. Insightful dietary interventions can help stimulate healthy digestive processes, allowing foods to more effectively nourish the body and provide strength and energy. This is not done through extreme diets, but rather through a balanced offering of whole, organic, and well prepared foods that are eaten in a calm and relaxing setting.

Children can be involved in the meal preparation, or they might take part in the clean-up after the meal. The small jobs surrounding regular daily activities such as meal time, preparing for bed in the evening, and getting ready for the day in the morning, provide the child with ASD ordered and predictable routines. They can learn to gradually increase their levels of self-responsibility and learn to care for others through supportive gestures of help.

The therapeutic daily life of Camphill is intended to particularly provide a cohesive experience to offset the sensory fragmentation the ASD child experiences. As an example, for the child with ASD, touch can be painful. To ameliorate that pain, a child might be provided with a variety of options using natural materials in order to gain confidence with differing tactile experiences. These may include cutting wood, pushing wheelbarrows, digging in the soil, walking in the woods, building shelters out of branches, playing in water (as weather permits), swimming, cooking, kneading bread dough, and many more. Therapeutic massage, aroma baths, and warm compresses can activate the child's sense of touch without disturbing the pain receptors.

Children are encouraged to play in Camphill, and those with ASD who might have rigid, repetitive movements are encouraged to enter into shared games and events. Indoor games, outdoor games, group games, and team games are all considered important aspects of social life. Harmonious movement in encouraged through regular walks in nature, and social interaction skills are taught through ring games, music games, and group games.

The living spaces in Camphill are designed for low acoustic impact and calming visual appearance. Quiet spaces are considered as important as communal spaces, and children with ASD are allowed both the quiet and separate moments to compliment the more challenging communal moments.

For more specific and elaborated descriptions of daily life, therapeutic activities, and educational approaches in Camphill, please see Jackson, R. (Ed). *Holistic Special Education – Camphill Principles and Practice*. Edinburgh, Scotland: Floris Press, 2006.

Conclusion

Camphill community life offers a unique contribution to the options for approaches to Autism Spectrum Disorder, specifically:

The therapeutic daily life in Camphill addresses many of the needs for sensory integration necessary to balance the sensory fragmentation so many with ASD experience.

The impulse for social change and the communal life that is an essential part of Camphill life serves as daily social skills training and guidance through both implicit and explicit example.

All of these examples for children can appropriately be translated into the adult setting, providing an integrated, cohesive life for adults with ASD.

While the causes of autism are not fully known, we accept that both physical and spiritual genetics take their respective places as possible root causes of ASD.

Anthroposophy guides the spiritual life of the Camphill communities in which the spiritual nature of every individual is respected. The belief is that every individual, whether with ASD or without, has a healthy spiritual core and can learn if given an appropriate, individualised environment.

Camphill communities provide the protected setting needed for the integrated, therapeutic daily life, which is its signature, modern, cutting-edge therapy for autism.

For more information about Camphill Communities worldwide, please see http://www.camphill.org/

For more information about the Camphill Communities in the U.S., please see http://www.camphill.org/?cat=4

CARD ELEARNING AND SKILLS: WEB-BASED TRAINING, ASSESSMENT, CURRICULUM AND PROGRESS TRACKING FOR CHILDREN WITH AUTISM

BY DR. DOREEN GRANPEESHEH AND
DR. ADEL C. NAJDOWSKI

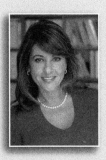

Doreen Granpeesheh, Ph.D., BCBA-D
Center for Autism and Related Disorders
19019 Ventura Blvd, 3rd Floor
Tarzana, CA 91356

Dr. Doreen Granpeesheh has dedicated over thirty years to helping individuals with autism lead healthy, productive lives. While completing her PhD in Psychology under Ivar Lovaas, she worked on the world-renowned 1987 study that showed a recovery rate of nearly 50 percent. Dr. Granpeesheh is a licensed psychologist in four states and is a Board Certified Behavior Analyst-Doctoral (BCBA-D). In 1990 Dr. Granpeesheh founded the Center for Autism & Related Disorders (CARD). CARD achieves success with every child through world-class treatment, staff training, curricula, and research. CARD provides services at 18 clinics in six U.S. states, as well as sites in Australia, New Zealand and partnerships in Dubai and Johannesburg. CARD employs over 800 staff and is a leading employer of BCBAs. Dr. Granpeesheh is on numerous Scientific and Advisory Boards for governmental and advocacy groups, and is the recipient of frequent honors, including the 2011 American Academy of Clinical Psychiatrists Winokur Award.

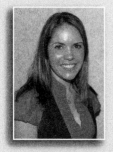

Adel C. Najdowski, Ph.D., BCBA-D

Dr. Adel Najdowski graduated from the University of Nevada, Reno in 2004 with her doctorate in Psychology. She is the co-creator of Skills™, a comprehensive assessment and curriculum for children with autism, and currently serves as the Director of the Skills department at the Center for Autism and Related Disorders. She has served children with autism for 16 years. Dr. Najdowski has taught multiple undergraduate and graduate level courses in psychology. She served on the editorial board for the Journal of Applied Behavior Analysis in 2009 and has been a National Board Certified Behavior Analyst (BCBA) since 2003. She has six first-authored publications, 18 co-authored publications, and has been an author on 63 presentations given at conferences. Her current research interests include teaching higher level skills to children with autism, assessment and curriculum design for children with autism, and feeding disorders.

CARD eLearning™ is a new web-based program for training individuals to deliver ABA-based intervention to children with autism spectrum disorders (ASD). Skills™ is a new web-based program for the assessment, curriculum design, and management of ABA-based intervention programs for children with ASD.

Center for Autism and Related Disorders

CARD eLearning and Skills were developed by the Center for Autism and Related Disorders, Inc. (CARD). CARD was founded by Dr. Doreen Granpeesheh in 1990 and provides behavioral intervention to approximately 1,200 individuals with ASD using an approach called applied behavior analysis (ABA). CARD currently has 19 offices across seven states within the United States, two offices internationally (New Zealand and Australia) and two affiliate sites (United Arab Emirates and South Africa). In addition to servicing children at these physical sites, CARD provides intervention to children on all continents using a consultative workshop model.

In the course of treating children for 20 years, CARD believes that children can recover from ASD and has published research on the recovery of children. While recovery is possible for a group of children with particular characteristics, it is not the only goal of intervention. Our goal is to help each child achieve the most they can and live life to the fullest potential.

Over the years, CARD has become well-known for their robust therapist training program and for having the most comprehensive curriculum for teaching skills to children with ASD in the world. Given the rising incidence of ASD, we have experienced a tremendous increase in the demand for CARD treatment services. This increase is what led to the development of both CARD eLearning and Skills. The two programs were created with the goal of helping as many children and their families affected by ASD as possible. It is our mission to provide global access to the highest quality of ABA-based intervention in the world. Both CARD eLearning and Skills can be accessed on the world-wide web at www.skillsforautism.com.

CARD eLearning

CARD eLearning is based on the didactic classroom portion of the therapist-level training provided at CARD for the last 20 years. The development of CARD eLearning was initiated in 2002 and the product was completed in 2010. Also, in 2010, research was published demonstrating that CARD eLearning is an effective tool for increasing academic knowledge of individuals on the principles and application of behavior analysis to the treatment of ASD.

CARD eLearning is an online training program designed to facilitate the provision of effective intervention for children with ASD by equipping users with foundational knowledge in autism, ABA and research-proven intervention techniques. CARD eLearning currently consists of 9 modules, equivalent to 40 hours of training. Each learning module focuses on a topic such as: "What is Autism?", "Applied Behavior Analysis (ABA)", "Skill Repertoire Building", and "Behavior Management." Each section of the CARD eLearning program is organized with teaching objectives, explanation of terms, examples of methodology, video demonstrations, printable study guides, online note taking, quizzes, and other learning tools.

Upon completion of CARD eLearning users are provided with a certificate of completion. Furthermore, organizations using CARD eLearning to train their staff can obtain reports about the performance of their staff. They can view the quiz and test scores of each user, determine which portions of the training were most difficult for the user to acquire by viewing how many times the user had to take a quiz to pass it, and compare the performance of staff with one another.

Skills

Skills is the online delivery of CARD's comprehensive assessment and curriculum and is also a globally accessible repository for data storage and analysis. While the CARD curriculum has been in continuous development and usage at CARD for 20 years (with new phases released annually), the development of Skills was initiated in 2003 and the product was completed in 2010. Skills involves four basic steps: (1) assess the child, (2) choose activities to teach, (3) start treatment, and (4) track progress.

FOUR STEPS

In the first step, the user interacts with the Skills assessment, which is not only the most comprehensive assessment of child development ever created but has also been demonstrated to have high test-retest and inter-rater reliability for its Language subscale. Using this tool, the user assesses the child's skill level across all areas of human functioning and across every possible skill that develops between the ages of 0 and 8 years.

The Skills assessment provides basic "yes" / "no" questions that are relevant to the child's chronological age. The questions are organized by eight developmental areas: social, motor, language, adaptive, play, executive functions, cognition, and academic skills. Within each of these developmental areas, questions are further organized by concepts (e.g., within the developmental area of "social skills" there are concepts such as "apologizing" and "initiating a conversation"). Questions are provided in the order of typical child development and are presented in an "intelligent" fashion in order to maximum efficiency.

Following completion of the assessment for any given developmental or concept area, users can view bar graphs depicting the percentage of skills in the child's repertoire in comparison to how he or she should be performing at his or her age. In addition, Skills provides users with a pool of available lesson activities directly linked to the areas identified (by the assessment) as needed to be focused on during teaching. This now enters into the second step of the Skills program wherein users choose activities to teach.

For the process of choosing activities, there are five tools available to help users make good choices. First, each lesson is assigned to a teaching level between 1 and 12, with level 1 being the most basic and 12 being the most advanced. Teaching should generally begin at lower levels before moving to higher levels. Second, activities are organized by the age in which they are observed in typical child development. Users should start by teaching younger skills before moving to older skills. Third, activities are presented and numbered (starting with 1 and moving forward) in the order in which one would usually teach them. Users should generally start by teaching activity 1 and progress forward in order. Fourth, each activity specifies the other activities that are considered prerequisites. Prerequisite skills should generally be mastered first. Finally, each activity is given one of three possible designations: (1) building block, (2) fundamental skill, or (3) expansion skill. Fundamental skills are the milestones and building blocks are considered steps toward learning fundamental skills. Building blocks are not required for every learner. Children who learn quickly might be able to skip past the building blocks whereas other children may rely on the building blocks for learning fundamental skills. Expansion skills are also not necessary for every child because they are not required for day-to-day functioning but can enrich a child's level of functioning within a particular skill area.

Once the user chooses lesson activities to place into the treatment plan, the user enters into the third step of the Skills program which is to start treatment. The user is now presented with an array of teaching materials to use during treatment. Each activity comes with a printable activity guide that provides step-by-step instructions, examples, teaching tips, and ideas for ensuring that what is learned is maintained and generalized in the child's daily life. The user is also provided with a series of printable handouts such as target checklists (e.g., targets for the activity of learning the recognition of emotions include "happy," "sad," "angry," etc.), teaching guides, worksheets, visual aids, and data tracking forms. In addition to all of these materials, users can view a short video clip of each activity being conducted by a therapist and child.

It is in the "start treatment" phase that the user has everything he or she needs to begin teaching, using the resources provided by Skills as well as the knowledge acquired from CARD eLearning. As the child learns and masters targets and activities, the user checks them off as being mastered within the Skills treatment plan. The action of checking off items automatically feeds data into the Skills database, generates printable bar graphs, and automatically plots data onto a multidisciplinary timeline.

The bar graphs show both progress within developmental and concept areas and depict a comparison between what skills the child had in his or her repertoire during the assessment and how far he or she has come during treatment. The multidisciplinary timeline is a line graph that shows the child's acquisition of targets and activities over time. The key feature of the multidisciplinary timeline is its ability to allow users to enter in other life events. With this ability, the child's entire treatment team (special educators, speech language pathologists, occupational therapists, medical doctors, etc.) can evaluate the effects of their interventions on child progress. For example, if the child starts a new biomedical intervention, it can be entered onto the timeline and its effects on the child's mastery of skills can be evaluated. Other behaviors and events can also be added including challenging behavior (e.g., stereotypy, tantrums, aggression, etc.) and events such as when the child's treatment hours change or the child is ill.

ANALYTICS

In addition to receiving graphs depicting the child's progress while using Skills, data in the Skills database can be used for the purposes of prediction of probable outcomes, team evaluation, and cost analysis. Given certain child parameters, Skills will be able to predict each child's expected best outcome from receiving ABA-based intervention in terms of his or her expected level of functioning as a result of treatment. Likewise, Skills will be able to predict how much of the Skills curriculum the child will learn given a hypothetical number of hours of treatment provided per week and in turn will be able to predict the length of time the child will need treatment at said number of hours in order to achieve the child's predicted best outcome.

In addition to predictive models at the child level, the analytics piece will allow interested parties to contrast the performance of children within the same treatment supervisor as well as to contract the performance of different treatment supervisors or treatment agencies with one another.

Given the child predictive model and the ability to conduct evaluations of the treatment team, treatment supervisors and agencies will be able to be given a ranking in terms of their effectiveness. Now, interested parties will be able to conduct a cost analysis on each case by correlating predicted best outcome for the child with supervisor/agency rankings.

SUPPORT

In addition to all of the features above that Skills offers, the website also comes with many tools for support. This includes a video library of "tips for success," navigational tutorials on every web page, support from a live expert, and a support community where users can ask questions, share ideas, and/or give praise.

Conclusion

In conclusion, CARD is among the largest autism treatment organizations in the world. CARD's state-of-the-art services, global reach, and comprehensive scope are matched by none. Two features that set CARD apart from others is our world-class training and insistence on a comprehensive application of ABA-based intervention to every imaginable skill a person with ASD may need to learn.

CARD is now in the position to share its 20 years of knowledge and expertise in providing treatment to children with ASD (and in many cases, recovering children with ASD) with the world. Neither quality nor quantity can be compromised in our mission to extend top-quality behavioral treatment to the maximum number of individuals with ASD possible. CARD eLearning and Skills have been released to achieve this mission and both self-improvement and fine-tuning will continue until this mission is accomplished.

CENTER FOR AUTISM SPECTRUM DISORDERS, MUNROE-MEYER INSTITUTE

BY DR. TIFFANY KODAK AND DR. ALISON BETZ

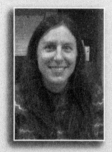

Tiffany Kodak, Ph.D.

Dr. Tiffany Kodak is an Assistant Professor in the Department of Pediatrics at the University of Nebraska Medical Center and Assistant Director of the Early Intervention Program in the Center for autism spectrum disorders at the Munroe-Meyer Institute. She graduated from Louisiana State University in 2006 with a Ph.D. in School Psychology. Dr. Kodak completed her graduate internship at The Marcus Institute in Atlanta, Georgia under the supervision of Drs. Wayne Fisher, Henry Roane, and Michael Kelley. Her post-doctoral fellowship was completed in 2006 under the supervision of Dr. Wayne Fisher. Her research has focused on several general topics, including the assessment and treatment of problem behavior, choice, behavioral economics, and skill acquisition with individuals diagnosed with autism and severe behavior disorders. She has published sixteen peer-reviewed research studies, and worked directly with individuals with developmental disabilities for fifteen years. Dr. Kodak is on the editorial board and served as the editorial assistant for the *Journal of Applied Behavior Analysis*, is a Board Certified Behavior Analyst (BCBA), and the recipient of the APA (Division 25) Applied Behavior Analysis dissertation award in 2006.

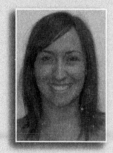

Alison Betz, Ph.D.

Dr. Alison Betz received a Master of Arts in Behavior Analysis from Western Michigan University, and her Ph.D. in Disability Disciplines with a specialization in Applied Behavior Analysis from Utah State University. She is currently completing a post-doctoral internship at the University of Nebraska Medical Center's Munroe-Meyer Institute. Her research interests and publications have focused increasing communication and social skills of young children with autism. She is currently focusing her research efforts on the assessment and treatment of severe problem behavior with individuals with disabilities. Other research interests include increasing the response variability of individuals with autism, the effects of token reinforcement, and schedules of reinforcement.

For more information about the programs in the Center for Autism Spectrum Disorders contact cawilli1@unmc.edu. To refer a child for services in the CASD, please fax (402) 559-5004 or email cawilli1@unmc.edu referrals, including child's name, date of birth, reason for referral, and contact information.

Munroe-Meyer Institute, University of Nebraska Medical Center

The Center for Autism Spectrum Disorders opened at the Munroe-Meyer Institute opened in 2006 as part of the University of Nebraska Medical Center. The center focuses on using the principles of behavior analysis to assess and treat child with autism and other developmental disabilities. The primary goal of the center is to improve the lives of children with autism spectrum disorders (ASD) and their families by: (a) providing comprehensive, state-of-the-art clinical services; (b) advancing knowledge about the causes of and treatments for ASD through systematic research; and (c) disseminating information about effective assessment and treatment through education, professional training, and consultation. There are three departments included in the Center for Autism Spectrum Disorders: Early Intervention Program, Severe Behavior Program, and the Pediatric Feeding Disorder Program. This chapter will focus on the Early Intervention and the Severe Behavior Programs.

Early Intervention Program

The emphasis of the Early Intervention Program within the Center for Autism Spectrum Disorders is to provide highly specialized services to children diagnosed with an autism spectrum disorder (ASD) between the ages of two and nine. The program utilizes assessment and treatment procedures based on the principles of Applied Behavior Analysis (ABA). Our program focuses on teaching (a) language, (b) academic and pre-academic skills, (c) appropriate social behavior, and (d) daily living skills (e.g., potty training).

In order to teach a variety of skills that are individualized to the specific needs of each child, it is the mission of the program to improve the quality of life for children with ASD and their families by providing empirically supported and comprehensive treatment services, developing and refining assessment and treatment procedures through systematic research, and promoting generalization and maintenance of acquired skills.

Program Description

The Early Intervention Program at the Munroe-Meyer Institute offers a continuum of services including evaluation, school consultation, clinic-based intervention, and home-based program development. Each child receives services based on his or her individual needs.

During therapy sessions, highly specialized techniques are used to teach children a variety of skills. Trained therapists conduct instructional procedures across settings ranging from individualized seat work, to naturalistic play interactions with adults and/or peers. A psychologist with specialty training in applied behavior analysis oversees all therapy sessions. Therapists record each occurrence of targeted skills, and the accuracy of the data is checked frequently. Session-by-session data are graphed, reviewed, and analyzed each day by therapists and supervising psychologists. Data are used to guide program development and refine the academic interventions.

Like many of their typically developing peers, children with ASD may not acquire skills through daily interactions in their home or school environment. To effectively teach children with ASD, tasks are broken down into small, measurable units, and each skill is practiced repeatedly until the child masters the skill. Some skills may serve as building blocks for other more complex skills (e.g., imitation, attending). Thus, we may begin working on more basic skills that allow children to acquire building blocks that prepare the child to learn more advanced skills and learn in a number of different environments. Once a skill is mastered, it is practiced periodically to make sure the child continues to maintain previously mastered skills over time. Parents are also provided with information and materials to work on mastered skills in the home environment. It is our goal for children to exhibit all newly learned skills in a variety of environments and with a variety of people.

If a child in the Early Intervention Program displays problem behavior that is of concern to the parents or school personnel, assessment and treatment procedures will be utilized to reduce the occurrence of the challenging behaviors.

Initial Evaluation. Children will be seen by a team of specialists with training and expertise in educational interventions. Some children may benefit from highly intensive early intervention, while other children may only require limited visits to our clinic or consultation between our staff members and school personnel. Our evaluation process may require an extended period of time because children respond differently to different academic instructional procedures. Our goal is to identify a number of instructional procedures that will result in the most rapid acquisition of targeted skills.

Treatment. Based on the needs of each individual child, a curriculum of academic, pre-academic, social, and language skills are developed. Targeted skills are worked on each day until the child reaches mastery criterion for the skill. Our model of intervention combines aspects of Discrete Trial Training, Natural Environmental Training, and Verbal Behavior. Treatment procedures may include Discrete Trial Instruction, Natural Language Paradigm, Incidental Teaching, Peer Mediated Strategies for social skills development, as well as a number of other empirically-validated procedures based on the principles of ABA.

Parent Training. Once an effective treatment is developed and the child has mastered some of the targeted skills, we train parents and other care providers to use the teaching strategies in other environments. The long-term success of the treatment depends on how accurately the program is carried out by parents, teachers, in-home aids, and other care providers. We encourage school personnel to participate in training as well. Our goal is to teach everyone who interacts with the child to use the instructional procedures that result in learning new skills and maintaining previously learned skills.

Severe Behavior Program

Approximately 10–15 percent of children with autism, developmental disabilities, and traumatic brain injuries engage in some form of destructive behavior such as aggression, self-injury, pica, or property destruction. The purpose of the severe behavior program within the Center for Autism Spectrum Disorders is to provide specialized services to individuals with autism and other developmental disabilities who display these destructive behaviors. It is often the case that children who do display these problematic behaviors pose a health risk for the child or to others, limit their learning and development, cause stress and hardship on their families, and may be at risk for long-term institutional care. Thus it is the mission of this program to improve the quality of life of the children who display destructive behaviors, and their families, by (a) providing the most advanced treatment services; (b) perpetuating the development and refinement of effective treatments of severe behavior through systematic clinical research; and (c) promoting the widespread dissemination of effective treatment technologies through highly specialized training and consultation.

Program Description

The severe behavior program provide specialized treatment to school-aged children (three to twenty-one years old) that display such severe destructive behavior that it poses a risk to self, others, or to the environment, and who cannot be safely managed or treated in a less-structured and intensive program. The program offers a continuum of services, including initial evaluation, outpatient services, day treatment, and parent/

caregiver training. An individualized program is created for each child, and that child moves through the program based on his or her personal needs.

Following the initial evaluation, during which the child and family meet with a team highly experienced in the assessment of severe problem behaviors and recommendations are given, the child may be referred to one of the following programs:

Day Treatment or Outpatient Services. Children with less severe behaviors are typically referred to outpatient therapy. With outpatient services, children are typically seen from one or two hours per day, one to five days per week. Children displaying more severe problem behaviors are typically seen in our day treatment program, in which the child is seen five or six hours, five days per week. Regardless of whether the child is referred to outpatient services or day treatment, the assessment and treatment of the problem behaviors are conducted in a similar manner.

All sessions are conducted in a specialized therapeutic environment that allows us to safely evaluate potentially dangerous behaviors. For each child, we begin therapy by conducting analog sessions that directly test the effects of specific environmental antecedent and consequences on the problem behavior. Data are collected on the targeted behaviors on computers by the therapists are reviewed by a licensed psychologists on a daily basis. The session data are then analyzed to develop and refine an individualized treatment for the child. Furthermore, all assessments and treatment components are evaluated systematically by using single-case research designs. This allows us to identify, refine, and replace ineffective components of the treatment plan.

Parent Training. The long-term success of the recommended treatment plan developed during therapy sessions is dependent on the accuracy of implementation by parents and caregivers. Thus, parent and caregiver training is a critical component of our program. Parent and caregiver training typically involves written and spoken instruction, modeling, behavioral rehearsal or role play, and systematic feedback during therapy sessions. Once the parents or caregivers demonstrate competency in implementing the treatment at the clinic, therapists then observe parents implementing the treatment in the home and other naturalistic settings. Furthermore, we provide treatment recommendations and training for the child's school or other caregivers.

CHELATION: REMOVAL OF TOXIC METALS

BY DR. JAMES B. ADAMS

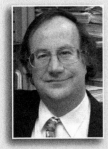

James B. Adams, Ph.D.

Professor
School of Mechanical, Aerospace, Chemical, and Materials Engineering
Arizona State University
PO Box 876106
Tempe, AZ 85287-6106
(480) 965-3316
(480) 727-9321 (fax)
http://autism.asu.edu

James B. Adams is a President's Professor at Arizona State University, where his research is focused on the causes of autism and how to treat it. He is also President of the Autism Society of Greater Phoenix, and is co-leader of the Autism Research Institute/Defeat Autism Now! Think Tank. His research includes toxic metals/chelation, nutrition (vit-amin/minerals, essential fatty acids, amino acids), neurotransmitters, and GI issues. He is the proud father of a daughter with autism.

Rationale: Many children with autism have a low amount of active glutathione, and a higher fraction of their glutathione is oxidized (inactive). Glutathione is the body's primary defense against mercury, toxic metals, and many toxic chemicals, so a low level of glutathione results in a higher body burden of toxins. Also, many children with autism had increased use of oral antibiotics in infancy, which alter gut flora and thereby almost completely stop the body's ability to excrete mercury. Normalizing glutathione, restoring gut flora, and removing toxic metals often results in reduction of the symptoms of autism.

Also, a major study by our group found that much of the variation in the severity of autism was associated with the level of toxic metals in the urine.

Preparation for Treatment: Prior to beginning chelation, it is important to first prepare the body for it. This includes:

1) Reducing exposure to toxins (by using organic food and reverse osmosis water, no mercury fillings, avoiding pesticides, etc.).
2) Improving levels of essential vitamins and minerals—see section on vitamins and minerals.
3) Improving glutathione levels—see section on glutathione.
4) Treating gut dysbiosis—see sections on gut treatments.

Testing:

It is difficult to assess toxic metal body burden. The best approach is to use a challenge dose of the relevant chelator (DMSA, DMPS, or possibly EDTA), and measure the level of toxic metals in the urine before and after taking it. A large increase indicates that the metals are present, and that the medication is helpful in removing them.

Hair, blood, and unprovoked urine testing only indicate recent exposure to toxic metals, and are *not* useful in determining past exposure. Children may have a high body burden but a low level in their current hair, blood, or urine.

The urinary porphyrins profile is a test of porphyrin production in the kidneys. Abnormal porphyrins may indicate an increased body burden of mercury, lead, or other toxic metals, but other factors such as oxidative stress might instead account for abnormal porphyrins, so the test results can be difficult to interpret.

Treatment: The chelation treatments I recommended include DMSA and DMPS, and possibly TTFD. These treatments should only be done under physician supervision, with regular evaluation of kidney and liver function and white blood cell count. All of the treatments except IV-DMPS can be done at home. DMSA is best for removing lead, and DMPS is best for removing mercury.

Length of Treatment: It is recommended to measure the amount of toxic metals in urine (preferably in a first-morning urine sample) before starting treatment. Then, every month or so, collect urine for about 8 hours after DMSA or DMPS treatment, and measure levels of toxic metals again. When the levels are within the lab's reference range (which is for people NOT undergoing chelation), then the chelator has probably removed most of the metals that it is able to. Since DMSA and DMPS bind to different metal differently, it is probably useful to use one until it urinary excretion is low, and then switch to the other. It may be useful to do a challenge dose every six months or so, as lower, maintenance doses may be helpful.

DMSA (dimercaptosuccinic acid): Oral DMSA is approved by the FDA for treating lead poisoning in children. Some of the compounded rectal suppositories also appear to increase excretion of toxic metals, but the transdermal forms do not measurably increase excretion of toxic metals.

Safety: DMSA only slightly affects excretion of most essential minerals, so a basic mineral supplement can compensate for this. The exception is that the first dose of DMSA removes a significant amount of potassium (equivalent to that in a banana), and that is not included in mineral supplements, so one or two servings of fresh fruit or vegetables should be consumed to restore potassium levels. DMSA also significantly increases excretion of cysteine, so that should be supplemented before and/or during therapy.

DMSA has a small chance of increasing liver enzymes or decreasing blood cell count, so those should be monitored during treatment. A major research study published by our group found that DMSA was generally very safe, and was highly effective in removing toxic metals, improving glutathione, normalizing platelets (a marker of inflammation), and possibly beneficial in reducing the symptoms of autism.

DMPS (2,3-dimercapto-1-propane-sulfonic acid): DMPS is not approved by the FDA, but a physician may have it legally compounded for IV, oral, and rectal use, all of which increase excretion of toxic metals. The transdermal form does *not* appear to increase excretion of toxic metals.

Safety: DMPS slightly increases the excretion of some essential minerals, so a basic mineral supplement is recommended to compensate for this loss. It is unknown if it causes a loss of potassium. DMPS has a small chance of increasing liver enzymes or decreasing blood cell count, so those should be monitored during treatment.

TTFD (thiamine tetrahydrofurfuryl disulfide): A small pilot study of TTFD (used as a rectal suppository) resulted in some increase in excretion of arsenic and possibly other metals, and also significant reduction of autistic symptoms. The transdermal form may also work, although more study is needed.

Safety: TTFD appears to be very safe, with animal studies at high doses finding no evidence of toxicity.

More info: Anyone considering chelation therapy is urged to read the Defeat Autism Now! Consensus Report on Treating Mercury Toxicity in Children with Autism, available at www.autismresearchinstitute.com. This report provides more detailed advice on pretreatments, treatments, dosages, and safety.

ARI Survey of Parent Ratings of Treatment Efficacy:

	% Worse	% No Change	% Better	Number of Reports
Chelation	2%	22%	76%	324

Research:

There is substantial evidence to suggest that many children with autism suffer from exposure to mercury, and probably other toxic metals and toxic chemicals. The data includes:

1) A literature review by Bernard S et al. showing that the symptoms of autism were very similar to those of people suffering from infantile exposure to mercury poisoning.

2) A study by James et al. found that children with autism had low levels of glutathione, which is the body's primary defense against mercury.

3) A large study by Nataf et al. found that over half of children with autism had abnormal levels of a porphyrin in their urine that highly correlates with a high body burden of mercury.

4) A study by Bradstreet et al. found that children with autism excreted three to six times as much mercury as did typical children when both were given DMSA.

5) A baby hair study by Holmes et al. found that children with autism had unusually low levels of mercury in their baby hair ($\frac{1}{8}$ normal), suggesting a decreased ability to excrete mercury. A replication study by Adams et al. found similar, although less dramatic, differences. The Adams et al. study also found that children with autism had much higher usage of oral antibiotics than did typical children, which is important because usage of oral antibiotics almost completely stops the body's ability to excrete mercury.

6) A small pilot study by Adams et al. found that children with autism had twice as much mercury in their baby teeth than did typical children, suggesting that they had a higher body burden of mercury during their infancy, when the teeth formed. That study also found that children with autism had a much higher usage of oral antibiotics during their infancy, similar to their baby hair study.

7) Two studies of airborne mercury, in Texas and in the San Francisco Bay Area, found that the amount of mercury in the air correlated with the incidence of autism.

8) There have been nine epidemiological studies of the link between thimerosal in vaccines and autism. Four published studies by the Geiers have consistently found that children who received thimerosal in their vaccines had a two to six times higher chance of developing autism than those who received thimerosal-free vaccines. Four published studies by groups affiliated with vaccine manufacturers have failed to find a link, and one was inconclusive. Three of the studies were conducted in other countries where the usage of thimerosal is much less and the incidence of autism is much lower, so those results have limited relevance to the U.S.

CRANIOSACRAL AND CHIROPRACTIC THERAPY: A NEW BIOMEDICAL APPROACH TO ASD

BY DR. CHARLES CHAPPLE

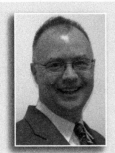

Charles W. Chapple, D.C., F.I.C.P.A.

Advanced Chiropractic Health Center
360 E Irving Park
Roselle, IL 60172
(630) 894-8778
www.drchapple.com

Dr. Charles W. Chapple completed his undergraduate studies at Nazareth College of Rochester, New York, receiving a bachelor's degree in biology before earning his doctorate degree in chiropractic from the National College of Chiropractic in 1991. Dr. Chapple holds many post-graduate certifications in areas such as chiropractic pediatrics (Fellowship in International Chiropractic Pediatric Association), acupuncture, applied kinesiology, and spinal rehabilitation. Dr. Chapple's studies have also encompassed treating neurological challenges involving children with developmental and learning delays, such as Sensory processing disorders: ADHD to Autism. A portion of his Roselle, Illinois practice focuses on the noninvasive benefits of chiropractic and craniosacral therapy to address retained primitive reflexes and sensory processing disorders. Dr. Chapple has a son on the spectrum, and thus finding solutions for individuals diagnosed with ASD is both a professional focus and a personal passion.

One has only to imagine themselves in the uncharted surroundings, where their frame of reference is skewed not only for all that they hear, see, touch, taste, and smell (the far senses) but also for their body awareness, movement, and balance (the near senses). These are challenges common to sensory processing disorders, which encompass a continuum of conditions ranging from attention deficit hyperactivity disorder (ADHD) to autism spectrum disorder (ASD) (See Figure 1).

Although the extent of these challenges can vary within the spectrum of disorders, their expressions can also provide many indicators for productive therapy, particularly

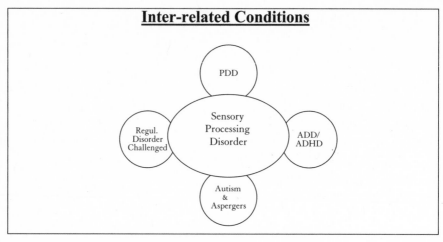

Figure 1.

when applied to the relationship between the nervous system and biomechanics. Individuals on the spectrum often give indications of areas within their nervous system in need of attention, through biomechanical manifestations (See Figure 2).

The central nervous system (CNS) and the facilitation of the biomechanics of its intimately related boney and membranous protective network (i.e. the cranium, the spine, and their attachments) through chiropractic, and craniosacral therapy (CST)

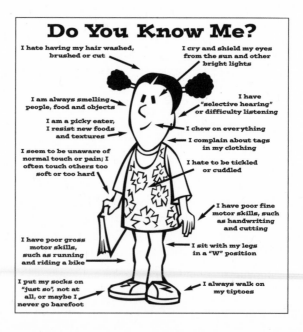

Figure 2.

Primitive-Postural Reflexes

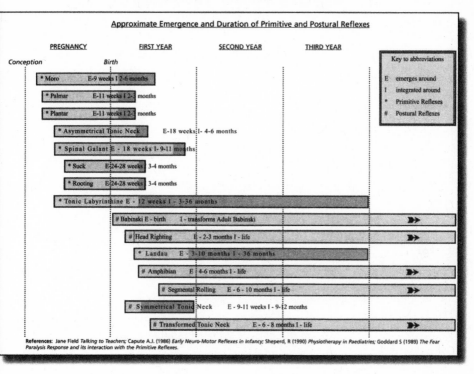

Figure 3.

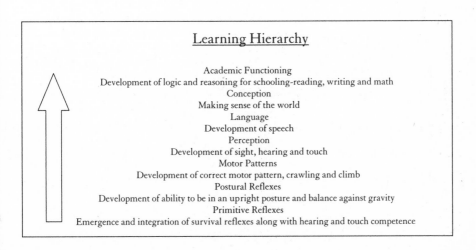

Figure 4.

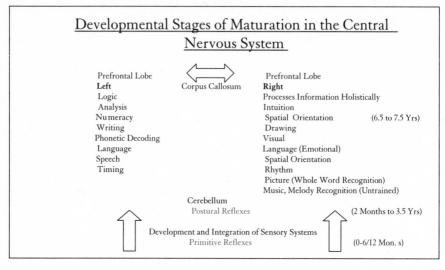

Figure 5.

enable a profound link through improved motor input to sensory system regulation necessary for brain communication and development. This motor to sensory to brain connection works towards benefiting the functional interaction between an individual's internal and external environments. More simply, movement grows the brain, and chiropractic and CST fine tune movement. The CNS is the circuitry that—along with many other amazing functions—connects an individual to their senses, and the senses to their reflexes.

The recognition that reflexes and sensory processing cannot be separated is significant in benefiting individuals with diagnoses on the spectrum, especially when considering the *primitive reflexes*. Often these individuals on the spectrum are caught in a "sensoreflexive no-man's-land", where they remain under the involuntary control of the *retained primitive reflexes* instead of the voluntary control of their *postural reflexes* (See figure 3). Further correlations have been drawn between motor development and academics (See Figure 4), as well as the necessity of first fostering the integration of primitive to postural reflexes in order for subsequent appropriate right- and left-brain communication and their relevant developmental stages (See Figure 5). Authorities in this field state that reflex profiles which are moderately to severely imbalanced would require specialized teaching and attention to motor imbalances, as well as a reflex stimulation/inhibition program in order to achieve sustained long-term improvements in development. Facilitating these functions of the CNS is critical to enabling *brain* to *body* interactions.

Brain Structures Involved in Autism and Anatomical Landmarks

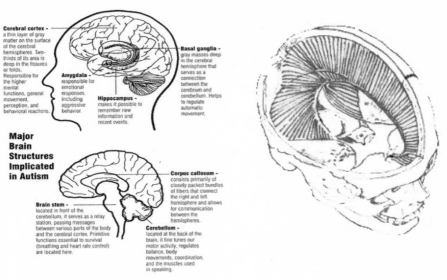

Cerebral cortex - a thin layer of gray matter on the surface of the cerebral hemispheres. Two-thirds of its area is deep in the fissures or folds. Responsible for the higher mental functions, general movement, perception, and behavioral reactions.

Amygdala - responsible for emotional responses, including aggressive behavior.

Hippocampus - makes it possible to remember new information and recent events.

Basal ganglia - gray masses deep in the cerebral hemisphere that serves as a connection between the cerebrum and cerebellum. Helps to regulate automatic movement.

Major Brain Structures Implicated in Autism

Brain stem - located in front of the cerebellum, it serves as a relay station, passing messages between various parts of the body and the cerebral cortex. Primitive functions essential to survival (breathing and heart rate control) are located here.

Corpus callosum - consists primarily of closely packed bundles of fibers that connect the right and left hemisphere and allows for communication between the hemispheres.

Cerebellum - located at the back of the brain, it fine tunes our motor activity, regulates balance, body movements, coordination, and the muscles used in speaking.

Figure 6.

Recognizing how our sensory system gathers information to regulate sensory input and knowing how an individual responds to particular sensory stimuli, can suggest a biomechanical approach to improve communication between the body's structure and function. For example, if an individual self-stimulates by rocking their head from side to side, particularly when stimulated by sound, this could indicate an improper regulation of the cranial nerve responsible in part for perception of sound and balance. So, this individual's rocking could be an attempt to self-regulate the sensory system as a result of difficulty with sound or balance, or both. Therefore, treatment would be intended to address the biomechanics in common to this cranial nerve and brain stem, such as the areas including but not limited to the temporal and adjacent cranial bones, cervical spine, and sacrum. Also the familiarization of the brain structures involved in ASD and their relation to the protective boney and membranous network which surrounds them is of great utility in treatment (See Figure 6).

Chiropractic and CST are gentle and noninvasive, hands-on approaches that assist the communication of the CNS, which is essential to both an individual's interaction with the surroundings and quite possibly to appropriate behavior. Benefits are intended through both these approaches' ability to access the body's circuitry in order to reduce or remove the interference upon it. The stimulation of motor input through chiro-

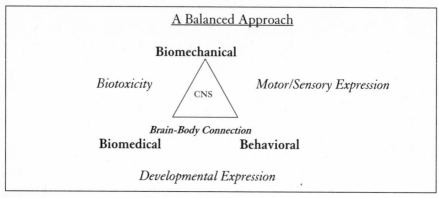

Figure 7.

practic and CST facilitates sensory input, which drives brain function and development. Therefore, both chiropractic and CST should be considered as an integral part of a balanced approach for treatment (See Figure 7).

Chiropractors identify a biomechanical complex of functional and/or structural and/or pathological articular changes that compromise neural integrity and may influ-

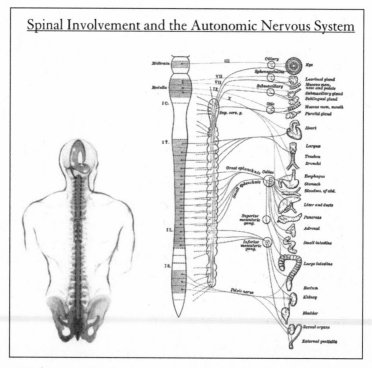

Figure 8.

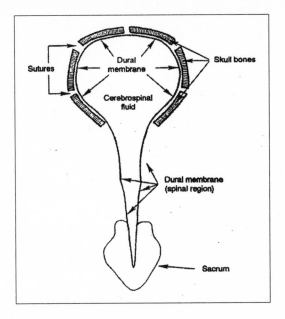

Figure 9.

ence organ system function and general health (See Figure 8) (called *subluxations* as an academic term), and utilize gentle spinal pressure techniques called *adjustments* to reduce or rid this complex. This biomechanical complex is characterized by:

- Irregular boney mechanics or spinal misalignment
- Nerves imbalances
- Muscle irritations
- Tissue inflammation
- Degenerative wear

CST focuses on relieving pressure on the brain and spinal cord through manual pressure techniques used at the cranium and sacrum. The CST system consists of membranes and cerebral spinal fluid, which protect the CNS (See Figure 9). Restrictions in this system are detected, and corrections are identified through manual monitoring of the craniosacral rhythm (CSR). Subluxations, as well as variations in the CSR (6–12 bpm), could indicate any number of motor, sensory, reflex, or neurological impairments, as well as causes of pain.

Healthcare practitioners are challenged to quantify variations of CNS communication within SPD conditions.

Frequently conventional tests appear unremarkable. Noninvasive tests such as infrared thermography (IF) and surface EMG (sEMG) can accompany a thorough history, exam, and other clinically relevant testing in order to illustrate altered CNS demands.

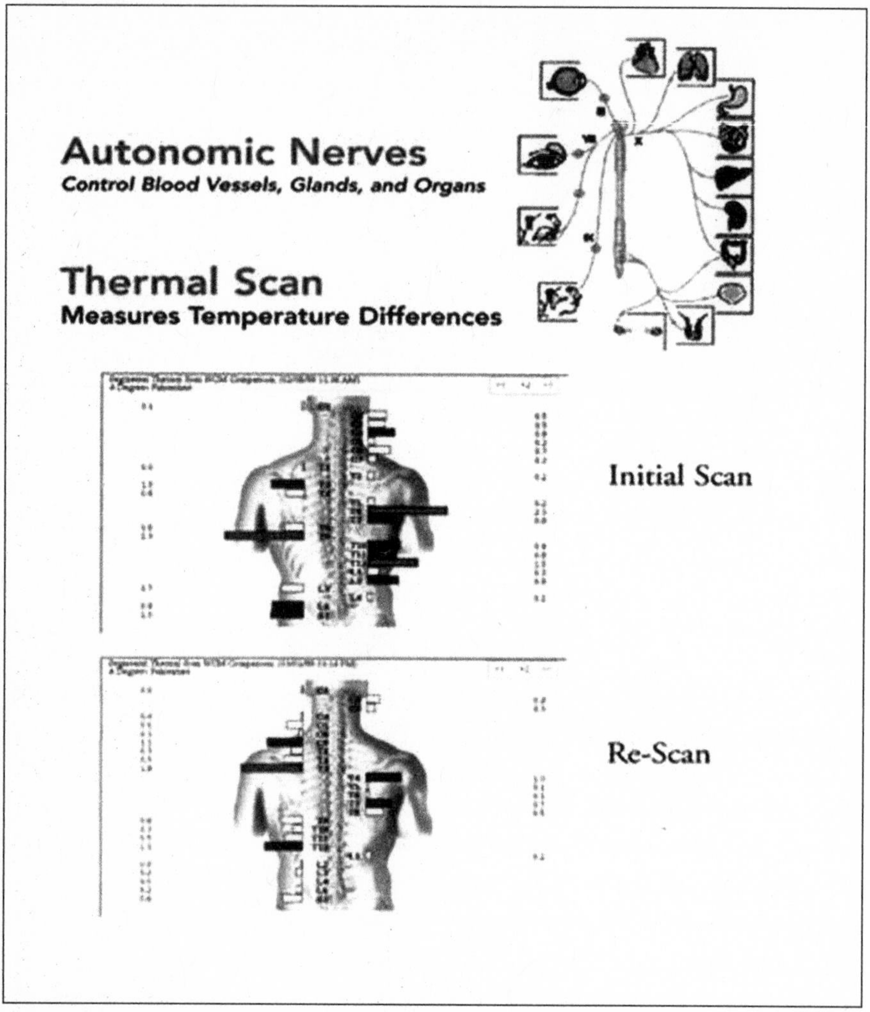

Figure 10.

Infrared thermography measures temperature variations along the spine as indications of imbalances in the autonomic nervous system, which can result from altered biomechanical complexes within the CNS (See Figure 10).

Chiropractic adjustments and CST work to restore more appropriate motor, sensory, reflex, and neurological input and improve motor to sensory to brain communication, therefore working within the body and not outside it.

Although there is no health care that is guaranteed or without risk, chiropractic and CST are among the safest and most effective approaches in benefiting the CNS, and therefore hold great potential as an integral part of a balanced approach in benefiting individuals challenged with SPD: ADHD to autism.

DANCE/MOVEMENT THERAPY

BY MARIAH MEYER LEFEBER

Mariah Meyer LeFeber, MA, LPC, R-DMT, DTRL

Hancock Center for Dance/Movement Therapy
16 N. Hancock St.
Madison, WI 53703
(608) 251-0908
www.hancockcenter.net
mariah@hancockcenter.net
info@hancockcenter.net

Mrs. LeFeber is a dance/movement therapist and licensed profes-sional counselor living in Madison, Wisconsin. She embodies her love of movement in both individual and group treatment for children affected by autism and mental illness. Beyond her passion for the healing power inherent in dance/movement therapy, Mrs. LeFeber further pursues her love of dance by teaching yoga for children and performing with a modern dance company.

Movement is a language. For children affected by autism, movement may be the only language they can rely on. Children with autism often have limited verbal abilities, making it extremely difficult for them to reach out to others (Hartshorn et al., 2001). When words fail, dance/movement therapy fosters a child's ability to relate, communicate, and connect on a nonverbal level.

Dance/movement therapy (DMT), which uses movement as a "universal means of communication," is a valuable form of communication for children with autism, especially those with underdeveloped speech skills (Erfer, 2005, p. 196). Dance/movement therapy provides the space for these children to explore and discover their bodies, while unlocking their potential for creativity. Children are encouraged to find themselves in a supportive environment where there is no "right" way to express or create (Canner, 1968).

As defined by the American Dance Therapy Association (ADTA), dance/move-ment therapy is "the psychotherapeutic use of movement as a process which furthers the emotional, social, cognitive, and physical integration of the individual" (American

Dance Therapy Association, 2008). Dance/movement therapy is an effective form of treatment for people with developmental, medical, social, physical, and psychological impairments (Levy, 2005). This expressive therapy is a bridge, linking creative expression through movement with psychological theory (Kestenberg et al., 1999).

Dance/movement therapy emerged in the 1940s in the United States. Marian Chace, also known as "The Grand Dame" of dance/movement therapy, led the emerging field. Through her work teaching dance to people with varied abilities, Chace recognized the profound impact of the movement on various facets of her student's lives, and began to bridge her work in dance to the world of Western medicine. In 1942, Chace was asked to bring this work to St. Elizabeth's Hospital in Washington, D.C. Here, psychiatrists also realized the benefits of this expressive and healing movement. In 1966, the American Dance Therapy Association formed, with Chace as the first president (Levy, 2005).

A second wave of dance/movement therapists emerged in the 1970s and 1980s. During this period, dance/movement therapy sparked the interest of many professionals, and therapists began experimenting with the use of the form with a variety of populations—including autism. In the midst of this, dance/movement therapy was also officially categorized as a form of psychotherapy.

In application, dance/movement therapy fosters socialization and communication in clients who otherwise might find it difficult to relate. The ability to engage fully through nonverbal activity sets dance/movement therapy apart from other forms of therapy. It creates an affirming environment for clients, where they are able to experience the value of belonging. Ultimately, dance/movement therapy provides both a bridge for contact and a medium for reciprocal communication for children with autism (ADTA, 2008).

A few basic principles form the guiding theory of dance/movement therapy. These overarching tenets of the field include the belief that: behavior is communicative, personality is reflected through movement, changes in movement will eventually lead to changes in personality, and the larger an individual's movement repertoire, the more options individuals have when it comes time for them to cope with the environment (Kestenberg et al., 1999; Meekums, 2002). The actual practice of dance/movement therapy relies on the observation of movement behavior as it emerges in relationship, more specifically the therapeutic relationship between client and therapist. Dance/movement therapists are trained to understand, reflect, and eventually expand on the nonverbal expression of their clients (Adler, 2003). A consistent, supportive and accepting atmosphere is used to begin the process of relationship formation, along with the following: mirroring (reflecting rhythms, patterns, and vocalizations expressed by the client), eye contact, touch, vocalizations, props, and rhythmic body action (ADTA,

2008; Erfer, 1995). In particular, props can be helpful with this population because they are very concrete and tangible, thus serving as a connecting medium between client and therapist.

In addition to the mirroring technique mentioned above, the approaches of both attunement and shape-flow adjustment (from the Kestenberg Movement Profile, one of many movement-analysis systems utilized by dance/movement therapists) help build the therapeutic relationship and augment the therapist's ability to make clinical choices. As described by Loman (1995), "attunement is based on sharing qualities of muscle tension, and Shape-Flow Adjustment is based on a similarity of breathing patterns and shape of the body between individuals" (p. 222). Within the therapeutic relationship, attunement builds a sense of empathy between therapist and client, while shape-flow adjustment builds trust in the relationship (Loman, 1995).

A constant priority, the initial and overarching goal for dance/movement therapists working with autism (or with any population) is to reach out and meet a client at his or her functioning level. Once this relationship has been established, it serves as a consistent guiding principle behind the work and emerges in the balance between the physical and relational. In the dance/movement therapy setting, relationships occur as a byproduct of the body in action and physical movement flourishes because of the trust built within the therapeutic relationship. When the physical and relational aspects of the work are in balance, movement truly can serve as a language for universal communication.

When building treatment goals, each child with autism presents with specific needs and challenges, yet a handful of goals are generally applicable. The first of these goals is increasing sensory motor and perceptual motor development, directly targeting the motor deficits often faced by children with autism spectrum disorder (ADTA, 2008; Erfer, 1995). By working from both a functional and expressive standpoint, dance/movement therapists can use simple vocabulary and movement to stimulate perceptual, gross, and fine motor skills. An example of this is teaching children the perceptual concept of "in and out" by having them physically step inside of a space (i.e., a hula hoop) and then outside of that same space. Through the gross motor movement, the children experientially learn the concept, which can then be generalized to other areas.

The second goal for dance/movement therapists is to help clients improve their socialization and communication skills. As the therapeutic relationship builds, clients increase their ability to interact as part of a group and communicate (verbally or nonverbally) within that group. Steps toward these goals include: increasing eye contact, participating in shared rhythmic activities with engagement (and independently whenever possible), recognizing and responding to group members, increasing proximity to the group, decreasing a need for interpersonal distance, developing trust, and forming an understanding of "self" as opposed to the "others" outside of the self (ADTA, 2008).

Although these social and communication goals can be met through several modalities, dance/movement therapy is unique because the steps towards these goals can all be experienced on a kinesthetic level. For example, in group rhythmic activity, group members move together with similar rhythms, intensities, and physical tensions. This extension of movement throughout the body helps a client to integrate what may be a fragmented sense of self (Levy, 2005). Moving small movements into total body activity helps build cohesiveness and a sense of grounding, not only for the person as an individual, but also for their identity as a group member. The similar rhythmic and movement patterns allow each client to feel that they belong on a nonverbal level.

Thirdly, building off of the growing understanding of self vs. others, dance/movement therapy works to foster body awareness and nurture a client's personal self-concept. By reflecting a child's movement nonverbally and then translating what is seen into simple language (i.e., mirroring the child in moving their head side to side, while verbalizing "I see you moving your head"), the dance/movement therapist positively verbalizes how the child appears, inherently improving his/her body awareness or body image. The simple verbalizations, or the "noticing" of what is going on, also help to structure the experience for the participant (Loman, 1995). As an added benefit, this verbalization of action naturally increases the movement repertoire of the client (applicable to goal one), as he/she is exposed to not only the conscious experience of his/her own movement but also that of the others in the room.

"Body image is one of the most fundamental concepts in human growth and development and one that appears to be lacking in children who are autistic" (Erfer, 1995, p. 197). Standing behind this concept, body awareness and a positive body image are imperative as the two combined form a foundation for a basic understanding of the self. Not only does the development of body awareness parallel sensorimotor development, the movement experience also helps children to orient to their space, their own bodies, and the others in the room. This orientation occurs on both an internal (self to self) and external (self and others) level. Because body image is formed from input from the vestibular, kinesthetic, proprioceptive, visual, and tactile systems, movement is an all-encompassing medium for the development of an individual's self-concept (Erfer, 1995).

A 1985 research study conducted by Enid Wolf-Schein, Gene Fisch, and Ira Cohen studied the use of nonverbal systems in children with autism and mental retardation. The study came to the conclusion that "dance/movement therapy should be considered an intervention for persons with both autism and mental retardation since there are indications that deviations in nonverbal behaviors do contribute to the overall pathology of the individuals" (Wolf-Schein, Fisch & Cohen, 1985, p. 78). This serves as an example of one of many studies indicating the potential for healing when combining dance/movement therapy and autism.

In more recent years, neuroscientists have been increasingly interested in the presence and impact of mirror neurons on mental health and relationships. Regarding this research, Cynthia Berrol notes, "a keystone of the therapeutic process of dance/movement therapy, the concept of mirroring is now the subject of neuroscience. The domains of mirror neurons currently under investigation span motoric, psychosocial and cognitive functions, including specific psychological issues . . . " (Berrol, 2006, p. 303). Dance/movement therapy inherently engages this mirror neuron system in the brain, for both those moving and those witnessing the movement of others. Since autism possibly relates to deficiencies in the mirror neuron system of the brain, dance/movement therapy has the potential to unlock and develop some of these deficient areas through the process of movement.

Risks and side effects related to dance/movement therapy are minimal. Movement may not be the preferred modality for expressing or relating for all individuals, although many who are open to trying the format find that it is a truly accessible approach to therapy. Like with any kind of movement, a person must be cautious and only do what is safely within their physical means in order to avoid any physical harm to self or others, within the process.

The American Dance Therapy Association (ADTA) is the professional organization for dance/movement therapists in the U.S. and beyond. To learn more about the field or find a dance/movement therapist in your area, visit the website at www.adta.org or contact the national office by phone at (410) 997-4040.

DIETARY INTERVENTIONS FOR AUTISM: DIFFERENT APPROACHES

BY KARYN SEROUSSI AND LISA LEWIS, PH.D.

Adapted from the book, *The Encyclopedia of Dietary Interventions for the Treatment of Autism and Related Disorders* (2008) by Karyn Seroussi & Lisa S. Lewis, Ph.D. (available at www.dietaryinterventions.com)

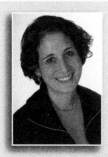 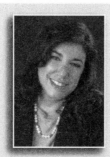

Karyn Seroussi and Lisa S. Lewis, Ph.D.

The Autism Network for Dietary Interventions: www.autismndi.com *The Encyclopedia of Dietary Interventions for the Treatment of Autism and Related Disorders*: www.dietaryinterventions.com

Karyn Seroussi is the author of *Unraveling the Mystery of Autism and Pervasive Developmental Disorder*, the story of her son's autism recovery through dietary and other biomedical interventions. Lisa S. Lewis, Ph.D. is the author of *Special Diets For Special Kids, I & II*, the foremost books on gluten- and casein-free diets for children with disabilities. In 1995, Karyn Seroussi and Lisa Lewis created an international parent network that has educated thousands about dietary and biomedical interventions for autism spectrum disorders. Thirteen years, three books, countless conferences, and over fifty thousand emails later, they decided to put it all together. In 2008, they gathered the sum of that knowledge and co-authored *The Encyclopedia of Dietary Interventions for the Treatment of Autism and Related Disorders* (www.dietaryinterventions.com).

The Two-Tack Rule:

If you are sitting on a tack, it will take a lot of aspirin to make you feel better. If you are sitting on two tacks, removal of one tack will not result in a 50% improvement.

—Dr. Sidney M. Baker, Defeat Autism Now! Co-founder; Author, Detoxification & Healing

Different Approaches: "The Diets"

The underlying problems in autism spectrum disorders usually have many layers. Opioid peptides from dairy and gluten may be just part of what is affecting your child. You may not see much improvement until all of the offenders have been addressed.

What to Remove?

Dietary intervention in autism is usually referred to as "the GF/CF diet," but most children seem to need modifications that go well beyond gluten and casein free regimens. It is not unusual to hear a parent in the online support groups say that their child is on a "GF/CF/soy-free/corn-free/egg-free low-oxalate diet, with probiotic foods and limited sugars."

Therefore, it's no wonder that people have begun to refer to most of these dietary interventions simply as "GF/CF diets" or "gluten-free and restricted diets." As public awareness of celiac disease and gluten intolerance increases, this is probably the easiest explanation one can give.

There is much conflicting information on the Internet and on various support lists about which diets are "best." When one child does extremely well on a specific regimen, caregivers may become convinced that his diet will work just as well for other children, sometimes to the point of fanaticism. This can serve to inspire others, but it can also result in pressing for inappropriate adherence to one regimen when another might actually be more suitable.

Experience has shown that most people on the autism spectrum will benefit from a diet that is strictly free of gluten and dairy; therefore, the removal of these should be considered the foundation for dietary interventions. Additional changes are almost always needed for optimum improvement, but one size does not fit all. Every parent's goal is to find the ideal removal or rotation of foods for their child that will provide maximum benefit without being unnecessarily restrictive.

The most commonly restricted foods include gluten, dairy, corn, soy, yeast, oxalates, sugars, and starches. Other principles may apply, such as the use of probiotic foods, healthy fats, organic foods, and the restriction of food additives and artificial colors.

The most common dietary principles currently in use come from the Specific Carbohydrate Diet, developed by Elaine Gottschall, the low-oxalate diet introduced to the autism community by Susan Owens, and the Body Ecology Diet, developed by Donna Gates. None of these diets were originally developed to address autism spectrum disorders, so they usually must be modified to suit a child's individual needs. Detailed descriptions can be found in the *Encyclopedia of Dietary Interventions* by Karyn Seroussi and Lisa S. Lewis, Ph.D.

Gluten

Gluten is a protein found in members of the grass family including wheat, spelt, barley, rye and triticale. Gluten can also be found in products derived from these grains, such as malt, grain starches, hydrolyzed vegetable/plant proteins, textured vegetable proteins, soy sauce, grain alcohol, some natural flavorings, and some of the binders and fillers commonly found in vitamins and medications (see below). In their pure form oats do not contain gluten, but commercial oats are almost always contaminated with wheat.

Avoiding Gluten: This can be a challenge for two reasons. One is that it takes some time to become familiar with the rules of the diet and the lifestyle changes that are involved. The other problem has to do with getting your child on board; many children with autism will eat only wheat-based foods, such as bread, muffins, pretzels, crackers, noodles, and breaded chicken or fish (nuggets and fish sticks). At first, it may be hard to persuade a child to try anything new.

However, most people get the hang of the diet in a week or two, and many good substitutes are now available for traditional wheat products. There are commercially available gluten-free breads at many supermarkets and at all health food stores. Crackers without wheat or gluten are also widely available, made from grains, rice, and even nuts. If your child likes pasta, there are many excellent gluten-free alternatives; they come in different shapes and sizes and can be used in any recipe. Gluten-free baking, once you get the hang of it, is an economical way to prepare your family's favorite baked goods at home.

It is a good idea to accustom your child to meat, fish, and chicken prepared simply, either baked, broiled, or grilled. However, many children start the diet eating only breaded, fried "nuggets." You can prepare these by making your own breading out of acceptable cereals, flours, or ground nuts. Most commercially prepared and fast-food versions are unacceptable.

Be aware that ingredients change in prepared foods, and that what was acceptable six months ago may not be so anymore. It is a good idea to learn to read labels, and to call companies for information whenever you are unsure about an ingredient or food.

When you are avoiding gluten, it is important to know about "hidden" sources. For example, most of these diets allow coconut and dried fruits, but some brands contain traces of gluten. Look for fruits that have no sulfites (added to preserve color and retard spoilage), especially if phenols are a problem. Be aware that raisins sold in canisters may have traveled down a conveyor belt that was dusted with flour to prevent the fruit from sticking together. Because the flour is not an "ingredient" it does not have to be listed on the package.

Many foods are labeled "wheat free," but that does not mean they are gluten free. When in doubt, call the manufacturer. Almost all packaged foods have a toll-free number or website on the label. Find out whether they can guarantee that the product is free from gluten. If it's not, make sure to let them know that this will affect your decision to use the product.

"Hidden" gluten can also be found in some unexpected places, such as the glue on envelopes, Dixie cups, ground spices (some use flour to prevent clumping), appliances, fast-food fryers, and tropical fish food.

Foods and Ingredients That Always Contain Gluten:

Barley

Barley Grass
(can contain seeds)

Barley Malt

Beer

Bleached Flour

Bran

Bran Extract

Bread Flour

Brewers Yeast

Brown Flour

Bulgur (Bulgar
Wheat/Nuts)

Bulgur Wheat

Cereal Binding

Chilton

Club Wheat

Common Wheat

Couscous

Dextrimaltose

Durum wheat

Edible Starch

Tabbouleh

Teriyaki Sauce

Textured Vegetable
Protein - TVP

Triticale

Einkorn

Emmer

Farina

Farina Graham

Filler

Flour

Fu

Germ

Graham Flour

Granary Flour

Groats

Hydrolyzed Wheat
Gluten

Hydrolyzed Wheat
Protein

Hydrolyzed Wheat
Starch

Kamut

Malt

Malt Extract

Malt Flavoring

Malt Syrup

Udon

Unbleached Flour

Vegetable Starch

Wheat Flour Lipids

Wheat Germ

Malt Vinegar

Matzo Semolina

Mir

Pasta

Pearl Barley

Rice Malt (if barley or
Koji are used)

Rye

Seitan

Semolina

Semolina Triticum

Shot Wheat (*Triticum
aestivum*)

Small Spelt

Spelt (*Triticum spelta*)

Spirits (Specific Types)

Sprouted Wheat or
Barley

Hydrolyzed Wheat
Protein

Strong Flour

Suet in Packets

Wheat Grass (can
contain seeds)

Wheat Nuts

Wheat Protein

Whole-Meal Flour

Milk and Dairy

Milk consists of 87.4 percent water, 3.5 percent protein, and between zero and 3.7 percent fat. We all grew up with the idea that milk is a healthy food, and are naturally reluctant to take it out of our children's diets. But is it really good for everybody?

All mammal mothers feed their infants milk, but humans are the only mammal that ingests the milk of an unrelated species, and continues to do so long after weaning. This may be why dairy is one of the eight foods to which those with food allergies most frequently react.[1]

Although most American children get their required calcium and vitamin D from milk, there are many other sources for these vital nutrients. Therefore, pediatricians who insist that milk is necessary for good health are misinformed. Many perfectly healthy children do very well without it. In fact, many cultures consider cow's milk unfit for human consumption. Cows have evolved to produce milk that is most beneficial to its intended recipients: calves. The milk of every type of mammal has striking differences in composition, with variation in the contents of fats, protein, sugar, and minerals. Each evolves to provide optimum nutrition to the young of its own species.

Although milk is rich in calcium, it may not be the best way to obtain this mineral. Cow's milk contains 1200 mg of calcium per quart, compared to 300 mg per quart of human milk. Despite this difference, studies have shown that nursing infants absorb more calcium than those fed cow's milk-based formulas.[2] This seems to be due to the fact that cow's milk is much richer in phosphorus, a mineral that can combine with calcium in the intestines and prevent its absorption. (This is another reason to avoid drinking soda pop, which is extremely high in phosphorus.) Finally, research has shown that cow's milk protein intolerance (CMPI) is associated with a very high frequency of multiple food intolerance and allergic diseases.[3]

We all know that growing bones and teeth need calcium, but most of us have no idea where else to get these important minerals. Green vegetables such as kale, collards, and bok choy are excellent sources of calcium, with the added benefit of being low in oxalates (spinach, though high in calcium, should be avoided if oxalates are a problem). Certain fish, like salmon and perch, are also good sources of calcium, but take care to buy fish that is not high in mercury or other environmental toxins. A mere tablespoon of molasses contains 172 mg of calcium (as well as iron), so if yeast is not a big problem it is a good choice for sweetening baked goods. Some nuts, beans, and seeds (like sesame seeds) are rich in calcium, but they should be ground for best absorption. Calcium-fortified orange juice is equivalent to a glass of milk, although it is very high in fructose (fruit sugar). Finally, if a child will not eat enough nondairy sources of calcium, there are many good supplements available. Because vitamin D is required to properly absorb calcium, a good supplement will contain both.

With all these problems, why would anyone want to feed their children dairy products? First, it is hard to fight back years of thinking that milk is "the perfect food." The necessity of milk is perpetuated by every advertising medium currently in use, so it is certainly understandable that most parents believe that it is their duty to feed their children as much cow's milk as possible. Despite all the celebrities who sport "milk mustaches," dairy is not necessary for good nutrition, and can actually be harmful for some children.

How to Avoid Dairy: Removing dairy from the diet is not as difficult as it sounds, but you need to understand a few basic principles. First of all, you must remove *all* sources of dairy. This includes obvious sources such as butter, cheese, cream cheese, and sour cream, but it also includes some "hidden" sources. There are several packaged foods that surprisingly contain some form of milk protein, such as canned fish and bread. Even soy and rice cheeses generally contain some form of casein or sodium caseinate. It is imperative that you learn to read and understand labels, and that you continue to check them each time you buy a food. Food manufacturers often switch out ingredients due to price or availability, so a once-trusted item must be considered suspect until you have double-checked the ingredients. In many cases, food manufacturers are allowed to use up old food labels even if minor changes have been made in the ingredients. If you think you see a reaction to a food that formerly produced no problem, call the company to verify that the ingredients listed are indeed correct. If not, you can inform them that you will no longer be able to use the product, and that you will be sharing this information with others who have the same dietary requirements. Customer feedback will sometimes persuade them to revert to an older recipe.

Foods to Avoid (always contain dairy):

Butter	Casein/caseinates
Cheese (all types)	Lactose
Skim milk	Milk chocolate
Whole milk	Yogurt
Buttermilk	Kefin
Powered milk	Ice cream/ice milk
Evaporated milk	Cream
Condensed milk	Sour cream
Goat's milk	Cottage cheese
Sheep's milk	Whey

Foods to Be Wary Of (often contain dairy):

Baked goods (even if GF)	Chicken broth
Bologna	Creamed vegetables
Broth (canned)	Margarine/buttery spreads
Candy	Mashed potatoes
Canned foods	Nougat/caramel/toffee
Salad dressings	Pudding/custard mixes
Candies	Scrambled eggs
Cakes/cake mix	Soy cheese
Chewing gum	Tuna fish (canned)

Keep in mind that "non-dairy" does not mean milk-free. It is a term the dairy industry invented to indicate less than 0.5 percent milk by weight, which could mean fully as much casein as whole milk.

Support Groups

If you are new to dietary interventions, you will find it to be a valuable use of your time to join a support group. There may be one in your area, but if not, there are some wonderful groups online. Those who have never been on an online support group will be amazed at how quickly their questions can be answered, and at the quality of support they can get from others who are more experienced. Just remember, every child is different, and what worked for your child may not work for all.

Some of the most popular autism-diet groups include:

Gluten-Free/Casein-Free Diet (GF/CF):
www.yahoogroups.com/group/gfcfkids

The Specific Carbohydrate Diet (SCD):
www.yahoogroups.com/group/pecanbread

The Low Oxalate Diet (LOD):
www.yahoogroups.com/group/Trying_Low_Oxalates

The Feingold Diet: www.yahoogroups.com/group/Feingold-Program4us

The Body Ecology Diet: www.bedrokcommunity.org

DIETARY INTERVENTIONS FOR AUTISM: SPECIFIC CARBOHYDRATE DIET

BY JUDITH CHINITZ

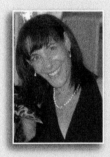

Judith Hope Chinitz, MS, MS, CNC
New Star Nutritional Consulting
(914) 244-3646
www.newstarnutrition.com
judy@newstarnutrition.com

After her son's diagnosis with autism in 1996, Judith Chinitz has spent the last fifeen years searching for answers. After saving her son's life through diet, and seeing firsthand the healing power of food, Judy earned a second master's degree in nutrition after having previously worked as a special education teacher. Currently she is continuing her studies at Columbia University's Institute for Human Nutrition. Judy is the author of We Band of Mothers: Autism, My Son, and the Specific Carbohydrate Diet, which also contains commentary by Dr. Sidney Baker. She also assisted Dr. Baker in founding Medigenesis, an Internet-based, interactive medical database.

I n the original Hippocratic Oath, treatment of the sick is not mentioned until the first sentence of the third paragraph: "I will apply dietetic measures for the benefit of the sick according to my ability and judgment; I will keep them from harm and injustice." Yet while even thousands of years ago there was recognition of the fact that food is the fundamental basis for health, providing the very building blocks of our bodies and the fuel to keep us alive, there is no mention of diet in the oath that our modern doctors take upon graduation.

In the world of autism, however, progressive thinkers like Dr. Bernard Rimland (the founder of the Autism Society of America and the Autism Research Institute) many years ago recognized that children with developmental issues were physically sick and that nutrition could play a role in healing them. The right diet, in fact, often ends up being the foundation stone that all other biomedical and educational treatments rest upon.

At the time of writing this chapter, the Autism Research Institute's data of parent reports on treatment has 71% of children showing improvement from what I have found to be—in my 15 years as the parent of a son with autism and as a nutritionist - the single best treatment for autism spectrum disorders. That is, the Specific Carbohydrate Diet. In fact, SCD now ranks as the number one dietary treatment. In my personal experience, the success rate of bringing about major global improvements via SCD is probably closer to 90%. And science is now providing more and more answers as to why this is the case.

At the Defeat Autism Now! Conference in April, 2010, Dr. Jeremy Nicholson, an eminent researcher at Imperial College in London, presented a paper he had just published in the *Journal of Proteome Research*[1]. He and his colleagues examined the organic acids in the urine of 39 children with autism and compared the results with those from controls, and found multiple abnormal metabolites that could only be produced by abnormal gut bacteria. The concluding words of his talk were something along the lines of, "Almost every abnormality we find in children with autism—the digestive issues, the immune system irregularities—can be explained by damage to the developing gut flora."

The human body contains approximately 10 trillion cells—and 100 trillion microbes. Our microscopic flora outnumber us 10 to 1. We are more other than we are ourselves. Our intestines contain billions and billions of bacteria that are absolutely crucial to health—and to life itself. At birth, we are meant to begin to acquire our "old friends" (as those in the field now refer to our synergistic microscopic residents) who will help us digest our food, make vitamins for us, keep pathogens from populating our digestive systems, develop our immune systems by regulating the process whereby we learn to differentiate good from bad, and self from non-self. 70% or so of our immune system is our digestive systems. Most germs enter through the nose and mouth and our first line of defense, therefore, are the immune defenses centered there. Developing a healthy population of old friends means developing a healthy body.

There is copious research supporting the fact that our good flora is responsible for the normal development of our immune systems, which happens mainly in the first 2 years of life. For example, a recent paper published in the Proceedings of the Nutrition Society[2] states, "Commensal bacteria are important in intestinal homeostasis and appear to play a role in early tolerance to foreign antigens….Dysregulation of this balance can contribute to the pathogenesis of numerous inflammatory conditions such as inflammatory bowel diseases." That is, a disruption of the development of the gut flora leads to a dysregulated immune system and potentially to gut inflammation.

And now, research is also beginning to provide proof that these same intestinal microbes are responsible for normal development as well.

On January 31, 2011, just a week before the writing of this chapter, a paper was published in the Proceedings of the National Academy of Science[3]. Researchers compared the development of control mice, which were exposed to typical microbes from birth, to a group of mice who were raised in a germ free environment. The latter group showed clear developmental abnormalities as adults. Interestingly, if the germ-free mice were exposed to normal microbes early enough in development, they too developed into normal adults. However, if the microbes were introduced when the mice were already grown, no improvement was noted. The study rightly concludes that this is an animal experiment and may not apply to human beings…But it's certainly safe to say the data are incredibly compelling.

Just a few years ago, another paper was also published in the Proceedings of the National Academy of Science[4] in which inflammation was induced in rats via injection of lipopolysaccharides, which are the toxins from pathogenic bacteria. The researchers write, "We hypothesized that peripheral inflammation leads to increased neuronal excitability arising from a CNS immune response." As predicted, the rats developed, "…a marked, reversible inflammatory response within the hippocampus, characterized by microglial activation and increases in TNF-alpha levels." Inducing inflammation via exposure to toxins from bacteria causes inflammation in the brain…at least in rats. Coincidently—or perhaps not so coincidently—such microglial activation has also been found in those with autism. "We demonstrate an active neuroinflammatory process in the cerebral cortex, white matter and notably in the cerebellum of autistic patients," writes Drs. Vargas and colleagues[5] as just one example of research in this area.

We know then that the brains of those with autism appear to have abnormal activation of the microglia (the immune system of the brain) and for years we've also known that individuals with autism appear to have abnormal gut flora. For example, in 2005 research was published in the *Journal of Medical Microbiology*[6] which showed high levels of clostrial species in the guts of people with ASD: "The faecal flora of ASD patients contained a higher incidence of the Clostridum histolyticum group…." The paper goes on to say, "Clostridia are recognized toxin-producers, including neurotoxins. Theoretically, toxic products may be over-expressed in the autistic gut, which may lead to increased levels in the bloodstream and thus exert systemic effects."

To repeat then what we know: we know that individuals in this current epidemic appear to have abnormal gut flora. We know that it is possible that toxins from these bacteria are causing systemic effects. We know that toxins from bad bacteria can certainly cause inflammation in the gut, and even inflammatory bowel diseases. We know that in rats, toxins from bacteria cause activation of the microglia, and thus inflammation in the brain. And finally, we know that in mice at least, early disturbances of normal gut flora can cause developmental abnormalities. So, while we cannot draw any definitive conclusions at this point, the evidence is mounting almost daily that bacterial dysbiosis plays an enormous part in this current autism epidemic.

So, what can we do to improve the gut flora of our children?

Refer back to the article in the *Journal of Medical Microbiology*: "Strategies to reduce clostridial population levels harboured by ASD patients or to **improve their gut microflora profile through dietary modulation** may help alleviate gut disorders common to such patients."

There is both considerable evidence that inflammatory bowel disease is associated with abnormal gut flora and also a large body of research published on the benefits of a diet low in complex carbohydrates/sugars when treating inflammatory bowel disease. One example: in 2000, a paper appeared in the *Israeli Medical Association Journal*[7] which concludes, "Combined sugar malabsorption patterns are common in functional bowel disorders and may contribute to symptomatology in most patients. Dietary restriction of the offending sugar(s) should be implemented before the institution of drug therapy." Back even in the 1990s, researchers found a positive association between high sucrose (white sugar) consumption and inflammatory bowel disease—and a negative correlation between fructose (the monosaccharide simple sugar found in fruit) and IBD.[8]

A recent article in the journal *Nutrition*[9] lays out the best treatments we have to date for curing a small intestine bacterial overgrowth. Therapies involve, among other things, probiotics and a diet low in foods that ferment (i.e. feed bacteria). "Therapy is usually directed toward reducing the bacterial load with antibiotics, but altering the functional properties of the microbiota by reducing or **changing the supply of fermentative substrate** or by the use of probiotics are promising alternatives."

This is the definition of the Specific Carbohydrate Diet.

Decades of scientific research is presented in the book which lays out the fundamentals of the Specific Carbohydrate Diet, *Breaking the Vicious Cycle*[10], by Elaine Gottschall. In the five plus years since Elaine passed away, more and more evidence has piled up providing substantiation for her premise that the removal of complex carbohydrates from the diet can markedly help diseased intestines, and in many cases bring about complete remission of inflammatory bowel diseases.

Before proceeding to explain how to implement SCD, it is vitally important to make clear that even individuals with no overt bowel symptoms can benefit from the diet. If your child is on the autism spectrum, the likelihood is that he or she has abnormal gut flora. Often parents—and we nutritionists—are stunned by the improvements made by even high functioning children who seem absolutely healthy. The only way to know if SCD is going to help is to do it.

How does SCD work? The prevailing belief is that bad bacterial microbes produce toxins irritating to the lining of the digestive system, which cause the tissue to try to protect itself by secreting mucus. (All gut bacteria, good and bad, produce acids in the process of fermentation.) A lot of bacteria mean a lot of acid. Now think about your runny nose when you have a cold. Once covered by a thick layer of mucus, the intestines are unable to break down complex carbohydrates. The necessary enzymes (secreted by the enterocytes of the intestines) cannot reach the food, leaving the undigested carbohydrates (sugars which cannot be broken down into digestible form) to fester and feed the bad bacteria. 50% of carbohydrate digestion occurs on the brush border of the small intestine. Our intestines can only absorb single molecule sugars, like glucose and fructose, which supply energy to every cell in our bodies. All that undigested sugar (from the incompletely digested di-saccharides (2 sugar molecules attached together) and poly-saccharides (long strings of sugar molecules such as found in starches) feeds the bacteria, leading to an increase in the overgrowth….which in turn produce more toxins…which leads to more mucus…which leads to worse digestion…. which leads to more food for more bacteria….

Elaine's Vicious Cycle.

To quote directly from *Breaking the Vicious Cycle*:

"In various conditions, a poorly-functioning intestine can be easily overwhelmed by the ingestion of carbohydrates which require numerous digestive processes. The result is an environment that supports overgrowth of intestinal yeast and bacteria…. The purpose of the Specific Carbohydrate Diet is to deprive the microbial world of the intestine of the food it needs to overpopulate. By using a diet which contains predominantly 'predigested' carbohydrates, the individual with an intestinal problem can be maximally nourished without over-stimulation of the intestinal microbial population."

By keeping nearly all complex carbohydrates out of the digestive system, the aberrant bacteria are starved to death. Of course, at the same time you're replenishing the gut with good flora in the form of probiotics: SCD legal homemade yogurt and/or store-bought probiotics (which are available from a host of retailers).

SCD stops the vicious cycle of malabsorption and microbial overgrowth by removing the microbes' food: sugars, specifically di- and poly- saccharides. Single molecule sugars, like those found in fruit, vegetables and honey do not require digestive processes, but are immediately absorbed by the intestine. Therefore, even diseased intestines can absorb them so that they are not available to feed the bad flora. Inflammation decreases as the bad microbial population dies out, toxin levels go down and digestion improves.

SCD absolutely does work and often it works miracles. Someday, in the not too distant future it will hopefully be accepted as what it is: **a fundamental treatment for bowel disease.**

The Specific Carbohydrate Diet involves the removal of any food that contains di- and poly- saccharides (that is, double and multiple chains of sugars). "Illegals" (as they're called by SCDers) include white and brown sugars, lactose (the sugar found in milk), maple syrup, all grain and all starch Permitted are proteins (eggs, meats, poultry, fish, certain dairy products (which have been fermented long enough that no sugars are left)), fruit, most vegetables (except the starches, like potatoes) and honey. Cookies, bread, cakes can be made with a variety of other flours rather than wheat: nuts, coconut, and fruit flours. There are legal substitutes for most well-loved foods, but parents must understand that the French fries and Skittles are out. Instead, you will be feeding your child only foods that are nutrient rich, wholesome and actually good for them. (There is a fairly comprehensive list of legal/illegal foods on Elaine's website: www.breakingtheviciouscycle.info .)

If your child is already a good eater—a rare thing in the ASD population—then switching to SCD won't be a problem. The foods are delicious. If, however, your child is a chicken- nuggets-and-French-fries-only kid, it may be a better idea to begin the diet slowly to avoid negative situations for both of you. As the parent of a child on the autism spectrum, your life is stressful enough. Fighting over every single bite of food at every meal for what could be weeks is not a good idea. I work with my clients to come up with individual plans based upon tolerance levels, parental choice, what the child is currently eating, and so forth.

For difficult children, we will often start by substituting one food at a time. For example, if your child loves cookies, make some SCD legal ones and replace the old favorites. Three or four days later, make your next substitution. Continue this pattern for the next month or two and before you know it, your child will not only be entirely SCD legal, but you will have gotten rid of all the junk food in your house.

If you live close to a good health food store, you will be able to buy nuts free of additives and can grind them into nut flours if you want to start SCD right away. To make things easier though, many high quality nut flours are available via the Internet. www.digestivewellness.com and www.lucyskitchenshop.com both are great resources for SCD flours and other products.

Don't start SCD until you are comfortable with the foods you have in the house or you'll just end up frustrated. Good preparation will make the transition much easier. The first step: It is absolutely crucial to read Elaine Gottschall's book if you're considering SCD. She provides an eloquent and easy-to- understand explanation of the history of the diet and the decades of science that support its efficacy, as well as providing some of the best SCD legal recipes. *Breaking the Vicious Cycle* is available via Amazon. com and BarnesandNoble.com, as well as through some of the SCD websites. It is THE formative work on the diet and I for one consider it nothing less than monumental in its importance.

Elaine and I planned to write a book together about SCD, autism and her journey with the diet. Tragically, she died just as we got started with her project. I carried on alone and in 2007 published, *We Band of Mothers: Autism, My Son and The Specific Carbohydrate Diet.*[11] (available via Amazon.com) The book is both a guide for managing SCD with children on the spectrum, but also a tribute to Elaine who was truly a towering human being. (In her crusade to help people suffering with bowel disease, she touched millions of lives. *Breaking the Vicious Cycle* is translated into 7 languages, and has sold well over a million copies.)

There are many wonderful cookbooks available and multiple websites devoted to SCD legal products, yogurt machines, yogurt starter, and so forth.

www.lucyskitchenshop.com (which sells superior quality almond flour, cookbooks, a yogurt machine and starter and other great products).

www.digestivewellness.com (which sells kosher SCD products, nut flours, apple chips, etc.).

www.scdrecipe.com—This website is owned by Raman Prasad, who is also the author of two wonderful SCD cookbooks. Raman, a former colitis sufferer, was cured via SCD and, being a fabulous cook, has collected many great recipes. His site also provides news updates, links, and other great resources.

www.scdiet.org/ - A library of SCD information, including news, links, recipes, and so forth.

One very important thing to know before you start SCD is that there are a series of regular regressions that may occur. No one knows why and not every child undergoes these regressions - but most do. Please remember: **the regressions are temporary. Do NOT stop the diet. You are doing nothing wrong!** The children tend to come out of the regressions better than ever. (For more information on the regressions, please refer to *We Band of Mothers*.)

One crucially important note: SCD is NOT a low carbohydrate diet. Unlike the Atkins diet, which limits the amount of carbohydrates consumed each day, SCD limits only the TYPE of carbohydrates eaten. Be sure to give you child plenty of fruit and vegetables every day, legal fruit juices and honey (assuming there is no significant yeast issue). I make it a rule that a carbohydrate must be given with every meal, even if it's just a snack. So if you are giving your child chicken nuggets for dinner, you must also have her eat some steamed carrots and an apple. (Someone reading this undoubtedly just had the thought, "My child eat an apple and carrots! That will happen when hell freezes over!" I have worked with hundreds of children and every last one of them learns to eat fruit and vegetables. It is not only possible: it is guaranteed, as long as you decide they will.)

When the body is deprived of carbohydrates (which provide glucose, the body's energy source), it will begin to break down protein, and eventually fat, to get the required energy to operate. During this process, ketones are released which are highly acidic. For multiple reasons this is extremely unhealthy in the long term. It is absolutely vital that you find ways of getting fruit and vegetables into your child several times per day to avoid ketosis.

Even if your child has food allergies—even to nuts—SCD is still a possibility. Granted, it's not easy. But it is most certainly do-able. Instead of using nut flours we use pumpkin seed, coconut, mango or bean flours all of which work well. Again, no matter what the dietary restriction, SCD is manageable.

The beauty of the SCD is that it is not only incredibly nourishing (there is no junk food allowed) but more, it is truly a healing diet. After a few years, many individuals can successfully go back to eating a completely unrestricted diet. Elaine Gottschall recommended staying on SCD for a year after the last symptom had vanished. The time required for healing varies radically from person to person, and diet is a slow heal. It takes several years even in the best cases. However, it is also entirely safe, healthy, and works almost all the time. SCD has the weight of what science we currently have supporting it. While the task may seem daunting, hundreds and hundreds of parents have succeeded in making radical improvements in their children's health and autistic symptoms through improving their gut microbes. You can too.

Most of all, you don't ever want to look back with regret and think, "If only…"

DRAMA THERAPY

BY SALLY BAILEY

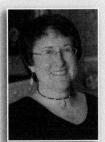

Sally Bailey, MFA, MSW, RDT/BCT

129 Nichols—CSTD Department
Kansas State University
Manhattan, KS 66506-2301
(785) 532-6780
sdbailey@ksu.edu
www.dramatherapycentral.com

Sally Bailey is an associate professor in the Theatre Department at Kansas State University where she directs the drama therapy program. She is the author of three books: *Wings to Fly: Bringing Theatre Arts to Students with Special Needs, Dreams to Sign: Bringing Together Deaf and Hearing Audiences and Actors,* and *Barrier-Free Theatre.* She has worked with clients on the autism spectrum using drama therapy for the past twenty-five years. Her chapter on "Theoretical Reasons and Practical Applications of Drama Therapy with Clients of the Autism Spectrum" was recently published in *The Use of the Creative Therapies with Autism Spectrum Disorders.* She is a past president of the National Association for Drama Therapy and recipient of NADT's Gertrud Schattner Award for distinguished contributions in the field of drama therapy.

Drama therapy applies techniques from theatre to the process of psychotherapy. The focus is on helping individuals grow and heal by taking on and practicing new roles, creating new stories through action, and rehearsing new behaviors which can later be implemented in real life. Drama therapy involves participants in informal drama processes (games, improvisation, storytelling, role play) and/or formal products (puppets, masks, plays/performances) to help clients understand their thoughts and emotions better, improve behavior, and learn social interaction skills.

Drama therapy is effective because it involves action methods which can be rehearsed or repeated until a skill is learned. An embodied, concrete experience makes skills easier for clients on the autism spectrum to grasp, remember, and implement (Bailey, 2007, 2009b). While literature on autism suggests that people with ASD are not creative and have little interest in connecting with others, drama therapists find that the ASD clients they work with are imaginative, highly motivated to participate in dramatic activities, and crave social connection, but are not sure how to make those connections. Drama therapy helps in this connection process as drama is all about human relating and relationships.

Neuroscientists looking at the arts, learning, and the brain have discovered that the arts are motivating for children because they create conditions in which attention can be sustained over longer periods of time (Posner, Rothbart, Sheese, & Kieras in Ashbury & Rich, 2008). An additional benefit of the arts, particularly drama, is that participants receive feedback in the process of enacting a scene from the other actors, and from the audience, as well as afterwards when the group discusses the scene and/ or when they replay the scene with corrections (Bailey, 2009a; Jensen & Dabney, 2000; Posner et al., 2008).

Temple Grandin (2002), a professor of animal science who has autism, says when she was growing up, she viewed many cultural customs and behaviors of neurotypical people as ISPs—Interesting Sociological Phenomenons. Role play can be the perfect way for people with ASD to come to a better understanding of the neurotypical world's ISPs. Practicing putting themselves in another person's or character's shoes can become the first steps toward understanding how the rest of the world feels, thinks, and relates; a way to begin developing and testing out a theory of mind.

Drama strongly engages the mirror neuron system in actors and audiences alike (Blair, 2008; McConachie, 2008). There are neuroscientists who suspect that autism may relate to deficiencies in the mirror neuron system (Ramachandran & Oberman, 2006) and others who believe that our empathic abilities and our abilities to learn cognitively and emotionally through observation relate directly to our mirror neurons (Iacoboni & Daprette, 2006; Iacoboni, et al., 2005; Oberman & Ramachandran, 2007). If this is true, then drama therapy could be extremely effective in promoting repair of weaknesses and disconnections in the mirror neuron system.

Drama therapy has been developed by a wide variety of practitioners. Most trained originally in theatre, then after recognizing the healing powers of drama, trained in psychology and psychotherapy. Early 20th century: Jacob L. Moreno in Austria and the U.S.; Peter Slade in the U.K.; Vladimir Iljine and Nikolai Evreinov in Russia. Late 20th century: Gertrud Schattner, Eleanor Irwin, David Read Johnson, Renee Emunah, and Robert Landy in the U.S.; Sue Jennings and Marian Lindkvist in the U.K. (Bailey, 2006).

Beginning in the early 20th century, drama was used by occupational therapists in hospitals and by social workers in community programs to teach clients social and emotional skills through performing in plays. The field began to integrate improvisation and process drama methods, emerging as a separate profession in the 1970s. In relation to treatment of clients on the autism spectrum, drama was one of the very first techniques used. Hans Asperger, the German doctor who first described Asperger's syndrome in 1944, created an educational program for the boys he was treating which involved speech therapy, drama, and physical education (Attwood, 1998). Sister Viktorine, director of the program, was killed when the ward on which she was working was destroyed in an allied bombing attack in World War II, so no record of exactly how she used drama survives (Attwood, 1998). At the very least, this early use of drama indicates an appreciation for the strengths it offers as an intervention. Currently, many drama therapists across the U.S. and internationally are involved in the use of drama therapy with children, teens, and adults on the autism spectrum.

Success rate

Grady Bolding (2007), a drama major at Kansas State University who is on the autism spectrum, says about his experience in theatre, "The world of theater helped bring me out of my shell, since I got free crash courses in interpersonal communications with every script. Today, I speak like anybody else" (Bolding, 2007, p. 3). He reports that his theater training has helped him learn how to make eye contact, show emotional expression during conversations, and read the emotional messages in others' voices and body language. He credits the characters that he has played on stage and the script analysis work he has done in classes with teaching him how to carry on a conversation off-stage. He has been able to take that understanding and apply it to the real people he encounters in everyday life. He says, "I can interpret the way someone else is feeling somewhat—just a little bit now. Back then [before drama training], people were just objects" (Personal communication, 2009).

A participant in The Spotlight Program, one of many dramatic arts programs springing up around the country for students with ASD, attests to this when he says, "I've gained friendships and learned new games, how to be more mature and how to interact with others" (North Shore ARC, 2008, p. 1). Another says, "I've learned to recognize myself in others" (North Shore ARC, 2008, p. 2).

When the drama activities are led by a trained drama therapist who knows how to target specific therapeutic goals, even more success can be achieved. The mother of an adolescent with ASD who I worked with told me:

I have seen the child we knew was inside, but which we rarely saw at home, come out on stage. . . . On stage she is at her most confident, most assertive, her most centered self. Being in the plays gives her something *entirely* her own. She decides for herself—she chose to participate, she helps write the play, she decides what role she's going to play. . . . In class you model appropriate and respectful behavior for the children and they pick it up and model your behavior back. You treat the children as young adults and you listen to their ideas. They learn by your actions how to treat others with respect. . . . Most adults tell our children to be quiet—they don't want to hear what they have to say. But [in drama therapy] what they have to say matters. . . . It's very hard for kids with special needs to have a large group of friends. They tend to be very isolated. I see her involvement [in drama therapy] as a great social experience. . . . At the end of the year she has created and maintained many social relationships and she has a sweet taste in her mouth, looking forward to *next* year (Personal communication, 1993).

Depending on the age, functioning level, and abilities of the client, drama therapists also use puppets, sandtrays, role play, masks, and many other dramatic activities to help clients safely and meaningfully practice new communication, social, and expressive skills.

Risk and/or side-effects

Drama is not for everyone, just as basketball is not for everyone. Not every person who is on the autism spectrum will want to participate in drama, but more may want to than might at first be suspected. See the documentary *Autism: The Musical* if you have doubts. If a client is open and willing to participating in drama therapy, there are no risks or negative side effects.

The National Association for Drama Therapy (NADT) is the professional organization for drama therapists in the U.S. and Canada. To find a drama therapist in your area, you can contact the NADT office at nadt.office@nadt.org or 571-333-2991 or you can send out a request on the Dramatherapy Listserve by e-mailing dramatherapylst@listserv.ksu.edu.

EARLY START DENVER MODEL

BY DR. SALLY ROGERS, DR. LAURIE VISMARA,
AND DR. GERALDINE DAWSON

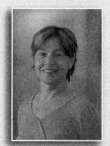

Sally J. Rogers, PH.D.

The M.I.N.D. Institute
2825 50th Street
Sacramento CA 95817
(916) 703-0264
sally.rogers@ucdmc.ucdavis.edu

Dr. Sally Rogers is a developmental psychologist and a professor of psychiatry at the M.I.N.D. Institute, University of California Davis. She has spent her career studying cognitive and social development in young children with disabilities. She has published over 150 papers, chapters, and books. Her current research focuses in three areas: developing effective interventions for infants and toddlers with autism that families and professionals can deliver, earliest identification of autism in infancy, and imitation abilities in ASD. The intervention model that she developed with Geri Dawson, the Early Start Denver Model, is internationally known, and the book, *Early Start Denver Model For Young Children With Autism: Promoting Language, Learning, And Engagement* (The Guilford Press, 2009) and accompanying instrumentation for this approach have been recently published.

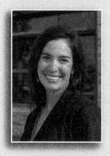

Laurie A. Vismara, PH.D., BCBA-D,
Assistant Professional Researcher, Department of Psychiatry
and Behavioral Sciences, School of Medicine

Dr. Laurie Vismara is an assistant research scientist with UC Davis Department of Psychiatry and Behavioral sciences and is a board certified behavior analyst. She specializes in conducting treatment research with young children with autism and their families. Her work examines treatment efficacy and effectiveness in autism using the Early Start Denver Model (ESDM), as well as developing a coaching curriculum and parent education model for immediate provision of intervention to at-risk infants and toddlers. More recently, she has examined the use of telemedicine for servicing families and training community-based professionals to implement the ESDM. Her work in implementation research related to professional and parent training has been published in numerous articles, including the *Journal of Autism, Journal of Positive Behavior Intervention, and Journal of Autism and Developmental Disabilities*. She also reviews for periodicals such as the *Journal of Early Intervention, Journal of Child Psychology and Child Psychiatry, Journal of Positive Behavior Support, Journal of Speech and Language Hearing Research*, and *Topics in Early Childhood Special Education*.

The ESDM[1] is based on a fusion of two well known approaches. First is the Denver Model, a comprehensive affective and developmentally based early intervention approach for preschool age children with autism originally developed by Rogers and colleagues.[2-3] The nature of the teaching interactions and the curricular priorities are heavily influenced by Stern's[4] model of infant interpersonal development and its successive developmental phases of the emerging social relationship between the infant and the caregiver.

The second is Pivotal Response Training (PRT). It involves a naturalistic application of applied behavior analysis to develop language and social skills, and has extensive empirical support developed by Laura Schreibman and Robert Koegel in the 1970s and '80s. [5-6]

An emphasis on eliciting strong positive emotion throughout interactions reflects Dawson and colleagues'[7] hypothesis that autism involves a fundamental deficiency in social motivation related to a lack of sensitivity to social reward. The resulting lack of social engagement, if not changed, can not only alter the course of behavioral development in autism, but also affect the way neural systems underlying the perception and representation of social and linguistic information are developed and organized.

History of development

The Denver Model began with a grant from the U.S. Department of Education to Dr. Rogers in 1981, and its effects as a group preschool intervention were first examined in a series of papers examining pre-post test data.[8, 3, 2] Significant accelerations in developmental rates of young children with ASD were found in several developmental areas, including cognition, language, reduction in autism symptoms, symbolic play, and social engagement. As a group, the children with autism doubled their developmental rates while in active treatment. Four independent replications of the model carried out in rural Colorado school districts[9] demonstrated significant accelerations of developmental rates within six months of implementation of the Denver Model. These studies suggested that the Denver Model has the capacity to affect development in many areas.

The first study of the Denver Model as an individually delivered intervention used a single subject design and randomized minimally verbal children to either the Denver Model or the PROMPT treatment.[10] The delivery involved one hour of individual treatment and parent training weekly, and daily one-hour home parent practice sessions for twelve weeks. Eighty percent of children acquired functional speech at a frequency of from ten to two hundred words per hour demonstrated in generalized probe sessions involving only natural communication interactions. A recent study of parent-delivered ESDM has also documented the efficacy of parent delivery in rapid acquisition of words, imitation, and social engagement. [11]

Success rate

The most recent study[12] involved 48 toddlers with ASD between eighteen and twenty-four months of age, randomly assigned to one of two groups: (1) The intervention group received, on average, twenty-five hours of the Early Start Denver model weekly, for two years; and (2) a community group who received community-based treatments. Groups did not differ at baseline in severity of autism symptoms based on ADOS scores, gender, IQ, or SES. Analyses documented that the intervention is effective for increasing children's IQ and receptive and expressive language ability, with results evident after only one year in intervention. After two years, children in ESDM showed a statistically significant average increase in overall learning composite scores (similar to IQ) of 17.6 points, whereas the control group showed an average increase of 7.0 points. Similar outcomes were also evident on receptive and expressive language, and on parent reports of communication, daily living skills, and motor skills. Longer-term follow-up studies are ongoing. In the last three published studies, acquisition of useful, communicative multiword speech has occurred with 80–90 percent of children enrolled in ESDM, in both parent-delivered intervention and twenty-five-hour per week home visitor intervention.

Content of intervention: developmental objectives

Each child's plan is defined by (1) **a set of short-term objectives** that represent what is to be taught over a twelve-week period and (2) **a set of activities** carried out daily to teach the objectives. The objectives are derived from a curriculum assessment carried out each twelve weeks using The Early Start Denver Model Curriculum Checklist.[1] The Curriculum Checklist covers the following ten domains: receptive communication, expressive communication, social interaction, imitation skills, cognitive skills, play skills, fine motor skills, gross motor skill, independence/behavior, and joint attention.

Process of intervention: teaching procedures

There are both general and specific aspects to the teaching process. General aspects of the teaching process, quantified in the ESDM Fidelity Tool, 1 involve the use of varied, naturalistic, child-initiated activities in which to embed instruction because of the empirically demonstrated gains in spontaneity, motivation, maintenance, and generalization that this kind of teaching supports for skills in which there are intrinsic reinforcers.[13-14] These are specified in the fifteen teaching behaviors assessed on the fidelity tool. Adults freely choose materials and activities in which to teach the targeted objectives to maximize attention and motivation, while considering the child's preferences and learning style.

Joint activity routines[15] are the vehicle for teaching. A joint activity routine involves a series of interactions between child and adult that allows for a shared activity to be begun, developed, elaborated, and completed. Inside a joint activity, objectives from at least two different developmental domains are taught. A joint activity routine typically lasts from two to five minutes, and involves multiple acts by both therapist and child. The materials and activities are generally chosen by the child, though the adult may offer choices and suggestions. Learning opportunities occur approximately every ten to fifteen seconds during treatment interactions. Transitions between activities are responsive to children's needs for a change and are carried out in a fashion that fosters child independence, motivation, and choice.

Tailoring the treatment: Response to Intervention (RTI)

A systematic decision process is used to "tailor the treatment," by systematically altering teaching procedures to improve progress if children are not progressing rapidly. This decision tree allows for the entire "toolbox" of teaching practices demonstrated to be effective for children with autism to be used if needed, but it prescribes **how** and **when** to alter teaching processes. While the teaching process favors naturalistic teaching, varied activities, intrinsic reinforcers, and shared control, no empirically supported teaching approach is "off limits."

Role of the family

Parents are an integral part of the intervention, influencing objectives, curriculum, and teaching practices. Parents are coached to fidelity in the ESDM intervention teaching approach to build their skills in incorporating the Early Start Denver Model approach in their natural caretaking and family routines as well as play activities throughout the day with their child. The goal of parent coaching is to empower parents via skill acquisition to promote a satisfying parent-child relationship and sense of parent competency and to generalize the skills across all daily family activities.

Risks or side-effects

The use of child choice, curriculum assessment, and decision tree minimize risks or side effects involving poor progress, child stress, and unwanted behavior because the approach can be tailored to each individual child's preferences, needs, and learning styles. The flexible delivery style (group education, parent delivery, 1:1 intensive, and 1:1 weekly therapy models) allows for the approach to fit into many different delivery systems. One risk involves cultural specificity. ESDM has not been tested outside of the U.S. and outside of highly skilled directed settings.

Innovative New Studies

A current randomized controlled trial study of web-based intervention is being carried out by Laurie Vismara, PhD, at the UC Davis MIND Institute. In this study, parents of young children with ASD will access a secure, multimodal interactive website about the ESDM Parent Curriculum,[16] a set of practices intended to be adopted and implemented by parents in their homes and throughout their daily play and caretaking activities. The website will feature real-time video sharing, live conferencing, and multimedia instructional documentation including videotaped learning modules, audio-annotated video reviews, and traditional text-based documentation. The goal of this application of telemedicine within a comprehensive multimedia approach is to provide parents with evidence-based intervening practices for addressing the developmental needs of their 18–48-month-aged child with ASD while tracking and organizing information specific to parents' mastery and child developmental changes. If such an approach is helpful to parents, it would demonstrate the promise and utility of innovative technologies for enhancing and accelerating the pace of autism research and treatment.

The need for intervention options that go beyond 1:1 live interaction with a therapist is becoming more and more obvious. Despite the increased awareness that early intervention significantly improves developmental outcomes,[17-20] there are numerous challenges to delivering high quality, empirically supported interventions to children with ASD and their families.[21-23] Barriers may include costly and time-intensive programs, long waiting lists, and few providers with specialized knowledge about ASD interventions limiting families' access to preventative mental health services in general and parenting services in particular.[21-22, 24-25] Two variables—an increase in the number of people seeking services due to increased diagnosis of ASD and increased public understanding of the importance of early intervention—coupled with the barriers to access cited above challenge researchers, policy makers, and service providers to find ways to disseminate systematic and effective strategies directly to families.[26-27]

Telemedicine (also called "telehealth" and "telepractice") involves the application of communication technologies to enable specialists to consult and deliver professional services in real time over a geographical distance.[28] These may be one solution for helping bridge the gap between families in need of ASD intervention and service delivery. For example, parents would be able to access remote technology (e.g., computer-based video conferencing software and the internet) from their home to receive live coaching from a specialized treatment provider while interacting with their child. Such an approach would allow information to be integrated in the child's most natural environment and among the people most familiar to the child. Further, remote access to intervention has the ability to provide families up to 24-hour support from any location and may save money and time to both parents and professionals.[29] This is the need that led to the current study.

A second current study involves a multi-site replication of the Dawson et al. 2010 examination of the Early Start Denver Model. The current study involves approximately 100 children between the ages of 12 and 24 months, in three very different geographic sites in the US. This study uses and the design and measurement strategies described in the Dawson et al 2010 paper, and asks the critical replicability question: Can an independent group replicate the original study and its positive findings? This large, methodologically rigorous, randomized controlled study will end in 2012.

ELEVATED MALE HORMONES: THEIR ROLE AND TREATMENT IN AUTISM SPECTRUM DISORDERS

BY DAVID A. GEIER, LISA SYKES, AND DR. MARK R. GEIER

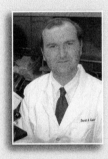

David A. Geier

Mr. Geier is vice-president of the non-profit 501(c)(3) Institute of Chronic Illnesses, Inc., vice-president of the non-profit 501(c)(3) CoMeD, Inc., and president of MedCon, Inc. He has been a research scientist at the National Institutes of Health in the Laboratory of Biochemical Genetics. David has co-authored more than 60 peer-reviewed medical studies, with more than 20 peer-reviewed studies on the relationship of genetic, biochemical and hormonal changes in autism. As a result of Mr. Geier's extensive research, he has been invited to present to the Institute of Medicine of the U.S. National Academy of Sciences on two occasions, and he has been invited to present to professional medical and scientific societies worldwide. David has patents pending for the treatment of patients diagnosed with autism. David was selected by Maryland Governor O'Malley in October 2009 to serve a 3-year term as a member of the Maryland Commission on Autism.

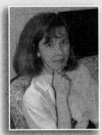

Rev. Lisa K. Sykes

Rev. Lisa Sykes serves as the associate pastor of Welborne United Methodist Church, Richmond, Virginia. She graduated from the University of Virginia, where she was an Echols Scholar, and from Princeton Theological Seminary. She has served the Virginia Annual Conference of the United Methodist Church for almost 20 years. Lisa's son Wesley was diagnosed with autism in 1998 and with mercury poisoning in 2000. Lisa is president of CoMeD, Inc., a 501(c)(3) nonprofit dedicated to the elimination of mercury from medicine. She is also the author of Sacred Spark, the compelling true story of her quest to restore the light in her son's eyes while igniting a global debate about autism and childhood vaccines.

Mark R. Geier, MD, PhD, FACMG, FACE, ABMG
ASD Centers, LLC
14 Redgate Ct
Silver Spring, MD 20905
Phone: (301) 989-0548
Fax: (301) 989-1543
mgeier@comcast.net
www.autismtreatmentclinics.com

Dr. Geier received his MD and PhD in genetics from George Washington University. He is a Fellow of the American College of Medical Genetics and is a Fellow of the American College of Epidemiology. Dr. Geier is board certified as a genetic counselor by the American Board of Medical Genetics and is a Founding Associate Member of the American College of Medical Genetics. He has been in clinical practice for over 30 years. He was a researcher in the Laboratory of General and Comparative Biochemistry at the National Institute of Mental Health, National Institutes of Health for 10 years. Dr. Geier has published more than 100 peer-reviewed academic articles, including more than 20 on the cause and treatment of ASD. His extensive research has resulted in him being invited to address the Institute of Medicine of the U.S. National Academy of Sciences on six occasions. In addition, he was invited to provide expert testimony to the Government Reform Committee of the U.S. House of Representatives. Dr. Geier has also presented to the Vaccine Advisory Committee of the FDA. Dr. Geier has patents pending for the treatment of patients diagnosed with autism.

Many clinical conditions occur in males more often than females, including autism spectrum disorders (ASDs), dyslexia, specific language impairment, attention-deficit hyperactivity disorder (ADHD), and early onset persistent antisocial behavior (Auyeung et al., 2009). The fact that these conditions occur more often in males than females suggests an obvious but only recently recognized association between these conditions and the "male" hormones (i.e., the androgens). In fact, ASDs have even been described as the result of an "extreme male brain" by psychologist, Dr. Simon Baron-Cohen (Baron-Cohen, 2002). While Dr. Baron-Cohen made this observation based on social deficits and attributes of individuals diagnosed with an ASD, the accuracy of his description may be more than skin deep. From behaviors to biomedical markers, elevated androgens correlate with many aspects of ASDs.

The higher occurrence of ASDs among males is well established. Children diagnosed with an ASD have a ratio of 4:1 (male:female), and the ratio is as high as 9:1 for those with a diagnosis of Asperger's syndrome. Recent evidence supports the suggestion that elevated androgen levels are related to the development of autistic traits. For example, scientific studies have found that elevated levels of androgens are correlated with problems in the following areas: poor eye contact, obsessive-compulsive behaviors, deficits in social interaction, delayed language development, and problem behaviors such as hyperactivity, poor attention, impulsivity, aggression, self-injury, and tantrums. In addition, elevated androgens were shown to be associated with reduced empathy and increased systemizing (Auyeung et al., 2009).

Examination of individuals diagnosed with conditions associated with high androgen levels revealed that these individuals present with an increased frequency of autistic traits in comparison to controls. For example, examination of individuals diagnosed with congenital adrenal hyperplasia, which is a genetic disorder that causes excessive adrenal androgen production beginning prenatally in both males and females, revealed that these individuals show masculinization (i.e., biological development of sex differences and changes that make a male body different from a female body, with most of the changes being produced by androgens) of performance in activities such as spatial orientation, visualization, targeting, personality, cognitive abilities, and sexuality, as well as exhibit significantly more autistic traits than unaffected controls (Knickmeyer et al., 2006). In addition, children diagnosed with premature adrenarche (i.e., a significant surge in androgen levels associated with puberty, occurring too early for the chronological age of the child) in comparison to children with on-time adrenarche revealed a significant increase in autistic traits, including social withdrawal and other social problems, problem behaviors, reduced language development, and information processing deficits (Dorn et al., 1999). In some cases of boys with undescended testicles, the administration of testosterone treatments resulted in the development of autistic traits and, in a few instances, clearly contributed to the individual being diagnosed with an ASD; this dramatically demonstrates the association between androgens and ASDs.

Further, a study of androgen levels in the families of individuals diagnosed with an ASD revealed an increased frequency of conditions associated with elevated androgens among family members in comparison to families without individuals diagnosed with an ASD. One study revealed that families with an individual diagnosed with an ASD had an increased medical history of reproductive cancers, tumors, or growths in the ovary, uterus, breast, or prostate relative to the families of the controls. In addition, the females in those families with a relative diagnosed with an ASD were also shown to have increased problems with their menstrual cycle (Ingudomnukul et al., 2007).

Consistent with the observed correlation between the clinical symptoms of ASD and elevated androgens, a series of studies have substantiated elevated levels of androgens in individuals diagnosed with an ASD. One method of study has focused on the use of finger length ratio between the 2nd and 4th digits (index and ring fingers) as an accurate measure for fetal testosterone. Studies researching fetal hand development have observed the sex difference in the ratio of the lengths of the 2nd and 4th digits in fetuses between 9 and 40 weeks of gestation. This 2nd-to-4th-digit ratio was observed to correlate with fetal testosterone levels measured in amniotic fluid samples. Similar digit-length ratios associated with elevated fetal testosterone levels were also found in children with autism compared to typically developing children. This pattern extended even to the siblings and parents of children with autism (Manning et al., 2001). In other words, a family containing at least one child diagnosed with an ASD is likely to have elevated testosterone levels in most if not all its members, including the females.

Further, a series of clinical studies examined symptoms and blood levels of male hormones in individuals diagnosed with an ASD relative to neurotypical individuals and found elevated androgens accelerated sexual development in a significant percentage of children with an ASD. In one study, 1-in-3 prepubertal-age children diagnosed with an ASD had symptoms of abnormally early male puberty (i.e., precocious puberty/premature puberty) and elevated blood testosterone levels (Tordjman et al., 1997).

Premature puberty is characterized by sexual development before the age of 8 in girls, and age 10 in boys. In girls, premature puberty is characterized by the development of breasts and by hair growth under the arms and in the genital region. The onset of ovulation and menstruation also may occur. In boys, the condition triggers the development of a large penis and testicles, with spontaneous erections and the production of sperm. Hair grows on the face, underarms, and the pubic area, and acne may become a problem (Geier et al., 2010).

While the early onset of puberty may seem fairly benign, in fact, it can cause problems when hormones trigger changes in the growth pattern, essentially halting growth before the child has reached normal adult height. Furthermore, children with this condition look noticeably older than their peers and may feel rejected by their friends and socially isolated. Adults may expect these children to act more maturely simply because they look so much older. Many of these children, especially boys, are much more aggressive than others their own age, leading to behavior problems (Geier et al., 2010).

Offering additional confirmation of the association between androgens and the diagnosis of an ASD, another study observed that more than 80% of individuals diagnosed with an ASD have elevated levels of androgens. Surprisingly, the girls diagnosed with an ASD had even higher androgen levels relative to age- and sex-matched controls than the boys diagnosed with an ASD (Geier & Geier, 2007; Schwarz et al., 2010). Females have testosterone as do males, but usually the levels of androgens in girls are lower than in boys. In further studies of girls diagnosed with an ASD, their significantly elevated androgen levels were associated with abnormally increased hair growth, sexual dysfunction, irregular and painful menstrual cycles (in some cases with significant bleeding), delayed onset of menstrual cycles, severe acne, epilepsy, and tomboy behaviors (Knickmeyer et al., 2006; Ingudomnukul et al., 2007). Moreover, other investigators concluded that children diagnosed with an ASD, both male and female, had profoundly increased androgens, and that these levels were associated with a significant increase in abnormally early puberty characterized by unusually high androgen levels (Majewska et al., 2010).

The importance of identifying elevated androgens among individuals diagnosed with an ASD is that it may offer important insights into the treatment of these patients. Since elevated androgens correlate with the development of many autistic traits, and individuals diagnosed with an ASD have increased clinical symptoms and increased blood levels of androgens, some clinicians reasoned that treatment therapies designed to significantly lower male hormones in individuals diagnosed with an ASD may result in significant clinical improvements in autistic traits (Geier & Geier, 2005). In practice, therapies purposed and utilized to accomplish this in the treatment of individuals diagnosed with an ASD have helped to significantly lower the overall production and/or block the function of androgens.

Some research studies have used animal model systems. For example, investigators used an anti-androgen medication called cyproterone acetate, which reduces the function and production of androgens, in the treatment of self-injurious behaviors and aggression in lab monkeys. These investigators observed that, as blood levels of androgens decreased in lab monkeys, there was a corresponding decrease in self-injurious behaviors and aggression (Eaton et al., 1999). Similarly, other investigators have used an anti-androgen medication called leuprolide acetate, which reduces the production of male hormones, in the treatment of anxiety, hyperexcitability, depression, impaired social interaction, and obsessive-compulsive behaviors in several lab animal species (Uday et al., 2007; Umathe et al., 2008a-d; Umathe et al., 2009; Gaikwad et al., 2010). Also, some investigators have found that leuprolide acetate administration resulted in improvements in cognition (Bryan et al., 2010).

Other studies have pursued human clinical trials of anti-androgen medications to positively impact such things as aggression and obsessive-complusive disorder. One study revealed that anti-androgen medication administration significantly lowered the blood levels of the androgens and was accompanied by significant reductions in outward-directed aggression, inappropriate sexual desire/function, anger, and anxiety (Loosen et al., 1994). Similarly, a small research evaluation administered anti-androgen medication to six male patients, all of whom were suffering from therapy-resistant obsessive-compulsive disorder. During the course of the trial, five out of six patients experienced considerable improvement. This finding supports the idea that anti-androgen medications may be effective in the treatment of those who are diagnosed with obsessive-compulsive disorder and have a positive effect on neurological function (Eriksson, 2007).

Finally, other investigators have reported on the use of leuprolide acetate administration to individuals diagnosed with an ASD. Leuprolide acetate administration to these patients significantly lowered their androgen levels and resulted in very significant overall clinical improvements in their socialization, sensory/cognitive awareness, and health/physical/behavior skills, with few nonresponders and minimal adverse clinical effects from the therapy. Giving these individuals leuprolide acetate also produced significant clinical reductions in hyperactivity/impulsivity, stereotypy, aggression, self-injury, abnormal sexual behaviors, and/or irritability. In addition, these individuals experienced improvements in focus, sleep cycle, and gastrointestinal function (Geier & Geier, 2006; Geier & Geier, 2007).

In considering the in-use safety of anti-androgen medications, the medicines with the least side effects and the most-characterized side effect profiles the medicines of choice have been on the market for many years; these include leuprolide acetate and cyproterone acetate. There are many individuals who have received these medications for many years for the treatment of conditions such as prostate cancer, female reproductive problems, and premature puberty without serious adverse effects. Furthermore, previous long-term follow-up of individuals receiving leuprolide acetate therapy in the treatment of premature puberty for many years revealed its administration was not associated with long-term reproductive dysfunction or impaired physical development (Tanaka et al., 2005). Finally, the administration of anti-androgen medications to individuals diagnosed with an ASD is not intended to deprive the individual of their sexuality nor to alter their normal developmental trajectory, but rather to regularize a process that was proceeding in an abnormal fashion and producing adverse effects and, thereby, improve the health of the patient and reduce the clinical symptoms associated with abnormally elevated androgen levels.

To illustrate the possible outcomes of anti-androgen therapy in a patient with an ASD, the following case study is provided.

At the age of 8, a boy diagnosed with an ASD began to exhibit sexual behaviors, masturbating frequently. He was developing hair on his legs and had been characterized by hyperactivity for years, requiring Clonidine to sleep and Tenex in order to function during the day. Even with these medications, his waking hours were characterized by incessant movement. He was averse to being touched, and his eyes did not stop to focus on any one point or event. He had chronic gastrointestinal problems, and, being nonverbal, he was failing to communicate using any of the assistive technologies offered to him.

Two months prior to his 9th birthday, he was given a test dose of leuprolide acetate. After administration, he went outside and began to swing on a tire swing using his feet to push a neurotypical behavior never seen before. He also was able to sit still and watch television with his eyes focused on the screen. Subsequent doses at the prescribed level of leuproide acetate resulted in the child seeking out touch and affection from his parents, focusing with greater clarity at different depths of field, an increase in receptive language, amelioration of gastrointestinal problems, the nearly complete disappearance of hyperactivity, and the development of a normal sleep cycle. Consequently, this child was able to be taken off both Clonidine and Tenex, which were prescribed for problems with hyperactivity and sleep cycle.

The child underwent anti-androgen therapy until the age of 13, when he entered puberty at an age typical of his sibling. During the course of treatment, this child made significant strides in being able to type on a keyboard and successfully communicate. There was breakthrough verbal language, but this was very limited. The child is now in high school and doing age-level work in some subjects.

For patients with more violent tendencies, the use of leuprolide acetate has increased their personal safety, the safety of their family members and, in some cases, has enabled the individual to be placed is a less restrictive environment.

Clearly, the potential of anti-androgen therapy holds tremendous promise for the treatment of an individual diagnosed with an ASD, contributing to the quality of their life by directly targeting a key biomedical indicator when it is elevated beyond the normal reference range. Screening all individuals with ASDs for elevated androgens and assessing this elevation relative to the individual's family may produce not only treatment options for ASDs and other androgen-related conditions, but also an understanding of why these conditions occur and who may be at risk. Routine screening of all persons with an ASD for elevated androgens is highly recommended as a standard part of the initial clinical assessment, and appropriate treatment should be initiated for those with elevated androgens.

ENZYMES FOR DIGESTIVE SUPPORT IN AUTISM

BY DR. DEVIN HOUSTON

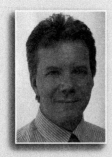

Devin B. Houston, Ph.D.

www.houston-enzymes.com
(866) 757-8627

Dr. Devin Houston founded Houston Enzymes in 2001 after many years of enzyme research in academia and industry. He invented the first enzyme product targeted to the autism community in 1999, and has since improved on that first effort. Dr. Houston continues to educate the public on enzymes and speaks on a regular basis at many autism conferences and parent groups.

The term "enzyme" refers to a broad class of specialized proteins that catalyze chemical reactions. Without enzymes these reactions would not occur or proceed at a rate not conducive to sustaining life. As catalysts, enzymes are not destroyed during the reaction. This allows a very small amount of enzyme to perform a large amount of work.

Digestive enzymes are a subset of enzymes specialized to break down foods after ingesting. These enzymes are necessary to derive nutrition from food. Specialized enzymes exist for different food proteins, carbohydrates, and triglycerides. The end result of their action is the provision of amino acids, glucose, and short-chain fatty acids to the body for production of compounds required for human metabolism.

The human body provides a fair amount of different enzymes for digestion, mostly from the pancreas and cells lining the gut wall. The bulk of the enzyme work occurs within the first part of the small intestine, or duodenum. It is here that protease enzymes begin the process of breaking proteins into smaller fragments called peptides, and carbohydrase enzymes start cleaving large carbohydrates into simple sugars. The duodenum and rest of the small intestine are also the site of absorption of nutrients into the systemic circulation.

Enzymes are present in raw foods but only in amounts sufficient to degrade the food over a period of several days. Many feel that enzymes in raw foods can supplement the digestion of food. Since digestion occurs within hours, not days, the actual contribution of food enzymes towards digestion is minimal. Enzymes can be supplemented in much more concentrated form. Fermentation of certain nonpathogenic fungi produces prodigious amounts of enzymes. Specific enzymes can be selected for production by altering the conditions under which the fungi are grown. The enzyme is then purified from the fungi, through many biochemical procedures resulting in a homogenous enzyme protein containing no fungal residue. The concentration of these enzyme blends is increased some billionfold over what is found in raw foods.

Many doctors have noted that children with autism often have gut problems. Inflammation can be a major problem. Tissues that are inflamed are damaged. Damaged cells don't produce enzymes, therefore, many children with autism may present with deficiencies in some enzymes until the gut is healed and operating normally. Malabsorption may present as well. Food intolerance and outright food allergies may also manifest in these children.

The most common food intolerance plaguing those with autism appears to be related to food proteins producing opioid-like peptides during digestion. Wheat and dairy products containing gluten and casein, respectively, are especially noted for producing exorphin peptides after contact with pepsin and elastase enzymes during the digestive process. This is a normal occurrence during digestion, however, some with autism exhibit stereotypical behaviors after ingesting wheat or dairy foods. One school of thought is that there may be an inappropriate interaction between opiate ligands and their receptors, however, this has not been substantiated. However, many parents found that diets that restrict wheat and dairy seemed to diminish the behavioral problems. The gluten-free/casein-free diet (GF/CF diet) is strongly recommended by many health care givers to their patients struggling with autism. The diet is not easy and requires a major lifestyle change for the patient and often the entire family.

Attempts were made in the 1990s to find an enzyme that would address the "peptide problem." Only when several protease enzymes were combined with a specific peptidase enzyme called dipeptidyl peptidase IV, or DPP-IV, was a degree of success obtained. DPP-IV was a known enzyme but not documented in commercially available enzyme blends until 1999. DPP-IV specifically degrades exorphin peptides and is produced by human gut cells. The fungal form is acid-resistant, as are most fungal enzymes. The actions of DPP-IV provide a possible mechanism of action and rationale for using protease enzyme supplements as a possible alternative to the GF/CF diet.

With the exception of alcohol, water, B vitamins, and some drugs, very little is absorbed from the stomach. Proteins and peptides are not absorbed until the food mass enters the small intestine. The stomach does not empty its contents into the duodenum until approximately two to three hours after ingestion. This provides a window of opportunity for addressing the problem proteins before their break down and absorption can occur in the small intestine. Plant-based enzymes are quite acid-resistant, unlike their pancreatic counterparts, and so may start working on foods within the stomach once in solution. A potent formulation of appropriate protease and peptidase enzymes can alter the pattern of protein breakdown such that exorphin peptides are not produced. If such peptides are produced, DPP IV peptidase can specifically degrade the exorphin peptides prior to food moving into the gut. However, the proper approach is to combine the DPP IV with other potent proteases to present a two-pronged attack: 1) change the manner in which the parent protein is broken down and, 2) use DPP IV to degrade any peptides that happen to form. It is interesting to note that this same approach is being used to develop an enzyme-based therapy for celiac disease.[1]

Enzymes may be helpful in other ways for those with autism. Keeping the gut free of undigested material prevents putrefaction that may lead to pathogenic bacterial blooms and yeast problems. Gas and bloating may be minimized by using carbohydrase enzymes such as lactase and alpha-galactosidase. Some vegetables contain carbohydrates such as stachyose and raffinose that are difficult for humans to digest. The human gut lacks the enzymes to degrade carbohydrates that become a food source for gas-producing bacteria. Alpha-galactosidase enzyme supplements can make up for the deficiency and ease the bloating. Chronic diarrhea may also be helped through the addition of enzymes such as amylase and glucoamylase that degrade starchy foods.

Other enzymes, such as xylanase, may modify some plant polyphenolic compounds by removing certain sugar groups that are attached to these compounds within the plant cells. These "phenolic compounds" are sources of antioxidants and other nutritional substances, and may play a role in modifying oxidative stress.[2] Removal of the sugar groups allows absorption of many polyphenolics and their subsequent metabolism by human cells.[3]

Enzymes are very likely one of the safest dietary supplements available. No upper limit has been established for dosing of any food-grade enzyme. No amount of plant-based digestive enzyme has been found to cause toxicity or side effects. Dosing of enzymes is not based on body weight or age as most of the ingested enzyme stays in the gut and is eliminated or broken down in the colon by microbial proteases. Enzymes are optimally given at the beginning of each meal to allow more contact time with the food in the stomach. Enzymes will not interfere with most medications, unless the medication is made of protein, carbohydrate, or triglyceride.

Well-controlled studies of enzyme use for the digestive problems associated with autism will eventually happen. The long history of safe use of enzymes in the food industry, however, should provide optimism and encouragement to try enzyme supplements without worry of significant side effects.

HOW ENZYMES COMPLEMENT THERAPEUTIC DIETS

BY KRISTIN SELBY GONZALEZ

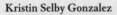

Kristin Selby Gonzalez

Director of Autism Education, Enzymedica
752 Tamiami Trail
Port Charlotte, Fl 33953
1-888-918-1118
www.enzymedica.com
www.facebook.com/kristinselbygonzalez
www.twitter.com/KSelbyGonzalez

Kristin Selby Gonzalez is the Director of Autism Education for Enzymedica, which is a leading enzyme manufacturer. She is also a national spokesperson, educator, radio show host and writer within the autism community. Kristin serves on the editorial team of the magazine Autism Science Digest. In addition, she is the mother of an eight-year-old boy with autism. Kristin has been working with her son for over six years and has seen him progress from very withdrawn with no language to a playful and interactive boy who now speaks in five-word sentences. She possesses an extraordinary body of knowledge and experience with both educational and biomedical interventions for autism, including enzyme therapy, dietary intervention, sensory integration, and play therapy. She speaks to parents and professionals across America at national autism conferences. She volunteers her time for the non-profits AutismOne, Autism Hope Alliance, and the Autism Treatment Center of America. Kristin holds a Bachelor of Arts degree in Elementary Education and Theater Arts.

First, I think it is best to define what enzymes are and what role they play in our bodies. Technically enzymes are proteins that act as catalysts. More commonly, enzymes are known as the workers of the body and have many different functions and jobs. All living things produce enzymes, and these enzymes all work within a specific pH and temperature range. It has been said by Dr. Edward Howell that we have thousands of enzymes and perhaps some enzymes that we have yet to discover. I often think of our bodies like the deep sea as we are continuing to discover new things and there is so much that is still unknown to us. Enzymes are responsible for every function we do such as blinking our eyes, moving our arms, and digesting our foods.

Digestive enzymes are produced by our bodies, found in raw foods, and sold as nutritional supplements. There are four groups of digestive enzymes: protease, which breaks down proteins; amylase, which breaks down carbohydrates; lipase, which breaks down fats; and cellulase, which breaks down fibers. From the moment food enters the mouth, enzymes start to go to work. As we chew we begin to activate enzyme activity. As food travels to our stomach, then to our small intestine, and then through our large intestine, there are enzymes there assisting with breaking up the food all along the way. Visualize your digestive tract as somewhat of a conveyer belt. Imagine as the first bottle drops at a bottling factory there is a worker to oversee that it lands upright; then the bottle travels down to where the liquid will be added and there is a worker there overseeing that; the bottle still needs to be capped off . . . well, you can see where I am going with this. Enzymes work in a similar fashion as each one has a specific job and purpose.

As I mentioned previously, digestive enzymes are also found in raw food. It was Dr. Edward Howell, author of *Enzyme Nutrition*, who illustrated what would happen if someone were to pick an apple from a tree and leave it on the kitchen counter for two weeks. Some of us might say the apple would rot, and that would be correct in a sense. Mother Nature supplied that apple with enough enzymes to digest itself. So, it would only make sense that the fresher the apple, the more enzyme activity the apple would provide to help you digest it when you eat it.

Digestive enzymes are also found in a supplemental form that can be purchased at a health food store. A person would typically take this type of enzyme supplement with the first bite of food. Taking a digestive enzyme with a meal allows for the enzymes to aid proper digestion by breaking down foods into valuable nutrients for the body. Why take an enzyme supplement? Our bodies may send us certain signs or signals to let us know we may have an enzyme deficiency. Indications of a possible enzyme deficiency include gas, bloating, acid reflux, heartburn, constipation, diarrhea, particles of food visible in the stool, skin rashes, and more. We need to become better detectives in figuring out the causes of these signs and listen to what our bodies are trying to tell us.

Now, let's talk about therapeutic diets as I have often heard that some believe supplemental enzymes can replace a therapeutic diet. I wish that were true, but in most cases it just isn't. Supplemental enzymes and therapeutic diets are what I like to think of as the "dynamic duo," working synergistically in the body for optimal results. For the majority of those who have sensitivities, they should consider looking into a clean diet, a good digestive enzyme, a good probiotic, and a good omega fatty acid supplement. In my own son's case, even though I had him on the cleanest diet imaginable, I still needed to give him a good digestive enzyme to help break down food. My son was constipated and would only have a bowel movement every three days until we figured out how to help his body absorb the nutrients he was taking in by his food. Many other children have constipation for longer periods of time—sometimes dangerously so, including possible impaction and reabsorption of toxins. Anything that is not broken down by the gut can, in essence, putrefy and feed bad bugs that have pathological physiological effects and sometimes negative cognitive consequences. Also, the brain also needs to receive nutrients. By giving my son a diet that his healing tummy could handle, appropriate for each level in the process, and combining this with the use of a good digestive enzyme, probiotic, and omega supplement, we have seen wonderful results.

What does this mean in terms of children with autism learning and functioning well? Imagine if you have tried to learn algebra while you had a headache or a stomach ache. It would be quite difficult. We focus so much of our time on different educational and other therapies that often we overlook the foundational importance of healing and sealing the gut. Other therapies are more successful when a child feels healthy and is free of pain. And when foods are broken down completely causing less irritation to the gut and resulting in fewer undigested substances entering the bloodstream, then fewer substances cause allergic-type reactions that affect the immune system and, consequently, the nervous system, thinking, and learning. Furthermore, I think that everybody would agree that everyone thinks and functions better when nutrients are absorbed to be utilized for the many cognitive and other processes of the body.

There are many different levels of digestive sensitivities for individuals on the autism spectrum. Some are truly allergic to specific foods, while others may show signs of intolerance to foods (an adverse reaction to a food not associated with an allergy and, therefore, not shown on an IgG allergy test). What is important to look for when trying to discern digestive sensitivities are behaviors and physical signs such as dark circles under the eyes, red cheeks, red ears, rashes, hyperactivity, lethargy, sweating, aggression, mood swings and/or sleep issues. I recommend keeping a food diary, which can be very beneficial when trying to pinpoint food intolerances. When discovering which diet works best for an individual on the spectrum, it is crucial not to give up and keep searching until you find one that works. Sometimes taking it one step at a time and eliminating one food at a time can be easier for you and your child. This way you can really see how each food affects your child.

At the end of the day there is not one thing that works for every child ultimately it takes trial and error to see what is best for each individual. We do know that no matter how healthfully you eat, if your digestive system isn't breaking down and absorbing the nutrients in your food, then the body can't function and operate to capacity. When the gastrointestinal system is operating properly, this benefits our immune system, our energy level, and our emotional and physical well-being. I think that the quote by Jean-Anthelme Brillant-Savarin (1755-1826) says it best: "Digestion, of all the bodily functions, is the one which exercises the greatest influence on the mental state of an individual."

THE FLOORTIME CENTER

BY JAKE GREENSPAN AND TIM BLEECKER

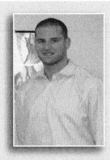

Jake Greenspan
jake@dirss.com

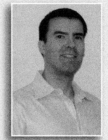

Tim Bleecker
tim@dirss.com

The Floortime Center™
4827 Rugby Avenue,
Bethesda, MD 20814
301-657-1130
info@dirss.com

Jake Greenspan and Tim Bleecker are the co-directors of The Floortime Center™ in Bethesda, Maryland. The Floortime Center is a child development center specializing in the use of the DIR®/Floortime™ model. With the help of Dr. Stanley Greenspan, they developed evaluation and intervention programs based on all aspects of the DIR model. Since the start of The Floortime Center in 2004, they have worked with over 900 families, and have presented 1 to 4 day workshops for various health and educational organizations.

Workshops include:
  -Training the entire Special Ed. District of Maui, HI in DIR/Floortime
  -Working on an ongoing basis with 5 Special Ed. Schools throughout the U.S..
  -Training numerous special needs organizations in DIR/Floortime

Floortime is a developmental approach that focuses on strengthening the whole child through improving the ability to regulate their nervous system, to attend to their environment, to relate with a broad range of emotion, to communicate physically and verbally, and to think logically—the developmental ladder. Mastering these functional capacities in the developmental ladder enables children, and all of us, to learn, to socialize, and to think. This happens first at basic levels and eventually at higher levels of abstract reasoning. By using the principles of the Floortime approach, parents and other caregivers can help a child progress to higher and higher levels of social and emotional cognition.

It is the social interactions that start at birth that help wire the brain so that we learn from new experiences and move up the developmental ladder. Children with Autism have difficulty learning through social interactions and from their environment. Floortime harnesses children's motivation so that their thinking ability can build on the richness of human interaction and new experiences.

Floortime is based on three main principles:

- To follow the child's lead identify emotional interests;
- To challenge the child to move up the developmental ladder; and
- To expand on those challenges in a dynamic fashion so that the child is always creating and experiencing something new.

Following the child's lead allows us to join their world and establish a mutual trust. Once we have established that trust, we can gradually draw the child out of his world and into ours. By joining him and discovering what interests and motivates his, we can learn which of his interests will hold his attention sufficiently for his play partner to eventually challenge—to create a game around activity or toy that involves him in a relationship and provides new experiences. If the child invites you into his world and is happy to have you join in, it may not be necessary to become more challenging right away. However, if a child is more avoidant or self involved often joining the activity is insufficient for connecting with them. We need to challenge children to climb the developmental ladder voluntarily. This means that we create challenges, based on using their developmental capacities, which they are motivated to overcome.

Through following a child's lead we can also identify sensory activities that his body and nervous system need to function at a higher level. Whether he is on a swing, trampoline, or ball, we can gain an understanding of the types of stimulation that help regulate his nervous system. Without having a regulated nervous system, a child will have difficulty interacting and be willing to have new experiences. If we have rhythmic patterns in our activities where we start and stop and start and stop, always paying attention to the child's response to us, we will see that children will begin to attend and engage and even begin to interact—exactly what the child needs to reach higher levels. Because of the importance of a regulated nervous system in the early stages, Floortime will emphasize movement and physical activities during those interactions, and consequently, Floortime may seem different when helping a child work on the earlier developmental milestones than when working on the later ones.

Example 1—Johnny

Two-year old Johnny came into the office for the first time, upset and clinging to his mom. According to his parents, he had a problem with transitions: he didn't have the problem at home, only at new places. They also said that he had problems playing with toys appropriately and didn't look at or communicate with them.

Once we settled into a play room, Johnny began moving from object to object, looking at each one for a second before moving to the next. In this very fragmented and disorganized manner, he moved around the room, not engaging with any person. Once he had made many circuits around the room, he began a particular self-stimulatory behavior—finding small objects, looking at them very closely, and waving them in front of his eyes. In further talking with Mom and Dad, I learned that he liked to play games that involve tickling and moving through space, such as being tossed up the air. However, if left on his own, he tended to find small objects that move, and wave them in front of his face or spin them.

In order to follow his lead it was important to understand his sensory system to know which sensations he enjoyed and which to be cautions of. As I observed Johnny moving around the room and talked with his parents, I learned that he had under-reactive tactile, proprioceptive and vestibular systems. That is, he needed and would sometimes seek out certain touch, pressure and movement. He also exhibited a sensitive visual-spatial system: he had difficulty understanding the organization of new spaces and could get overloaded and distracted by lots of visual detail or changes to familiar details.

While we were talking, Johnny, true to form, had picked up a piece of ribbon and was waving it in front of his face. To join the play, Dad got down on the floor near Johnny (but not right in front of him) and picked up one of the ribbons that Johnny had discarded. Dad waved it in the air and said with excitement, "Wow, I'm waving this ribbon. Look at it move. This is great!" Dad's enthusiastic ribbon waving elicited a quick glance from Johnny, but nothing more. He immediately turned back to his own ribbon. Unfortunately following Johnny's lead with high affect was insufficient to establish shared attention. Johnny was too self-involved.

I instructed Dad to become a little more playfully obstructive with Johnny and gently involve himself in the ribbon that Johnny was waving. First, Dad used the same high affect and enthusiasm to describe his intended actions, saying, "Oh boy, look at your ribbon, I want to see that one! I want to get it." Again, his enthusiasm gained little response. Since it was important for Johnny to understand what Dad was going to do, I coached Dad to reach in very slowly and to have his fingers crawl up Johnny's leg like a spider. As Dad moved up Johnny's body toward the arm with the ribbon, Johnny glanced at Dad and moved the ribbon away. Dad, giving a positive affective response to Johnny's reaction, said, "Oh, you don't want me to get that ribbon!", and let his hand fly backward.

Dad continued this same pattern of explaining his actions, providing tactile sensation (tickling) with his fingers crawling toward the ribbon and always accepting and responding to Johnny's response. As Dad persisted, saying, "I want to see that ribbon. Here I come…", Johnny began to look at him, sometimes with a little smirk flitting across his face as Dad reached for the ribbon and Johnny moved it away. Dad had enticed Johnny to play a game. Dad continued to challenge Johnny by reaching for the ribbon, but he also expanded on the challenge by moving further away from Johnny. In this way, as he said, "I'm coming to get that ribbon!" Dad could start at one end of the room and move slowly to the other side, all while Johnny was watching and anticipating when to move the ribbon away as Dad came nearer.

Over the next month Johnny's parents did hours of these games each day in 20 minute increments at home. The toy that Johnny would be interested in would change and so did the challenges mom and Dad provided. They reported that Johnny actually let them start to play a tug of war with different toys and eventually let them take the toy as he chased them to get it back. The more they played these games and challenged a little more each time, the more Johnny enjoyed these games, especially because he always won. His attention, connection to his environment and engagement with his parents improved significantly, which allowed us to start challenging him to use more complex communication.

Example 2—David

David was four-years old when he and his parents came to see me. His parents were concerned about his aggressive behavior and limited language. They reported that it was difficult for David to interact with them for any period of time. He was always bouncing around the room and became easily upset if they tried to start an activity with him.

This pattern quickly repeated itself at the clinic. David wouldn't sit still and, when approached, ran away. Mom and Dad resorted to leading him by the arm to an activity. When Mom playfully pulled him to the toy castle and began playing, he became agitated and hit her. He just wanted to continue running around the room, which he did with a big smile on his face.

I asked David's parents to change the way they were trying to engage with David. Instead of introducing an activity that he wasn't interested in, they could join his activity, that is, his running around the room. At first, they simply chased him around the room, which David seemed to enjoy. After about five minutes, I coached them to playfully challenge him by becoming a human fence with their arms stretched out so when he was in the corner, he had to figure out how to 'escape.' He began his escape by scooting under their arms. Mom and Dad quickly regrouped and put their arms lower so that he had to climb over their arms. When Mom asked David, "What should I do with my arm now?" David excitingly responded with, "Move arm!" Enjoying the escape game, David then ran to another part of the room so they could capture him again. During this game David's parents noticed him giving them more smiles and eye contact and using more language. He did not have another aggressive outburst, such as his hitting Mom earlier, for the rest of the 45-minute session.

David's parents learned that his body needed certain inputs such as movement and deep pressure (that is, vestibular and proprioceptive inputs). David became more regulated, emotionally connected and interactive with his parents when they followed his lead and gave him the sensory inputs, such as movement, that his body needed. Over the next few months David's parents were able to turn these simple chase games into more complex games. They incorporated stuffed animals that both chased and were chased in simple imaginative play. Slowly, David's back and forth interactions became longer and included more language. He also had a significant decrease in negative behaviors because his parents were constantly giving him the sensory support he needed by joining his active world.

The key to David's success was his parents' learning the Floortime principles that helped them 1) join him in his preferred activities (ones that helped him regulate his sensory system), 2) playfully entice him to stay connected for longer periods of time, and 3) eventually challenge him to expand his play and interactions. Gradually David increased his language and progressed to higher levels of thinking.

Example 3—Sally

Sally was diagnosed with autism at the age of three. By age seven she was still self-absorbed, unable to expand her usage of language and ideas, and lacked interest in creating relationships. Her favorite activity was scripting: repeating memorized segments, such as lines from a favorite movie, in her case, Disney movies. Her concerned parents reported that Sally preferred to be self-absorbed in her fantasies rather than interact with them or her older sister.

At home Sally would go to the corner of the room with the same toys and repeatedly reenact a scene from a movie or favorite TV show. She ignored Mom and Dad when they tried to join her play. Although she had some meaningful language, she used rote language in most of her interactions. Additionally, she craved certain movements and would often spin herself in a circle. She also easily became overloaded by her sensory environment such as loud noises and many types of tactile inputs.

Typically, Mom and Dad had tried to get Sally's attention by using a loud, excited voice. They had not realized that increasing the volume would overwhelm her sensitive auditory system and create less interaction. Her parents also had attempted to stop her scripted activities by trying to involve her in a different activity that they thought she would enjoy. This strategy rarely worked and Sally always went back to her scripts.

Mom and Dad started using Floortime therapy in order to find a way to reach Sally and help her develop stronger relationships with her family. Their goal was to learn how to join her play by following her lead while not overwhelming her sensitive sensory system.

A Floortime therapist coached Sally's parents on the fundamentals of joining her scripted activities—basically to pretend to be the characters in her Disney dramas. Mom and Dad were surprised by this suggestion because they thought that this would reinforce her scripting behaviors. The therapist suggested that Dad get on the floor with Sally, follow her lead and join her script by becoming the prince in her movie. Sally did not seem to mind Dad joining in because he did not try to introduce a different activity. He was also coached to use a quieter voice and move at a slower pace.

Over the next few sessions Sally began to enjoy having her parents become the different characters in her dramas. She initiated play sessions by telling Mom, Dad and her older sister which characters she wanted them to be. Within a few weeks Mom and Dad began gradually challenging Sally to expand her play. For example, they had their character do something slightly different from the usual scripted storyline. Sally did not become avoidant or self-absorbed because her parents helped her expand her play at her own individual pace.

Mom and Dad learned to tailor their interactions to Sally's unique profile so they could join her world and help her climb the developmental ladder. They also became aware of her unique auditory and tactile sensitivities so they could keep her regulated, join her play and eventually challenge her to expand on her ideas and language. After a year of intensive Floortime therapy Sally looks forward to having other people join her play. She often develops new and creative ideas and rarely depends on her scripts. She is also starting to show some interest in playing with her peers at school. Sally still has areas that need work, but most importantly she now enjoys connecting with her parents and sister with warm smiles and is not self-absorbed in her own world.

More professionals are agreeing that a parent centered approach is ideal for children with autism. Floortime strengthens the most important relationships in a child's life, it gives the parent control over their child's development, and it integrates into everyday life. As a result Flootime helps children progress all the time, not just when in a therapy session. Floortime has the ability to improve the core deficits of autism of relating and communicating and can be applied to children of all ages and developmental abilities. Floortime never assumes that there is a limit to what children with autism can achieve, and instead continues to challenge each child to rise to their true developmental potential.

FOOD SELECTIVITY AND OTHER FEEDING DISORDERS IN AUTISM

BY DR. PETULA VAZ AND DR. CATHLEEN PIAZZA

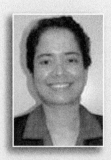

Petula C. M. Vaz, Ph.D.

985450 Nebraska Medical Center
Omaha, NE 68198-5450
(402) 559-8863
Fax: (402) 559-5004
pvaz@unmc.edu

Dr. Petula Vaz is an Assistant Professor at the Center for Autism Spectrum Disorders, Munroe-Meyer Institute at the University of Nebraska Medical Center. Her primary research interests are in the area of pediatric feeding disorders. Dr. Vaz is a licensed and certified speech-language pathologist. She is also a certified provider of VitalStim therapy for swallowing disorders. Dr. Vaz received her Ph.D. from Ohio University specializing in dysphagia and voice disorders. She has extensive predoctoral, doctoral, and postdoctoral research and clinical training in swallowing and feeding disorders. Dr. Vaz has several years of graduate and undergraduate level teaching and clinical mentoring experience.

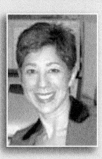

Cathleen C. Piazza, Ph.D.

Cathleen C. Piazza received her Ph.D. from Tulane University. She is Professor of Pediatrics and Director of the Pediatric Feeding Disorders Program at the University of Nebraska Medical Center in Omaha, and she previously directed similar programs at the Marcus Institute in Atlanta and at the Johns Hopkins University School of Medicine in Baltimore. Dr. Piazza and her colleagues have examined various aspects of feeding behavior and have developed a series of interventions to address one of the most common health problems in children with disabilities. Her research in this area has been among the most systematic in the field and has firmly established behavioral approaches as preferred methods for assessment and treatment. In her roles as clinical, research, and training director, Dr. Piazza has mentored a large number of interns and fellows who have gone on to make significant contributions to the field. Highly regarded for her general expertise in research methodology, Dr. Piazza is currently editor of the *Journal of Applied Behavior Analysis*.

Introduction

Feeding disorders in children involve the inability or refusal to consume sufficient amounts of liquid and solids to meet hydration and nutritional needs. Feeding problems occur in up to 90 percent of children with autism (Kodak & Piazza, 2008), and over 60 percent of these children exhibit selective eating behavior (Twachtman-Reilly, Amaral, & Zebrowski, 2008). The high incidence of pediatric feeding problems in children with autism have led some researchers to suggest that feeding difficulties in infancy may be an early sign of autism (Keen, 2008; Laud, Girolami, Boscoe, & Gulotta, 2009; Twachtman-Reilly et al.). The triad characteristic of autism—impairments in social interaction, communication deficits, and repetitive or stereotyped behavior—usually remain undetected during the first year of a child's life and are frequently missed until the child's second birthday. The presence of feeding disorders with selective eating behavior in children could potentially be a diagnostic precursor of autism. Therefore, early identification and management of feeding disorders in children is crucial. In addition, failure to address feeding disorders in a timely manner may lead to malnutrition and dehydration that may hinder physical growth and brain development, and it may also lead to other serious medical conditions such as failure to thrive, and even death.

Pediatric Feeding Disorders Program

The Pediatric Feeding Disorders Program (PFDP) at the University of Nebraska Medical Center's Munroe-Meyer Institute is one of the leading pediatric feeding disorders clinical, research, and training centers in the country. The assessment and treatment strategies used in the program focus on an interdisciplinary, empirical approach to feeding problems. A major component of the assessment and treatment strategies are based on the principles of applied behavior analysis, but the integration of the expertise of other disciplines such as medicine, speech, and occupational therapy, and nutrition are critical as the majority of feeding problems in children have a multifactorial etiology (Rommel, De Meyer, Feenstra, & Veereman-Wauters, 2003). The PFDP is well recognized for its commitment to high quality, interdisciplinary clinical care, to the teaching of health professionals, and to research related to pediatric feeding disorders. Dr. Piazza, the director of the PFDP, and her team have presented and published numerous research papers in this area.

Philosophy

The PFDP's interdisciplinary team consists of physicians, psychologists, nurse practitioners, nutritionists, speech-language pathologists, occupational therapists, physical therapists, social workers, feeding behavior technicians, and aides. Parents and caregivers are active participants in the child's feeding program. Research suggests that interdisciplinary treatment such as the type provided by the PFDP is the most effective and appropriate method of treating children with severe feeding problems (Cohen, Piazza, & Navathe, 2006; Kerwin, 1999; Volkert & Piazza, in press) including children with autism.

Program Structure

Children with autism between the ages of zero and twelve years with feeding problems of varying severity that compromise growth and/or nutrition are seen at the PFDP. Children over the age of twelve years are considered for admission to the program on a case by case basis. The PFDP has three different levels of service where the intensity of services provided vary along a continuum: a day treatment program, an intensive outpatient program, and an outpatient program. Children whose feeding problems are life-threatening or who have not progressed sufficiently with less frequent therapy are good candidates for the day treatment program. Children attending the day treatment program receive daily intensive therapy from Monday through Friday from 8:30 AM to 5:00 PM for approximately eight weeks. The program involves intensive feeding therapy sessions five to six hours per day, nutritional monitoring, and caregiver training. Once children have met their goals in the day treatment program, they are transitioned to the intensive outpatient program. The intensive outpatient program is for children who continue to require services after the day treatment program or whose feeding problems would respond to less intensive therapy. The intensive outpatient component of the program involves therapy sessions three to five days per week for approximately one to four hours per day. Once a child's treatment is stabilized in the intensive outpatient program, he or she is then transitioned to the outpatient program to maintain treatment gains, and progress the child to age-typical eating patterns. In the outpatient program, children are typically seen once or twice a week for approximately one to three hours of therapy. Depending upon the severity of the child's feeding problem, the entire course of treatment (i.e., to progress the child to age-typical feeding) may take up to two years.

Program Development and Monitoring

During the admission, the interdisciplinary team and the parents/caregivers develop specific goals for the child, which are the focus of assessment and treatment. Thus, all assessments and treatments are goal oriented and data driven. Common goals include increasing caloric intake, increasing acceptance and consumption of solid food and liquids, decreasing supplemental feedings (e.g., gastrostomy [G-] tube feedings), increasing texture and variety of consumed foods, decreasing inappropriate mealtime behavior, and caregiver training. The long-term goal of the program is for the child to become an age-typical eater. The team meets at least once a day to discuss the data and to revise the assessment and/or treatment plan as necessary. The program differs from the traditional interdisciplinary team model in that individual, discipline-specific (pull-out) therapy is not provided. Instead, the team develops a protocol that is individualized for the child. This protocol is followed by everyone who feeds the child. Therefore, the feeding therapy occurs during meals, in the presence of solids and/or liquids, under very specific conditions that have been developed beforehand by the entire team.

Assessment

The initial evaluation begins with the caregiver feeding the child as he or she would at home. Data are collected on child and caregiver behavior, which include how the caregiver prompts the child to eat and how the caregiver responds to child-appropriate and -inappropriate behavior. The child's responses to various textures and type of food and liquids and use and need for types of utensils are assessed. These data are used to develop hypotheses about current environmental events that may maintain child-appropriate and -inappropriate behavior and the child's current level of oral motor skills. Children with high levels of inappropriate behavior during caregiver-fed meals participate in a functional analysis (FA) to determine how specific environmental events affect child behavior (Piazza, Fisher, Brown, et al., 2003). The results of the FA result in a specific, prescribed treatment for the child.

Children with high levels of inappropriate behavior in the presence of specific foods or textures often participate in a food-preference (Munk & Repp, 1994) or texture-preference assessment (Patel, Piazza, Layer, Coleman, & Swartzwelder, 2005; Patel, Piazza, Santana, & Volkert, 2002), respectively. A hierarchy of food or textures the child refuses to eat is developed. The results of the assessment are used to develop individualized treatment protocols to facilitate the acceptance of target foods or textures as indicated.

Treatment

Individualized treatment protocols consistent with current research literature are developed that meet specific needs of these children. For example, a treatment based on negative reinforcement is used with children whose inappropriate behavior is maintained by escape from presentations of liquids or solids. Typical negative reinforcement-based treatments include providing a break following appropriate behavior (e.g., acceptance, swallowing) and elimination of escape for inappropriate behavior (escape extinction; Gulotta, Piazza, Patel, Layer, 2005; Kelley, Piazza, Fisher, Oberdorff, 2003). A treatment based on positive reinforcement is used with children whose inappropriate behavior is maintained by attention. Typical positive reinforcement-based treatments include providing attention or tangible items following appropriate behavior (e.g., acceptance, swallowing) and the elimination of attention for inappropriate behavior (attention extinction; Bachmeyer et al., 2009; Piazza, Patel, Gulotta, Sevin, Layer, 2003; Reed, Piazza, Patel, et al., 2004).

These types of treatments typically focus on increasing acceptance of food and decreasing inappropriate behavior. However, there may be other variations of these treatments that are implemented for children who show resistance to escape and/or attention extinction, such as blending preferred and nonpreferred foods together to increase acceptance of nonpreferred foods (Mueller, Piazza, Patel, Kelley, & Pruett, 2004; Piazza, Patel, Santana, et al., 2002); fading or altering some component of the mealtime environment gradually (Freeman & Piazza, 2002; Patel, Piazza, Kelly, Ochsner, & Santana, 2001) for a child who is cooperative with some aspect of the feeding situation, but not others; preceding presentation of a food or liquid with a low probability of acceptance, by a food or liquid with a higher probability of acceptance (Patel, Reed, Piazza, et al., 2006) for a child who demonstrates acceptance of some foods or some aspect of the feeding situation (e.g., acceptance of an empty spoon) but not others.

Increases in acceptance for some children might be accompanied by increases in expulsion (spitting out food). Such a response would necessitate the addition of treatment components designed to reduce expulsion. For example, the therapist might re-present expelled food (Sevin, Gulotta, Sierp, Rosica, & Miller, 2002). The therapist also might evaluate how texture of food affects expulsion (Patel, Piazza, Santana, et al., 2002). Some children hold or pocket accepted food, a behavior known as "packing." There are a variety of treatments used to reduce packing and increase swallowing. One treatment involves "redistribution" of packed food with a spoon or a Nuk brush to place packed food back on the child's tongue (Gulotta, Piazza, Patel, et al., 2005). In other instances, it may be necessary to reduce the texture of one or more food items (Patel, Piazza, Layer et al., 2005).

Caregiver Training

Research studies have shown that caregivers can be trained successfully to implement treatment protocols (Mueller, Piazza, Moore, et al., 2003; Najdowski, Wallace, Doney, & Ghezzi, 2003; Werle, Murphy, & Budd, 1993). The long-term success of a feeding program depends on the accuracy with which caregivers follow through with treatment procedures. Therefore, once an effective treatment is identified, caregiver training to monitor treatment integrity is a crucial final component of treatment.

Outcomes

Our empirically based, interdisciplinary treatment program is highly effective. The program has an 86 percent success rate with severe feeding problems (based on outcome data collected in the PFDP at the Kennedy Krieger and Marcus Institutes, where Dr. Piazza was the director). The costs associated with behavioral treatment are significantly less than those associated with alternative means of nutrition such as G-tube feeding. Data from studies on treatment of feeding disorders suggest that treatment of feeding problems results in improved quality of life for the child and family, reduced overall health care usage and costs, and reduced family stress.

GASTROINTESTINAL DISEASE: EMERGING CONSENSUS

BY DR. ARTHUR KRIGSMAN

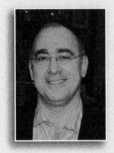

Arthur Krigsman, MD

148 Beach 9th Street
Far Rockaway, New York 11691
(516)239-4123

Dr. Krigsman is a pediatrician and board-certified pediatric gastroenterologist. He has extensive experience in the evaluation and treatment of gastrointestinal disease in children with autistic spectrum disorder and participates in the growing field of research designed to better understand GI disease in this group of children. He has presented his findings in peer-reviewed journals and has shared his experience at scientific and lay meetings, and at a congressional hearing dealing with autism and its possible causes.

The presence of chronic gastrointestinal (GI) symptoms in children with autism spectrum disorder (ASD) has been well established. Prospective reviews of the frequency of these chronic and often intense GI symptoms, based upon thoughtful questioning of the parents, reveal that they occur in as many as 70-80% of ASD children. The GI symptoms in these children are of a wide variety and include abdominal pain, diarrhea, constipation, abdominal distention, and growth failure ("failure to thrive"). In my experience with over 1400 such patients, I have often heard the parent state, "I can live with the autism, but I can't stand to see my child suffer with pain and severe constipation." Because the communicative and behavioral aspects of autism are the most obvious, and because the GI symptoms frequently begin during infancy (prior to the onset of the behavioral and cognitive problems), parents are often unaware of the impact of the GI problems on their child's health until years later.

Historically, when parents do finally bring these GI complaints to the attention of their general practitioner or pediatric gastroenterologist, their significance is often minimized or dismissed. There are many reasons for this, including lack of familiarity with the GI diseases frequently seen in ASD, uncertainty on the part of the physician about how to properly proceed in the evaluation of these diseases, and long-standing beliefs in the medical world that GI symptoms in the "mentally handicapped" are mysterious and poorly defined, similar to what is observed in many patients with mental retardation. Lastly, the political controversy and unending media misinformation swirling around the three scientists who were the first to describe bowel disease in ASD patients has given rise to doubts in some academic circles as to whether anything is really wrong at all with the bowels of these children.

Fortunately, the GI problems of children with ASD are now getting attention. First was a full-day conference jointly sponsored by NASPGHAN (North American Society for Pediatric Gastroenterology, Hepatology, and Nutrition), the American Academy of Pediatrics, and Autism Speaks. It was dedicated solely to further our understanding of the GI disease in these children. In addition there are two consensus statements published in a January 4, 2010 supplement to the journal *Pediatrics,* offering guidance to clinicians as to how best evaluate gastrointestinal symptoms within the setting of ASD.

The two most important points to keep in mind are that (a) GI symptoms should be evaluated no differently in children with ASD than they would in neurotypical children, and (b) problem behaviors may be the sole manifestation of a gastrointestinal problem. Let us explore these two statements.

The presence of chronic (i.e., long-standing) GI symptoms demands medical evaluation. The fact that the child has autism is merely an interesting sidebar item. The clinical story typically begins with the parents' concern over the chronicity and intensity of their child's GI symptoms. It is this that brings them to the pediatrician or gastroenterologist. The symptoms typically consist of any, some, or all of the following:

- abdominal pain
- diarrhea (defined as unformed stool that does not hold its own shape but rather conforms to the shape of the container/nappy/diaper that it is in)
- constipation (defined as infrequent passage of stool of any consistency or passage of overly hard stools regardless of frequency)
- soft-stool constipation
- painful passage of unformed stool
- rectal prolapse
- failure to maintain normal growth
- regurgitation
- rumination
- abdominal distention
- food avoidance

An additional layer of complexity appears when there is an observed correlation between the intensity of the GI symptoms and the level of cognitive-behavioral dysfunction. Parents will often say that they can predict their childs on any given day based on how their stool looks. In the non-ASD world of pediatric gastroenterology, the GI pathology responsible for these varying symptoms is often difficult to determine from the symptoms alone. The same holds true in the ASD patient group. In both cases, numerous underlying GI problems can cause these symptoms. In my experience with ASD children, the following diagnoses have been endoscopically confirmed and determined to be causing some or all of these symptoms:

- eosinophilic esophagitis (EoE)
- esophageal hypereosinophilia (EH)
- reflux esophagitis
- Candida esophagitis
- esophagitis of unknown origin
- Barrett's esophagus
- peptic gastritis
- eosinophilic gastritis
- lymphocytic gastritis
- autoimmune gastritis
- gastric ulcer
- gastropathy of unknown origin
- *Helicobacter pylori* gastritis
- peptic duodenitis
- duodenal ulcer
- white-spot (micro-erosive) duodenitis
- *H. pylori* duodenitis
- non-specific enteritis
- celiac disease
- non-specific colitis
- Crohn's disease

Of course, ASD children may suffer from the same common GI ailments as neurotypical children (e.g., constipation, reflux, transient stomach virus infections, etc.), so a GI complaint in an ASD child does not automatically suggest the presence of the above-mentioned diagnoses. It is certainly appropriate to undertake a trial of empiric (that is, treatment of a suspected disorder without prior confirmation of the true diagnosis) therapy for any of the common childhood GI problems (e.g., reflux, constipation, etc.). However, if the symptoms prove resistant to conventional empiric therapies or if the suspected diagnosis is that of a chronic disorder that will require long-term treatment (i.e., inflammatory bowel disease), empiric therapy is inappropriate and contraindicated. The fact that most ASD children experience chronic GI symptoms, and that most ASD-GI-symptomatic children have demonstrable causal pathology of the types listed above, has led many to conclude that GI pathology occurs with increased frequency in ASD children when compared to neurotypical children. This is certainly the conclusion I have drawn in working with these children.

The approach to evaluating these chronic symptoms should be the same as those employed to diagnose and treat neurotypical children. Established diagnostic algorithms exist for all of the above-mentioned symptoms and include a careful taking of the history, physical examination, blood tests, stool tests, urine tests, abdominal imaging studies, nutritional assessment, and assessment of growth patterns. These tests should be designed to cover as broad a spectrum of potential diagnoses as possible, including metabolic diseases such as mitochondrial disorders. Needless to say, these tests are most useful when they provide strong evidence of a specific diagnosis. However, more often than not, even the most comprehensive non-invasive evaluation does not shed light on the cause of the symptoms in the ASD-GI patient. These are the cases that usually require direct visualization of the GI tract via endoscopy. Endoscopy not only provides direct visualization of the lining of the GI tract but also the ability to obtain a small sample of tissue (biopsy) for microscopic examination by a pathologist. The recent introduction of wireless capsule endoscopy (commonly referred to as the "pillcam") allows direct visualization of the small intestinal lining not accessible to more conventional endoscopy and has contributed greatly to our understanding of bowel disease

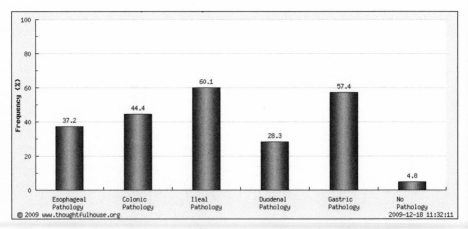

Frequency by Anatomic Location of Various GI Pathologies in ASD-GI Symptomatic Children Undergoing Endoscopy and Colonoscopy. Performed by Arthur Krigsman, MD. 2003-2009. Reported by Independent Pathologists (Mount Sinai Hospital NY, Lenox Hill Hospital, NY, and CPL Labs, TX.)

in ASD children. ASD-GI patients who have undergone diagnostic endoscopy and biopsy frequently have more than one of the diagnoses listed above, and the precise order in which they need to be treated, as well as the nature of their relationship to each other, has to be further studied.

For the most part and for the sake of simplicity, the various diagnoses of the esophagus and stomach depicted above are also seen in the neurotypical population but the ASD-associated enterocolitis (ASD-EC) present in the majority of ASD-GI patients, and well described in the medical literature, appears to be unique to ASD patients. (The exception to this appears to be a focal enhanced gastritis described only within the population of ASD-GI patients.) Because of this, established treatments for the esophageal and gastric (stomach) diagnoses exist, but the best treatment for the ASD-associated enterocolitis is unknown. It is uncertain whether treatment of non-specific enterocolitis may also treat some of the esophageal and gastric pathology. Much work needs to be done in this area. It does seem clear, though, that ASD-associated enterocolitis is, in many cases, a chronic disease. Because academic interest in the area of autism-associated bowel disease is increasing, it will be interesting to see the results of clinical trials aimed at determining the treatment outcomes of a variety of pharmaceutical and dietary interventions for autism-associated enterocolitis. Many researchers believe that these clinical trials should include established therapies for other inflammatory bowel diseases (IBDs) such as Crohn's disease and ulcerative colitis. The rationale for this

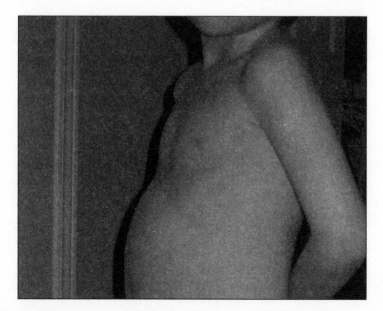

Abdominal Distension in a Child with Autism Associated Enterocolitis

is that preliminary data demonstrate an interesting overlap between the clinical presentation, laboratory findings, and endoscopic/histologic findings of autism-associated enterocolitis and IBDs. As in Crohn's disease, the symptom presentation of ASD-associated enterocolitis may consist of abdominal pain, diarrhea, abdominal distention, and growth retardation. Interestingly, constipation and difficulty in passing soft or unformed stools is a frequent presenting symptom in ASD-associated enterocolitis though this is not thought to be typical of the symptoms of Crohn's disease (though there are reports of just such presentation in Crohn's disease as well). Abdominal x-rays of ASD children presenting with chronic GI symptoms characteristically show fecal loading, meaning a colon loaded with stool. The colon in these patients does *not* typically appear distended on x-ray, thus providing reassurance that there is no obstruction. Obstruction would represent a medical emergency and requires urgent medical attention. In such cases, the patient is quite ill and toxic looking. The constipation most typical in ASD-GI children is best referred to as "soft stool constipation." This means that the child will go many days (often up to a week or more) without a bowel movement. During this period, the abdomen becomes progressively more distended. Parents often report that the progressive retention of stool correlates with progressive worsening in the child's *behavior* (e.g., "stimming," aggression, self-injurious behaviors, hyperactivity) and *cognition* (i.e., focus, processing, thought, and language, etc.). The stool that is finally produced after many days is semi-formed or unformed and is often produced only with great straining.

Other interesting overlaps in the clinical presentation of ASD-associated enterocolitis and Crohn's disease exist as well. Disturbance in growth patterns is often noted at presentation. Interestingly, even after all other gastrointestinal symptoms are resolved with the appropriate medications and diet, disturbances in growth patterns often persist. The deviation from normal growth can affect linear growth (height),weight, or both. Preliminary data indicate that this growth delay occurs despite adequate caloric intake and in the absence of any evidence of malabsorbtion. However, in some patients, there may indeed be a component of GI disease related malabsorbtion. There are reports of decreased bone mineralization in ASD children, independent of their being on any specific restrictive diet. In addition, reports of duodenal brush border enzyme deficiencies (not associated with known genetic defects) in ASD-GI patients further suggests a possible underlying mucosal inflammatory process that may contribute to growth retardation.

Overlap in laboratory testing between ASD-associated enterocolitis and IBD includes the finding of an elevated erythrocyte sedimentation rate, C-reactive protein, and platelet counts as well as the presence in the stool of lactoferrin, calprotectin, and lysozyme. The latter three stool markers are considered specific for the presence of intestinal inflammation. The relative frequency with which these markers of inflammation are present in ASD-associated enterocolitis as compared to IBD has not yet been determined. Perhaps most interesting in terms of laboratory overlap is the frequent presence of elevated IBD-specific serologic markers. These markers are serum antibodies to both bacterial and fungal gut flora that are statistically associated with the presence of IBD and are rarely found in the non-IBD population. It is important to point out that these markers are *not* considered to be a diagnostic test for IBD. They are most appropriately used when a clinician is trying to distinguish Crohn's disease from ulcerative colitis and when attempting to determine the likelihood of particularly aggressive forms of Crohn's disease.. However, their frequent presence in ASD-GI children suggests that a similar mechanism of disease might be present there as well and provides potential avenues of further research.

In patients undergoing clinically indicated diagnostic endoscopy for the above symptoms, there is the frequent occurrence of a non-specific mucosal inflammation. The term "non-specific" indicates that the features seen under the microscope, though not normal, do not indicate the presence of a specific disease. It implies that the finding is not normal, but that many causes are possible. Though there are specific microscopic features of Crohn's disease that allow one to make a definitive diagnosis, it is not unusual for Crohn's disease patients to produce biopsies that are non-specific in nature. Such is the case with ASD-associated enterocolitis where the majority of the patients demonstrate non-specific findings upon biopsy. However, there are a number of ASD-GI children whose intestinal biopsies demonstrate the changes strongly suggestive of Crohn's disease.

These clinical, laboratory, and endoscopic/histologic overlaps provide strong preliminary support for clinical trials that investigate the efficacy of pharmaceuticals commonly used to treat IBDs. It is our hope that such clinical trials will be undertaken soon.

Moving on to the second of our statements made at the outset of this article, parents, physicians, and therapists must realize that difficult-to-treat ASD behaviors or behaviors that have not been responsive to standard behavioral interventions may be the *sole* manifestation of a GI diagnosis. This means that unprovoked aggression, violent behavior, and irritability may have an underlying GI cause, and this must be taken into consideration prior to the reflexive desire to begin a psychotropic drug such as risperidone (despite its FDA approval for the treatment of autism). Gastroesophageal reflux disease, gastritis/gastric ulcer, and constipation are just three examples of GI diagnoses that are known to cause such behavioral symptoms. In addition, poor focus and an inability to make significant academic or communicative progress despite intensive interventions may indicate the presence of treatable bowel disease that, once treated, can significantly improve the child's degree of disability. The concept of behavioral problems as a symptom of GI disease was strongly supported in the consensus article published in the January 4, 2010 supplement of the journal *Pediatrics*.

The take-home messages are as follows:

1. Treatable GI disease is exceedingly common in ASD.
2. The signs and symptoms that alert one to the possible presence of GI disease are both conventional (e.g., diarrhea, abdominal pain, etc.) and ASD-specific (e.g., behaviors, aggression, poor response to therapies, etc.).
3. The approach to the GI evaluation of these signs and symptoms should be no different from a child without autism.
4. Parents and therapists who note such signs and symptoms must strongly advocate for the child regarding the need for a comprehensive GI evaluation.
5. Treatment of GI disease should follow established treatment protocols for the particular diagnosis.
6. GI diagnoses unique to ASD require further study to determine best treatment practices.
7. Empiric treatment for common, transient childhood conditions is appropriate but should be halted if the patient demonstrates non-responsiveness.
8. Empiric treatment for suspected chronic disease in inappropriate and contraindicated.

HELMINTHIC THERAPY AND IMMUNE ABNORMALITIES

BY JUDITH CHINITZ

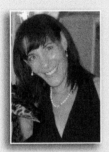

Judith Hope Chinitz, MS, MS, CNC

New Star Nutritional Consulting
(914) 244-3646
www.newstarnutrition.com
judy@newstarnutrition.com

After her son's diagnosis with autism in 1996, Judith Chinitz has spent the last fifteen years searching for answers. After saving her son's life through diet, and seeing firsthand the healing power of food, Judy earned a second master's degree in nutrition after having previously worked as a special education teacher. Currently she is continuing her studies at Columbia University's Institute for Human Nutrition. Judy is the author of *We Band of Mothers: Autism, My Son, and the Specific Carbohydrate Diet,* which also contains commentary by Dr. Sidney Baker. She also assisted Dr. Baker in founding Medigenesis, an Internet-based, interactive medical database.

Autism, Immune Abnormalities, and Parasite Therapy

In 1964, Dr. Bernard Rimland published his book, *Infantile Autism: The Syndrome and Its Implication for a Neural Theory of Behavior,* proving that autism was a physiological—as opposed to a psychological—condition. By the 1970s, researchers began to note immune system abnormalities in autistic children. In the 1980s, researchers such as Dr. Reed Warren, for example, demonstrated that those with autism had abnormal lymphocyte responsiveness (that is, their white blood cells don't respond normally to germs) and abnormal levels of various types of immune cells, including low levels of natural killer cells. (This means that children on the autism spectrum have a hard time fighting pathogens, like yeast, viruses, and bacteria.)

In 1998, Dr. Sudhir Gupta of the University of California, Irvine, published a paper in the *Journal of Neuroimmunology* entitled, "Th1–and Th2-like cytokines in CD4+ and CD8+ cells in autism." This paper states that the ". . . data suggest that an imbalance of Th1–and Th2-like cytokines in autism may play a role in the pathogenesis of autism."

To date, a few of the specific abnormalities found in individuals with autism include:

a.   In an unstimulated state, individuals with autism have higher levels of proinflammatory cytokines (chemical messengers of the immune system) than control groups.

b.   With stimulation of the immune system (i.e., with the introduction of pathogens), individuals with autism spectrum disorders (ASD) have markedly higher levels of proinflammatory cytokines than controls.

c.   Specific proinflammatory cytokines that have been found to be high in people on the spectrum include tumor necrosis factor-α (TNF-α) in both the blood and the gut; interferon gamma (IFN-γ) in both the blood and the gut; and higher levels of IL-12 in the blood.

d.   Individuals with ASD have lower levels of regulatory cytokines (those chemicals that turn off inflammation) like interleukin-10 (IL-10) than control groups.

e.   Brain specimens from subjects with autism exhibit signs of ongoing inflammation and abnormalities in immune signaling and immune function.

These proinflammatory chemicals appear to affect not just how these individuals respond (or don't respond) to disease-causing microbes; they also affect the health of the body in general, the digestive system and the function of the brain itself.

Dr. Martha Herbert, an Assistant Professor of Neurology at Harvard Medical School, and a pediatric neurologist at the Massachusetts General Hospital in Boston, a foremost authority on autism, has stated repeatedly that the brain is downstream from the digestive system, meaning that if the latter is compromised, the former suffers. The lining of our digestive system comprises about seventy percent of the immune system. Our bodily systems are not separate entities, but all parts of one whole. If one part is compromised, the rest are affected.

Also evident from the medical literature is the finding that many individuals with ASD have abnormal gut microbiota. What does this mean? The human body contains trillions of microbes, far more than there are cells in our bodies. No one really knows exactly what the composition of these microbes should be. However, we do know that there should be something like 400–500 different types of bacteria living in our intestines. Multiple researchers have now demonstrated that individuals with ASDs have not only abnormal amounts of bacteria living in their digestive systems, but also seemingly abnormal kinds as well. It's a chicken-and-egg scenario: abnormal gut microbiota leads to abnormal gut conditions compromising the immune system, but the reverse is also true. Abnormal immune functioning within the gastrointestinal tract will lead to abnormal microbiota.

In January of 2011, a paper was accepted for publication in the *Proceedings of the National Academy of Science*, entitled, "Normal gut microbiota modulates brain development and behavior." The researchers found that mice raised in a germ free environment, devoid of normal gut microbes, had highly abnormal development when compared to normal peers. If normal microbes were introduced early enough in development, as adults the two groups were indistinguishable. However, introducing normal flora to an adult germ-free population did not remediate the developmental abnormalities. They conclude: "Our results suggest that the microbial colonization process initiates signaling mechanisms that affect neuronal circuits involved in motor control and anxiety behavior." Of course this study was done on mice and animal models do not always translate into the same meaning for humans. However, these data are certainly compelling.

That our "old friends," the microflora that live in and on us, are absolutely crucial to normal, healthy life, is accepted fact. That disturbances in this biome early in life can affect the development of the immune and central nervous systems looks more and more likely.

The hygiene hypothesis, which was first proposed about twenty years ago, conjectures that we have become "too sterile." With the advent of germ theory a century ago (the recognition that many diseases arise from specific germs), we have concentrated our efforts on eradicating bacteria, yeasts, and parasites from our environment and ourselves. However, the fact is that many species of these organisms were normal parts of human flora for all of evolution, and without our old friends, we may have tipped our immune systems into a chronic state of imbalance.

So, where does this leave us? Many individuals with autism have abnormal gut microbiotia and abnormal immune functioning. How best to handle this is not yet known. Many doctors focus on killing off the bad stuff—antibiotics for bad bacteria, antifungals for Candida, etc. And this helps . . . sometimes. Another line of thought though is to shift the immune system and gut back into normalcy by *adding* good flora and fauna, rather than, or as well as, subtracting bad—especially when the lines between good and bad may be more blurred than originally thought.

Enter Parasites

The presence of helminths was natural and endemic for the evolving humanoid species up until seventy-five or so years ago. We lived on and with the soil, and thus our intestines were filled not only with bacteria and yeasts, but protozoa and other parasites too—including helminths. Helminths are a family of parasitic worms that include roundworm, hookworm, tapeworm and whipworm, among others.

With our current anti-germ way of thinking, many are immediately horrified when they first think about "infecting" themselves with parasites. "Aren't parasites bad?" is the typical first question from those first learning about this form of therapy.

Well, yes, they certainly can be. A 20-foot tapeworm living in your intestines might be considered undesirable. Then again, we are all very well aware of the health benefits of yogurt, with its live bacteria. Do you equate this with purposefully eating salmonella? Like bacteria, some parasites are good and some are bad. And like bacteria, some are perhaps meant to be in us. And like bacteria, the amount matters. An absence of good bacteria in the gut will seriously compromise the health of the individual. More and more research suggests that an absence of good parasites is a major factor in the development of certain disorders.

Perhaps most fascinating of all, several papers were published in 2010 pointing to the fact that the bacteria of our intestines seem to work synergistically with helminths. Dr. Joel Weinstock, a preeminent researcher of helminths role in disease, who is now at Tufts University in Boston, recently looked at a mouse model of inflammatory bowel disease and found that helminthic infection actually positively altered the bacterial content of the gut. He concludes, "These data support the concept that helminth infection shifts the composition of intestinal bacteria." In fact, researchers at the University of Manchester in England found that a certain type of helminth is reliant upon the microflora of the intestine to reproduce. When the number of bacteria in the mice intestine were reduced, so were the number of hatched helminth eggs: "Critical interactions between bacteria (microflora) and parasites (macrofauna) introduced a new dynamic to the intestinal niche…" It appears that mammals evolved carrying an entire complex, inter–and intra-dependent ecological system within them.

In 2007, Dr. Kevin Becker of the National Institutes of Health, published an article in *Medical Hypotheses* entitled, "Autism, asthma, inflammation, and the hygiene hypothesis." Dr. Becker concludes, "Altered patterns of infant immune stimulation may hypersensitize the early immune system not toward allergic sensitivity and bronchial hypersensitivity but to inflammatory or cytokine responses affecting brain structure and function leading to autism. It is well documented that immune cytokines play an important role in normal brain development as well as pathological injury in early brain development. It is hypothesized that immune pathways altered by hygiene practices in western society may effect brain structure or function contributing to the development of autism."

The idea that a loss of our natural helminth population may be playing a factor in the etiology of autism is becoming more wide spread. Dr. William Parker, of Duke University, is researching helminths' effects on health. He recently published a paper on the topic, *Reconstituting the depleted biome to prevent immune disorders*. He writes, "Not only must the effects of biome depletion on a particular generation be considered, but the epigenetic effects on future generations may be profound….For example, the association of autism with inflammation and the epidemic nature of this disease in post-industrial societies point toward The Biome Depletion Theory." Dr. Parker goes on to say:

> We cannot escape the biology imposed by our evolution, and the medical science of the future will take that fact fully into account. At present, we need to direct intensive research toward biome reconstitution. The approach needs to be devised systematically rather than piecemeal. We need to know which organisms to utilize, and when and how to utilize them. We need to know the safety and efficacy of biome reconstitution for various conditions, including which hyper-immune conditions can be cured versus which can be prevented but not cured by biome reconstitution. We need to know the effects of biome reconstitution not only on one generation, but on subsequent generations. We must determine if new technologies are needed to reduce potential side effects of helminth colonization. In short, we need to know how to reconstitute our biome and keep that biome healthy. It is time for a paradigm shift in the enterprise of biomedical research and subsequently of medicine. Our evolution and our resulting biology require it.

As Dr. Parker correctly points out, there are too many unanswered questions. But we do have some good information already. Research thus far has shown that certain helminths raise levels of regulatory cytokines (those chemicals that turn off inflammation) and they lower levels of inflammatory cytokines, including TNF-α. That is, helminths may do exactly what is needed to improve the immunological functioning of individuals on the autism spectrum. There have now been several clinical studies done on individuals with asthma, allergy, multiple sclerosis (MS), and inflammatory bowel disease. Results have varied depending on the disease and the type of parasite tested and of course may have been affected by the length of the trial and the dosages used. However, multiple trials have now demonstrated significant positive effects of helminths on these disease. Anecdotally, many people have now benefitted enormously from therapeutic doses of parasites for diseases such as MS, inflammatory bowel disease, asthma and allergy, Samter's triad, Sjögren's syndrome, and of course autism.

Over the last two years or so, more and more parents have put their children on courses of TSO, which are porcine (pig) whipworm ova (eggs). As these are not native to humans, they live for only two to three weeks in the human gut. Anecdotal reports have been astounding, to say the least. The children are showing global improvements, which are sometimes dramatic. The incidence of negative side effects is extremely low, and consists of nothing more than reports of increased hyperactivity, some agitation, and sleep disturbances.

My son Alex is fifteen years old, and profoundly autistic. In 2002, an endoscopy/colonoscopy showed that he had horrific bowel disease (colitis) and his immune system was so compromised that to live he required intravenous immunoglobulin (IVIG human antibodies) IVs for seven years. I first read of parasite therapy and the hygiene hypothesis (the idea that we are too sterile, too devoid of normal microbiota) in 1999, in an article in *The New York Times*, which described the work being done with TSO by Dr. Weinstock, who at that time was at the University of Iowa. He had tested these worms in seven individuals with inflammatory bowel disease, and had six of them enter remission. The seventh also dramatically improved. I tried to get the University of Iowa to treat Alex, but they refused as he fit none of their criteria. It took me eight years of waiting to be able to get TSO for him, but when I finally did (in October, 2007) Alex's response was as dramatic as I always knew it would be.

Within ten weeks his perpetual stomach bloating began to disappear. His evening screaming attacks stopped as the pain from the gas subsided. His mood become more and more stable—he was happy almost all the time. The changes were remarkable, and this in a child who has rarely responded to any treatment.

Now, many children with autism have responded extraordinarily well to TSO: improved digestive functioning, increased language and cognition, improved social skills, better mood and mood regulation, and more. The average amount of time it takes to begin to observe the changes is about twelve weeks. Some children, however, have certainly taken longer, even up to eighteen weeks. TSO is taken orally: small vials of saline solution containing the invisible ova are drunk every two to three weeks. However, TSO is so expensive at the moment that it is beyond the reach of many families, especially considering that it must be done continuously.

Because of the expense, I looked for other parasites that would do the same and cost less. Alex (as do several other children on the spectrum), now hosts human whipworms (*Trichuris trichiura*) and 50 hookworm, *Necator americanus*. Within eight weeks of his first dose of hookworm, Alex (who at the time was fourteen years old) demonstrated the ability to read for the first time. Currently he is slowly but surely making his way through the *Hooked on Phonics* computer reading program, for the first time in his life has written several letters independently, is doing addition problems—this from a child who, 3 years ago, had never even identified a shape or color. What I have seen in terms of cognitive, behavioral and gut benefits is not exclusive to Alex. Many children with autism now have some form of helminth and have shown similar patterns of global improvement.

Hookworm and whipworm cannot reproduce directly in their host. They live in the intestines and lay eggs, which are passed out in stool. Under certain specific environmental circumstances, the eggs then mature to an infective stage, at which point they can enter the host. (When we lived without modern plumbing and hygiene practices, stool would end up on soil or in water.) Thus, there is no danger of being "infested." If any adverse symptoms do occur, the worms can be destroyed with a dose or two of an anti-parasitic medication, such as Albendazole.

That said, there have not yet been any formal studies done on children with autism, and not even that many on adults with other issues. Those contemplating trying this therapy should be aware that it is untested, not approved by the FDA and that no one can guarantee safety 100 percent. (Then again, this is true for almost all therapies for autism, both accepted and alternative.) For those of you with children over 18 years of age, Mount Sinai Hospital, in New York City, has been recruiting for some time now to do a study on adults with autism and TSO. At the time of writing this though, the study had not yet begun. I live in hope though that some day soon, my revisions of this chapter will contain the results of real clinical trials in our population.

Parasites like TSO are not prescription medications. They are natural substances, purchased on one's own through companies like Ovamed (www.ovamed.org). However, it is a wise idea to proceed only with a doctor's approval and guidance, since Albendazole is a prescription. (TSO will die in two to three weeks anyway, but it is always best to proceed with reasonable caution.)

There is far more we don't know than we do about the immunological causes of autism, the events that have triggered the abnormalities, and mostly the way to remediate the condition. We don't even know if these abnormalities are the cause of autistic symptoms, and if they are the culprit, exactly what mechanisms caused the developmental problems. However, as the parent of a son with autism, and as a clinician, I find it criminal that when I type the words "autism" and "inflammation" into the PubMed database, I get a response of a total of 18 papers published in all of 2010. (Just to put that into perspective, in just January and February of 2011, 38 papers were published on male pattern baldness.) Science is meaningful and crucial—but it moves too slowly to help our children now. Parasite therapy may seem radical to many, but after fifteen years of battling my son's tremendous immune and digestive disorders, and after many years of following the research on the topic, I made the decision (the right one, as it turns out) to proceed. My philosophy was beautifully expressed by Dr. Herbert at the Autism One conference in Chicago, in May, 2008: "When faced with prolonged scientific uncertainty, use your best judgment."

THE HOLISTIC APPROACH TO NEURODEVELOPMENT AND LEARNING EFFICIENCY (HANDLE)

BY CAROLYN NUYENS AND MARLENE SULITEANU

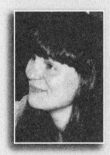
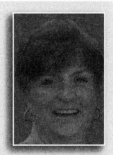

Carolyn Nuyens and Marlene Suliteanu, OTR/L

The HANDLE Institute
7 Mt. Lassen Drive, Suite B110
San Rafael, CA 94903
(415) 479-1800
www.handle.org

Carolyn Nuyens, executive director of The HANDLE Institute, has extensive personal and professional experience in the autism community. She is a Certified HANDLE Practitioner and Instructor. She traveled to India in 2005 with the creator of HANDLE, Judith Bluestone, to introduce HANDLE to the autism community there.

Marlene Suliteanu, OTR/L, also a Certified HANDLE Practitioner and Instructor, with a therapy practice in Oceanside, California, is Judith Bluestone's sister. Judith authored *The Fabric of Autism: Weaving the Threads Into A Cogent Theory* as a semi-autobiographical, in-depth explanation of how HANDLE understands autism.

No two individuals diagnosed with autism present with exactly the same concerns or behaviors. Therefore nothing about HANDLE is arbitrary, standardized, or self-limiting. This article presents both what knowledge HANDLE practitioners share with others who would attempt to help folks on the spectrum, and how the unique HANDLE principles and practices differ from those others.

Characteristics, Commonalities

Although each person on the spectrum is unique, neurodevelopmental characteristics shared by many individuals with autism are:

1. Hypersensitivities, especially auditory, tactile, and vestibular—which means bothered by sounds and irritated by imposed touch sensations (think: seams in socks, tags in shirts, hugs and kisses), and "gravitational insecurity" because the vestibular system tells us how gravity is acting on our bodies.

2. Low muscle tone (throughout the body)—which is about the readiness to respond to task challenges, of which the first and uncontrollable one is gravity itself; and it's what we use to modulate movements (how fast, how hard, etc).

Another experience shared by many on the spectrum: digestive disorders. HANDLE practitioners consider it likely that hypersensitive ears contribute to that, because the jaw is next to the ears. When chewing anything sounds very loud (which it does if our ears are hypersensitive), we avoid chewing, and thus don't start the digestive process soon enough for the stomach to know what enzymes to create. This is only one simple example of how irregularities in one system can cause irregularities in others. There are typically multiple contributing factors to digestive problems that individuals on the spectrum experience.

A commonality considered vital is *language*, especially related to interpersonal relationships and as it affects how some professionals gauge intelligence. Producing intelligible and appropriate language is probably the most complex task anyone achieves: it requires oral-motor precision and learned patterns of movement, and all of that must happen synchronized with breathing. Remember that auditory issues and low muscle tone recur among many individuals on the spectrum; either or both can limit effective spoken communication. Adding in the need to partner right hemisphere (ideas) with left hemisphere (words and sentence structure) complicates the more "physical" elements significantly.

There is a crucial one not yet named: *stress*. When life is difficult—proportional to how challenged anyone feels at any given time—there is an internal experience of stress. For essentially everyone on the autism spectrum, the body/brain baseline level of stress is very high. Anything added to systems already struggling to create and maintain stability can be overwhelming. "Anything" can mean perfumes, crowds (especially of children), household cleaning products, even medications, and always includes performance and behavioral expectations beyond the person's ability.

Because HANDLE practitioners know that, they understand that a "tantrum" or "meltdown" is actually a call for help, a plea to notice that the stress level has overflowed its container. A word of caution to family members: Try to identify what pushed your loved one beyond endurance—and don't expect it to always be the same thing. It could be noise in high-ceilinged supermarkets; or maybe it was the crowds, or smells, or any combination of these things. Always trust that there *is* a precipitating cause.

Who Provides HANDLE Services? Where?

The HANDLE Institute (in San Rafael, CA) confers the credential of Certified HANDLE Practitioner on individuals who have completed (1) a sequence of post-graduate intensive and explicit training programs; (2) a supervised internship, the duration of which is not time-based but competence-based and therefore varies in length from nine months to several years; and (3) an exam for which there are no "right" answers, but rather engaging the intern in processing and reasoning from the HANDLE perspective, and to applying neuroscience creatively and always individually. There are also Certified HANDLE Screeners, but their clientele are usually not on the autism spectrum.

The practitioners represent diverse backgrounds: there are educators, counselors, occupational therapists, a chiropractic neurologist, and others from diverse fields of endeavor. There are practitioners on every continent. Two Canadian provinces have certified practitioners: Ontario and British Columbia. The environment in which HANDLE services occur varies too, but has in common the interpersonal relationship foundation of nonjudgmental respect, and a "physical" manifestation of the core HANDLE premise: stressed systems to do not get stronger. So each site in which you encounter a HANDLE practitioner will strive to minimize sensory disturbance. Practitioners even wear only all-natural clothing without dramatic patterns or harsh colors, and no scents. The site limits auditory or visual distractions. Work surfaces are wood. And you won't find reflective surfaces like mirrors.

What Is a HANDLE Program?

Although there are slight variations specific to the practitioner and the site, basically the program consists of a three-part start-up sequence, followed by six about-monthly Program Review visits.

The start-up sequence:

1. Evaluation

The HANDLE Practitioner provides a comprehensive and sensitive evaluation (usually employing the copyrighted Learning Foundations Inventory) involving interactive tasks; assessment of specific neurodevelopmental functions; and an extensive interview of client, plus in some cases parents and other caregivers, to gather information about particular concerns such as health problems, nutrition, sleep, and pertinent details of the developmental history. The initial evaluation is typically scheduled for two hours, but varies depending on the complexity of the situation and the client's participation.

The HANDLE practitioner observes the individual's response patterns during this unique series of tasks and rapport-building activities. The client's responses are never judged, and do not result in any scores or diagnostic labels. Instead, the responses provide information to help the practitioner see how the body/brain system is working. The practitioner analyzes how the client takes in, processes, and uses information. Seemingly perplexing behaviors come together like pieces of a puzzle, as the HANDLE practitioner analyzes both the individual systems and how the systems interact with each other.

Among the functions and systems considered are:
- Olfaction and gustation (smell and taste)
- Tactility and kinesthesia (touch and movement)
- Vestibular functions (balance, proprioception, muscle tone)
- Visual functions (including visual tracking, convergence, accommodation, and specific light sensitivity)
- Oral motor functions (dental factors, speech articulation)
- Hearing and auditory processing (sequence, syntax, meaning)
- Reflex inhibition and differentiation of movement/response
- Rhythm and timing
- Lateralization (right-versus-left)
- Midline crossing and interhemispheric integration
- Receptive and expressive language skills
- Visual discrimination and memory
- Visual-motor integration
- Visual-spatial processing
- Temporal-spatial organization
- Attentional priorities

2. Instruction: *Neurodevelopmental Profile and Recommended Program*
The practitioner assembles the findings of the evaluation into a chart of those interactive and interdependent sensory-motor systems: what's serving him/her well, and how it does; and what's getting in his/her way, interfering with efficient function. This image is the Neurodevelopmental Profile.

Based on that Profile, the practitioner recommends an initial program of seemingly simple activities, each of which is complex neurologically and addresses several aspects of what interferes with the client's ability to satisfy life's demands efficiently. Two examples: a Crazy Straw, used as instructed, supports focused vision, even bowel and bladder continence, as well as the more obvious oral motor skills; Face

Tapping stimulates the trigeminal nerve to integrate all five senses, affecting speech and auditory sensitivity (especially important to folks on the spectrum). Nutritional recommendations may be made, as well as suggestions for environmental or lifestyle changes to improve functioning and reduce stress.

HANDLE routes each person toward his/her full potential with an individualized program of activities that require virtually no special equipment, to gently enhance functioning. The client is guided through each activity to help his/her brain/body system process and organize information more efficiently. Each HANDLE program is customized for effective implementation in the client's home or other supportive setting. The program usually requires less than a half hour daily to complete, doesn't have to be done all at once, or even in a certain order. Some activities may require support from a helper.

The HANDLE practitioner gives the client whatever materials are needed to do each activity, including written instructions. Both the assessment and the presentation are recorded and the client receives a copy as a DVD.

Among the key distinctions of a HANDLE program is the one principle guiding every kind of sensory-motor activity and other recommendation. It is called Gentle Enhancement. The objective of each recommended activity is to provide organized stimulation without producing stress. Weak, disorganized, damaged, or immature systems need to be "gently enhanced." The parent or caregiver is taught to recognize the signs of a stress state change and deal with it in an effective manner; and the client learns how to identify how the body conveys its needs, to respect them too. Gently enhanced systems get stronger; stressed systems shut down. It's a near-reflexive way that the brain fulfills its primal directive, namely to keep us safe. Honoring the body's signals of what input it can use and what exceeds its tolerance—at all times—earns from the body a comparable kind of respect: the client stabilizes, to enable him/her to function more efficiently.

3. Fine-tuning Follow-up

A week to ten days later the client returns to the practitioner to assure reliable familiarity with everything that was taught: *why* as well as how to implement the program independently. During this one- to two-hour appointment the practitioner watches the client perform all the activities in the program, making corrections or adjustments as needed. Just as importantly, the client is encouraged to give feedback about the program and what was experienced. Often it surprises clients and families that changes can have occurred within that first week, and the practitioner asks about those changes. Video recordings made of all clinical sessions provide the client and caregiver a tool for easy reference at home.

Program Review Visits

After approximately one month of the client-family's implementing the recommendations, they return to the practitioner to determine whether changes that have occurred
due to the neurological reorganization, the creation of neural connections, and/or the
kinesthetic learning warrant different activities. Often the initial program establishes
prerequisites to higher level challenges. This sequencing logic applies thereafter. That
is, as the client implements HANDLE recommendations, changes occur; those changes
represent gains in systems that previously interfered with function; now those systems
can accept additional challenges, toward full functional interaction with the other systems of the body.

Program reviews are usually scheduled every four to six weeks, depending upon
client needs. Some clients choose to receive off-site program reviews, via Skype, or
through e-mail discussion and videotapes/DVDs.

What Changes Can You Expect From a HANDLE Program?

The most frequent report of post-HANDLE behavior changes are "more calm" and
"sleeps better." Other gains: toilet training, eye contact, hair washing, balance, organization, focus—etc.!— including communication skills, both receptive and expressive
language. Given the vast diversity among clients, there is no way to predict changes
precisely. What always happens is gains in the interactive dynamism of all the sensory-
motor systems, and that in turn, enables more efficient functioning, which means less
stress. Combining the strengthened sensory-motor interaction with the client applying
the principle of Gentle Enhancement, and it's easy to understand how a reduced stress
level generalizes. Less stress clearly looks like a "more calm" life, and can allow the
client to sleep better; it also often means better digestion, and a stronger immune
system, thus less susceptible to illness.

A Book About HANDLE

You can find a more extensive explanation of how HANDLE understands autism, in
The Fabric of Autism: Weaving the Threads Into A Cogent Theory, by Judith Bluestone.

HOMEOPATHY—THE HOUSTON HOMEOPATHY METHOD

BY CINDY GRIFFIN AND LINDYL LANHAM

Cindy L. Griffin, DSH-P, DIHom., BME, BCIH, DCNT, FBIH

Homeopathy Center of Houston
7670 Woodway Drive, Suite 340
Houston, TX 77063
(713) 366-8700
www.HomeopathyHouston.com
Info@HomeopathyHouston.com

Ms. Griffin is President/Co-Founder of Homeopathy Center of Houston, and Regent and Instructor of Homeopathic Clinical Studies for Houston School of Homeopathy in Houston, Texas. Trained in sequential and classical homeopathy, and biomedical approaches to autism, she is a regular conference speaker at Autism One, National Autism Conference, and has spoken at international conferences in Australia and Canada. She has authored a four-year curriculum on Sequential Homeopathy, as well as many magazine articles on autism, homeopathic self-care for flu, vaccine injury, women's health, and sits on the editorial board of the Journal of the American Association of Integrative Medicine. She is Board Certified in Integrative Medicine by the American Association of Integrative Medicine. Many children have recovered from autism under her oversight, including her own son, who recovered from Asperger's syndrome with the Houston Homeopathy Method. She and Lindyl Lanham have created the only sequential homeopathic method for autism based on the vaccine injury/biomedical/gut-brain model of autism.

Affiliations and Certifications:
- Board Certified in Integrative Health, AAIM
- Diplomate of College of Natural Therapies, AAIM
- Editorial Board Member, JAAIM
- Board Member, Texas Health Freedom Coalition Steering Committee
- Member Texas Complementary and Alternative Medicine Association
- Fellow of the British Institute of Homeopathy

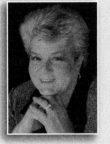

Lindyl Lanham, DSH-P, BS Sp.Ed., BCIH, DCNT

Homeopathy Center of Houston
7670 Woodway Drive, Suite 340
Houston, TX 77063
(713) 366-8700
www.HomeopathyHouston.com
Info@HomeopathyHouston.com

Ms. Lanham is Vice President/Co-Founder of Homeopathy Center of Houston, and primary creator of the Houston Homeopathy Method of Sequential Homeopathy for Autism and ASDs. Their method is the original and only sequential homeopathic method worldwide to be designed around the vaccine injury/biomedical/gut-brain model of autism. She has coauthored a number of articles that have appeared in several autism magazines including *The Autism File*, and *The Autism Perspective* and has been interviewed numerous times for VoiceAmerica and Autism One Radio, among others. She is a regular speaker at Autism One, has spoken at the National Autism Conference, as well as the MINDD conference in Australia and the NuPath conference on homeopathy and autism in Canada. Lindyl worked with autistic children as early as 1972, and continues to focus on autism as her primary specialty. She has seen many children with autism fully recover using the Houston Homeopathy Method under her direction and direct consultation. She is board certified in Integrative Medicine, and is the mother of a son recovered from Tourette's syndrome with the Houston Homeopathy Method and natural medicine.

Affiliations and Certifications:
• Bachelor of Science in Special Education
• Board Certified in Integrative Health, AAIM
• Diplomate of College of Natural Therapies, AAIM

Standing on the shoulders of giants, the Houston Homeopathy Method incorporates the best applications of homeopathic remedies into a cohesive, comprehensive and effective complex method gaining improvements and even full recoveries in children with autism. Sequential homeopathy provides the infrastructure of the approach, clearing the damage of physical, chemical, medical and emotional traumas. Working in reverse chronological order, these traumas are addressed by the use of well-researched, and often bio-medically confirmed, homeopathic remedies appropriate to each event.

References to the Law of Similars can be found in ancient Egyptian papyrus and Greek medical documents, but Samuel Hahnemann, M. D. (1775–1843), is the genius behind modern day homeopathy. His multiple editions of *The Organon* still today provide the guidelines for classical, constitutional or sequential homeopathy.

For over two centuries, homeopathic medical treatment has brought about recovery from acute and chronic health issues for millions of people worldwide in a rapid, gentle and permanent way. Until the 1920s homeopathy accounted for approximately

25 percent of all medicine practiced in the United States. Its renowned use has been long acknowledged throughout the world as a major medical therapeutic approach. In many European communities homeopathy is recognized alongside conventional medicine as an alternative mainstream medical approach.

Homeopathy is founded upon the Law of Similars, *Similia similibus curentur*, or "like cures like" (Gk. *hómoios* = similar to and *páthos* = suffering.) Dr. Hahnemann observed from his experiments with cinchona bark, used as a treatment for malaria, that the effects he experienced from ingesting the bark were similar to the symptoms of malaria. He therefore reasoned that, as a fundamental healing principle, homeopathic remedies must be able to produce symptoms in healthy individuals similar to those of the disease. Upon further experimentation, he realized that by inducing a similar "artificial disease" through the use of a tiny and diluted amount of a substance (a homeopathic remedy) that recovery would follow. For example, peeling an onion causes the eyes to burn, sting, itch and water. These same symptoms are relieved by the use of homeopathic *Allium cepa* (red onion) during a cold or allergy attack.

Over time, Hahnemann discovered that smaller amounts achieved greater therapeutic benefit, and that diluted amounts of substances actually were the most therapeutic while doing no harm. Most homeopathic remedies today, made from minerals as well as botanical and biological sources, are considered "micro-doses" or "nano-doses" of the source substance and are made in pharmaceutical laboratories under current international standards called current Good Manufacturing Practices (cGMP.)

Most homeopaths believe:

- Healing = wholeness.
- True healing is self-healing—living creatures naturally seek balance and health
- Homeopathy's role is to augment the rebalancing and healing process

However, while there are as many ways of practicing as there are homeopaths, two diverse philosophies in the homeopathic world stand out: classical and sequential.

Classical homeopathy focuses primarily on the "Totality of Symptoms" and finding the single remedy that most completely covers all of the client's symptom-pictures. The classically trained homeopath goes into great depth exploring the mental as well as the physical symptoms and searching extensively for the one remedy that appears to envelop not only the greatest number of symptoms but also the greatest number of characteristics composing the client's constitution. The chosen remedy should address the predominate symptoms as well as predominant characteristics and should be prescribed according to minimal dosing laws.

While being first classically trained, the sequential homeopath not only looks at the client symptom-picture, but also at a detailed history of traumatic events. Strongly influenced by the work of Constantine Hering M. D. (1800–1880), the "father of American homeopathy," and author of "Hering's Laws of Direction of Cure," sequential homeopaths focus primarily on the etiology by close examination of the client's history believing that illness occurs when the immune system is compromised or stressed by traumatic events and is no longer functioning optimally. The immune system is charged with resisting and responding to invaders and impacts from physical, chemical and emotional traumas. However, eventually these traumas can weaken the resistance and bring about physiological changes in the body's regulation resulting in illness. Sequential homeopathy uses homeopathic remedies to allow the body to "return to the scene of the crime" and address the damage left behind, harness the resources of the immune system to resist and destroy the offenders in a reverse chronological sequence, allowing the restoration of equilibrium and true health. Employing the natural balancing mechanisms of elimination, respiration, and inflammation (heat which will kill bacteria or viruses) the body will return to homeostasis (balance). Once balance is restored, the body can then reestablish wholeness (self-healing).

With its basis in the sequential therapy work of Jean Elmiger, MD, broadened by an updated view of the use of isopathy (the use of a homeopathic remedy made from an actual pathogen or chemical toxin in order to aid the natural detoxification or clearing of that pathogen or toxin,) the Homeopathy Center of Houston immediately recognized sequential homeopathy as the perfect causation-based starting point for autism. The sequence of homeopathic "clearings" peels away each individual layer comprising the client's personal history of drug, chemical, physical, vaccine, or emotional insults and exposures, all arranged event by event in reverse chronological order according to the client's history, or timeline. Each individual trauma is "cleared" encompassing all the effects of its impact—this means, for instance, that clearing any single event includes the use of multiple remedies derived from carefully chosen homeopathic remedies, as well as isopathic remedies made from pathogens and toxic chemicals included in the insult, to facilitate the immune system as it rebalances or clears itself in order to heal.

Sequential homeopathy is uniquely able to spur the release of cell memories, toxins, viruses, and bacteria trapped in cells, allowing a reduction of the burdens and demands on the immune system over time. Autism is largely viewed as a collision between genetic predisposition and environmental and vaccine insults. Sequential homeopathy can reduce the body burden, while supporting the natural healing processes to undo the damage left behind through this clearing process, in a natural systematic manner.

As a holistic approach, sequential homeopaths consider the emotional state as well as the physical state. In autism, when a child has limited or no speech, remedies that address processing and release trapped emotions can become a major contributor to recovery. If a child processes pent up feelings through dreams or artwork or behavior, the result will always lead to further improvement. Physical healing frequently follows emotional release and healing. Whether recent or farther back historically, as they apply to the event being addressed, emotional healing plays a key role in the child's current level of comfort as well as long-term recovery. Of all ASD therapies, only sequential homeopathy can offer emotional support without the use of drugs.

At the heart of the Houston Homeopathy Method's infrastructure lie vaccine injury and its reversal. While controversial among the medical discussion of autism, parents of children with autism very frequently report that their child regressed significantly after the administration of one or more vaccines. During the process of clearing each individual child's vaccine record, it is not unusual to see a child briefly regress significantly when their regressive vaccine is cleared, followed by a fairly immediate and often dramatic improvement overall. This would tend to support the parent's assertions that the particular vaccine truly contributed largely if not wholly to the child's autism. This phenomenon has been observed repeatedly in hundreds of children who have worked with the Houston Center.

The Homeopathy Center of Houston homeopaths have necessarily gone beyond Hahnemann, Hering and Elmiger in their work with autistic children. Homeopathic analysis of a case typically relies upon a reporting by the client of the most subtle intricacies of their complaints. Because autistic children have limited or no verbal abilities, the Houston homeopaths turned to biomedical research in autism in order to determine what stereotypical behaviors may indicate. Children with autism do not have the benefit of a normally functioning gastrointestinal tract, and because over 70 percent of the immune system resides in the gut, the immune system is also dysfunctional. This means that more supportive remedies must be employed with these children on a daily basis.

Searching for homeopathic solutions to 21st century problems, the approach embraced oligotherapy, gemmotherapy, homotoxicology, cellular reprogramming therapy and German biological medicine. Many of these forms of homeopathic remedies are fast-acting in the area of pain reduction, but with a long-term effect of supporting and improving the efficiency of the entire detoxification and healing process. Most of these children have a history of gut pain, whether expressed or not. Head banging, sudden tantrums, strange posturing and picky eating are all indications of gut discomfort. Proprietary, autism-specific homeopathic combinations developed at the Homeopathy Center of Houston have reduced and relieved gut pain quickly and permanently in many of the children while working through their timelines to the causational issues. After many years of research and study in the biomedical world of autism, a successful case-taking method has been developed to interpret the presenting symptoms as observed by the parents and reported during the monthly consultations.

The uniqueness of the Houston Method is its focus on the vaccine injury, biomedical, gut-brain model of autism, and its application of multiple homeopathic approaches to reverse the problems of autism. The method is systematically designed for that model, yet highly individualized by the practitioners to address each child's needs. This has created a program with a more consistent positive response from autistic children than with classical or sequential homeopathy alone and is accomplished without the use of pharmaceuticals, chelation agents, or large amounts of supplements.

Within the first year, with optimum compliance, approximately 75 percent of the parents report significant improvements in their autism and a small number even report recovery. Most of the recovered children required two to three years of work with the center. Some very difficult and intractable cases have shown encouraging and ongoing improvements.

While many therapies involve an inherent risk of permanent regressions, homeopathy in any form cannot bring on a new pathology. It can only bring to the surface healing processes or detoxification of offending agents and the underlying symptoms those agents caused. The most concerning issues faced at the center involve short-term regressions during the detoxification and clearing period. These are usually symptoms brought on during the mobilization and elimination of toxins, or are temporary healing responses—the body's natural means of rebalancing itself. Typically short-lived, and followed by improvements soon after, some of these regressions may happen intermittently for several months, or even last for a week or more. These can include rashes, fevers, or behavioral regressions. However, these resolve, or wax and wane through the process. A worst-case scenario involves one client who repeatedly broke out in a measles-like rash which at one point covered his body for almost ten days. He also developed an intermittent lack of appetite and other regressive behaviors. While the rash was unpleasant to see, after each event, the rash disappeared, the regressions abated, his speech and focus improved and his diet expanded.

Just one of the many recovered cases involves a seven-year-old boy whose parents had tried many biomedical therapies prior to coming to Homeopathy Center of Houston, some of which caused significant worsening, and others caused significant emotional trauma, such as being strapped to a papoose board during lengthy testing procedures or IV chelation. Once he began the Houston Method, each month he experienced a brief, mild worsening of one or two behaviors for a few days at the "peak of the clear," or an occasional mild rash. Each of these mild regressions or physical symptoms was then followed within a few days by marked improvements in speech, eye contact, interaction, or cognitive and academic function. At almost exactly one year after starting the program, he was functioning with no help in school, had caught up to grade level academically, fully recovered his speech and was indistinguishable from any other normal eight-year-old boy in his class—except for his amazing intellectual curiosity!

Development of the general Houston Homeopathy Method was begun by Cindy Griffin, DSH-P, DIHom., BCIH, DCNT through her general practice, where she expanded on Elmiger's original sequential therapy. Her current area of special interest is the effects of glutamate and strep on OCD and aggression. The Houston Homeopathy Method for Autism and ASDs was introduced and has been constantly updated and greatly expanded from Cindy's earlier work by Lindyl Lanham, DSH-P, BS Sp.Ed., BCIH, DCNT when the practice began to see autistic children in 2002. Lindyl's background included work with blind, deaf and autistic children as early as the 1970s at the Texas School for the Blind's Deaf-Blind Annex, followed by ten years as a special education teacher. Later she homeschooled her two sons, the younger being diagnosed with Tourette's syndrome at the age of eight. He has since 90 percent recovered from the tic disorder through homeopathy, has received his baccalaureate degree and is currently in graduate school. The practice was later joined by Julianne Adams, DSH-P, BCIH, BA Psych, who brought to the method a tireless desire to research strep, nutritional and homeopathic products, and to improve on the method from a holistic viewpoint. Jenice Stebel, DSH-P, DIHom, BCIH has contributed research on the treatment of parasites and strep, as well as being well versed in several special diets for autism. Lynn Rose Demartini, RN, DSH-P, LMT, BCIH, DCN has brought a great deal of medical insight from her years in practice in public health, emergency medicine, massage therapy and as a life-long student of several other holistic therapies. While all homeopaths follow the same basic approach, The Houston Homeopathy Method of sequential homeopathy continues to grow and improve through regular case conferences, and a devotion by all its practitioners to continuing education and research. All practitioners are Board Certified in Integrative Medicine by the American Association of Integrative Medicine (AAIM). Cindy Griffin and Lindyl Lanham are Diplomates of the AAIM College of Natural Therapies, and Lynn Demartini is a Diplomate of the AAIM College of Nursing.

HOMOTOXICOLOGY AND BEYOND

BY MARY COYLE

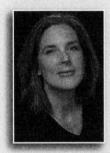

Mary Coyle, D.I.Hom

Real Child Center
1133 Broadway, Rm. 1015
New York, NY 10010
(212) 255-4490
www.realchildcenter.com

Mary Coyle, D.I.Hom, has been consulting with families of children with autism for over 12 years, and in 2009, founded the Real Child Center in New York City. She works in collaboration with a number of DAN physicians, neurologists, naturopaths, nutritionists, classical homeopaths and chiropractors in the surrounding NY area. She received a BSc from the Univ. of Washington, and obtained her Diploma in Homeopathy in 2000. She has been personally trained by some of the experts in the field, including Jean Elmiger MD, creator of Sequential Homeopathy, and author of "Rediscovering Real Medicine," and German naturopath, Dr Andreas Marx. Along with her colleague Sandra Stewart, Mary conducted a MPI teleconference entitled, "Autism Solutions," and is co-creator of the Stewart-Coyle Holistic Practitioner Course. For two years she hosted an Autism One radio show covering bio-energetic healing, and has presented at LIA, Autism One and the NAA in New York City.

As more research is devoted to the science of environmental health, toxicology, and epigenetics, the public is gaining vast new insights into how and why toxic exposures (both exogenous and endogenous) effect the health of our children. Perhaps the question, "Is your child in the autistic spectrum?" might one day be replaced with, "How toxic is your child?"

Toxins and their impact on human health were indeed the passion of Germany physician Dr. Hans-Heinrich Reckeweg, who developed the theory of Homotoxicology over 60 years ago. Through integrating two well-established healing systems, the principles of homeopathy (like cures like) and medical science, Reckeweg developed a

systematic approach designed to stimulate the body's own defense mechanism to produce and promote self-healing and self-regulation.

Derived from three words, "homo" meaning man, "toxico" meaning toxin, and
"logy," from the Greek word, and "logos" meaning study, thus homotoxicology means
the study of toxins on humans. And functioning as a holistic approach, homotoxicology
is not designed to simply focus on just one particular pathogen or toxic metal, and then
shoots to kill. Instead, it suggests to systemically supports the body's physiologically
which allows it to effectively manage its own pathology.

Toxins and How they Relate to the Child with Autism

A national human adipose tissue study determined that most, if not all, humans carry a
toxic body burden of at least 250 chemicals. No matter how pristine a lifestyle *we think*
we're living, there's simply no way of escaping them. Equally disturbing, this toxic load
doesn't just sit quietly in our biological terrain. Scientific studies show but a portion
of that toxic load is passed-down transgenerationally, from mother to fetus, and even
expressed through breast milk. As one out of every four American child is now diagnosed with a chronic illness, researchers and lay people alike are inquiring more than
ever as to the etiology of this health crisis. What role does this ever-increasing barrage
of environmental toxins potentially play into the dramatic increase in not just autism,
but chronic illnesses and autoimmune diseases as well?

Traits Versus Syndromes

To answer that question some researchers suggest we look to our wildlife. Theo
Colburn, Senior Scientist of the World Wildlife Fund, cited in her acclaimed book,
"Our Stolen Future" that scientists research trends in our wildlife by identifying and
observing *traits* such as, IQ decrements, behavior aberrations, and physical malformations. However, when it comes to investigating human health, the model shifts to *syndromes,* which are then translated into diseases or disorders, such as multiple sclerosis,
asthma, diabetes, ADHD and Autism. Identifying syndromes simplifies and standard-
izes illness to assist the medical community to determine the most appropriate pharmaceutical, surgical, etc. intervention. But the rise in autism and the common ailments
many seem to share, such as gastrointestinal stress, gut and brain inflammation, food
sensitivities, and immune dysfunction, have pushed the scientific and ASD community
beyond the classic syndrome/pharmaceutical model. Parents of children with autism
are continually re-inventing the word "detox" and discovering new and innovative
ways to restore their child's health. Homotoxicology is quickly becoming one of those
primary methods.

The Green Movement and Autism

There's no doubt about it, the public is willing to pay more to keep the chemicals out. In only the last several decades, the word "organic" has popped-up all over the consumer marketplace—attaching its name to everything from bedding to bug spray. Parents of children with autism, along with their physicians, are rolling up their sleeves, and digging deeper than ever before to uncover their child's toxic load–testing hair, saliva, urine, stools, and blood for all kinds of chemicals, heavy metals and pathogens. Undoubtedly, identifying the toxic load of these children, other than just the routine serum lead levels provided through yearly check-ups, has provided valuable insights and potential therapeutics for many children with autism.

Homotoxicology and Beyond Begins with the Terrain

One of the primary goals of homotoxicology is simply to supply the body with enough strength and fortitude to ignite the healing process. In other words—to dump the junk. Analogous to this thinking is to imagine a tree covered with fungal over-growth. We spray that tree with a fungicide, and if we're lucky, it might never show up again. If we're not lucky, it grows back. In which case, we spray again. If the fungus stubbornly returns, we often take more aggressive measures. The unfortunate side-effect is that with each subsequent, and more robust, fungicide treatment, the tree becomes more compromised. The fungus becomes more opportunistic, and now we're functioning in a vicious downward spiral towards disease.

A more green, or holistic, approach is to supply the tree with the necessary tools to garner adequate vitality to manage its own fungus. With proper light, mineral- rich soil, clean air and water, etc. the tree might now have what it takes to manage its own fungus. Of course, this is a much more difficult route than merely dousing it with chemical sprays. In addition, if one critical aspect is amiss, such as not providing the tree with sufficient light, the fungus may grow back. As they say in Chinese medicine, you have to surround the dragon, or it will always be chasing its tail. The same hold true with homotoxicology.

Needless to say, minimizing as many stressors as possible will expedite the autistic child's healing process: Reducing EMF exposures, determining food sensitivities, healing gut dysbiosis, creating enough down-time, are just a few challenges to be resolved as we surround the dragon. No easy task in this ever-increasing toxic and stressful world.

Beginning the Journey of Homotoxicology

In his model, Dr. Reckeweg has broken-down all diseases, and categorized them under three processes.

- Excretion of the toxin: Such as diarrhea, skin eruptions, mucous, fever, cough
- Deposition (deposits) of the toxins: Such as warts, hemorrhoids, cysts
- Degeneration through the actions of the toxins: Such as Autism, diabetes, MS, lupus, neoplasms

Reckeweg viewed disease as the body's *meaningful* biological response to homo-toxins; and its attempt to remove them. He refers to toxins as homotoxins (toxins derived from by the body itself, environmental pollution or pharmaceutical interventions). The primary focus being the cause (homotoxins) that is distressing the system, and not just the symptoms.

Table of Homotoxicosis

Essential to the effectiveness of homotoxicology is the unblocking of the enzymatic system. Enzymes act as catalysts for the mobilization, and excretion of the toxins. To avoid confusing a healing reaction for a disease state, Reckeweg developed The Six Phases Table. The Table acts as a guide to understanding the various psychological and physiological changes one works through during the process of removing the toxins. Many practitioners of homotoxicology feel that understanding these reaction modes is essential to the therapy's success.

The Excretion, inflammation, Deposition Phase are in the Humoral Phases. This occurs when the enzymes have remained intact, enabling the progression towards the natural removal of toxins (termed Regressive Vicariation) through the various excretion pathways. The toxins have not yet reached a saturation point, and remain in the extracellular tissues. The primary pathways of elimination include the skin, liver, kidney intestines, mucous membranes and lymphatic system. The secondary pathways include the nose, lungs, stomach, genitals, bladder and pancreas.

The Impregnation, Degeneration and Neoplasm phase are in the Cellular Phases. This occurs when damage has been done to the enzymatic system and therefore, the toxins cannot be completely eliminated, leading to the development of deterioration (termed Progressive Vicariation). A saturation point of the toxin(s) has been reached, and the toxins have begun penetrating the cells.

The Child with Autism and the Table of Homotoxicosis

It's not uncommon to hear parents remark that their child with autism has never, or no longer, mounts a fever. Or that their skin is pale and translucent, even during the summer months. That their eyes are dull with dark circles underneath, and the pupils are often dilated. That undigested food is often found in the stool, or that they are chronically constipated. Or that they never stop moving (aka—wired but tired). According to Six Phases Table, the child with autism might fall somewhere between the Impregnation and Degeneration Phase. This is no surprise, as recent research has uncovered a sub-population of ASD children suffering from mitochondrial distress, and lack the proper cellular metabolism to efficiently perform necessary metabolic functions. In short, it appears that there's just not enough tiger in the ASD child's tank.

The Flow System and the Child with Autism

At the turn of the century, biologist Ludwig Von Bertalanffy, described every living system (man, bird, slug) as systems of flowing elements, designed to gain and maintain balance. According to the tenets of homotoxicology, substances which disrupt the flow system (homotoxins) will inevitably cause disease. Reckeweg stated "Illness is the expression of the action of the greater defense system against homotoxins, or the organism's attempt to compensate for the damage caused by homotoxins." How the body effectively, or ineffectively, deals with these homotoxins can relate back to disturbances in the flow system. Reckeweg developed his chart to monitor the reactions through the Six Phases Table. If the "flow system" is severely blocked, reducing sufficient energy production, this could result in metabolic acidosis, creating an acid environment. This becomes a perfect breeding ground for the proliferation of microorganism (think back to the tree analogy), and the biological terrain is disrupted. Toxic waste products and microforms poison the body, thus increasing acidity. This further increases opportunistic microorganism, and decreases cellular energy—and increases inflammation. And the vicious cycle continues . . .

Homotoxicological Remedies

Homotoxicological products activate what Reckeweg called the "greater defense system," which is a collective biological response to react, neutralize and eliminate homotoxins. Some of these products include drainage remedies, which are complex preparations, (mixtures of homeopathic and herbs). Drainage remedies are usually organ-specific, designed to drain the liver, kidneys, lymph, adrenals, colon, etc. Other remedies include homeopathic cellular supports products designed to supply the body with the vitality it needs to stimulate organ systems and immune function. Low-potency homeopathic formulations specially geared for each individual, such as nosodes and sarcodes, are also primary tools employed in homotoxicology. In essence, biotherapeutic support products assist the body's physiology to move the toxins out, as well as facilitate more efficient blood flow, which instigates faster healing.

AND BEYOND . . . .

Functioning as the template, and working in the systematic fashion, homotoxicology can incorporate other health strategies (which support the biological terrain) into its matrix to maximize therapeutic results. If a child is hovering in the degeneration phase, most practitioners of homotoxicology would consider it wise to starting-off slowly, so that you may move quickly down-the-road. This is accomplished first through property drainage of the eliminative pathways, and concentrating on supplying the body with adequate cellular energy and support. Rebuilding with proper supplementation and nutritionals is also an essential step before integrating more physically challenging interventions.

Tracking Progress

What are some things to look for as your child begins to rebound in a positive direction through the Six Phases Table? Some parents have reported better eye contact; improved receptive and expressive language; happier and more interested in life and new things; more comfortable in their own skin; more integrated and grounded; sleeps longer and more deeply; improved bowel movements; tans and/or sunburns in the summer; catches the family cold or flu (garbage in, garbage out); makes more connections physically, emotionally and cognitively; gains weight and height; better gross and fine motor skills. Some have even remarked that their child no longer seems to be functioning in "survival mode," and is simply not as stressed-out, and therefore, more available to learn. Lab tests are also excellent vehicles for tracking and verifying these improvements.

The Evidence

One of the more notable articles includes, "Critical Review and Meta-Analysis of Serial Agitated Dilutions in Experimental Toxicology," where it states that, "Four of five outcomes meeting quality and comparability criteria for meta-analysis showed positive effects from SAD preparations." (SAD meaning serial agitated dilutions.). Authors include Dr. Wayne B. Jonas, former Director of the Office of Alternative Medicine at the National Institutes of Health.[1]

Where Would Homotoxiciology Fit Into Your ASD Child's Plan?

In consider homotoxicology analogous to a degreasing agent. Addressing cellular toxicity is like taking the grease off cellular walls to enable subsequent therapies to stick just that much better. Many parents have experienced different results using the tenets of homotoxicology. Some have reported amazing gains, while others cited slow-but-steady improvement. And then of course, there are those who are just non-responders. Our family found homotoxicology in 1995 after our son was diagnosed with autism. Looking for a therapy centered around removing toxins without *negatively impacting the active immunity*, homotoxicology resonated with our thinking and desire the find a safe, yet effective means of restoring his health and removing the blockages. He's make remarkable progress ever since.

A Final Thought

In the early years, while desperately searching for someone to rescue our son from the abyss of autism, a very smart mom gave me some very sound advice. She warned me of the peril of latching on to a guru. Keeping a watchful eye, and performing regular lab tests to track and tweak my son's program, put me firmly in the driver's seat. Don't be intimated to pick the brains of physicians, therapists and parents–as you, and your trusted team, continually make tough decisions as to what to put in, and take out, of your child's therapy cart. And thanks to recent breakthroughs in neuroscience proving that the brain is always changing itself–at *any* age, we are now armed with the scientific evidence that utilizing strategies to elevate health, coupled with the right physical, emotional and cognitive stimulation- there's plenty of reason to stay hopeful.

INTEGRATED PLAY GROUPS MODEL

BY DR. PAMELA WOLFBERG

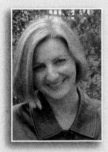

Pamela Wolfberg, Ph.D.

Autism Institute on Peer Relations and Play
Integrated Play Groups Training,
Research and Development Center
www.AutismInstitute.com or www.wolfberg.com
info@wolfberg.com

Associate Professor/Director, Autism Spectrum Program
Department of Special Education
San Francisco State University,
1600 Holloway Avenue
San Francisco,
CA 94132,
(415) 338-7651.
Wolfberg@sfsu.edu

Pamela Wolfberg, Ph.D. is Associate Professor and Director of the Autism Spectrum program at San Francisco State University and co-founder of the Autism Institute on Peer Relations and Play.. She received her doctorate from the University of California, Berkeley. As originator of the Integrated Play Groups (IPG) model, she leads research, training and development efforts to establish inclusive peer socialization programs worldwide. She is widely published and the author of *Play and Imagination in Children with Autism* and *Peer Play and the Autism Spectrum: The Art of Guiding Children's Socialization and Imagination*. She is the recipient of several distinguished awards for her scholarship, research and service to the community.

Integrated Play Groups (IPG) is an empirically validated model for promoting socialization, communication, play, and imagination in children on the autism spectrum, while building relationships with typical peers and siblings in natural settings. (Wolfberg, 2009, 2003) The model is grounded in current theory, research, and practice pertinent to addressing core challenges in autism that affect both social and representational aspects of play. Embedded in this model are methods for observing, interpreting, and building on children's play interests and social communicative abilities, and for designing environments conducive to social and imaginative play.

Conceptually, the IPG model is described as multidimensional, encompassing developmental and ecological features that are framed in sociocultural theory. (Vygotsky, 1966; 1978) In practical terms, an IPG brings together children with autism (novice players) in mutually engaging play experiences with more capable peer play partners (expert players) while guided by a qualified adult facilitator (play guide). Each IPG is individualized as a part of a child's comprehensive educational and therapy program. IPG programs take place in natural settings, including in the home, school and community. Group members range from three to five players with a higher ratio of expert to novice players. Each group meets twice weekly for thirty to sixty minutes sessions over a twelve-week period, or longer. Play sessions are tailored to the unique interests, developmental capacities, and sociocultural experiences of child participants.

Drawing on finely tuned assessments, the IPG intervention (guided participation) provides a system of support for maximizing each child's developmental potential and intrinsic motivation to play, socialize, and form meaningful relationships with other children. Equal emphasis is placed on guiding the typical peers to be more accepting, responsive, and inclusive of children who may present differing ways of playing communicating and relating to others. Moreover, novice and expert players are encouraged to mediate their own play activities with as little adult guidance as possible.

The IPG model was created by Pamela Wolfberg, Ph.D. (Associate Professor and Director of the Autism Spectrum Program, San Francisco State University, and cofounder of the Autism Institute on Peer Relations and Play). In its early conception, Dr. Wolfberg worked in close collaboration with Adriana Schuler, Ph.D. (Professor Emeritus, SFSU) and Therese O'Connor, MA (Co-founder of the Autism Institute on Peer Relations and Play). Over the years, the model has continued to evolve and expand, owing to the collective efforts of many other remarkable professionals, family members and the children themselves participating in local, national and international training, research, and development initiatives.

The IPG model was first initiated as a pilot research project in an urban elementary school, with a small grant from the San Francisco Education Fund. (Wolfberg, 1988) Based on the preliminary success of this project, the IPG model was expanded through a model demonstration and research project that was supported, in part, through a grant from the United States Department of Education. (Wolfberg & Schuler, 1992) In 2000, the Autism Institute on Peer Relations and Play (www.autisminstitute.com) was established as a center for IPG training, research, and development. Opportunities for IPG training, research, and development are also offered as a part of the Autism Spectrum Graduate Program (Project Mosaic) at SFSU (www.sfsu.edu~autism), and in conjunction with our other major research projects with support from Autism Speaks (Wolfberg, Turiel & DeWitt, 2008) and the Alexander von Humboldt Foundation. (Julius & Wolfberg, 2009)

A wide range of professionals and family members have received initial preparation for applying the practices of the IPG model in inclusive settings. To become fully
qualified to formally deliver the IPG model as a program or service with an official
endorsement (i.e., certification) from the Autism Institute on Peer Relations and Play
requires intensive training and supervision at the advanced level. Advanced training
comprises a competency-based curriculum that draws on the foundational book: *Play
and Imagination in Children with Autism* (Wolfberg, 2009) and the IPG Field Manual
Peer Play and the Autism Spectrum: The Art of Guiding Socialization and Imagination.
(Wolfberg, 2003)

Currently, the IPG model is being adopted by increasing numbers of schools and
organizations at the local, national, and international level. The expansion of programs
around the globe coincides with the IPG model having gained widespread recognition as among established research-based practices for children on the autism spectrum. (see for example: California Department of Education, 1997; Iovannone, 2003;
National Autism Center, 2009) This is consistent with the recommendations of the
National Research Council, (2001) which has ranked the teaching of play skills with
peers among the six types of interventions that should have priority in the design and
delivery of effective educational programs for children on the autism spectrum.

To address the growing need to support diverse learners on the autism spectrum
and their families, extensions of the IPG model are also emerging through collaborative efforts. Incorporated into the model are such innovations as sensory integration,
drama, art, video and other creative activities of high interest for children as well as
teens. (see for example Bottema, 2008; Fuge & Berry, 2004; Neufeld & Wolfberg, 2009;
Wolfberg & Julius, 2009; Wolfberg, McCracken & Tuchel, 2008) Another current initiative is focused on universal playground design and programming that supports the
unique social, imaginative, and sensory needs of children on the autism spectrum in
mutually engaging experiences with peers and siblings. (Wolfberg, 2010) These newer
efforts are currently at various stages of development and investigation.

Success Rate

The IPG model has an established and growing research base documenting ample evidence of a high success rate. A series of small- and large-scale studies have been and are
currently being conducted to evaluate and replicate the IPG model. (Gonsier-Gerdin,
1993; Lantz, Nelson & Loftin, 2004; Mikaelan, 2003; O'Connor, 1999; Richard & Goupil,
2005; Wolfberg, 1988; 1994; 2009; Wolfberg & Julius, 2009; Wolfberg & Schuler, 1992;
1993; Wolfberg, Turiel, & DeWitt, 2008; Yang, Wolfberg, Wu & Hwu , 2003; Zercher,
Hunt, Schuler & Webster, 2001) Most investigations have been focusing on the effect of
the intervention on the social, communication, and play development of children with

autism, representing diverse abilities (mild to moderate to severe), ages (three to eleven years), settings (community, home, school) , geographic locations (Asia, Europe, North America) and languages (English, French, German, Chinese). Social validation measures assessing parent perceptions of the impact of the intervention on their children with autism have also been included.

Overall, outcomes for the children with autism consistently show relative gains in social, communication, and play development. Specifically, decreases in isolate and stereotypic play have been noted, along with collateral gains in increasingly socially coordinated play and representational play (functional and pretend). Language gains also have been noted in several cases. Further, the evidence suggests that skills may be maintained after adult support is withdrawn. The data also supports evidence of generalization beyond the specific IPG across peers/siblings, settings, and social activity contexts.

The attitudes, perceptions, and experiences of the expert players have been explored through observation and interviews with play guides and the children themselves. Findings to date suggest that the peers developed greater sensitivity, tolerance, and acceptance of the novice players' individual differences. They also articulated a sense of responsibility as well as an understanding of how to include the less skilled players by adapting to their different interests and styles of communication. Novice and expert players also reported having fun while forming mutual friendships extending beyond the IPG.

Risk and/or side-effects

There are no known risks or side effects associated with the IPG model when implemented with fidelity.

INTEGRATIVE EDUCATIONAL CARE

BY DR. MARY JOANN LANG

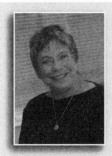

Mary Joann Lang, PhD

Beacon Day School
588 N. Glassell Street
Orange, CA 92867
(714) 288-4200
(714) 288-4204 fax
www.beacondayschool.com

Dr. Mary Joann Lang founded Beacon Day School in June 2004 for students with autism spectrum disorder (ASD) and related disabilities. Dr. Lang also founded Beacon Autistic Spectrum Independence Center, an in-home therapy-based program for children with ASD. Throughout her career, Dr. Lang has worked with children diagnosed with ASD and has lectured widely on the topic. She has been involved with the care of children for more than 25 years, first as a nurse practitioner and educator, then as an educational psychologist. Dr. Lang has many professional publications.

In 1988, Dr. Lang graduated from the University of Southern California with her PhD in educational psychology. A Diplomate of the American Board of Neuropsychology, Dr. Lang has been a practicing, licensed neuropsychologist since 1991. A member of several professional organizations, including the National Academy of Neuropsychology, Dr. Lang is also an associate professor at Azusa Pacific University.

Using an innovative model that will enhance learning is critical to academic, social-emotional, and motor development. An integrated approach to learning will provide students with more learning opportunities and thus be able to generalize their knowledge, social skills, and motor ability. Understanding this approach is critical to educational planning. The goal of education in a student's life needs to focus on the whole child versus simply the results of standardized testing, which may skew the teacher's perspective of the student's ability.

In order to understand the whole child, the following areas need to be considered in planning for a child's education: cognition, educational achievement, adaptive behavior, social roles, health, and context. Since schools primarily look at cognitive functioning and academic achievement in terms of placement, teaching strategy, and therapies, these cognitive functions need to be understood in greater depth.

Definition and Need

Traditional models of education are not effective for children with an autism diagnosis as they have challenges in communication, adaptive behavior, social skills, and self-regulation. Behavior issues arise because of these deficits. Integrated educational care has been gaining new ground in recent years. An integrated educational model is necessary for children with autism in order for them to reach their highest potential. A model like this looks at both strengths the child possesses and challenges they face. Understanding these will help to identify areas in need of support, informing the educator as to how to enhance the child's learning environment.

An integrated educational model focuses on many different subjects and goes beyond the traditional classroom that uses textbooks to teach children concepts and ways of doing things. For example, Beacon Day School uses this approach in teaching students with autism and related disabilities. At Beacon Day School, integration is used on two different levels: 1) integrating necessary therapies such as speech and language, physical, and occupational therapy into the student's day; and 2) integrating academic skills in order to enhance generalization.

This integrated educational model incorporates flexible schedules and student groups in order to cater to individual learning and what the individual child needs most. Rather than looking at just the student, an integrated curriculum focuses on all the facets that connect and influence the world of the student. In an integrated educational model, the focus is on cognition (attention, memory, language, visual/spatial functioning, reasoning, and coping strategies), educational achievement, adaptive behavior, social skills, and health, with all of these examined within the context of the child's home, school, and community. With all of this in mind, the focus can be on the whole child and the surrounding spheres of influence.

The concept of integrated curriculum has been around for quite some time, but has only recently been applied within the educational setting. According to Humphreys, Post, and Ellis (1981), integrated educational care is "one in which children broadly explore knowledge in various subjects related to certain aspects of their environment" (pp.11). In this sense, learning and teaching are seen in a holistic view that is interactive. Within an integrated educational care framework, there are many levels of integration. It can include implementing objectives that overlap with goals listed on the child's Individualized Education Program (IEP), implementing model lesson plans that involve activities across assessments, enriching or enhancing students' abilities through specific activities that focus on communication skills and ways of relating to others through community based instruction, and implementing assessment activities that examine a wide range of functional capacities (Palmer, 1991). An integrated model with this basis will provide students with unified knowledge, while still encouraging them to learn new things. With an integrated educational model centered on these principles, the student will be prepared for lifelong learning.

Educational Planning

As was mentioned previously, in order to understand the whole child, the following areas need to be considered in planning for a child's education: cognition, educational achievement, adaptive behavior, social roles, health, and context. It is important to understand how these areas function, what behaviors and symptoms arise due to challenges in these areas, and what interventions and accommodations can be utilized to help the child grow in these areas.

Cognition

Cognition involves many different areas of functioning that include: attention and information processing, sensory-motor function, language, executive function, memory and learning, social skills, and emotional function. Parents and teachers need to be aware of the individual child's limitations in these areas and emphasize their strengths that will help them overcome these limitations.

ATTENTION AND INFORMATION PROCESSING

In order to function in everyday life and complete schoolwork successfully, a child needs to have good attention and information processing abilities. Attention involves selective attention (choosing what to listen to), shifting attention (moving from one stimuli to another), divided attention (splitting attention between two things), and sustained attention (staying focused on one thing for a long period of time). If a child has poor attention and information processing, they may have difficulty initiating focus, sustaining focus, and maintaining a train of thought. Difficulties in processing information may involve the need for repetition of instructions and an extended time to complete assignments and tasks.

Therapies and accommodations that are focused on these two areas of functioning should start with structuring the learning environment and eliminating distractions. This involves a set routine/schedule so that the child knows what is expected each day. Different sheets can be developed, such as note sheets and flow charts, in order to help the child visualize and take in information as well as keep information manageable and in limited quantities to avoid information overload.

SENSORY-MOTOR FUNCTION

This area of functioning includes a child's gross–and fine-motor skills. Gross-motor skills involve large muscles working to accomplish a task and include balance, body posture, and coordination. Fine-motor skills involve more specific ways of functioning, such as holding a pencil and writing letters. While some children with autism may be particularly strong in this area, many have great difficulty with these aspects of functioning due to underdeveloped muscles. Examples of difficulties in this area include sensitivity or lack of sensitivity to touch and textures, poor pencil grip, poor hand-eye coordination, impaired speech, and poor balance.

Physical activities should be encouraged for children with autism in a structured setting. Occupational and physical therapists can aid in helping children with autism to develop gross-and fine-motor skills. Additionally, sensory integration therapy can help by implementing a sensory diet, focusing on sensory-based activities, and applying pressure to joint areas in order to provide a calming and soothing environment.

LANGUAGE

Language involves many different ways of communicating, including speech, listening, reading, writing, and interpreting information. Different ways of processing language include auditory processing (understanding speech sounds), oral expression (linguistic competencies and oral vocabulary), and receptive language (listening to and interpreting information). Challenges in any one of these areas associated with language can result in not listening, difficulty with word problems, limited vocabulary, and difficulty with interpreting information.

Visual cues can be incorporated in order for lessons and instructions to be well received by the child. Careful attention should be paid to words and meanings in order to increase vocabulary. Study sheets, outlines, and note pads can be incorporated to aid in attention and learning of new words and meanings. Time extensions may be necessary for tests and assignments in order to make sure the child is optimally learning the material. Necessary information should be reinforced and repeated to stress importance.

EXECUTIVE FUNCTION

Executive function is considered to be the "conductor" of many different cognitive processes. It involves planning, organizing, flexibility, abstract thinking, rule acquisition, and self-regulation. Children with autism have a difficult time organizing, multitasking, and prioritizing information. They have difficulty planning for due dates of homework assignments and dates of upcoming tests.

Teachers, parents, and mental health professionals should provide children with autism structure in their daily activities. They can be taught responsibility for personal items through reminders and modeling done by the adult. Organizational tools can be provided that will help the child gain more order and control in their assignments and general life.

MEMORY AND LEARNING

Memory is comprised of four different groups: short-term memory (recall up to a minute without rehearsing material), long-term memory (information remembered for a long time), working memory (separation of different information such as visual and verbal), and comprehensive knowledge (information that is rehearsed and able to be recalled). These aspects of memory make it possible for the individual to receive, recall, store, and hold information. Challenges in this area take the form of inattention, inability to recall information, frustration, and difficulty following long, detailed directions.

Interventions may involve repetition of information to increase storage of information. The teacher should break up information into small parts and provide cues to assist in recall of information. Lists and charts can help students to remember information. The learning environment should be relaxed in order to alleviate pressure.

SOCIAL SKILLS

Positive ways of relating to others aid in developing friendships and avoiding being mistreated by others. Social skills involve communication, tone of voice, sense-of-humor, and the ability to take on another person's perspective. Nonverbal social skills are also important and involve active listening, relaxed manner, and confidence. Individuals with autism tend to lack social skills, including difficulty recognizing social cues and being unaware of boundaries.

Different recreational activities like clubs and sports teams can help facilitate communication and development of friendships. The environment should be enjoyable and non-threatening to boost communication skills.

EMOTIONAL FUNCTION

Being able to regulate one's emotional state helps to prevent an over–or under–reaction in a situation. Instances that may bring about an emotional reaction are requests to complete assignments, reacting to separations, and relational conflicts. Challenges in this area may include: blaming others for problems, tantrums, pulling away from others, clinging to others, frustration, and restlessness.

Discussing thoughts, feelings, and behaviors could help in regulating emotion. Role-playing different situations can help prepare an individual for an emotionally-charged situation. Teaching children to discuss their feelings helps them feel understood. The student should be able to retreat to a calm area that avoids overstimulation.

Educational Achievement

Individuals achieve at different rates. Individual education plans can help identify areas in which a child needs to grow as well as areas of strength. Outlining specific areas of need will help the team to collaborate on what interventions to use for the student. Teaching strategies and interventions are tailored to the individual child's strengths that can help them overcome areas of weakness.

Adaptive Behavior

Adaptive skills are necessary for helping a child thrive within their home, school, and community. Having the skills to adjust one's behavior in a particular environment or situation will help to prevent disruptive behavior. This can be achieved through community-based activities, vocational activities, and implementation of coping skills.

Participation, Interactions, and Social Roles

Understanding one's role in society and ways of acting appropriately are synonymous with social skill development. Specialized guidance can help children learn how to interact appropriately with others. Team building activities can help children understand ways of relating to others and recognize the perspectives of others.

Health

Individuals with autism have a variety of health issues that include allergies and seizure disorders. These issues can hinder educational progress. Teachers should be aware of medical conditions the child is suffering from and stay current on their medical treatment plans through collaboration with the family and primary care physician. Dietary interventions and implementation of medicines may be used to help with health issues.

Context

Intervention should be implemented in the home, school, and community environments. Continuity of care is important in enhancing overall development. This can be a time of learning and collaboration among parents, school staff, and health professionals.

Even with the best intentions and interventions, disruptive behaviors may occur in the classroom. The best intervention strategy for managing behaviors is applied behavior analysis (ABA). Behaviors may occur that might inhibit the use of an integrated model in the classroom. Therefore, some effective classroom environmental strategies need to be considered. There are several examples that include:

- Establishing rules and expectations for appropriate classroom behavior.
- Developing rules and procedures that are practiced by students with the help of teachers.
- Making students aware of the rewards for following the rules as well as the consequences if they do not.
- Create a warm and inviting learning environment.
- Implement a daily educational schedule that provides structure to the classroom.
- Design and model positive alternatives to challenging behaviors.
- Monitor behavior and, if problems arise, alter interventions to meet the needs of the student.

Beacon Model for Integration

Consideration of challenges in functioning aids in the establishment of a supportive environment that enhances self-esteem, recognizes individual strengths, and identifies areas in need of support. Parents, teachers, children, and professionals should work as a team in order to try to achieve established goals. Growth and learning occur at all times of the day and positive reinforcements should remain consistent throughout the day, both at school and at home. Conferences, IEP meetings, home visits, and informal meetings should all be utilized to enhance communication and collaboration between team members.

Regular reports about behavior and performance in school should be provided to parents. It would also be helpful for parents to share information about the child's behavior outside of school. Progression in all areas of development is dependent upon structure and consistency in the home, school, and community.

The child is understood in context. This means that each area of development: communication, social skills, motor skills, academic accomplishment, and others will be related to the cognitive functions discussed above (memory, emotions, attention, language, visual-spatial skills, executive function, and health) to ensure that all is functioning in a way that promotes development. A main focus is on identifying areas in need of growth and support that affect the overall performance of the child. Attention to detail is important, especially when looking at specific areas of cognition.

Autism influences cognitive, emotional, physiological, and social development. Each area needs to be addressed when looking at the whole child. Therapies and interventions are selected for the individual child so that they can function at their best within the home, school, and community. An integrative model that focuses on the whole child in context goes beyond what the IEP addresses and looks at all of the contributors to the diagnosis of autism. Identifying these will help the team to develop positive ways of influencing the child's overall condition. As one area of functioning improves, other areas will follow in the path towards positive developmental growth.

Why Integrate?

An integrative educational model provides an opportunity for collaboration among students, teachers, and parents. It engages students in the learning process and is an exciting change to the traditional educational model. Approaching the whole child promotes continuity in functioning across a wide range of contexts. The integrative educational model is designed to be enjoyable and motivating, not only for the student but for their surrounding support system as well. Gaining support from the community and utilizing resources within the community encourages development of a partnership and erases stigmas. The goal is to promote optimal functioning of the individual student in many developmental areas in order for the student to thrive within the home, school, and community.

INTESTINE, LEAKY GUT, AND AUTISM: IS IT REAL AND HOW TO FIX IT (INCLUDING WITH PROBIOTICS)?

BY DR. ALESSIO FASANO

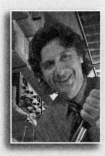

Alessio Fasano, MD

University of Maryland School of Medicine
Mucosal Biology Research Center and Center for Celiac Research
Health Science Facility II, Room S345
20 Penn Street
Baltimore, MD 21201
(410) 706-5501
Fax. (410) 706-5508
afasano@mbrc.umaryland.edu

Dr. Fasano is Professor of Pediatrics, Medicine, and Physiology at the University of Maryland School of Medicine and is the Director of the Mucosal Biology Research center at the same Institution. Dr. Fasano was born in Italy, where he completed is training as a pediatric gastroenterologist. In 1993, he was recruited at the University of Maryland and founded the Division of Pediatric Gastroenterology and Nutrition. In 1996, he established the Center for Celiac Research, a unique facility that offers state-of-the-art research, teaching, and clinical expertise for the diagnosis, treatment, and prevention of celiac disease. Dr. Fasano's research program encompasses both basic and clinical areas, including bacterial pathogenesis, intestinal pathophysiology, and prevention and treatment of both acute and chronic diarrheal diseases. In recent years, Dr. Fasano's research has focused on intercellular tight junctions (TJ) pathophysiology and its role in the pathogenesis of autoimmune diseases, with special emphasis on celiac disease. Dr. Fasano has published more than 170 peer-reviewed papers and his research quality and creativity is further reflected in the filing of more than 160 patent applications, many of which are approved. He is an elected member of the American Society for Clinical Investigation. Because of his translational science, he has been awarded several prizes, including the 2005 Innovator of the Year Award, the 2006 Best Academic/Industry Collaboration Award, the 2006 Entepreneur of the Year Award, the 2007 America's Top Doctor's Award, and the 2009 Researcher of the Year Award. His research has been funded by the National Institutes of Health since 1995. Dr. Fasano has been a permanent member of the NIH study section, and continues to serve as an ad hoc reviewer.

The Intestine and ASD

The human intestine is a deceptively complex organ. It is lined by a single layer of cells exquisitely responsive to stimuli of innumerable variety, and is populated by a complex climax community of microbial partners, far more numerous than the cells of the intestine itself. Under normal circumstances, these intestinal cells form a tight, but selective barrier to "friends and foes": microbes and most environmental substances are held at bay, but nutrients from the essential to the trivial are absorbed efficiently. (1,2) Moreover, the tightness of the epithelial barrier is itself dynamic, though the mechanisms governing and effecting dynamic permeability are poorly understood. What is becoming increasingly clear is that a leaky gut is associated with a large number of local and systemic disorders, including autism spectrum disorders (ASDs). (3)

ASD and Diet

ASDs are heterogeneous neurodevelopmental disorders that affect approximately 1 percent of the general population. (4) It is generally agreed that there are multiple causes for ASD, with both genetic and environmental components involved. Gastrointestinal (GI) symptoms are frequently experienced by subjects with ASD, but their prevalence, nature, and therefore best treatments, remain elusive. (5,6) The most frequent GI symptoms experienced by subjects with ASD include constipation, gastroesophageal reflux, gastritis, intestinal inflammation (autistic enterocolitis), maldigestion, malabsorption, flatulence, abdominal pain or discomfort, lactose intolerance, enteric infections, etc. Of the almost fifty treatments proposed for ASD, seven (antifungal therapy, chelation, enzymes, GI treatments, intestinal parasite therapy, nutritional supplements, and dietary options for autism) are specifically focused to the GI tract, and they will be addressed in detail in other parts of this book. It is worthwhile to note that in a recent survey conducted by the Autism Research Institute involving more than 27,000 parents of autistic kids, avoidance of gluten (~9,000 cases) and/or casein (~7,000 cases) were the most frequent treatments implemented in their children, with a better : worse ratio of 30:1 and 32:1, respectively.

Intestine, Microbiome, and Leaky Gut

A possible unifying theory to "connect the dots" of all the factors mentioned above would link changes in gut microorganisms ecosystem with leaky gut, passage of digestion products of natural food, such as bread and cow's milk that would activate immune inflammatory cells that cause inflammation both in the intestine (autistic enterocolitis) and the brain (ASD). Alternative to the inflammatory hypothesis, it has been proposed that the defect in the intestinal barrier in ASD patients allows passage of neuroactive peptides of food origin into the blood and then into the cerebrospinal fluid, to interfere directly with the function of the central nervous system (CNS). No matter which of the two theories turns out to be correct, changes in intestinal microbiome and the consequent leaky gut seem to be the common denominators. Therefore, it would be logical to consider manipulation of the gut microbiome as the most effective intervention to treat ASD. Among the different strategies currently available to change the gut microbiome, the use of probiotics seems to be the most promising and feasible long-term intervention.

Definition of Probiotics

Probiotics are nonpathogenic bacteria that are claimed to have several beneficial effects related to their capability to either reduce the risk or treat a series of diseases. (7) Most probiotics are bacteria, which are small, single-celled organisms. Bacteria are categorized by scientists with genus, species, and strain names. For example, for the probiotic bacterium *Lactobacillus rhamnosus* GG, the genus is *Lactobacillus*, the species is *rhamnosus*, and the strain is GG. Most probiotic products contain bacteria from the genera *Lactobacillus* or *Bifidobacterium*, although other genera, including *Escherichia*, *Enterococcus*, *Bacillus*, and *Saccharomyces* (a yeast) have been marketed as probiotics. The requirements for a microbe to be considered a probiotic are simple. The microbe must be alive when administered, must be documented to have a health benefit, and must be administered at levels shown to confer the benefit. Probiotic products should be safe, effective, and should maintain their effectiveness and potency through the end of product shelf life.

Formulation of Probiotics

Once destined for commercial use, these bacteria are purified, grown in large numbers, concentrated to high doses, and preserved. They are provided in products in one of three basic ways: (8)

- as a culture concentrate added to a food at medium levels, with little or no opportunity for culture growth
- inoculated into a milk-based food (or dietary supplement) and allowed to grow to achieve high levels in a fermented food
- as concentrated and dried cells packaged as dietary supplements such as powders, capsules, or tablets, and delivered at a range of doses

Probiotic bacteria have a long history of association with dairy products. This is because some of the same bacteria that are associated with fermented dairy products also make their homes in different sites of the human body. Some of these microbes, therefore, can play a dual role in transforming milk into a diverse array of fermented dairy products (yogurt, cheese, kefir, etc.), and contributing to the important role of colonizing bacteria. Dairy products may provide a desirable "probiotic delivery vehicle" for several reasons. To date, however, there is little research on the impact of delivery vehicle and probiotic efficacy for any of the possible formats. This is an important area for future research.

The table below lists some commercial strains currently sold as probiotics. (9) Species are listed as reported by manufacturer, which may not reflect the most current taxonomy. Note that to be legitimately called a "probiotic," a strain must have undergone controlled evaluation for efficacy. The strains listed in this table may or may not have been adequately evaluated. The purpose of this table is to give the reader a sense of what is commercially available, not to provide recommendations for probiotic strain use.

Strain	Commercial products	Source
L. acidophilus NCFM *B. lactis* HN019 (DR10) *L. rhamnosus* HN001 (DR20)	Sold as ingredient	Danisco (Madison, WI)
Saccharomyces cerevisiae (boulardii)	Florastor	Biocodex (Creswell, OR)
B. infantis 35264	Align	Procter & Gamble (Mason, OH)
L. fermentum VRI003 (PCC)	Sold as ingredient	Probiomics (Eveleigh, Australia)
L. rhamnosus R0011 *L. acidophilus* R0052	Sold as ingredient	Institut Rosell (Montreal, Canada)
L. acidophilus LA5 *L. paracasei* CRL 431	Sold as ingredient	Chr. Hansen (Milwaukee, WI)
B. lactis Bb-12	Good Start Natural Cultures infant formula	Nestle (Glendale, CA) Chr. Hansen (Milwaukee, WI)
L. casei Shirota *B. breve* strain Yakult	Yakult	Yakult (Tokyo, Japan)
L. casei DN-114 001 ("*L. casei* Immunitas")	DanActive fermented milk	Danone (Paris, France)
B. animalis DN173 010 ("Bifidis regularis")	Activia yogurt	The Dannon Company (Tarrytown, NY)
L. reuteri RC-14 *L. rhamnosus* GR-1	Femdophilus	Chr. Hansens (Milwaukee, WI) Urex Biotech (London, Ontario, Canada) Jarrow Formulas (Los Angeles, CA)

Strain	Commercial products	Source
L. johnsonii Lj-1 (same as NCC533 and formerly *L. acidophilus* La-1)	LC1	Nestlé (Lausanne, Switzerland)
L. plantarum 299V	Sold as ingredient; Good Belly juice product	Probi AB (Lund, Sweden); NextFoods (Boulder, Colorado)
L. rhamnosus 271	Sold as ingredient	Probi AB (Lund, Sweden)
L. reuteri ATCC 55730 ("Protectis")	BioGaia Probiotic chewable tablets or drops	Biogaia (Stockholm, Sweden)
L. rhamnosus GG ("LGG")	Culturelle; Dannon Danimals	Valio Dairy (Helsinki, Finland) The Dannon Company (Tarrytown, NY)
L. rhamnosus LB21 *Lactococcus lactis* L1A	Sold as ingredient	Essum AB (Umeå, Sweden)
L. salivarius UCC118		University College (Cork, Ireland)
B. longum BB536	Sold as ingredient	Morinaga Milk Industry Co., Ltd. (Zama-City, Japan)
L. acidophilus LB	Sold as ingredient	Lacteol Laboratory (Houdan, France)
L. paracasei F19	Sold as ingredient	Medipharm (Des Moines, IA)
Lactobacillus paracasei 33 *Lactobacillus rhamnosus* GM-020 *Lactobacillus paracasei* GMNL-33	Sold as Ingredient	GenMont Biotech (Taiwan)
L. plantarum OM	Sold as Ingredient	Bio-Energy Systems, Inc. (Kalispell, MT)
Bacillus coagulans BC30	Sustenex, Digestive Advantage and sold as ingredient	Ganeden Biotech Inc. Cleveland, OH)
Streptococcus oralis KJ3 *Streptococcus uberis* KJ2 *Streptococcus rattus* JH145	ProBiora3 EvoraPlus	Oragenics Inc. (Alachua, FL)

Safety of Probiotics

Although the safety of traditional lactic starter bacteria has never been in question, the more recent use of intestinal isolates of bacteria delivered in high numbers to consumers with potentially compromised health has raised the question of safety. The safety of lactobacilli and bifidobacteria has been reviewed by qualified experts in the field. The general conclusion is that the pathogenic potential of lactobacilli and bifidobacteria is quite low. This is based on the prevalence of these microbes in fermented food, as normal colonizers of the human body, and the low level of infection attributed to them. However, reports of association of lactobacilli and bifidobacteria with human infection (commonly endocarditis) in patients with compromised health suggest that these microbes have rare opportunistic capability.

In many countries, the use of probiotics is not regulated by legislation comparable to that applied to drugs. Hence, the use of probiotics has become widespread despite the fact that their efficacy in clinical practice is not based on solid scientific evidence. For this reason, probiotics are often catalogued as "alternative" therapies.

Efficacy of Probiotics

While the initial use of probiotics was based on anecdotal reports of their beneficial effects, we have more recently witnessed a series of more rigorously designed clinical trials documenting the potential use of probiotics for the treatment of a variety of pediatric disorders, including enteric infectious diseases, allergic and atopic disorders, and intestinal inflammatory diseases. The two most studied probiotics are lactobacillus GG and bifidobacteria BB12, and there have been a large number of studies with these organisms in the pediatric population, with consistent good safety data (lack of side effects) but mixed efficacy. The inconsistent positive therapeutic results may be related to the fact that each probiotic organism has different effects, and therefore they cannot be used indiscriminately for each disease. Indeed, different conditions may be triggered by different microbiota composition and therefore may require different probiotics to be effectively treated. By performing more detailed studies to link gut microbiota composition to certain conditions, such as ASD, we will be able to decipher the host-microbe cross talk and, therefore, we will be able to customize probiotic treatment for specific conditions (i.e., personalized medicine). Another strategy that may complement the use of probiotics is the treatment with prebiotics. Prebiotics are nondigestible oligosaccharides (i.e., sugars), which pass through the intestine into the colon, where they are fermented by the colonizing bacteria. (7). The fermentation products, short-chain fatty acids, produce an acid milieu, which facilitates the proliferation of health-promoting bacteria.

Despite the fact that in a recent survey involving 539 primary pediatricians, 19 percent of them suggested the use of probiotics for the treatment of their ASD patients, (9) no well-designed studies have been conducted to justify their routine use in autism. Ideally, all treatments should be based on principles of evidence-based medicine proving the efficacy of treatment judged on the basis of the strength of evidence, including randomized, controlled clinical trials, which are at the peak, followed by cohort studies, case control studies, and then case reports.

Probiotics are available in the United States in foods, dietary supplements, and medical foods. There are no drugs approved for human use in the United States. In the past few years, the diversity of food products containing probiotics has expanded considerably. Not all products, even those claiming to be "probiotic," deliver adequate levels of probiotic microbes that have been documented to have health benefits. Nevertheless, probiotics represent very promising strategies and, therefore, it would be desirable to perform well-designed, multi-center studies to establish the microbiota of ASD patients in order to choose the proper probiotics to reestablish a healthy gut ecosystem able to decrease or completely ameliorate the clinical presentations of ASD.

INTRAVENOUS IMMUNOGLOBULIN (IVIG)

BY DR. MICHAEL ELICE

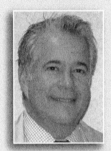

Michael Elice, MD

Autism Associates of New York
77 Froehlich Farm Boulevard
Woodbury, NY 11797
info@autismny.com
(516) 921-3456

Dr. Elice is a board-certified pediatrician and has been in practice for thirty years. Dr. Elice is a graduate of Syracuse University and the Chicago Medical School. He completed his pediatric residency at the North Shore University Hospital in Manhasset, New York. He has academic teaching positions and is on the staff of North Shore University Hospital and Schneider Children's Hospital. He is an associate professor of pediatrics at the New York University Medical School and the Albert Einstein School of Medicine. He is on the medical advisory board of the New York Families for Autistic Children (NYFAC) and is a member of the National Autism Association New York Metro Chapter. He has lectured at Defeat Autism Now! conferences around the country.

Autism spectrum disorders (ASDs) are currently defined as a syndrome of impaired social interaction, impaired communication skills, and restricted repertoire of activity and interests. The diagnoses contained within the spectrum range from attention deficit disorder (ADD), with hyperactivity (ADHD), obsessive compulsive disorder (OCD), tic disorders (such as Tourette's syndrome, aka TS), pervasive developmental disorder, not otherwise specified (PDD–NOS), and oppositional defiant disorder (ODD). These diagnoses are usually made prior to age three years, and have been on the rise over the past thirty years. The current statistics released by the Centers for Disease Control (CDC) and state health departments report the incidence of autism is 1:58 to 1:110 children, depending on geographic location, making autism spectrum disorders one of the greatest epidemics in pediatric medicine.

Intravenous immunoglobulin (IVIG) therapy has been used for common variable immunodeficiency syndrome (CVID), a disorder characterized by low levels of serum immunoglobulins and increased susceptibility to infections. The variability refers to the degree and type of immunoglobulin deficiency the patients had. Most individuals with CVID present first with recurrent bacterial infections. The underlying biomedical etiologies on children with autism have been under investigation. Genetic disorders possibly associated with epigenetic activity may lead to an increased incidence of multiple system disease in these children. Certain subsets of these children have a high incidence of immunological abnormalities and autoimmune disease. They also have markedly decreased serum immunoglobulin levels and impaired antibody responses. Based on the immunological abnormalities, a number of trials of IVIG have been utilized in autistic children. Gupta et al., in an open clinical trial, administered IVIG to ten children aged three to twelve years at four-week intervals for six months. Evaluations from the IV infusion nurse, physician, parents, and therapists showed clinical improvement in most of the patients. Younger patients showed greater improvement. Plioplys treated ten autistic children, ages four to seventeen years, with IVIG, four times every six weeks and found similar results. Delgiudice-Asch et al. administered IVIG monthly for six months to five autistic children. The sensory response Ritvo-Freeman scale showed a clinically meaningful response.

Based on this information, new research in autism spectrum disorders dictates the measurement of serum immunoglobulins, B and T cell lymphocyte levels, and anti-streptococcal antibodies. Patients who have received immunizations against polio, measles, diphtheria, tetanus, and strep pneumoniae may have low or absent antibody levels to one or more of these vaccines indicating a degree of immunodeficiency.

A subgroup of patients with OCD, ADD/ADHD, and tics or Tourette's syndrome has been identified who share a common clinical course characterized by dramatic symptom exacerbations following group A beta-hemolytic streptococcal (GABHS) infections. The term PANDAS has been applied to these patients, signifying Pediatric Autoimmune Neuropsychiatric Disorders Associated with Streptococcal Infections. The clinical symptoms are characterized by presence of the OCD and/or tic disorder, prepubertal onset of symptoms, intermittent exacerbations, neurological abnormalities such as motoric hyperactivity, adventitious movements, and the temporal association of the symptom exacerbations and GABHS infections.

In the 1980s, studies of childhood onset OCD and parallel investigations of rheumatic fever and its associated symptoms suggested a useful model of pathophysiology of these symptoms. It was thought that in certain children, susceptibility to genetic disorders possibly associated with epigenetic and transposon activity may lead to an increased incidence of multiple symptom disease in these children. Thus, certain strains of GABHS incite the production of antibodies that cross-react with central nervous system cellular components to cause inflammation of the basal ganglia in the brain resulting in these neuropsychiatric symptoms. Nearly 75 percent of these patients have symptoms of childhood onset OCD, worries about harm to self and others, violent images and behaviors, and ritualistic behaviors. These symptoms commence about four weeks prior to onset of the adventitious chorea-like movements, leading to the speculation that OCD might occur as a sequel of strep infections.

In a study by Swedo, et al. of fifty children meeting the PANDAS criteria, 40 percent met the DSM-IV (*Diagnostic and Statistical Manual of Mental Disorders, Fourth Edition*) criteria for ADHD, 18 percent ODD, 28 percent anxiety disorder. Exacerbations of OCD/tic symptoms were also accompanied by emotional lability and irritability, tactile/sensory defensiveness, motoric hyperactivity, messy handwriting, and symptoms of separation anxiety; a unique constellation of symptoms. The treatment for PANDAS is currently being studied including prophylactic antibiotics to prevent recurrent streptococcal infections and IVIG therapy. The children demonstrated dramatic improvements in OCD symptoms, anxiety, depression, emotional lability, and global functioning based on global change scores (41 percent). In contrast, placebo administration was associated with little or no change in overall symptoms severity. Side effects were limited to the duration of the procedure and included dizziness, nausea, and headache. In most cases, the discomfort occurred only during the first or second infusion and often persisted for twelve to twenty-four hours. Over 80 percent of patients who received IVIG remained much or very much improved at one-year follow-up, with their symptoms now in the subclinical range of severity. These results are particularly impressive in light of previous reports of the intractable nature of pediatric OCD and tic disorders. Long-term outcome studies in OCD have found less than one third of the patients with clinically meaningful symptom improvements.

In 2005 Boris, et al. published a study showing beneficial response of IVIG therapy in autistic children to whom 400 mg/kg IVIG was administered each month for six months. Baseline and monthly Aberrant Behavior Checklists were completed on each child in order to measure the child's response to IVIG. The participants' overall aberrant behaviors decreased substantially soon after receiving their first dose of IVIG. Total scores revealed decreases in hyperactivity, inappropriate speech, irritability, lethargy, and stereotypy (stimming, repetitive behaviors). This led to a reasonable rationale ratio to utilize IVIG therapy in children with autism.

The procedure of intravenous infusion of immunoglobulin is quite simple. The serum is sent to the doctor's office and remains frozen until the patient arrives, to ensure freshness. The volume to be infused is set up in a calibrated mechanical pump that begins the infusion at a slow rate to make sure the patient is tolerating the infusion. Depending on the volume to be infused, which is based on the weight of the patient, the procedure usually takes four to five hours.

Several days before the infusion, the patient receives information regarding premedication and hydration. Premedication might consist of oral ibuprofen and Benadryl at home or approximately one hour before arriving at the office. Sometimes it is necessary to administer IV Benadryl or Valium to relax the patient so that the IV catheter can be placed. This is a simple procedure, much like venipuncture to draw blood from a vein. The difference is that a catheter, a plastic extension of the needle, is threaded into the patient's vein and remains there for the duration of the procedure. The catheter allows a bit more flexibility of movement, so the patient may be more comfortable. In our office, the patient has the option of lying on an exam table with a comfortable backrest and pillow so they can sleep through the infusion or in a reclining chair so they can read or watch TV or a DVD of their choice. We encourage parents to bring these items for the comfort of the child.

A trained IV nurse is always present and will monitor vital signs; i.e., temperature, blood pressure, and pulse, as well as monitor the pump to be certain the infusion is proceeding efficiently. In the unlikely event that the patient demonstrates vital sign alterations or any other problem, the nurse will assess and report to the supervising physician. A crash cart for CPR/medications is always available. Thus far, we have never had any such incident.

Once the procedure is completed, the catheter is removed, instructions for at-home care are given, and the patient is discharged. There is a small possibility that the patient may develop fever, malaise, nausea, or headaches. These are rare and can be dealt with additional ibuprofen or Benadryl. The patient is instructed to make an appointment for the next monthly infusion. After the first infusion, seeing how simple it actually is, parents and children are very comfortable with the experience.

The treatment for common variable immunodeficiency characterized by low levels of serum immunoglobulins is similar to that of other disorders such as PANDAS. Intravenous immunoglobulin (IVIG) has led to improvement of symptoms. IVIG is a plasma product formed by taking antibodies from thousands of donors. The plasma undergoes processing for mixing, antibody removal, chemical treatment, and filtration to remove viruses, and then is freeze dried. This extensive processing dictates the high cost of the infusion, which is approximately $4,000 per child. This varies depending on the weight of the patient calculated based on 1 gram/kg of weight.

Intravenous immunoglobulin replacement combined with antibiotic therapy has greatly improved the outcomes of patients with PANDAS, CVID, and other autism spectrum disorders. The aim is to keep the patients free of infectious disease and to prevent the ensuing chronic inflammatory changes that may occur as a consequence of this immune system dysregulation. In our clinical practice, we have many children who have received IVIG. Based on anecdotal reports of parents, educators, and therapists, there have been improvements in focus and attention, and decreases in OCD/tic behaviors. In addition, these children—who are often sick with strep throats and other illnesses—have sustained longer intervals of health, compared to their previous history. Most recently, one of our patients visited Disney World, where he had been at least twenty times in his life. His older brother got strep throat and was treated with appropriate antibiotics. Forty-eight hours later, the patient became violent, started screaming, could not sleep, and was basically out of control. Within twenty-four hours of starting antibiotics, his behavior improved dramatically. Like "apples to oranges," said his father. This underscores the value to prophylactic antibiotics and IVIG which is the next step in treating this "autistic twelve-year-old male."

The results of these investigations, as well as clinical response noted in our practice, suggest that IVIG is highly beneficial to a subgroup of patients with tics and obsessive-compulsive symptoms. However, they do not provide support for routine use of immunomodulatory agents in OCD and tic disorders. IVIG is a potent immunological therapy. A NIH Consensus Statement asserted that the risks involved in the use of IVIG are minimal.

Other articles have confirmed their safety, after two decades of experience. Latov et al. reported that IVIG is used in the treatment of immunological diseases that affect the entire neuroaxis, including the brain, spinal cord, peripheral nerves, muscles, and neuromuscular junction. In prospective, controlled, double-blind clinical trials, IVIG was found to have proven efficacy in Guillain-Barré syndrome, chronic inflammatory demyelinating polyneuropathy, multifocal motor neuropathy, and dermatomyositis. It was found to probably be effective in myasthenia gravis and polymyositis, and possibly effective in several other neuroimmunological diseases. Further studies are needed to evaluate the use of IVIG for neuroimmunological diseases in which its efficacy is suspected but not proven and to elucidate its mechanisms of action.

Ongoing Results

The year 2010 was a successful one for intravenous gamma globulin therapy in our practice. We treated five patients age 7 to 15 years, all males. Their clinical presentation of ADHD, OCD and tics suggested the etiology of their behaviors was PANDAS. Laboratory values confirmed hypogammaglobulinemia (low IgG levels), elevated AntiStreptolysin O Antibodies (ASO) and elevated Anti DNAse B Antibodies. There was a past history of strep infections but none of the patients had recent strep illnesses according to the parents.

IVIG was administered monthly over the course of six months. The dosage was calculated in a range of 0.4 to 1.0 gram per kilogram of body weight. The rate of the infusion never exceeded 100gms. per hour. Some of the infusions lasted for 8 hours.

Premedication varied from patient to patient. Most were given Ibuprofen and Benadryl prior to arriving at our office. Depending on the individual, IV benadryl, toradol, solumedrol or valium was given to keep the patient calm and in some cases diminish the exacerbation of choreiform movements and tics. The tics varied from motoric behaviors to vocal/verbal sounds and repetitive speech. A physician or nurse was present with the family at all times. There were no adverse reactions observed other than an occasional complaint of headache. In one patient who was non verbal headache pain was assessed based on his repetitive hitting his head and throwing his head into the back of the chair.

Vital signs were assessed at regular intervals to insure stable blood pressure, pulse and temperature. None of the patients experienced any alterations in these modalities.

Parents completed the Aberrant Behavior Checklist (ABC) before the first infusion and after the sixth infusion. The total 'before' and 'after' scores were compared as a percent change and is reported below.

PATIENTS

Patient #1—G.I. 7 year old male. Score change = behaviors actually increased 9%. However, the changes were noted in language since he progressed from non verbal to speaking, although inappropriately. Tantrums and adverse behaviors increased but were age appropriate since they occurred when he didn't get what he wanted where previously he didn't respond. He no longer required antibiotic prophylaxis for strep infections. He is now reading, writing and doing mathematics on an age appropriate level. He is more compliant and follows directions.

Patient #2—A.S. 12 year old male. Score change = 25% reduction in aberrant behaviors.

Most significant changes were decreases in aggression, temper outbursts and self-injury.

Recurrent body movements (chorea) involving shaking extremities and stereotypy diminished significantly. Attention, obedience and compliance with instructions improved. He was able to sit for longer periods of time and is showing more positive social reaction to others.

Patient #3—C.G. 15 year old male. Score change = 88% improvement

This was one of our more difficult cases. This fully developed teenager lost language and the ability to control motor and vocal tics to the extent that he couldn't sleep at night or sit still during the day. Between the fifth and sixth infusion, family noticed less hyperactivity and bizarre behavior. Choreiform movements diminished. Less staring blankly into space, repetitive speech and self-talk as use of language reemerged. Most significantly, he no longer has tantrums, stereotypical behaviors and restlessness. He doesn't cry or bang his head. Hand ticking and erratic mood changes have been reduced to a minimum. He is definitely more socially aware as expressive language reemerges.

Patient #4—C.D. 9 year old male. Score change = 38% improvement.

Most significant change in this child was in the diminishing of repetitive speech which was an obstacle to his progress in school. Choreiform movements, restlessness, stereotypy and bizarre behaviors all decreased. Hyperactivity, including running and jumping, distractibility and self-talking decreased as well. Social interaction with peers and adults and attention span increased.

Follow-up laboratory investigation showed normalization of IgG levels and the absence of ASO and AntiDNAseB antibodies.

Although the results of the ABC Checklists were not scored to assess true statistical significance, parent observation and reporting, physician observation and patient responses all support the effectiveness of IVIG treatments in these individuals. As the physician who examines them at regular monthly intervals, I can attest to these clinical improvements. As new double blind, placebo controlled studies are under way at the National Institute of Mental Health, it is still important to document evidence based observational improvements on a case by case basis.

LOW DOSE NALTREXONE (LDN)

BY DR. JAQUELYN MCCANDLESS

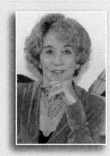

Jaquelyn McCandless, MD

www.lowdosenaltrexone.org

Jaquelyn McCandless MD is certified by the American Board of Psychiatry and Neurology and licensed in Hawaii and California, and has specialized in the bio-medical treatment of autism for the last twelve years. Dr. McCandless initiated the Defeat Autism Now! Physicians' Clinical Training in 2003, and is the author of the first clinical biomedical treatment book for autism, *Children with Starving Brains, a Medical Treatment Guide for Autism Spectrum Disorder,* first published in 2002, latest and 4th Edition published in February 2009, by Bramble Books.

In the last eleven years of working with children with autism spectrum disorder, I have learned—along with my colleagues in the Defeat Autism Now! organization focused on the biomedical aspect of autism—that children with this diagnosis are immunocompromised. This is shown by their inability to self-detoxify and low gluta-thione levels and abnormal immune parameters compared to neurotypical children. I conducted a private clinical study in 2005 on a medication to assess its help for immune status, a very low dose of an FDA-approved generic (1997) drug called naltrexone, an opioid antagonist used for adult opioid and alcohol addiction at usual doses of 50 mg or more per day. Studies over a decade earlier on full or higher dose naltrexone showed benefit in autistic self-injurious behavior (SIB) but at that time the connection between opioids and our immune systems was not widely known or understood. Autism researchers were hoping to counteract the opioid effects of casein and gluten with the opioid antagonism offered by naltrexone, rather than subjecting children to dietary restriction (GF/CF diets). Panksepp, Shattock and other early researchers noted variably better results with low doses; studies on higher doses were more equivocal in children, and noncompliance due to the bitterness of the drug posed a problem for autistic children, most of whom could not swallow capsules. After it was learned that most cases of SIB were due to pain from gut inflammation, which children were unable to describe, appropriate anti-inflammatory and other treatments for this gut condition decreased the use of naltrexone for SIB.

For private clinical studies in response to my request for a suitable transdermal form of low dose naltrexone (LDN), molecular pharmacologist Dr. Tyrus Smith then (2005) at Coastal Compounding Pharmacy in Savannah GA created a very effective transdermal cream compounded with emu oil. This allowed easy adjustment of dosing (some of the smaller kids did better with only 1.5 mg), the bitter taste was no problem, and the pleasant cream made in oil from the emu could be put on the children's bodies while they slept. The cream is put into syringes, with 0.5 ml providing 3 mg for children or 4.5 mg for adults; most adults prefer capsules; both are equally effective. Our use is of an ultra-low dose of pure naltrexone, less than 1/10 the recommended dose of 50 mg usually used for addiction, called low dose naltrexone, or LDN; it must be compounded (3 mg for children, 4.5 mg for adults) for "off-label" use to get these tiny doses. In private unpublished research studies I found that sixteen out of twenty children (80 percent) increased their CD4+ count in sixteen weeks of LDN usage and 70 percent of twenty-eight parents of children with autism raised their CD4+ count. LDN has shown itself to be a non-toxic, effective immune enhancer, non-addicting, inexpensive (cost for month's supply of transdermal cream or oral capsule $25–$40, depending upon where you get it), and extremely easy to use (one capsule OR one transdermal application at bedtime, only once, daily). Many thousands of children with autism have been or are using LDN since I introduced it to the autism community in 2005; 75 percent of a 200-parent assay at that time rated LDN "overall beneficial." Though children are often prescribed this medication for immune benefit by their doctors, what parents appreciate most is increase in cognition, language, and socialization. I have dozens of letters and posts of grateful fathers telling me LDN has finally given them a relationship with their child and mothers who tell me that for the first time their child is playing with their siblings. Though many things about autism are heartbreaking, one of the saddest is the isolation and aloneness these children have. Very often they can be seen playing by themselves, seemingly preoccupied with an inner life or with repetitiously manipulating or lining up toys or objects, while totally oblivious of other children on a playground playing and relating.

History of LDN: Naltrexone is an extremely safe drug that was originally approved by the Food and Drug Administration in 1984 as a treatment for heroin, opium, and alcohol addiction due to its effectiveness in blocking the opioid receptors in the brain that drive the craving for these drugs. The dosage used is usually 50 mg/

day for these disorders, and there is a current study using similar dosages to treat obesity. A New York physician, Bernard Bihari MD, in working with hospitalized AIDS patients in 1985, was giving some patients naltrexone to help addiction craving issues while they were being treated for AIDS. Cravings were helped, but their immune systems were responding negatively; he learned from a researcher at Penn State, Dr. Ian Zagon, that in his research work with canines, naltrexone actually helped the immune system more as the dose was lowered. Dr. Bihari did lower the dose, and determined that ideal dosing to help immunity was much lower than the dose needed for addiction therapy. Because naltrexone was able to block opioid receptors, it also was effective at blocking the reception of opioid hormones that are produced by brain and adrenal glands, including endorphins and enkephalins (specific types of endorphins that occur at the body's nerve endings and act as transmitters). Many of our body's tissues have receptor sites for endorphins, including nearly every cell in the immune system. This makes naltrexone an ideal treatment for managing pain, boosting immune function, and in many, boosting mood. Some parents call it the "happy cream," many noting that for the first time ever, after starting it, their children wake up happy. Dr. Bihari discovered naltrexone was able to accomplish these benefits in a low dose (between 1 to 4.5 mg, rather than 50 mg) taken once a day at bedtime, and the dose used most frequently for children under 100 pounds is 3 mg.

Since Dr. Bihari's discovery, LDN has been shown to have benefit for a wide variety of illnesses related to low immune function besides HIV/AIDS, including virtually every known cancer, as well as chronic fatigue syndrome, fibromyalgia, gastrointestinal disorders (celiac disease, colitis, Crohn's disease, irritable bowel syndrome), lupus, multiple sclerosis (MS), Parkinson's, rheumatoid arthritis, psoriasis, amyotrophic lateral sclerosis, and Alzheimer's disease. Many MS and other autoimmune patients have been on this medication for many years without progression of their disease, and the general consensus is that those with serious diseases such as MS and metastatic cancer should take LDN indefinitely. Some children with autism have been on LDN for two to four years, ever since I introduced it to the autism community in 2005 (including my beloved granddaughter Chelsey, adorning the cover of my book, and inspiration for all my work in autism).

Although naltrexone is non-toxic and virtually free of side effects, occasionally it can cause sleep problems or hyperness during the first week or two of its use. If sleep problems persist, reducing the dose from 4.5 mg to 3 mg or in children from 3 mg to 1.5 to 2 mg is often helpful. The primary contraindication for LDN is the use of narcotic pain medications, and in children taking steroids, usually for gut inflammation, I request they not start LDN until they are down to 10 mg or less a day of prednisone on their way to going off steroids completely. It is not advised to administer LDN to someone who is taking immunosuppressants, as they will tend to counteract and neither be optimal.

As an effective, non-toxic, non-addicting, inexpensive behavioral and immuno-enhancing/modulating intervention, LDN is joining our biomedical arsenal to help more and more children recover from autism as well as helping many persons both adult and children with autoimmune diseases including HIV+ AIDS, MS, Crohn's, fibromyalgia, and cancer, or any disease that is caused by immune/autoimmune impairment or endorphin deficiency. Currently used in ultra small doses as an "off-label" FDA approved medication, LDN must be physician-prescribed and also compounded for the tiny dosing required. The filler medium carrying the medication is very important—it is required, in order to provide most benefit to be hypoallergenic and immediate-release to get the "jumpstart" for the brain to send the message out to the adrenal and pituitary glands to tell them to make endorphins. As to the carrier, I personally prefer emu oil for transdermal use and avicel for capsule preparations.

For more information on LDN, see www.lowdosenaltrexone.org, or you may join Autism_LDN@yahoogroups.com, and see www.LDNAfricaAIDS.org on my research on LDN for HIV/AIDS in Africa.

MEDICINAL MARIJUANA: A NOVEL APPROACH TO THE SYMPTOMATIC TREATMENT OF AUTISM

BY DR. LESTER GRINSPOON

Lester Grinspoon, MD

Harvard Medical School
35 Skyline Drive
Wellesley, MA 02482
www.marijuana-uses.com
www.rxmarijuana.com
lester_grinspoon@hms.harvard.edu

Dr. Lester Grinspoon is a professor of psychiatry emeritus at the Harvard Medical School and a well published author in the field of drugs and drug policy. He has authored more than 190 articles in scientific journals and ten books, including *Marihuana Reconsidered* (Harvard University press 1971, 1977, and American archives press classic edition, 1994) and *Marijuana, the Forbidden Medicine* (Yale University press, 1993, 1997), now translated into fourteen languages. Dr. Grinspoon is a frequent lecturer on drug policy issues and has appeared as an expert witness before legislative committees in many states and numerous committees of the U.S. Congress. In 1990 he received the Alfred R. Lindesmith Award for Achievement in the Field of Scholarship and Writing from the Drug Policy Foundation in Washington, DC.

Drugs have a place in treating autistic symptoms, but their uses are limited. Antipsychotic drugs and mood stabilizers may help autistic patients who repeatedly injure themselves. The older conventional antipsychotic drugs have serious side effects on body movements; the novel or atypical drug risperidone (Risperdal) has shown a glimmer of promise in recent research. Anticonvulsants may be useful in suppressing explosive rage and calming severe anxiety. About 20 percent of autistic people have epileptic seizures, and some researchers have suggested that unrecognized partial complex seizures, which cause changes in consciousness but not muscular convulsions, are one source of autistic behavior disturbances. In several control studies, selective serotonin reuptake inhibitors (SSRIs) have been found to relieve depression and anxiety and reduce compulsive ordering, collecting, and arranging. Unfortunately, little is known about the long-term effects of drugs in autistic children, and no known drug has any effect on the underlying lack of capacity for empathy and communication.

With the explosive growth of interest in exploring the medicinal capacities of marijuana, some courageous parents, dissatisfied with the usefulness and toxicity of the above mentioned drugs, and desperate to find pharmaceutical means of relieving their children of some of the harsh symptoms of autism, have been experimenting with oral doses of cannabis. The following anecdote was provided by Marie Myung-Ok Lee who teaches at Brown University. She is the author of the novel *Somebody's Daughter* and is a winner of the Richard J. Margolis Award for Social Justice Reporting.

My son J, who is nine years old, has autism. He's also had two serious surgeries for a spinal cord tumor and has an inflammatory bowel condition, all of which may be causing him pain, if he could tell us. He can say words, but many of them don't convey what he means.

J's school called my husband and me in for a meeting about J's tantrums, which were affecting his ability to learn. Their solution was to hand us a list of child psychiatrists. Since autistic children like J can't exactly do talk therapy, this meant sedating, antipsychotic drugs like Risperdal (risperidone).

As a health writer and blogger, I was intrigued when a homeopath suggested medical marijuana. Cannabis has long-documented effects as an analgesic and an anxiety modulator. Best of all, it is safe. A publication by the Autism Research Institute described cases of reduced aggression, with no permanent side effects.

After a week on Marinol, which contains a synthetic cannabinoid, J began garnering a few glowing school reports. But J tends to build tolerance to synthetics, and in a few months, we could see the aggressive behavior coming back. One night, at a medical marijuana patient advocacy group, I learned that the one cannabinoid in Marinol cannot compare to the sixty in marijuana, the plant.

Rhode Island, where we live, is one of fourteen states where the use of medical marijuana is legal. And yet, I hesitated. Now we were dealing with an illegal drug, one for which few evidence-based scientific studies existed precisely because it is an illegal drug. But when I sent J's doctor the physician's form that is mandatory for medical marijuana licensing, it came back signed. We underwent a background check, and J became the state's youngest licensee.

The coordinator of our medical marijuana patient advocacy group introduced us to a licensed grower, who had figured out how to cultivate marijuana using a custom organic soil mix. The grower left us with a month's worth of marijuana tea, glycerin, and olive oil—and a cookie recipe. We paid $80.

We made the cookies with the marijuana olive oil, starting J off with half a small cookie. J normally goes to bed around 7:30 PM.; by 6:30 he declared he was tired and conked out. As we anxiously peeked in on him, half-expecting some red-eyed ogre from Reefer Madness *to come leaping out at us, we saw instead that he was sleeping peacefully. Usually, his sleep is shallow and restless.*

When J decided he didn't like the cookie anymore, we switched to the tea. After two weeks, we noticed a slight but consistent lessening of aggression. Since we started him on his "special tea," J's face, which is sometimes a mask of pain, has softened. He smiles more. For the last year, his individual education plan at his special needs school was full of blanks because he spent his whole day in an irritated, frustrated mess. Now, April's report shows real progress, including "two community outings with the absence of aggressions."

The big test has been a visit from Grandma. The last time she came, J hit her. This time, she remarked that J seems calmer. As we were preparing for a trip to the park, J disappeared, and we wondered if he was going to throw one of his tantrums. Instead, he returned with Grandma's shoes, laying them in front of her, even carefully adjusting them so that they were parallel. He looked into her face, and smiled.

It's strange, I've come to think, that the virtues of such a useful and harmless botanical have been so clouded by stigma. Meanwhile, in treating J with pot, we are following the law—and the Hippocratic Oath: First, do no harm. The drugs that our insurance would pay for—and that the people around us would support without question—pose real risks to children. For now, we're sticking with the weed.

How is J doing now, four months into our cannabis experiment? Well, one day recently, he came home from school, and I noticed something really different: He had a whole shirt on.

Pre-pot, J ate things that weren't food. J chewed the collar of his T-shirts while stealthily deconstructing them from the bottom up, teasing apart and then swallowing the threads. His chewing become so uncontrollable we couldn't let him sleep with a pajama top (it would be gone by morning) or a pillow (ditto the case and the stuffing). The worst part was watching him scream in pain on the toilet, when what went in, had to come out.

Almost immediately after we started the cannabis, this stopped. Just stopped. J now sleeps with his organic wool-and-cotton, temptingly chewable comforter. He pulls it up to his chin at night and declares, "I'm cozy!"

Next, we started seeing changes in J's school reports. At one August parent meeting, his teacher excitedly presented his June-July "aggression" chart. For the past year, he'd consistently had thirty to fifty aggressions in a school day, with a one-time high of 300. The charts for June through July, by contrast, showed he was actually having days—sometimes one after another—with zero aggressions.

I don't consider marijuana a miracle cure for autism. But I do consider it a wonderful, safe botanical that allows J to participate more fully in life without the dangers and sometimes-permanent side effects of pharmaceutical drugs, now that we have a good dose and a good strain. Free from pain, J can go to school and learn. And his violent behavior won't put him in the local children's psychiatric hospital—a scenario all too common among his peers.

We have pictures of J from a year ago, when he would actually claw at his own face. That little child with the horrifically bleeding and scabbed face looks to us now like a visitor from another world. The J we know now just looks like a happy little boy.

We worried that "the munchies" would severely aggravate J's problems with overeating in response to his stomach pangs. Instead, the marijuana seems to have modulated these symptoms. J still can get overexcited if he likes a food too much, so the other day, we dared to experiment with doenjang, *a tofu soup that he used to love as a baby. The last time we tried it, a year ago, he frisbeed the bowl against a tile wall.*

We left J in the kitchen with his steamy bowl and went to the adjoining room. We heard the spoon ding. Satisfied slurpy noises. Then a strange noise that we couldn't identify. A chkkka bsssshhht doinnng! We returned to the kitchen, half expecting to see the walls painted with doenjang. *Everything was clean. The bowl and spoon, however, were gone.*

J had taken his dishes to the sink, rinsed them, and put them in the dishwasher—something we'd never shown him how to do. In four months, he'd gone from a boy we couldn't feed, to a boy who could feed himself and clean up after. The sight of the bowl, not quite rinsed, but almost, was one of the sweetest sights of my parental life. I expect more to come.

(Readers interested in a more detailed account of J's treatment with marijuana are referred to the section on Featured Patient Accounts on my Marijuana As Medicine website www.rxmarijuana.com).

Because autism is such a devastating and so far incurable disease and the available pharmaceutical products have such limited usefulness and serious side-effects, many parents—like Marie Myung-Ok Lee—seek out alternative therapies. I have had the opportunity to consult with and help a small number of these parents explore marijuana as a medicine, which can help to control some of the severe behavioral problems. (For the approximately one in five children with autism who suffer some sort of seizure disorder, it is important to note that marijuana is an excellent anticonvulsant, and was widely used as such in the last part of the 19th century and the early decades of the 20th.) Those who have persevered in the arduous process of both finding the correct oral vehicle and titrating the optimal dose, have been rewarded in more or less the same ways she has.

The first obstacle in the path of anyone who wishes to explore cannabis as a medicine is to overcome the widely held belief that it is a very dangerous substance. The misinformation campaigns of the United States government and such organizations as the Partnership for a Drug-Free America notwithstanding, marijuana is an unusually safe drug. In fact, after federal-court-ordered lengthy hearings before a Drug Enforcement Administration Law Judge, involving many witnesses, including both patients and doctors, and thousands of pages of documentation, Judge Francis L. Young in 1988 asserted that "marijuana, in its natural form, is one of the safest therapeutic active substances known to man . . . " Cannabis was much used in Western medicine from the mid-19th century until shortly after the passage of the Marijuana Tax Act of 1937, the first of the Draconian legislation aimed at marijuana. There has never been a recorded death attributable to marijuana. When it regains its rightful place in the U.S. pharmacopeia, it will soon be recognized as one of the least toxic medicines in that compendium. While there are no studies of the toxicity of cannabis in children, neither are there pediatric studies of the toxicity of risperidone and other conventional drugs used in the treatment of autism. However, to the extent that one can extrapolate the adult toxicity profiles of the antipsychotic drug risperidone and cannabis, the latter is the much safer drug.

It is often objected, especially by federal authorities, that the medical usefulness of marijuana has not been demonstrated by controlled studies, the rigorous, expensive, and time-consuming tests necessary to win approval by the Food and Drug Administration (FDA) for marketing as medicines. The purpose of the testing is to protect the consumer, by establishing both safety and efficacy. Because no drug is completely safe (nontoxic) or always efficacious, a drug approved by the FDA has presumably satisfied a risk-benefit analysis. The cost of doing the controlled studies necessary for FDA approval may run to about $800 million per drug, a cost borne by the drug company seeking it as a necessary prerequisite for the distribution of its patented product. Because it is impossible to patent a plant, pharmaceutical companies are not interested in developing this herbal medicine, and so far the cannabinoid products they have developed are not nearly as useful as whole herbal marijuana.

But it is doubtful whether FDA rules should apply to marijuana. First, there is no question about its safety. It has been used for thousands of years by millions of people, with very little evidence of significant toxicity. Similarly, given the mountain of anecdotal evidence which has accumulated over the years, no double-blind studies are needed to prove marijuana's efficacy. Any astute clinician who has experience with patients who have used cannabis as a medicine knows that it is efficacious for many people with various symptoms and syndromes. What we do not know is what proportion of patients with a given symptom will get relief from cannabis, and how many will be better off with cannabis than with the best presently available medicine. Here, large control studies will be helpful.

Physicians also have available evidence of a different kind, whose value is often underestimated. Anecdotal evidence commands much less attention than it once did, yet it is the source of much of our knowledge of synthetic medicines as well as plant derivatives. Controlled experiments were not needed to recognize the therapeutic potential of chloral hydrate, barbiturates, aspirin, curare, insulin, or penicillin. Furthermore, it was through anecdotal evidence that we learned of the usefulness of propranolol for angina and hypertension, of diazepam for status epilepticus (a state of continuous seizure activity), and of imipramine for childhood enuresis (bed-wetting) although these drugs were originally approved by the FDA for other purposes. Anecdotes or case histories of the kind presented here by Marie Myung-Ok Lee are, in a sense, the smallest research studies of all.

Anecdotes present a problem that has always haunted medicine: the anecdotal fallacy or the fallacy of the enumeration of favorable circumstances (counting the hits, and ignoring the misses). If many people suffering from, say, muscle spasms caused by multiple sclerosis take cannabis and only a few get much better relief than they could get from conventional drugs, these few patients would stand out and come to our attention. They and their physicians would understandably be enthusiastic about cannabis and might proselytize for it. These people are not dishonest, but they are not dispassionate observers. Therefore, some may regard it as irresponsible to suggest, on the basis of anecdotes, that cannabis may help some people with a variety of symptoms and disorders. That might be a problem if marijuana were a dangerous drug, but it is becoming increasingly clear that it is a remarkably safe pharmaceutical. Even in the unlikely event that only a few autistic children get the kind of relief that "J" gets, it could be argued that cannabis should be available for them because it costs so little to produce, the risks are so small, and the results so impressive.

While federal law is absolute in prohibiting the use of marijuana for any purpose, beginning with California in 1996, there are now fourteen states where it is possible to use it as a medicine, within specified limits. California, in addition to being the first state to make an accommodation to patients in need of cannabis, is also one of the states in which the legal interpretation of those needs and the means by which they can be filled is broad enough to satisfy the demands of patients with the wide variety of symptoms and syndromes for which this herb is useful. New Jersey, the latest state to adopt medical marijuana legislation, is unfortunately among the most restrictive. It is so restrictive, both with respect to the symptoms and syndromes for which a patient is allowed to use the drug and the means by which patients are allowed access to it, that only a relatively small percentage of the patients who would find marijuana more useful, less toxic, and less expensive than the conventional drugs they presently use will have access to it. Fortunately for her and her family, Marie Myung-Ok Lee lives in Rhode Island, where after presenting the appropriate credentials from "J's" physician, she was licensed to legally obtain marijuana. However, in most states patients or the people responsible for their care have to make, what for many of them, is a very difficult decision—whether to buy or grow cannabis outside of the law.

Beyond gaining access to marijuana, there are the problems involved in the preparation of this medicine in a form suitable for children. The most common way in which marijuana is used as a medicine is through inhalation of the smoke from a pipe, a joint, or a vaporizer. This is the preferred method for adults, because it makes it possible for the patients to precisely titrate the dose, because with this method of delivery they will perceive the therapeutic effects within minutes. However, inhalation is not an option for children who suffer from autism; for these patients, the best route for administration is oral, in the form of cookies, brownies, tea, etc. There are now available marijuana cookbooks from which a variety of edibles which appeal to children can be found. With ingestion, the therapeutic effects will not appear before one and a half to two hours, but the advantage is that they last for many hours. Beyond preparing the edible, are the challenges of determining the right dose (such as beginning with a fraction of a cookie and increasing the dose as needed), and establishing a schedule for taking the medication. These tasks will require some experimentation on the part of the parents, but with experience they will soon find the best recipes for their child, the ideal dose, and a workable schedule. Unfortunately, because there is presently no easy and available way of knowing with any precision the potency of any particular batch of marijuana, each newly prepared edible will have to be re-titrated, but with experience, caregivers will find this an increasingly less difficult task. It is also important to remember that cannabis is a very forgiving medicine; one would have to be considerably over the "ideal" dosage mark to cause any difficulty.

One way of minimizing what are usually minor therapeutic differences between one batch of cannabis and another is to try to use the same strain of marijuana every time an edible is prepared. At the same time, many patients who use marijuana as a medicine take advantage of the fact that there is a growing variety of available strains, each with slight differences in the percentages and ratios of the different therapeutic cannabinoids. This allows patients to empirically explore the different strains in an effort to identify the particular strain which appears to be the therapeutically most useful for their symptomatology.

The parents of autistic children carry a heavy burden. They are constantly challenged and frustrated by the child's inability to communicate, his impulsiveness, and his destructive and self-destructive behavior. They and other caregivers become emotionally drained and physically exhausted from the constant need for supervision. It is my hope that this paper will bring to the attention of many of these parents the possibility that there may be a new, if not officially or even medically approved, approach to their daunting challenge. While this approach may not work for all, it assuredly will do no harm.

MELATONIN THERAPY FOR SLEEP DISORDERS

BY DR. JAMES JAN

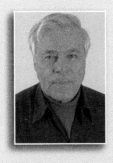

James E. Jan MD, FRCP(C)

Clinical Professor
Pediatric Neurology and Developmental Pediatrics
University of British Columbia
Senior Research Scientist Emeritus
Children's Hospital
Diagnostic Neurophysiology
4500 Oak Street
Vancouver, BC, Canada, V6H 3N1
jjan@cw.bc.ca

Dr. Jan is the author of over two hundred scientific articles and three books. As a child neurologist he worked with children who had various neurodevelopmental disabilities for more than forty years. In the early '90s he and his team introduced melatonin therapy for the sleep disorders of special needs children diagnosed with ASD, ADHD and various forms of intellectual deficits. This therapy is now used worldwide. Dr. Jan is semiretired now and no longer sees patients, but he teaches at the Children's Hospital and is involved in sleep research.

Melatonin (N-acetyl-5-ethoxytryptamine) is a small lipid and water soluble molecule which can readily enter all cells and bodily compartments. It is mainly derived from the pineal gland but it is also produced, in small amounts, in most tissues. Normally melatonin secretion into the bloodstream and spinal fluid begins in the evening, because darkness promotes its production and light inhibits it. Melatonin is thought to be present in all living organisms.

Research during the last fifty years, since its discovery, has shown that this hormone-like molecule has many important functions in the body. It plays a major role in sleep regulation, brain development, protection against toxins and it is a powerful antioxidant. It also synchronises metabolic activities and has shown beneficial effects on many diseases. Therefore, it is not surprising that there is a great interest in melatonin research among the scientific community.

Melatonin has been sold as an over-the-counter sleep aid since 1993 in the U.S. and since 2004 in Canada. It is synthesized commercially. Melatonin is produced from animal pineal glands is ineffective, dangerous, and fortunately not readily available. Melatonin products are sold in oral and sublingual tablets, capsules and in liquid forms. Some products, such as the sublingual tablets, capsules and liquid are called "fast-acting" because they act rapidly, but only promote sleep for three to four hours. Other, so-called "slow-release" products release melatonin slowly and promote sleep longer, for six to eight hours. These controlled-release tablets usually also contain fast-acting melatonin, therefore they are useful for treating both sleep onset and sleep maintenance difficulties. Melatonin is not a sleeping pill; in fact it is very different from hypnotic drugs. This natural sleep promoting substance is remarkably free from short- and long-term side effects, in contrast to hypnotics. Melatonin cannot be patented, because it is a naturally occurring substance, therefore any company may market it. Major pharmaceutical firms are not interested in investing money in researching it because, if they develop a better product, other companies can also sell it, and therefore the profits are limited. However, by modifying the basic formula, melatonin analogs have been developed, which are more expensive and do not appear to have an advantage over regular melatonin in sleep promotion. These analogs require prescriptions and cannot be sold over-the-counter.

History of Melatonin Therapy for Sleep Disorders

About twenty years ago our Melatonin Research Group at the Children's Hospital in Vancouver for the first time began using melatonin therapy for children with various neurodevelopmental disabilities and persistent sleep disturbances. Some children had severe intellectual deficits due to brain damage, autism spectrum disorders (ASDs), abnormal brain development, progressive neurological conditions and a variety of genetic disorders. Others had no intellectual disabilities but were diagnosed with attention-deficit/hyactivity disorder (ADHD) and anxiety disorders. For the most part, these sleep disturbances included difficulties falling asleep, frequent prolonged awakenings and early morning awakenings which were usually diagnosed as circadian rhythm sleep disorders. Early on we realized that children with severe neurodevelopmental problems responded similarly to melatonin therapy, whether their disturbed cognitive functioning was due to ASD, brain damage or maldevelopment of their brains. Therefore, their sleep disorders were not specific to their medical conditions but were related to their coexisting intellectual difficulties. It was puzzling as to why some children responded well to therapy whilst others did not but then it became clear that the treatment was only beneficial for those sleep disorders which were associated with low blood levels of melatonin or inappropriately timed pineal melatonin secretion. Frequent awakenings during the night were generally associated with low blood melatonin levels whereas difficulties falling asleep, without frequent awakenings, were most often related to delayed onset of pineal melatonin secretion. Early morning awakenings were sometimes due to low melatonin levels and, at other times, had neurological causes since the brain has different regulatory mechanisms for falling and staying asleep from those for waking up.

During the twenty years of our research we have not seen any significant short or long-term side effects or addictive properties and the effectiveness was not lost over time, as with hypnotics. Most importantly, better sleep was associated with improved health, behaviour and learning and in diminished parental stress.

Why Do We Need to Sleep?

Research has shown that sleep is needed for metabolic restoration of the brain and cognitive development. Inadequate sleep predisposes children to poor health, such as infections, obesity, diabetes and heart disease; also to disturbed behaviour and numerous cognitive and memory difficulties. Healthy sleep is especially important for the brain development of young children because several years of markedly poor sleep may cause irreparable damage to their growing nervous systems. Complete sleep deprivation in animal experiments results in death within a couple of weeks. Loss of sleep is markedly disturbing; in fact, forced sleep deprivation is a known form of torture.

The human sleep-wake cycle parallels day and night changes and in this cyclic process, our environmental contact tells when to sleep. This partially explains why 70 to 80 percent of special needs children with marked cognitive problems, who have difficulties understanding environmental cues, experience persistent sleep problems. Children with anxiety or ADHD may understand that it is time for them to sleep, but their over-excited brain circuits do not give the required signals to initiate pineal melatonin secretion until later and, as a result, they have delayed sleep onset. Oral melatonin bypasses this delayed signalling and generally promotes sleep within thirty minutes.

Sleep Research in Children With ASD

Surveys show that the majority of children with ASD experience sometimes lifelong sleep disturbances which are most stressful for them, their caregivers, and the entire family. Usually these sleep difficulties are falling asleep, frequent awakenings and early morning awakenings, therefore, they are circadian rhythm sleep disturbances. Several studies have shown that melatonin therapy has a high success rate and the treatment is now accepted worldwide. In the past in several publications on melatonin treatment, we have included children with ASD. Then in 2007 our group published a carefully designed study of controlled release melatonin therapy for fifty children with severe developmental problems. Out of this group, sixteen children had ASD. All sixteen children responded, completely or partially, to melatonin therapy.

For children with ASD, melatonin was most effective for delayed sleep onset, but it also promoted longer sleep maintenance without any side effects. Better sleep was associated with parent-reported improvements in health, behaviour and learning. Occasionally a reduction in anxiety and self-stimulating mannerisms was also noted because melatonin has anti-anxiety properties. Sleep promotion techniques were generally ineffective in our 16 children before melatonin therapy but afterward they responded better to sleep hygiene.

Parental observations were the best method of diagnosing and following the children's sleep difficulties. Blood, saliva, and urine tests for melatonin levels were available, but they did not offer practical benefits since even a short melatonin trial was more informative. Sleep diaries, actigraphs, which measure movements, or video tapes, were useful in documenting sleep patterns, but polysomnography was almost never necessary.

Side Effects of Melatonin Therapy

The labelling of some over-the-counter products indicates that melatonin should not be given to children or to pregnant women. This warning is based on misinformation. In fact, over the years melatonin treatment in numerous studies has not caused a significant adverse effect in children.

Several years ago, a letter to a medical journal suggested that melatonin therapy might trigger seizures. This was an incorrect observation; in fact melatonin has anticonvulsant properties. It was also claimed that this therapy during puberty is dangerous, which was again incorrect because in contrast to animals, the sexual development and sexual behaviours of humans are not affected by melatonin.

Toxicity has not been observed either even with the ingestion of high doses, and taking melatonin during pregnancy has not caused malformations in the fetus in numerous animal studies. The reason for this high safety profile is likely because normally we produce our own melatonin throughout our lives. Vivid dreaming is commonly noted, but, to the vast majority of people taking melatonin, this is not a problem. This molecule has immunological benefits and we have commonly observed less frequent respiratory infections during therapy.

Suggestions for Melatonin Therapy

The following suggestions may be useful when contemplating melatonin therapy:
- Ideally, a thorough medical evaluation would be beneficial because children with ASD may also have sleep disorders which do not respond to melatonin therapy, for example sleep apnea.

- If possible, healthy sleep habits should be established first because mild sleep difficulties will respond without melatonin therapy.

- Recording the child's sleep pattern (going to bed, falling asleep, awakenings, and associated behaviours) in a detailed diary for one to two weeks before and during the initial treatment period is very useful because any change in sleep would become easier to notice.

- Melatonin is an over-the-counter medication, therefore a prescription is not required in the U.S. and Canada. Nevertheless, it is better when a health professional supervises the treatment.

- Fast-release melatonin is more useful when the child has difficulties falling asleep without frequent awakenings. Slow-(controlled-) release formulations are the best for multiple awakenings with or without sleep onset delay.

- The oral dose should be given about thirty minutes before the desired bed time, and not several hours earlier, which is impractical. Melatonin may be mixed with a spoonful of jam, pudding, or ice cream. Tablets should not be chewed because then the controlled-release melatonin is converted into fast-release. This is the reason why smaller tablets for children are better than the larger ones which are generally marketed for adults.

- There is no advantage in using liquid melatonin unless the child has swallowing difficulties.

- There are no dose formulas which fit everyone as melatonin is not a sleeping pill. Starting with 1 to 3 mg is the best and then small incremental changes can be made every couple of days. Parents know their own children well, so they are in the best position to judge what the lowest and most optimal dose would be. Frequent awakenings are usually harder to treat than sleep onset delays and they often require higher doses, sometimes even up to 10 to 12 mg.

- Once the therapeutic threshold has been reached, additional doses do not result in deeper sleep. One cannot overdose a child into a toxic state, though large doses may cause temporary morning sleepiness.

- From time to time, when a child appears overly agitated, a larger dose may be given, or another dose could be administered one to two hours later. Repeating the dose in the middle of the night is only rarely helpful.

- Some children require melatonin replacement therapy for several months or years, others for life. Parents could stop the treatment every six to twelve months and, if the sleep problems recur, they could restart melatonin at the same dose. Melatonin can be stopped abruptly without causing any problems.

- In rare situations, when certain sleep centres of the brain are damaged, melatonin therapy is ineffective. When a child has early morning awakenings and melatonin does not fully help, a hypnotic drug is sometimes given as well. However, sleeping pills lose their effects with time.

- Melatonin may be administered during the day before medical tests (EEG, CT, MRI, and hearing evaluations) because it reduces the anxiety of children with ASD; therefore it makes them more co operative.

- Sleep hygiene should be continued, even when the melatonin therapy is successful.

- In our experience, when children are tired and sleepy, they are usually ready to go to bed and fall asleep. It is when they cannot fall asleep that they may exhibit difficult bedtime behaviours. In such situations, it might be wiser to treat them with melatonin first to correct their medical deficiency and then the difficult behaviours might diminish or even disappear. Certainly, behavioural therapies are more successful when the children are not exhausted.

MERIT: INTEGRATING ABA WITH DEVELOPMENTAL MODELS

BY JENIFER CLARK

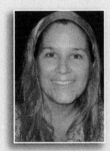

Jenifer Clark, MA, PhD (c)

New York, NY
212-222-9818
clarkjenif@aol.com
MERIT-consulting.org
JeniferClark.com

Jenifer Clark has been working with children and families for over fifteen years. She received her master's in psychology from NYU and is completing her Ph.D. in clinical psychology at CUNY. She has worked as an ABA therapist and consultant since 1992. She specializes in working with children with autism and has taught atypical development at Hunter College. Currently, she is the director of Boost!, an afterschool program for children with autism. This program focuses on teaching socialization and leisure skills to children on the spectrum, incorporating typical children as peers and social models. Ms. Clark is the co-founder and therapist for Sibfun, a support group for siblings of children with special-needs. She consults at special needs and typical schools and continues to consult with children and families.

Despite the wide base of empirical data that supports ABA in the treatment of autism, there are critics who express concerns over the impact that this treatment has on the emotional life of the child. Many argue that it is antithetical to design an intervention that would give a child with autism repeated experiences of having their distress ignored. Some are concerned about the impact these experiences have on a developing sense of self and the child's capacity to attach and increase relatedness. Parents can be put off by the data driven nature of the ABA methodology. Many families have shared with me their stories of seeking to embrace a more developmental model but feeling as if they are failing to offer their child much needed remediation during a critical period.

It is clearly the case that children with autism struggle with the concept that it is worthwhile to communicate their needs to another person. This being the case there *are* significant detrimental effects that can evolve from repeatedly ignoring distress. If a child with autism is deprived of the experience of having their feeling states acknowledged—which is a precursor to acknowledging feeling states in others—how will they develop this capacity?

In response to these growing concerns, pediatric neurologists and developmental specialists are increasingly encouraging parents to use a blended intervention to treat their child's autism. They are recommending that parents set up a program for their child that incorporates ABA and other more developmentally based approaches. Many parents are at a loss for how to accomplish this integration however. Therapists tend to be deeply committed to either one philosophy or the other and there is considerable resistance to working cooperatively. Additionally, the dominant methodologies developed from two very different philosophies and they frequently contradict one another at times in terms of how the intervention should proceed and how to interpret the behavior of the child.

Clearly there is a tremendous need for a treatment model which attends to autism in its entirety: one which successfully integrates the incredibly effective remediation, repetition and hierarchical teaching common to ABA with a developmental model that focuses on the equally important emotional development of the child. As ABA satisfies the need to remediate the core deficits of autism, *mentalization* emphasizes the need for a mutual acknowledgement of inner states. Mentalization describes the process in which we attend to the thoughts and feelings of another (Fonagy et al, 2002). Mentalization based therapies provide a way of conceptualizing our interactions with children with autism in a manner that consistently takes into account, and reflects back to them, their inner world.

An Integrated Model

MERIT–Mentalization Enhanced Remediation –an Integrated Treatment is a hybrid treatment approach. The MERIT model accomplishes emphasizes the structured and hierarchical teaching that is a crucial component of remediation while incorporating a mentalizing approach in all interactions with the child.

The three most important aspects of this model are providing mentalizing experiences to forge a relationship with the child, allowing mentalization to inform the treatment on a regular basis, and remediating the social-emotional areas that prevent the child from progressing in this area of development.

Forging the Relationship

In the initial phases of treatment the therapist engages in mentalization in order to understand and forge a relationship with the child. As the therapist comes to understand how this child thinks, learns and even how they cope with anxiety, all of this information will be influence how the therapist interacts with the child. This intimate relationship, which involves learning a child's likes and dislikes, as well as challenges and strengths, is, in fact, critical in using mentalization to treat autism.

It can be challenging to make sense of the inner life of a child with autism and therefore mentalization plays a pivotal role in the treatment. We cannot relate first-hand to a child who experiences sounds as painful and sensory issues as completely preoccupying. And yet, this process of being understood is an undeniably crucial aspect of development. A therapist must pose the question: How is this particular brain processing information? A therapist's job is to put him or herself in a child's place and to try to understand what it is the child is experiencing. A therapist must be able to determine the most constructive experiences to help a child with autism learn and be able to relate. This understanding will be a powerful guide to the therapy as well as a tremendous source of reinforcement and motivation for the child.

The Remediation

Traditional ABA programs that target areas such as verbal imitation, visual imitation, fine motor tasks and expressive and receptive language skills are incorporated into the treatment. The way in which concepts are introduced and the interactions before, during and after each discrete trial are profoundly influenced by the therapist-child relationship. This relationship is distinct from the relationship in some developmental programs in that the MERIT therapist will be directive. The MERIT therapist has an agenda and that is to remediate the areas of core deficit exhibited by that particular child. The heterogeneous nature of autism means that although all children with autism can be helped by remediation, it is dire that individual differences be taken into consideration. Failure to do so can result in disengagement both from the work and more importantly, from the therapist.

While engaged in their work, it is important that the child, despite their potentially limited capacity to understand language and gestures, feels understood. The therapist can increase communication through the use of language, gestures and visuals. Additionally, the work itself should evolve in such a way that it reflects an understanding of the child. Even if the child has a limited ability, initially, to process the world around them, presumably they can take in the experience of being less frustrated than they had been in their previous interactions with others. They can begin to trust that they can be successful. The nature of the relationship can be one of trust that nothing will be asked of this child that they cannot do (with some help). Ideally these interventions begin to remediate some of the areas of deficit which make it difficult to benefit from interactions with another or to process communication. The work builds upon itself. With each passing week the child develops more skills which allow him to better engage in social exchanges but in the meantime the relationship, which is critical to the work, is continually growing.

Remediating Social-Emotional Capacities

Some of the areas of deficit particular to autism, interfere with a child's ability to benefit fully from a mentalizing stance. *How can a child who can't perceive facial expressions benefit from his mother's warm smile? How can children with auditory processing deficits understand when they are being consoled? How can children who cannot attend to stimuli join their parents in reciprocal interactions?* These areas can be remediated to a measurable extent that will allow these children to gain more from formative interactive experiences.

Through remediation, children with autism can be taught to attend to the salient features in a social interaction, identify emotional states on faces and participate in social reciprocations. Once these types of skills have been established, they will allow the child with autism to begin to participate more in the social world, which will in turn fuel their emotional development.

The neurological differences experienced in autism, impact the perception and experience of the world. MERIT offers an opportunity to build these capacities through remediation, which in turn increases coping, ability to deal with drives, and expands understanding and sense of self.

For the child with autism, sensory input from the outside can often not be organized and is completely overwhelming to the nervous system. Many children with autism will avert their gaze or cover their ears in an attempt to reduce the influx of disconnected stimuli. There can be a sense that external input is fragmenting and assaultive. Their sense of cohesiveness is constantly being disrupted as a result of unintegrated environmental stimuli. Repetitive self-stimulation provides continuity of experience which is soothing, stable and reliable.

My model is increasing the capacity for symbolic representation and integration, and thereby allowing the child with autism to become more organized. It is not, in my view, a case of either ABA or developmental interventions but rather ABA moving towards and allowing for the success of more developmentally based approaches. Cognitive remediation for the difficulties with abstraction, generalization, and symbolization in autism allows for the development of cognitive structures in the context of a highly dynamic exchange. This is the basis for the development of symbolization and language.

The repetition seen in discrete trial learning is not merely the repetition of cognitive exercises, but is additionally the repetition and re-internalization of experiences with a responsive other. Along a developmental trajectory, a child with autism must build a basic capacity to achieve early concept formation such as same and different, categories and relationships. These are precursors to the development of language and the development of these skills is very organizing to the child with ASD. In the case of autism it is not that the case that these achievements cannot occur; they just fail to happen without appropriate intervention.

Jonathan: increasing the capacity for symbol formation

Jonathan was unable to match non-identical pictures (different pictures of dogs or crayons or cups). I moved to an earlier step and required him instead to match identical objects. I experimented with pictures of crayons. If the pictures were exact replications he was successful at this task but I soon realized that if the background was different (the crayon was placed on the table rather than the rug) or of the orientation was different, Jonathan did not recognize the crayon as the same crayon. Jonathan practiced matching crayons with a painstakingly simplified approach. Initially, I used pictures that were only slightly different. The crayon had the same background and the orientation was only changed slightly. Gradually I was able to introduce more significant differences between the pictures including completely different backgrounds and orientations. He was eventually able to match different colors and brands of crayons and understood that they too were crayons. I was able to teach Jonathan to match other non-identical objects and with each new target he was able to learn the objective with less and less practice. Finally Jonathan was able to match non-identical objects without a practice period. He had achieved a goal that is an important precursor to primitive figurative language.

Imagine the consequence of failing to remediate the skill deficit described above. Would Jonathan have the capacity to recognize his mother if she changed her shirt? If she was in a different context (at school rather than at home)? The relationship between the remediation and skills is complex but critical in optimizing the development of children on the spectrum.

Sebastian: distinguishing play from reality

Sebastian was a preschooler I worked with for a year. Although he had responded positively to the interventions designed to teach expressive and receptive language his symbolic play was still delayed. Concrete thinking is analogous to ASD and can make pretend play very frightening to the child with autism. Sebastian and I read the story of the 3 pigs and he enjoyed the pattern woven into the dialogue of the story. He quickly memorized the words and I thought that the story might allow a bridge into pretend play. Sebastian was having a playdate with another child and he was thrilled about the idea of playing "three little pigs". He was somewhat anxious but was enjoying reciting his lines as a "pig" and therefore went along with the game. His peer was the wolf and when it came time for her to blow the house down, Sebastian became hysterical. It was as if the little girl had transformed into the wolf.

Not wanting to abandon the idea that Sebastian could be taught to enter into the world of imaginative play, in a slow, systematic, safe way I began to introduce the concept of pretending. I made some games that had cards to choose. Each card had a character and you had to say something that character would say. The other person had to guess which card you had chosen. Sebastian liked this game very much. It was predictable and safe but it also had him beginning to realize that he could talk like a particular character and still be Sebastian. Just because he said "I live in a pineapple under the sea," he did not become Spongebob. From there we began to work on varied forms of charades, including a "who would sing this?" game and eventually we developed concepts of what characters in a particular role would do and say.

Using this systematic approach Sebastian was able to learn to engage in many forms of pretend play. By the time he was 5 years old, he regularly joined in with his typical preschool classmates in the pretend area and contributed to making up complex stories as they played varied versions of "family" and "dinosaurs". By allowing Sebastian a gradual entry to pretend play, I was able to help him to realize we remain in reality even when we venture into the world of pretend. This systematic process decreased Sebastian's anxiety, which had been overwhelming, and allowed him to benefit from the joy of pretend as well as all of the other skills that pretending enables typical children to develop.

These vignettes emphasize the need for an integrated approach. In both cases hierarchical learning, shaping and reinforcement were used to remediate a skill that interfered with a more relational aspect of development. Mentalization was used to understand the child's failure to develop a particular skill and that information in term informed the treatment. Both children required the task at hand to be broken down into its component parts before they could successfully acquire the new skill.

Conclusion

ABA and developmental models have proven success in treating children with autism. The future of autism treatment involves finding a way to integrate these proven methodologies that offers parents and treatment providers a clear and coherent philosophy regarding the treatment of children with autism. It is evident that there is a need for a treatment model that is well integrated and cohesive and at the same time inclusive and current with regard to what we know about the brain and neuroplasticity.

MERIT offers such an integration. MERIT takes into account the individual differences of the child as well as his unique learning style and importance is placed on working with the family to enhance the child's outcome. Autistic children's success hinges on the remediation of so many compromised areas of functioning and it is only when all of these core deficits are being addressed simultaneously and in a way that is fostering a connection to others that a child can enjoy optimal success.

METHYL-B$_{12}$: MYTH OR MASTERPIECE

BY DR. JAMES NEUBRANDER

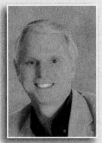

James A. Neubrander, MD, FAAEM

Comprehensive Neuroscience Center
100 Menlo Park, Suites 410 and 200
Edison, NJ 08837
(732) 906-9000; (732) 906-7888
www.drneubrander.com
www.neuro-center.com
www.IBRFinc.org

Dr. Neubrander trained in Pathology and Laboratory Medicine and is Board Certified in Environmental Medicine. He is the Medical Director of Autism Research for the International Brain Research Foundation and Medical Director of the Comprehensive Neuroscience Center in Edison, New Jersey. He serves on many scientific advisory boards dedicated to treating autism and neurodevelopmental disorders. He lectures many times each year at National and International Conferences and Physician Training Courses. His lectures are scientific, evidence-based, and emphasize newer treatments or modifications of established protocols that appear to enhance clinical outcomes beyond the results previously reported. He is the coauthor of several peer-reviewed articles, has been interviewed and filmed for many documentaries and television spots, has been referenced in many books written about autism, nutrition, and environmental medicine, and has been quoted innumerable times by scientists, researchers, clinicians, and lay persons, most notably for methylcobalamin, hyperbaric oxygen, and heavy metal detoxification.

Since the mid '90s, I was one of a handful of physicians who had been using the only two available forms of vitamin B$_{12}$, cyano-B$_{12}$ and hydroxy-B$_{12}$, to treat children with autism. We used these forms of B$_{12}$ because the majority of children with autism had an abnormal elevation of the organic acid known as FIGLU (formiminoglutamic acid). Though we believed we saw minor improvements by using B$_{12}$, we never saw anything remarkable. In the '80s and '90s, the Japanese had been studying the methyl form of B$_{12}$ for many disorders, none of which were autism. It was not until the late '90s that the methyl form finally became available in the United States, though it was not commonly used. In March of 2002, I became the first physician in the world to ever use the methyl form of B$_{12}$ in a child with autism. Amazingly, the child showed many significant changes.

The second child I treated, who previously used three- to four-word utterances, began speaking in six- to eight-word sentences within two weeks. Not only was he now talking, he was also interacting with everyone. This included his shocked school bus driver whom he tried to kiss, and his even more shocked crossing guard whom he started hugging and talking to every day! Such social interactions, especially spontaneously initiated, were something that he never did prior to methyl-B$_{12}$. His parents jokingly said that things might have been better for them before they started the shots, because then they had a little peace and quiet in the house and not all his constant chatter!

Now, more than a million dose evaluations later, the single most predictable treatment I have seen to positively affect more than 90 percent of children on the spectrum is methyl-B$_{12}$ injections if done according to the protocols I have continued to improve upon over the last seven years. Though shots are initially feared by most parents, they soon learn that the shots are painless, easy to administer, and give the greatest number of clinical responses when compared to oral, nasal, or transdermal routes of administration. Interestingly, prior to starting therapy, the majority of children who respond to methyl-B$_{12}$ injections have high normal to high levels of B$_{12}$ in their blood, rather than the low levels would be expected. The reason for this appears to be what I call "B$_{12}$ diabetes." Just as blood sugar builds up in the plasma of a diabetic because it cannot get into the cell, B$_{12}$ builds up in the plasma and does not get into the cell, possibly due to a transcobalamin transporter problem.

Methyl-B$_{12}$ is methylcobalamin. Every time you see the word "cobalamin," you can substitute the word "B$_{12}$." In the late 1920s, when vitamins were first discovered, they were called "*vital amines.*" Eventually the words were combined to form what we know today as "vitamin." When B$_{12}$ was discovered, it was called the "cobalt vital amine" because a cobalt atom is found deep within the molecule. The name was later shortened to be called the "*cobal*t vit*amin,*" what we know today as "cobalamin." The cobalamins represent a *family* of cobalt containing vitamins. To better understand this, consider "cobalamin" to be the last name of a family, analogous to "the Smiths." The different types of B$_{12}$ are analogous to the first names of each family member that identifies them from each other. For the Smiths, there could be Jennifer, Ashley, Megan, Michael, Matthew, or Jeremy. For the Cobalamin family, the individual family members are named Methyl, Adenosyl, Hydroxy, Cyano, Glutathionyl, and Sulfito. They each have their own jobs and assignments to do. The two senior family members of the cobalamin family are methyl-B$_{12}$ and adenosyl-B$_{12}$. Only these two forms have "coenzyme" properties that allow them to complete special assignments with specific enzymes found in the body, especially in the brain and mitochondria when we are discussing autism.

Methyl-B$_{12}$'s unique coenzyme activity unlocks the enzyme methionine synthase. Every time it is unlocked, methionine synthase transfers a methyl group to homocysteine allowing homocysteine to re-enter the methionine cycle. This reaction is vital for methyl groups to be passed from one molecule to the next, a process called transmethylation. For children with autism, the results of transmethylation are increased language, focus and attention, awareness, cognition, independence, socialization and interactive play, appropriate emotional responses, affection, eye contact, and improvements in gross and fine motor skills.

The science behind why methyl-B$_{12}$ works for autism is sound. The folate cycle, methionine-homocysteine cycle, and homocysteine-glutathione pathway are intricately interwoven in a delicate balance that exists to create and then pass along methyl groups, and to create glutathione, the body's most important intracellular antioxidant. The folic acid cycle receives premethylated folic acid molecules from food, vitamins, or from a folic acid recycling process. Premethylated folic acid molecules are presented to the MTHFR (methylene tetra hydro folat) enzyme to become methylated folic acid. Methylated folic acid donates its methyl group to "naked B$_{12}$" for it to become methyl-B$_{12}$. Methyl-B$_{12}$, in the presence of methionine synthase, passes its methyl group to homocysteine which then becomes methylated (or re-methylated) homocysteine, also known as methionine. Methionine then adds an adenosyl molecule to become S-adenosylmethione (SAMe), the "universal methyl donor." It is SAMe's job to transfer the methyl group (transmethylation) to many different types of molecules in the brain to produce the clinical results previously discussed. Once the methyl group has been transferred, the remaining molecule, S-adenosylhomocysteine (SAH) still retains the adenosyl group. Unfortunately, SAH blocks further transmethylation until the adenosyl group is removed, a process that requires adequate zinc, and at times the removal of dairy. Once SAH loses the adenosyl group, what is left is "naked" (or parent) homocysteine, devoid of methyl of adenosyl groups.

Depending on various factors, "parent homocysteine" will proceed one of two ways. When oxidative stress is under control, homocysteine will enter the methionine-homocysteine cycle just described. However, when oxidative stress is high, homocysteine will be shunted down the homocysteine-glutathione pathway to create glutathione, the body's primary intracellular antioxidant. Oxidative stress is a condition where "wild unpaired electrons" cause significant tissue and cellular damage before they find a mate. Antioxidants provide such mates.

Jill James, Ph.D., demonstrated that children on the autism spectrum had lower values of active glutathione than controls. Richard Deth, Ph.D., found that methionine synthase is critical for a special dopamine receptor and normal brain function. Dr. Deth also documented that many substances damage or block methionine synthase activity, including mercury, the infamous agent found in vaccines containing thimerosal.

With this scientific background, one can begin to understand how the administration of injectable methyl-B$_{12}$ works for children with autism from each of the three pathways previously described. In the folate cycle, the MTHFR enzyme is frequently mutated. This results in low production of the methyl groups needed to make methyl-B$_{12}$.

By injecting methyl-B$_{12}$, we bypass the problem. In the methionine-homocysteine cycle, the addition of methyl-B$_{12}$ allows more methyl groups to first be donated to SAMe and subsequently passed along to the crucial molecules in the brain that will reduce autistic symptoms. In the homocysteine-glutathione pathway, methyl-B$_{12}$ has been shown to help restore the critical balance between methylation and transsulfuration.

Since March of 2002, I have treated thousands of children on the autism spectrum and have personally monitored over a million doses in my clinic. My research has included the clinical responsiveness to all forms of commercially available B$_{12}$: cyano-B$_{12}$, hydroxy-B$_{12}$, adenosyl-B$_{12}$, and methyl-B$_{12}$. It has investigated the clinical responsiveness from all routes of administration: oral, sublingual, transdermal, nasal, intravenous, intramuscular, suppository, and subcutaneous. It has evaluated the clinical responsiveness from shots varying from weekly to daily, from various stock concentrations, and from different pH values. It has evaluated the clinical responsiveness when B$_{12}$ has been used in combination which other agents, most commonly folinic acid, glutathione, and/or N-acetylcysteine. It has investigated the clinical benefit and side effect patterns when used concurrently with TMG, SAMe, methionine, NAC, glutathione, B6, folic acid, folinic acid, 5-MTHF, DMG, ALA, etc. *In summary, from seven years of intense clinical research I cannot emphasize enough how much the right protocol matters. Which protocol is selected can make or break how effective the shots are for any given child.*

In my clinic, according to the protocols I have developed over the past seven years, I consistently find that the injectable form methyl-B$_{12}$ if far superior to any other route of administration when one considers the percentage of children who respond, the intensity of each response, and how many responses each child exhibits.

Key factors necessary to achieve maximum effectiveness are beyond the scope of this chapter. They include, but are not limited to the pH and concentration of the stock solution, the mcg/kg of the dose used, the frequency of the injections, the route of administration, and if given subcutaneously, the site of the injections, the evaluation tools used by the parents to report their findings, and the presence of selected key supplements reaching predetermined dosage ranges prior to implementing higher doses of methyl-B$_{12}$, or prior to increasing the frequency of the injections. The most common initiation protocol I use is a dose of 65 mcg/kg drawn from a stock solution of 25 mg/mL given at a ten-degree angle into the adipose tissue of the buttocks once every three days. A local anesthetic cream can be locally applied at the site of the injection.

As previously stated, the primary categories of improvement include increased language, focus and attention, awareness, cognition, independence, socialization and interactive play, appropriate emotional responses, affection, eye contact, and improvements in gross and fine motor skills. In my clinic, the frequency for at least some of these responses is 94 percent. The average number of responses is thirty to fifty out of a possible total of 135. Though the intensity of response can be very strong at times, the majority of parents report mild, mild-to-moderate, or moderate improvements. The positive effects build over 2½ to 4 years. Should the shots be discontinued prior to that amount of time, many children will regress. After 2½ to 4 years, many children can be weaned off their shots. 60 to 70 percent of children do better on daily shots, but only if certain key supplements are being taken at the recommended ranges provided in the Supplement Review Program as shown on my website.

Compounding pharmacies must make the injections. Depending on the pharmacy used, the shots usually range from $0.50 to $1.50 each. I only prescribe preservative-free shots in prefilled syringes rather than less expensive multi-dose vials that contain preservative. I do this because of two theoretical risks. First, injecting preservatives into children on the spectrum may exacerbate their inability to detoxify, something already known to be compromised in the majority of them because they have less glutathione than their peers. Second, even though alcohol swabs are to be used, the risk for Myco-plasma, bacterial, or viral contamination still exists, and I will not take that risk.

Best case anecdotal stories, including a section showing *Recovered Kids*, can be viewed in the video section of my website; www.drneubrander.com. One remarkable story is Caitlin's. Her mother was a speech pathologist who, while in training, refused to do a rotation to learn about autistic children because she wanted to have nothing to do with it. Unfortunately, when Caitlin was 2½ years old, Caitlin's mother was dev-astated when the doctor told her Caitlin was not just autistic, but severely so. Caitlin progressed very quickly from methyl-B$_{12}$ shots and fully recovered. Today, no one can tell she was ever autistic! Unfortunately, best case scenarios are unusual. The majority of patients show mild or moderate improvements which, as they follow my protocols for 2½ to 4 years, continue to improve.

Long-term use is safe as documented from pernicious anemia patients. Serious side effects do not occur. However, nuisance side effects are fairly common. The good news is that they usually pass within four to six months as the body adjusts to keep the good and delete the bad. Common side effects are hyperactivity, stimming, and mouthing objects. Occasionally sleep is disturbed though more often it improves. Side effects belong in two categories: positive-negative vs. negative-negative, and tolerable vs. intolerable. A common positive-negative side effect for young children is pinching or tantruming, as they become much more aware of what they want and ask for it in perfectly good "autism-ese." When you do not understand, they get upset and tantrum or pinch to get your attention so you will do what they want you to do. Now that they are much more aware of what they want, they also get upset and tantrum when you tell them to do something they don't want to do.

In summary, every child on the autism spectrum deserves a clinical trial of inject-able methyl-B$_{12}$ because it has proven to be an effective treatment for the majority of children on the autism spectrum, if done correctly.

MITOCHONDRIAL DYSFUNCTION AND ITS TREATMENT

BY DR. RICHARD E. FRYE

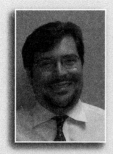

Richard E. Frye, M.D., Ph.D.

Department of Pediatrics
Division of Child and Adolescent Neurology and The Children's
Learning Institute
7000 Fannin—UCT 2478, Houston, TX 77030
Richard.E.Frye@uth.tmc.edu

Dr. Richard E. Frye received his M.D. and Ph.D. in physiology and biophysics from Georgetown University. He completed his residency in pediatric at University of Miami and residency in child neurology at Children's Hospital Boston. Following residency Dr. Frye completed a clinical fellowship in behavioral neurology and learning disabilities at Children's Hospital Boston and a research fellowship in psychology at Boston University. Dr. Frye also completed a M.S. in biomedical science and biostatistics at Drexel University. Dr. Frye is board certified in General Pediatrics and in Neurology with Special Competency in Child Neurology. Dr. Frye has been funded to study brain structure function in individuals with neurodevelopmental disorders, mitochondrial dysfunction in autism and clinical trials for novel autism treatments. Dr. Frye is the medical-director of the University of Texas medically-based autism clinic. The purpose of this unique clinic is to diagnose and treat medical disorders associated with autism, such as mitochondrial disorders and subclinical electrical discharges, in order to optimize remediation and recovery.

Recent studies have suggested that autism may be linked to dysfunction of the mitochondria—the powerhouse of every cell in our body. In addition to a lack of cellular energy production, mitochondrial dysfunction can affect both energy and non-energy producing metabolic systems since many metabolic systems feed their final biochemical products into mitochondrial pathways and/or derive their biochemical substrates from mitochondrial pathways. Furthermore, dysfunctional mitochondria can create reactive oxygen species that can damage the mitochondria and other important cellular components.

Those affected by mitochondrial dysfunction manifest non-specific symptoms including developmental delay, loss of developmental milestones (i.e., regression), seizures, easy fatigability, gastrointestinal abnormalities and immune dysfunction. In general, mitochondrial dysfunction affects body systems that have high energy demands such as the brain, gastrointestinal system and immune system. Some of the same body systems that are dysfunctional in mitochondrial disorders are also dysfunctional in autism. Recently studies have suggested that approximately 5% of individuals with autism have strictly defined mitochondrial disease while a larger number of individuals with autism might have less severe mitochondrial dysfunction.

Mitochondrial dysfunction is treated through four approaches: (1) precautions to prevent metabolic decompensation; (2) vitamin supplements to support mitochondrial function; (3) modification of the diet to optimize mitochondrial function; and (4) investigation of medical disorders associated with mitochondrial dysfunction..

Precautions:

Individuals with mitochondrial dysfunction should avoid physiological stressors such as fasting, extreme cold or heat, sleep deprivation, dehydration and illness. If an individual with mitochondrial dysfunction becomes sick, fever should be treated aggressively and good hydration should be maintained, potentially with intravenous hydration with carbohydrates if necessary. Certain drugs and environmental toxins which depress mitochondrial function should be avoided. For example, common toxins which inhibit mitochondrial function including heavy metals, insecticides, cigarette smoke and monosodium glutamate. Common drugs that inhibit mitochondrial function include acetaminophen, non-steroidal anti-inflammatory drugs, alcohol, some antipsychotic, antidepressant, anticonvulsant, antidiabetic, antihyperlipidemic, antibiotic and anesthetic drugs. Specific precautions are required for surgery and anesthesia.

Vitamin Supplementation

Vitamins may enhance mitochondrial enzyme function and may result in improved efficiency of energy generation. In addition, some vitamins serve as antioxidants, which may slow the progression of the mitochondrial dysfunction due to high amounts of reactive oxygen species. Standard supplementations for mitochondrial dysfunction include Co-Enzyme Q10 (5-15mg/kg/day), levo-carnitine (30-100mg/kg/day) and B vitamins. Typical B vitamins include thiamine (50-100mg/day), riboflavin (100-400mg/day), nicotinamide (50-100mg/day), pyridoxine (200mg/day) and cyanocobalamin (5-1000 mcg/day). Co-enzyme Q10 analogs, for example Ubiquinol, have better bioavailability than co-enzyme Q10, providing the same effect at 1/10th to 1/20th the dose. Acetyl-L-carnitine (250-1000mg/day) is a natural constituent of the inner mitochondrial membrane. Biotin (5-10mg/day) is an important cofactor for several mitochondrial enzymes, especially those that process fatty acids. Antioxidants useful for individuals with mitochondrial dysfunction include vitamins E (200-400 IU/day) and C (100-500 mg/day), alpha-lipoic acid (50-200 mg/day) and folic acid (1-10 mg/day).

Diet Modifications:

Some patients respond to frequent meals high in complex carbohydrates. For some patients an overnight fast can be enough to destabilize mitochondrial function. Such patients can be treated with complex carbohydrates such as corn starch before bedtime while some can be awakened in the middle of the night for a snack while others may require a feeding tube to receive feeding overnight. Other patients respond to low carbohydrate diets such as the ketogenic diet. The ketogenic diet should be initiated and monitored by an practitioner familiar with the diet as it can cause acidosis and exacerbate metabolic disorders is certain cases. Some patients respond to medium chain triglyceride oil supplementation since these fats do not require carnitine to be transported into the mitochondria.

Associated Medical Disorders

Individuals with mitochondrial disease have high rates of cardiac, gastrointestinal, endocrine, growth, vision and immunological abnormalities. Thus, such organ systems should be screened for dysfunction. Seizures and subclinical electrical discharges are relatively common in mitochondrial disorders, so practitioners should have a high index of suspicion for these abnormalities. Cerebral folate deficiency has been reported in both mitochondrial disorders and autism. This disorder can be easily treated with folinic acid so it should be strongly considered in individuals with mitochondrial dysfunction.

History of development

In 1962 two independent researchers linked dysfunctional mitochondria to medical disease. In the last thirty years, several dozen genetically-based mitochondrial disorders have been described — all of them rare. It is becoming increasingly recognized that mitochondrial dysfunction, as opposed to mitochondrial disease, may contribute to the development and progression of many common neurodegenerative diseases such as Parkinson's disease.

Although mitochondrial dysfunction in autism has only recently been more widely recognized, the first biochemical evidence of mitochondrial dysfunction was reported over twenty years ago. Dr. Mary Coleman from Georgetown University described an elevation in serum lactic acid in a subset of children diagnosed with autism. Over the past five years, others have confirmed elevations in lactic acid, as well as abnormalities in other metabolic markers of mitochondrial dysfunction in children with autism.

In general, milder mitochondrial dysfunction responds better to treatment than more severe dysfunction and treatment initiated sooner in the course of the disorder will probably be more effective than treatment initiated after long standing mitochondrial dysfunction. However, the success rate of treatment is very variable for several reasons. First, the efficacy of mitochondrial treatment, even for well-known mitochondrial disorders, has not been well studied. Second, the mitochondrial dysfunction identified in autism has not been well characterized and treatment for mitochondrial dysfunction in autism has not been well studied. Third, the benefit of treatment may not be obvious as treatment my simply prevent progression of symptoms rather than reverse symptoms. Fourth, any benefit from treatment may take several months to observe.

Most vitamins are well tolerated, even at high doses. Some children with autism may have behavioral side-effects from some vitamin. Thus, it is important to start vitamins one at a time so that any side-effects can be linked to a particular vitamin. Levocarnitine has been linked to behavioral disturbances, especially in children with fatty acid abnormalities. Pyridoxine has been suggested to result in peripheral neuropathy at high doses. Children should be carefully monitored when the ketogenic diet is started as the diet can worsen the metabolic acidosis associated with mitochondrial dysfunction.

For More Information

THE UNITED MITOCHONDRIAL DISEASE FOUNDATION

www.umdf.org

MUSIC THERAPY

BY LEAH KMETZ

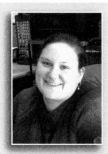

Leah Kmetz, MMT, MT-BC

titacleah@me.com

Leah E. Kmetz, MMT, MT-BC currently is employed by Fairfax County Public Schools in Northern Virginia and runs a private practice specializing in Autism. She is a graduate of both Slippery Rock University and Shenandoah Conservatory, in music therapy.

Music is heard many places that you'll go. It is so common in our society that many times we can drown it out if we are not paying attention. The music industry makes millions of dollars a year selling instruments, sheet music, CD's, concert tickets, and music merchandise to the general public. If music has such a strong pull in our everyday lives, why can't it change us? It does. We are not the people we were yesterday and many times music can influence who we are and what we do in the future, but for people who have special needs it can be much more powerful when engaging in music with a music therapist.

Merriam (1964) suggests that music has 10 functions people engage in, both as literate and non-literate cultures. These functions include emotional expression, aesthetic enjoyment, entertainment, communication, symbolic representation, physical response enforcing conformity to social norms, validation of social institutions and religious rituals, contributions to the continuity and stability of culture and the contributions to the integration of society. These functions help support the foundation of music therapy practice and reinforce the desired behaviors we look to improve in autism. While some of these functions are not related to the deficits in autism, many are strong links in to the improvement of a deficit area.

Kaplan (1990) suggests that the arts, and specifically music, serve as different functions in our lives. He suggests that they form knowledge, are collective possessions, are personal experiences, provide therapy, are a moral and symbolic force, have incidental commodity, are symbolic indicators of change, and link the past, present, and future together. Kaplan and Merriam differ in their ideas of functions, but there seems to be a link in understanding that music affects a person on not only a social level but also personal and subconscious levels.

The autism spectrum is a unique umbrella that groups people who have significant delays in social skills, communication and language, and a preoccupation with oneself and/or objects. (DSM IV, 2000) These delays can manifest at different frequencies and each case is unique. There is a high frequency of people with autism who develop a special relationship with music. This relationship can help promote the occurrence of physical, academic, or social skills. (AMTA 1999) Music therapy offers a structured goal orientated experience to help develop these skills in many people with autism, through a connective musical source.

Music therapy is the process of using musical games and activities to promote individualized goals based on the client's needs. This practice is both clinical and evidence based and is provided by a board certified music therapist who has completed training at an accredited university. Music therapists work on physical, cognitive, social, and emotional goals that are based from assessments made by the therapist. Through participation in both active and passive activities, clients' goals are both strengthened and generalized to other areas of living. Continual assessment occurs until the client is set for termination based on accomplishments of his/her goals, or the clinical team determines a termination point. (AMTA, 1999)

Deficits in autism are usually found in the areas of social skill development, communication and language skills, and a preoccupation in oneself or objects. Music therapy has the opportunity to engage clients in activities that provided teaching and support for desired behaviors. Because music is an enjoyable activity, clients are more likely to participate and respond by cuing and innate response. Music can provide multi sensory activities that engage interaction among the participants and a sense of security with the familiarity.

The following examples show you a few ways music therapists work with clients with autism. These are not the only activities, but generated for the clients particular needs.

Social Skills

Social skills are wide range of behaviors people exhibit towards others that are considered socially acceptable and can differ among groups of people. Common social skills include greeting people, keeping appropriate body space, and knowing when to talk in a conversation. These skills cover both non-verbal and verbal traits that are used in sync to engage in conversation between people.

Client A is working on greeting others. Client A is a 12 years old with autism. He has verbal skills, a large vocabulary and grade level reading skills, but only uses words when prompted by an adult. He is able to make eye contact but will not initiate a greeting. The music therapist and Client A read the social story together and then learn it as a song. This song is practiced many times over a few sessions along with activities that support greeting people he knows. Client A will practice greeting pictures of people he knows in music activities. At this time, no new pictures are introduced because the focus is just greeting people that we know. The music therapist will then work on incorporating skills during session and during transition times and when the client needs assistance will sing or hum the song to reinforce the desired behavior. Other people who work closely with the client can also be taught the song so that he will have the musical prompt as needed, until client A consistently greets others without prompts.

In this case, a social story is used that follows Carol Gray's format (2000). Sentences are carefully written to describe the situation the person will encounter and what specifically will or can be done. These sentences are usually short and give a desired behavior to the client that will help them understand and feel more comfortable when it happens. They also provide skills and tasks for them to complete to help the client be successful. The most important goal is that the client is given only one direction and supportive information is used to balance the story and the event. Once the story is read and understood, it is also taught as a song. When writing the song, it is important to keep the same words and phrases as the story and incorporating a new melody that the client will enjoy. Other music activities are used to follow up to support and generalize these new skills into their common vocabulary and life.

Another way to teach social skills in music is by practicing a technique that is focused around music. The client receives training during their music lesson so that they can be successful outside of the music lesson, like with social stories.

Client B is 13 years old with a very large vocabulary and social interaction skills, but lacks email and computer socialization skills. He is seen once weekly and plays piano well. Client B has set up an email account with his parents, but rarely checks his emails or doesn't answer them. Client B expresses that he knows they are there, but does not initiate response unless asked to in the email or by an onlooker. He has received music therapy services for 9 years. The music therapist and client B have established a system for sharing songs. When client B finishes learning a song, he is to record it and then send it via email to the music therapist. The music therapist sends back responses about the recording asking questions, or comments about the recording. Sometimes the therapist does not respond. During sessions emails are viewed and discussed and referred to as conversations in person. These discussions are based around the music that he performs and improving electronic dialogue.

Communication and Language Skills

Language skills develop from vocal skills, but can be difficult for some people. These skills can help one be more successful in attaining needs and becoming independent. Language can be difficult for some clients because of tactile or sound issues. Developing and engaging in language seem to be typical goals.

Client C is a five year old male with severe language delays. One of his goals is to be able to pronounce common words from his daily vocabulary sheet. Client B loves to hum and sing, but little verbal production or clear diction. Using his daily vocabulary sheet, songs are identified that contain these words. Client C and the music therapist sing the songs together. Small goals are set for the client to first imitate correct sounds of the words and then eventually over time, produce the correct word, with clear diction, and in the correct tempo. As sessions progress new words are chosen from the list and introduced in the sessions while reinforcing the previously learned words. The music therapist works to incorporate successful words into other songs to gain generalization.

Clients who have goals in communication can range from using language to respond to a non-linguistic system, such as sign language or picture communication. Communication is an essential part of life and when we can properly communicate our wants and needs can be met more easily.

Client D has limited verbal skills and often chooses to communicate in non-verbal ways. He has been offered picture cues and a PECS book to facilitate communication, but rarely chooses to use them. Client D loves to listen to music and often times seeks out his brother to play guitar. Once in music therapy, goals are set to use PECS for all communication. Client D is given cards to represent instruments and songs that he likes. During the session the therapist requires Client D to use the strips to communicate, with small phrases. When correctly communicating he is rewarded with the desired task and the session continues. As sessions continue and longer sentences are required and other activities that involve extra-musical words are required. As the other therapists and his parents introduce new words the music therapist also reinforces those words.

Cognitive skills

Cognitive skills are used to become independent adults and to help maintain a quality of life for people with autism. These skills are varied, but for people who respond well to music, these skills can become less stressful and sometimes less difficult when paired with music.

Client group E is a group of autistic students who are in the 7th and 8th grade. These students are seen in the school setting and working at completing their state assessments, but are having difficulty learning science terms. They are seen daily by a music therapist who works closely with their classroom teacher. The students were asked to identify parts of the plant and then explain the growth process. Client group D sings daily in music and enjoys learning new songs. They were taught the parts of the plants by using a melody to a previously learned song. Using exact wording from the classroom worksheets and keeping true to the order, students would use the song to identify the parts and eventually put them in order without assistance. By working through this song in music therapy, the classroom teacher felt the students quickly completed the activities for assessment and when students reached a difficult part she would remind them to sing the song which would inspire the students to become less confused about the process.

These techniques are only a sampling of what music therapists can do and change with the needs of each client. It is important to know that when working with a music therapist that the plan of treatment will be different for each client and will be tailored to fit their needs and their personal enjoyment. To find a music therapist in your area the American Music Therapy Association would like to help at www.musictherapy.org.

NEUROFEEDBACK FOR THE AUTISM SPECTRUM

BY DR. SIEGFRIED AND SUSAN F. OTHMER

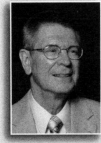

Siegfried Othmer, PhD
Susan F. Othmer

The EEG Institute
6400 Canoga Avenue
Suite 210
Woodland Hills, CA 91367
(818) 456-5975

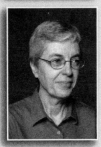

Siegfried and Susan F. Othmer were attracted to the emerging field of neurofeedback in 1985 to help with the epilepsy of their son Brian. If Brian were diagnosed today, he would surely also be labeled Asperger's, so his may have been the very first case in which a child benefited for his Asperger's from having training with neurofeedback. Siegfried Othmer is a physicist with long experience in aerospace research until he was drawn into the field of neurofeedback. Susan Othmer studied physics and neurobiology at Cornell until her Ph.D. research was derailed by her son's epilepsy. The Othmers have taught neurofeedback to thousands of professionals over the last 20 years in some 9 countries. The neurofeedback training instruments they either developed or inspired are used by more clinicians than any other. The Othmers have published research on neurofeedback in application to ADHD, mental retardation, addictions, chronic pain, and PTSD. Siegfried Othmer is co-author of the book *ADD: The Twenty-Hour Solution*. Siegfried Othmer is currently Chief Scientist at the EEG Institute in Los Angeles, CA. Susan Othmer is the Clinical Director. Their younger son Kurt is CEO of EEGInfo, a neurofeedback service organization for clinicians. Siegfried Othmer is also President of the Brian Othmer Foundation, under whose auspices neurofeedback services are being delivered worldwide to our veterans and active duty servicemen.

Neurofeedback is a highly promising emerging therapy for the autism spectrum. At issue here is a tool for the direct training of brain function, one that has already shown itself highly effective in addressing a wide range of "mental health" concerns. As has been the case for other therapies, its application to the autism spectrum has been complicated by the inherent complexity of the condition we confront. In the following, we recapitulate the development of neurofeedback for the autism spectrum and give some guidance to both therapists and parents with regard to the choices open to them.

Our own work with the autism spectrum using neurofeedback goes back some 25 years. In those early days of the field, the principal application of neurofeedback was to Attention-Deficit Hyperactivity Disorder (ADHD), but the very same procedures were clearly also helpful for a variety of other issues. So it came naturally to want to try these methods also with children on the autism spectrum. These early attempts were just as likely to make things worse as they were to make things better, so we quickly placed a virtual fence around autism and decided we did not know enough to venture there. Some years later, a few practitioners in our network reported some good results with newer techniques, so the door was once again opened to working with the autism spectrum.

Neurofeedback procedures have proliferated in kind over the years, and with a broader set of clinical tools, it was also possible to match up to a broader set of clinical challenges in the autism spectrum. The point was being reached where one could reasonably expect worthwhile progress with nearly all autistic children. At the same time, scientific understanding of the issues was advancing to the point where the neurofeedback work could now be understood in terms of an accepted model. Before going into more detail on the neurofeedback approach, it is helpful to have that model in mind.

Therapies for autism can be broadly lumped into approaches that address biomedical issues that lie in the causal chain and methods that attempt to ameliorate the behavioral consequences. At first blush, neurofeedback fits into the latter category, and indeed neurofeedback practitioners tend to belong to the "mental health camp." But in truth, this assignment is not a good fit at all. By addressing behavior at the level of the brain itself we are in fact opening up an entirely new terrain that does not fit comfortably either within the standard biomedical model or the standard mental health or behavioral model.

Looked at from the perspective of brain behavior, the most obvious shortcoming in autism lies at the level of integration of function. Moreover, this deficit is not uniform across functional domains but rather afflicts particularly our emotional core that allows us to function in socially-connected ways. At the level of the brain, even our emotional functioning is organized by neural networks. We already know that there are developmental flaws in the structural connectivity of these networks. Beyond that, however, there are also deficits in the functional connectivity that operates on this flawed architecture. If we just survey the structural deficits in the white matter, we find no reason to believe that emotional networks should be selectively impacted. At the level of functional connectivity, they clearly are. This is where neurofeedback comes in.

In this kind of training, we work to bring the neural network of emotional connectivity back online, among other things. We must necessarily operate within the limitations of what is available in terms of structural connectivity, but the good news is that emotional connectivity in the autistic child lies largely in the functional domain and is therefore clinically accessible to us. *EEG neurofeedback* allows us to do this efficiently. There is at present essentially no other comparable means to bring this about.

In addition to adopting the "brain perspective" on autism, it is helpful also to adopt the child's perspective for additional insights. What is the life experience of the autistic child who is not emotionally connected? We can gain insights into this by reflecting on other children who have severe attachment issues (often known by the term "Reactive Attachment Disorder"), for example, those who may have been raised in Chinese, Russian, or Romanian orphanages without the benefit of early nurturing. Such children live in extreme states of raw fear. We derive our sense of safety in the world from our early social relationships. In the absence of these comforting social bonds, the experience of life can be uncertain, capricious, and even threatening. The lack of assuredness in navigating one's world drives the nervous system toward heightened states of activation and arousal. The brain can never relax its vigilance because the child lacks the experience of a sense of safety. Even if the child presents as shut down, the internal state of that system is invariably one of high arousal—without apparent exception.

There is an even larger truth here. In the presence of various kinds of dysfunction, the brain will attempt to compensate by increasing activation generally. The effect may, however, be counterproductive. In any event, it imposes costs. We know very well what happens when we try to function in a highly agitated state. Brain function suffers. The larger principle at issue here is that problems in functional connectivity are not merely consequence. They are also the cause of yet further dysfunction. This is best visualized by reference once again to another affliction, namely Post-Traumatic Stress Disorder (PTSD).

In this condition, there may be nothing in the causal chain beyond the witnessing of a highly traumatizing event. Yet the lingering physiological consequences can devastate the rest of that person's life. In this case, we have no choice but to trace all these adverse consequences back to the original event, and all we have to work with is functional connectivity (which is demonstrably altered). There had been no physical injury, after all. Everything that occurred in that trauma experience lay in the functional domain at the outset. Very clearly, then, deficits in functional connectivity are quite sufficient to wreak all kinds of havoc with our physiology, and that is what also happens in the autistic spectrum.

The significance of this observation is that by addressing functional connectivity in autism directly, we are not only helping with the consequences of other biomedical deficits, we are also remediating an important element in the causal chain of dysfunction in its own right. This helps to make the case that neurofeedback should be an early intervention in the autistic spectrum. Given what we now know, we believe that it should be the very first thing undertaken by any family whose child is suspected of starting to exhibit autistic features. Families already involved in other therapies should consider folding neurofeedback in early as a high priority. But this is getting ahead of the story. Just what goes on in neurofeedback training, and how is it done?

Given the above model, it would be simple enough (at least in principle) to just characterize the deviations in functional connectivity and target those in training. The deviations are numerous, however, and one still needs a guiding principle to determine the appropriate order in which they should be addressed. And then one runs into the usual conundrum that some approaches help and others don't. So matters turn out not to be so simple at all. We have evolved a very different approach, one that starts with the observation already made above that the autistic child lives with an over-aroused nervous system, and that status does not do the child any favors.

In a kind of triage mentality, we find it most appropriate to move the child's brain out of emergency mode as the first order of business. "Calm the stressed and agitated nervous system" is the operative principle. This can be done relatively straightforwardly with essentially any autistic child, irrespective of level of functionality or of age. This strategy finds additional support in our work with servicemen coming back from Iraq and Afghanistan with PTSD and traumatic brain injury and in our work with children with severe attachment issues. All three of these classes of problems will be started with the very same neurofeedback approach because the initial objective is common to them all: it is to move the nervous system to a calmer and more controlled place. All three confirm for us that we are doing the right thing for each of them.

What actually happens in a session is as follows: The child sits in a large comfy chair in front of a large video screen. (Alternatively a young child may be held on a parent's lap or in a car seat.) Three electrodes are adroitly mounted on the child's scalp while the child is, hopefully, distracted by images on the screen. A skilled clinician can accomplish this task in about 30 seconds. The electrode leads are held out of the child's field of view. The images on the screen already relate to the "game" that the child will be watching for the feedback. This video game-like display encodes information derived from the child's EEG, so that the ebb and flow of game performance relates directly to a salient feature in the child's EEG. For example, the EEG variable may be reflected in the speed of a car or rocket or train. Other visual features in the image may be used as well to provide corroborative cues. Auditory feedback likewise encodes the information. And there is a tactile feedback module that also reflects the desired signal.

So the child experiences immersive feedback in which the relevant information is corroborated with appeals to different sensory systems.

Functional improvements are observed almost immediately, simply by virtue of this change of state in which the nervous system functions. Of course one needs to do a number of sessions in order to get the brain to acquire new habits of functioning. All the while, additional functional improvements continue to surface while others continue to consolidate. What has been learned here is that the matrix of functional connectivity is itself a strong function of the state of arousal of the central nervous system. The greatest and swiftest payoff for our efforts therefore lies in first tending to the brain's emergency mode of function into which it has escalated.

One can often witness the effect on the child within the very first session. Understandably, the child most commonly starts out terrified of the novelty of neurofeedback and at minimum suspicious of the electrodes about to be attached to the scalp. But almost as soon as the training gets under way, one can often see a kind of tranquility settle on the child's face and a certain composure descend over his body. The child may even become completely still, and some have been observed to shift to a meditative pose—all quite uncharacteristic of the child who was brought in by the parents just hours earlier. The child's brain will have noticed that the information presented on the screen in some way actually mirrors its own activity. It cannot help but be intrigued to see its own activity mirrored back to it in this fashion, and so it becomes engaged in the process. Once the brain is thus entrained into the experience, then of course the child readily goes along for the journey. One can even think of this as guided meditation for the autistic brain. It clearly relishes the experience, and those dreaded electrodes are long forgotten by the child.

The immediate payoff for the child is that he is just more comfortable in his own skin. The secondary payoff is in terms of emotional relating. This follows from the fact that affect regulation is intimately coupled to arousal regulation. Regulating the one influences the other and vice versa. In fact, we have chosen to target our emotional circuitry as the most direct way of training arousal regulation, taking advantage of this relationship. A third critical payoff is that the brain is progressively much more stable. In general, the child will then go through life more on an even keel. More specifically, this training can be very helpful for children whose autistic presentation is further complicated by a seizure disorder. In fact, epilepsy was the first clinical indication for which efficacy of EEG feedback was proved in animal and human subject research, so the focus on seizure susceptibility is appropriate. The story is consistent throughout: moving the child to better-regulated arousal states helps brain stability, and so does the re-normalization of connectivity relationships. Control of seizures then may open the door for enhanced cognitive function. We will have kindled a virtuous cycle in which every specific advance also promotes the overall objective of enhanced functionality.

Over time, the training process is repeated at various scalp sites in order to pursue other specific functional objectives, and in each case the training is shaped into its most productive course by the response of the child within session and across sessions. If everything goes as expected, the agenda gradually proliferates in terms of targeting and progresses on many fronts. Every feature of autistic behavioral presentation can be selectively targeted one after another. This is typically done in an order that emulates our original developmental sequence. Thus, for example, right hemisphere function is addressed before left-hemisphere function. The first placement is always on the right parietal region, which leads to profound bodily calming and to bringing the child into body consciousness and into awareness of large-scale spatial relationships, i.e., of the relationship of self to the outside world. Right prefrontal training targets emotional connectivity directly. And interhemispheric placement is specifically helpful for the instabilities such as seizures. Eventually, left-side training may be introduced for more specific purposes.

Right-hemisphere training is is quite commonly the key to the emergence of language because the right hemisphere is in charge of acquiring new skills. Language becomes a left-hemisphere function only once it becomes routinized. Moreover, the problem may not be language ability per se at all, but rather the very concept of communication itself. Once that concept is grasped, language may suddenly burst forth in fully formed sentences.

After a sufficient number of sessions to thoroughly establish the method for a particular child, it is often advisable to let parents take over the training at home, using a rented instrument, with ongoing remote supervision from the clinician. There is no obvious endpoint to the training, as the increasingly competent brain just continues to develop new competencies. Somehow our society needs to assure that every autistic child has the opportunity to expand his mental horizons with neurofeedback.

NEUROIMMUNE DYSFUNCTION AND THE RATIONALE AND USE OF ANTIVIRAL THERAPY

BY Dr. MICHAEL GOLDBERG

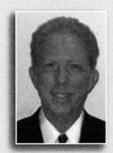

Michael J. Goldberg, MD, F.A.A.P
5620 Wilbur Avenue #318
Tarzana, CA 91356
(818) 343-1010
Fax: (818) 343-6585
office@neuroimmunedr.com
www.neuroimmunedr.com
www.nids.net

Dr. Michael J. Goldberg graduated from UCLA Medical School in 1972, after which he did his pediatric internship and residency at LAC + USC Medical Center, entering private practice in the San Fernando Valley in 1975. Since the early 1980s, his interest has focused on the development and treatment of immune dysregulation / neurocognitive disorders, including CFS/CFIDS and its particular connection to ADHD, in children and in adults. This interest has extended into the neurocognitive dysfunctional link between many children with autism/PDD and siblings or parents with ADHD and CFIDS.

He is actively pursuing collaboration with researchers to accelerate identification and potential new therapeutic modalities for these children. Dr. Goldberg is currently the founder and director of the neuroimmune dysfunction syndromes (NIDS) medical advisory board and research institute. Dr. Goldberg is also the author of *The Myth of Autism*.

Author's note: If you believe your child truly has a disorder called "autism" this chapter does not apply to you. If your child was ever affectionate (which excludes a child from the diagnosis of "autism" per Dr. Kanner) and you believe your child might be suffering from a true medical disease, then please continue.

Background and Rationale

The Centers for Disease Control and Prevention now says that one child in every 110 has an autism spectrum disorder (ASD), which represents almost 1 percent of births in this country; including one in every seventy-one males. New rates are already quoting one child in ninety-one. No genetic or developmental disorder in the history of written medicine has ever come remotely close to 1 percent of children, much less greater. No genetic or behavioral syndrome with such profound symptoms can increase at the rates cited above without being in reality a true medical disease. Reviews of ASD medical research over the last decade (or more) clearly point to a disease-mediated neurological dysfunction (or encephalopathy) likely triggered by an immune system, neuroimmune dysfunction with a probable chronic viral infection or reactivation component.

I began my medical career as a general pediatrician. Once in private practice, it was not long before I started noticing parents and then their children coming in with unusual presentations that we were not taught about in medical school. In the late 1980s, through research, conferences and presentations, it became clear we were looking at a neuroimmune-mediated process, a disease process that was throwing off the brain, the nervous system, and overall physical function of the adults being discussed and the children presenting in my practice. Family histories of these children repeatedly showed a high link to allergies and other immune-mediated disorders (e.g., rheumatoid disease, thyroid dysfunction, multiple sclerosis [MS], lupus, irritable bowel syndrome, and chronic fatigue syndrome) within the family. Clinical patterns were very similar to children with allergies I had worked with since becoming a pediatrician, but there was now a large neurocognitive dysfunctional component, fatigue, and often "mono-like" symptoms, along with the "normal" allergies, immune problems, etc. This increase and change in patterns is consistent with the fact that all immune-mediated disorders (e.g., allergies, migraines, lupus, MS, Alzheimer's, leukemia, lymphomas, and diabetes) have increased dramatically in children and adults over the last twenty-five+ years. What was the rare, mixed ADD/ADHD child has now become the majority.

Open to ongoing debates about environmental factors, global warming, and the ozone layer, there can be no real debate that something has changed and is quite different than when we were all growing up. This is certainly not the environment we were programmed for 200 or 2000+ years ago. A simplistic way to understand the linkage of all of this is that many adults and children (now even infants) are starting not at the "neutral" of many years ago, but are being born in an already "immune-stressed" state. Then, whether an adult, adolescent, child, or infant, a combination of additional stresses—even simple allergies, rashes, eczema, congestion and/or infection are factors in many of these children—adds up to a point where our neuroimmune system becomes dysregulated and dysfunctional.

Unlike the idea of autism sixty years ago, most of these children today are linked by the concept of a dysfunctional neuroimmune system, open to the high probability of secondary infection with chronic viruses. It became obvious that these children have a hyperreactive immune system, explaining many food and environmental sensitivities and often outright allergies. The NeuroSPECT (*single photon emission computed tomography*) scans on these children consistently reveal reduced blood flow in areas of the brain, particularly the temporal lobes. This reduced flow is secondary to a neuroimmune shutdown (similar to how we all feel when fighting a cold or other illness) but continuing on an autoimmune course (it continues to be shut down in an unregulated manner). This is a disease process, not developmental or prewired genetically.

Assessment

Currently, when a child comes in to my office for evaluation, I begin by looking at his or her symptoms as a pediatrician, a medical physician. As I review their history and medical records, I try to determine if they have been injured during pregnancy or delivery, if there has been any brain injury or damage. If I cannot find physiological damage and the child presents in this dysfunctional state called "autism," I will begin a further workup. This usually includes blood work (focused on the immune system, viral markers, food allergies, and normal pediatric markers), and a NeuroSPECT scan (not routinely needed). I am looking for markers and data that suggest an autoimmune or viral profile. Testing being done now is primitive compared to research protocols we will look at to fully define the complexities of this immune and viral process, but, thankfully, there are general markers that at least help point to problems and help define therapies. While minimal blood work should include an immune panel (CD4, CD8, natural killer cells, B cells), viral titers, immunoglobulins, and general pediatric health screens, review and history alone are often only consistent with a disease process that can only be immune or viral in origin. If indicated, I may request neurological testing or other subspecialty evaluation such as a pediatric endocrinologist since some of the children show thyroid or growth issues, reflecting a classical autoimmune, endocrine issue. I will obtain a NeuroSPECT scan if needed.

Intervention

The first step in therapy should be to remove foods or other supplements that may trigger reactions or act as stimulants to their immune system. When asked about what is the healthiest thing to build up a child's immune system, my first response is "remove the negatives." That is the key to helping the immune system stop reacting inappropriately and is the first step to beginning to let the immune system and body repair themselves.

Dairy (bovine protein) is the number one allergen in the world. So the first step I will always take is to remove all milk and dairy products. Wheat/grains are the number two allergen in the world. It is very important to limit carbs. Berries, strawberries, cherries, and other red foods—these may hype up many children, possibly fire off the immune system (which then literally attacks the brain). From there it depends on the child and their food screen (as a guide, never an absolute). Some children do need to be off nuts (many) or citrus (some), which are number 3 and number 4 in the allergy groups. Most of these children should avoid nuts. Nuts are highly allergenic, and they contain arginine, which feeds herpes viruses (and is often in many of the supplements given to the children).

If a viral or fungal process is identified by blood work or suspected strongly from history and the patient's course, I will treat with an antiviral or antifungal medication. The "reactivated" or chronic viral activity generally seems to be herpes related when it comes to the central nervous system, particularly the temporal lobes. In medical school we are taught herpes viruses like to go to the temporal lobes of the brain. The idea of retroviruses playing a potential role merely heightens the medical magnitude of the problem. Within the herpes family, the main pathogens are probably HHV-6, HHV-7, and HHV-8 (consider higher-order herpes virus), not classical herpes simplex I or II. Whether variants of cytomegalovirus, Epstein-Barr virus, or mutated versions are present is open to ongoing clinical investigation.

I have found that children who have a history of fine or gross motor problems or a history of regressive behaviors or skills and/or an abnormal electroencephalogram (EEG) have a significant higher probability of a concurrent complex viral process. While open to further research, presumably when a virus—or now retrovirus—is present, I believe it is probably secondary to the immune dysfunctional state rather than the primary cause.

If there is evidence of a virus, with strict diet control initiated, I will then turn to an antiviral (antivirals will not work adequately if one is consuming foods or supplements irritating or creating ongoing dysfunction within the immune system). Antiviral choices at this time should be limited to known "safe" (when monitored) antivirals, which include acylovir (Zovirax), valacyclovir (Valtrex), and *famciclovir* (Famvir). While there are other stronger antivirals that might be considered in new trials, this author believes the key remains to help the immune system become healthy, and then it can, in theory, handle viruses and even retroviruses. I will re-stress that to have any chance of success, one must think of the role of the immune system as a critical ally, not be stimulating or trying to force manipulate it; and then one must dose at full, appropriate (but not over) therapeutic levels without starting and stopping blindly.

After diet eliminations (eliminate immune system stressors as much as possible), evaluation of an antiviral (usual), antifungal (sometimes), then I begin to look at applying a selective seratonin reuptake inhibitor (SSRI). This is not to treat a child for "depression" or to control behavior, but rather to attempt to address the temporal lobe hypoperfusion being seen on the NeuroSPECT scan.

Do one step at a time, change only one variable at a time, allowing time to analyze and observe if each step is truly working/helping. I have also learned over many years to first focus on physical changes (e.g., sharpness, alertness, brightness in the eyes, and general health), then to analyze, look, and focus on developmental and educational progress, as "rehabilitation" of a child, never training.

Like any other person, any biological organism, there are multiple variables affecting the mood, actions, and attitude of a child. None of us would have been able to learn if we were sent to school chronically ill, with a foggy brain, often painful headaches, and body aches. It's time to think of these children as what they are, pediatric patients who are very ill, often crying because they are in pain. This is not "behavioral." When functioning and feeling well, like other children, these children grow and develop, obviously brighter, happier, and ready to learn.

It is time to revert to medical school training, go back to pediatrics, and help support a child within our abilities. In the meantime, as a parent trust your instincts (pediatric principle 101: "listen to the mothers"), and believe in yourself and your child. Again, believe in your child: believe they were born with potentially normal, often above normal intelligence; believe they can be helped, that they can potentially recover. Then it is time to begin the right fight, a battle you, your child, and your family have a right to believe you can win.

46

NUTRIGENOMICS AND OPTIMIZING SUPPLEMENT CHOICES

BY DR. AMY YASKO

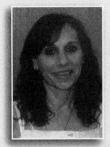

Amy Yasko, Ph.D., CTN, NHD, AMD HHP, FAAIM

Bethel, ME
(207) 824-8501
www.DrAmyYasko.com

Amy Yasko received her undergraduate degree in chemistry and fine arts from Colgate University and her PhD in the department of Microbiology, Immunology, Virology from Albany Medical College. Her postdoctoral work included fellowships in the Department of Pediatric Immunology and the Cancer Center at Strong Memorial Hospital, as well as the Department of Hematology at Yale Medical Center. Dr. Yasko was Director of Research at Kodak IBI as well as a principle/owner of several biotechnology companies including Biotix DNA and Oligos Etc., Inc. After receiving additional degrees as a traditional Naturopath and becoming a Fellow in Integrative Medicine, Dr. Yasko shifted her focus from biotechnology to natural medicine. With her knowledge in these various fields she developed a protocol including a nutrigenomic test used to aid in addressing such complex conditions as autism, chronic fatigue syndrome, and other chronic neurological issues. Through the use of herbs and supplements and biochemistry testing to chart client progress, many who follow her protocol have improved and have even recovered. Dr. Yasko has spoken at conferences hosted by the NY Academy of Science, is listed in Who's Who in Women, has received the CASD Award for RNA research in autism and has published numerous articles as well as chapters in books related to her more conventional work in biotechnology. At present she donates much of her time on her discussion group www.ch3nutrigenomics.com and offers advice and suggestions to the many who seek her help on their path to recovery.

I believe that autism is a *multifactorial condition,* meaning that a number of circumstances need to go awry simultaneously for autism to manifest. I often refer to my Princess Diana example . . . if the car wasn't speeding, if the paparazzi weren't chasing her, if they weren't in a narrow tunnel, if she had been wearing a seat belt . . . if you could eliminate any one of those factors then perhaps the end result would have been different. So too, I believe is the case with autism. I see and address autism as a multifactorial condition that stems from underlying genetic susceptibility combined with assaults from environmental toxins and infectious diseases. It has been shown in other instances that multifactorial diseases are caused by infections and environmental events occurring in *genetically susceptible individuals*. Basic parameters like age and gender, along with other genetic and environmental factors play a role in the onset of these diseases. Infections combined with excessive environmental burdens only lead to disease if they occur in individuals with the *appropriate genetic susceptibility*. I believe this is the case in autism, and using this theory to approach autism has resulted in positive improvements.

Personalized Genetic Screening

One clear, definitive way to evaluate the genetic contribution of multifactorial conditions is to take advantage of new methodologies that allow for personalized genetic screening. Currently, tests are available to identify a number of underlying genetic changes in an individuals' DNA.

The field of **nutrigenomics** is the study of how natural products and supplements can interact with particular genes to decrease the risk of diseases. By looking at changes in the DNA in these nutritional pathways it enables one to make supplement choices based on their particular genetics, rather than using the same support for every individual regardless of their unique needs. With a knowledge of imbalances in nutritional genetic pathways it is possible to utilize combinations of nutrients, foods and natural ribonucleic acids to bypass mutations and restore proper pathway function. The *methionine/folate pathway* is a central pathway in the body that is particularly amenable to nutrigenomic screening for genetic weaknesses. The result of decreased activity in this pathway causes a shortage of critical functional groups in the body called *methyl groups* that serve a variety of important functions.

Your Body's Editing Function

While the term may seem intimidating, a methyl group is actually just a group of small molecules, similar in size to the water molecule (H_2O). Water is a key to life as are methyl groups critical for health and well being. Methyl groups are simply "CH3" groups; they contain 'H' like in water and a 'C' like in carbon or diamonds. However, these very basic molecules serve integral functions; they are moved around in the body to turn on or off genes.

One way to look at the function of methyl groups is that it is analogous to the editing function on your computer. If we think about your body like a computer then you have just one computer that you need to maintain over the course of your life. The longer you have that computer the more outdated it will become. Over the course of a lifetime many of the keys may become stuck or broken. You may drop the computer and damage its function or spill your coffee on it. However, the editing function of the computer remains intact and compensates for these broken keys, misspelled words, and sticky space bars due to accidents of wear and tear. In the absence of this editing function, assume that these 'misspells' are accumulated in your body over the course of your life. If the editing function is impaired then you have no way to get around these misspelled words and other issues that affect your ability to function. Over your lifetime you will accumulate so many misspelled words, missed keys, etc. that at a certain point it would be impossible to read a 'document' amidst all of these mistakes. You can start to see why the proper functioning of the pathway that serves to edit your genes is so important. In addition to the editing of genes, this pathway also serves more direct roles in your body and is thus critical for proper function. While there are several particular sites in this pathway where blocks can occur as a result of genetic weaknesses, thankfully supplementation with appropriate foods and nutrients can help to bypass these mutations to allow for restored function of this pathway.

The Role of the Methylation Cycle in Your Body

The methylation cycle is the ideal pathway to focus on for nutritional genetic analysis because the places where mutations occur is well defined and it is clear where supplements can be added to bypass these mutations. In addition to its editing role, the function of this pathway is essential for a number of critical reactions in the body. One consequence of genetic weaknesses (mutations) in this pathway is increased risk factors for a number of serious health conditions. Defects in methylation lay the appropriate groundwork for the further assault of environmental and infectious agents resulting in a wide range of conditions including diabetes, cardiovascular disease, thyroid dysfunction, neurological inflammation, chronic viral infection, neurotransmitter imbalances, atherosclerosis, cancer, aging, schizophrenia, decreased repair of tissue damage, improper immune function, neural tube defects, Down's syndrome, Multiple Sclerosis, Huntington's disease, Parkinson's disease, Alzheimer's disease, and autism.

- **Inflammation, bacterial and viral infection**

    When you have bacterial or viral infections in your system it increases the level of inflammation in your body. This too relates back to this same *methylation cycle*. Increases in certain inflammatory mediators of the immune system due to infection such as IL6 and TNF alpha lead to decreases in methylation. Chronic inflammation would therefore exacerbate existing genetic mutations in this same pathway. The inability to progress normally through the methylation pathway as a result of methylation cycle mutations combined with the impact of viral and bacterial infections further compromises the function of this critical system in the body.

- **New cells and the immune system**

The building blocks for DNA and RNA require the methylation pathway. Without adequate DNA and RNA it is difficult for the body to synthesize new cells. New cell synthesis is needed to repair damaged cells, to maintain the lining of the gut, to make new blood cells as well as for your immune system that defends you against infection. T cells are a key aspect of your immune system and they require new DNA in order to respond to foreign invaders. T cell synthesis is necessary to respond to bacterial, parasitic and viral infection, as well as for other aspects of the proper functioning of the immune system. T cells are necessary for antibody producing cells in the body (B cells) as both T helpers and T suppressors are needed to appropriately regulate the antibody response.

- **Herpes, hepatitis and other viruses**

In addition, decreased levels of methylation can result in improper DNA regulation. DNA methylation is necessary to prevent the expression of viral genes that have been inserted into the body's DNA. Loss of methylation can lead to the expression of inserted viral genes such as herpes and hepatitis among other viruses.

- **Sensory overload**

Proper levels of methylation are also directly related to the body's ability to both myelinate nerves and to prune nerves. Myelin is a sheath that wraps around the nerve to insulate and facilitate proper nerve reaction. Without adequate methylation, the nerves cannot myelinate in the first place, or cannot remyelinate after insults such as viral infection or heavy metal toxicity. A secondary effect of a lack of methylation and hence decreased myelination is inadequate pruning of nerves. Pruning helps to prevent excessive wiring of unused neural connections and reduces the synaptic density. Without adequate pruning the brain cell connections are misdirected and proliferate into dense, bunched thickets. When nerves grow in this unregulated fashion it can cause confusion processing signals. *Synesthesia* occurs when the stimulation of one sense causes the involuntary reaction of other senses, basically sensory overload.

- **Serotonin, dopamine and ADD/ADHD**

Methylation is also directly related to substances in your body that affect your mood and neurotransmitter levels of both serotonin and dopamine. Methylation of intermediates in tryptophan metabolism can affect the levels of serotonin. Intermediates of the methylation pathway are also shared with the pathway involved in the actual synthesis of serotonin and dopamine. In addition to its direct role as a neurotransmitter, dopamine is involved in assuring your cell membranes are fluid and have mobility. This methylation of phospholipids in the cell membranes has been related to ADD/ADHD.

Membrane fluidity is also important for a variety of functions including proper signaling of the immune system as well as protecting nerves from damage. A number of serious neurological conditions cite reduced membrane fluidity as part of the disease process including MS, ALS, and Alzheimer's disease. In addition, phospholipid methylation may be involved in modulation of NMDA (glutamate) receptors, acting to control excitotoxin damage.

Methylation as One Piece of a More Complex Puzzle

In general, single mutations or *biomarkers* are generally perceived as indicators for specific disease states. However, it is possible that for a number of health conditions, including autism, it may be necessary to look at the entire methylation pathway as a biomarker for underlying genetic susceptibility for a disease state. It may require expanding the view of a biomarker beyond the restriction of a mutation in a single gene to a mutation somewhere in an entire pathway of interconnected function.

This does not mean that every individual with mutations in this pathway will be autistic or will have one of the health conditions listed above. It may be a necessary but not a sufficient condition. Most health conditions in society today are multifactorial in nature. There are genetic components, infectious components and environmental components. A certain threshold or body burden needs to be met for each of these factors in order for multifactorial disease to occur. However, part of what makes the methylation cycle so unique and so critical for our health is that mutations in this pathway have the capability to impair all three of these factors. This would suggest that if an individual has enough mutations or weaknesses in this pathway, it may be sufficient to cause multifactorial disease. Methylation cycle mutations can lead to chronic infectious diseases, increased environmental toxin burdens and have secondary effects on genetic expression.

By testing to look at mutations in the DNA for this methylation cycle it is possible to draw a personalized map for each individual's imbalances, which may impact upon their health. Once the precise areas of genetic fragility have been identified, it is then possible to target appropriate nutritional supplementation of these pathways to optimize the functioning of these crucial biochemical processes. As seen in the *diagram* below there are specific places in the cycle where support can be added. This support helps to bypass mutations in the pathway in a similar manner to the way you might take a detour on a highway. We can look at a mutation in this pathway as analogous to a collision that has totally shut down traffic going in one direction on a highway. Support to bypass mutations in this pathway is like taking an alternate route to avoid the accident on the highway. Thus, the use of key nutrients or foods can aid in helping to bypass methylation cycle mutations and help restore function to this pathway.

The Bottom Line

It has been my experience that viruses, bacteria, toxic metals and excitotoxins (like glutamate or MSG) also play a key role in the condition of autism. I do feel it is important to address these issues and to decrease the body's burden of metals and excitotoxins as well as eliminating bacterial and viral issues in the body. Restoring healthy gut function is another critical area of focus on the path to recovery. However, if we begin with a knowledge of our nutrigenomic weaknesses it makes it easier to address all of these aspects. While autism is a general term there are multiple levels of severity as well as a huge range of clinical presentations. Using nutrigenomic information takes into account that each child is an individual and needs to be seen as unique. This then allows for individualized supplement programs to target areas of weakness that customize support to address specific needs.

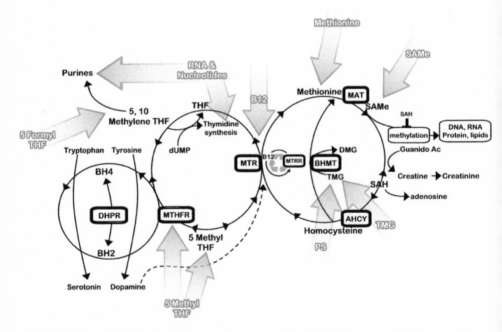

Methylation cycle indicating where supplements can be added to bypass mutations at specific points in the pathway. *Yasko, A. Pathways to Recovery. Bethel Maine: Neurological Research Institute, 2009. Page 143*

47

NUTRITIONAL SUPPLEMENTATION FOR AUTISM

BY LARRY NEWMAN

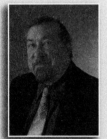

Larry Newman

Chief Operating Officer
Technical and Regulatory Affairs
Kirkman Group
6400 SW Rosewood St.
Lake Oswego, OR 97035
(503) 783-2704
lnewman@kirkmangroup.com

Larry Newman has been formulating nutraceuticals for autism and other developmental conditions for Kirkman Laboratories since 1999. As the chief operating officer for technical and regulatory affairs, he has worked with the leading physicians and clinicians in the special needs arena to develop science-based nutritional products that are utilized by patients with developmental disorders and special needs conditions.

Prior to his association with Kirkman, Larry ran the operations and technical departments of several large pharmaceutical, nutritional, and cosmetic companies, including IVC Industries, Hall Laboratories, Pharmavite Pharmaceutical and Bergen Brunswig Laboratories. He is experienced in developing all product types including liquids, tablets, capsules, creams, lotions and liquid pharmaceuticals.

Larry has a bachelor's degree from California State University and also attended USC school of pharmacy.

When we talk about cutting-edge therapies for autism spectrum disorders (ASDs), it is important to understand that no one type of therapy is effective for all persons with autism. Each individual has their own biochemical profile. What may be very effective for one autistic person may have no effect, little effect, or even a negative effect on another. The therapies we will be discussing here are those that have had a significant positive effect on an above average percentage of individuals over time.

A cutting-edge therapy is not purported to be a cure, but rather a treatment that consistently produces positive effects for those who try the therapy.

The most recent clinical work with autistic individuals indicates that a certain basic model with a defined set of priorities is the most logical way of implementing biomedical and nutritional interventions. This model allows parents or caregivers just getting started to set priorities and initiate a plan.

This chapter is mainly about how supplements will help the individual with autism. However, a discussion of the gut and diet establishes an essential foundation and is a necessary precursor to talking about supplementation. A properly functioning gut is better prepared to absorb nutrients and work in harmony with the immune and nervous systems, and an appropriate diet helps the gut and staves off detrimental immune and neurological effects.

Therapy #1—Clean up the Gastrointestinal Tract

It is well known and clinically documented that autistic individuals have a much greater incidence rate of gastrointestinal disorders than what is considered normal. A recent study done by Autism Speaks' Autism Treatment Network (ATN) reported that gastrointestinal (GI) symptoms occur in nearly half of children with ASD, and the prevalence increases as children get older. The results of this study were presented by ATN at the Pediatric Academic Societies annual meeting in Vancouver, British Columbia, Canada, on May 2, 2010. This study is extremely important in helping to set priorities in approaching autistic conditions. Patients with autism are medically ill, and addressing their gastrointestinal problems needs to be a first step.

In general, physicians have known for centuries that a well-functioning gastrointestinal tract and digestive system are crucial to good health. When digestion is working optimally, other organs and systems in the body have a better chance of working optimally as well. This is because the digestive system is responsible for processing the nutrients in our food, which in turn are used for growth, reproduction, development, tissue repair, healing, and organ function. In addition to providing fuel for the body through nutrition, the intestinal tract also plays an integral role in the functioning of the immune and nervous systems. The intestinal tract's relationship with neurological and cognitive function is often referred to as the gut-brain connection.

There are many distinct, recognizable signs of gastrointestinal disturbances, but as is often the case with autistic individuals who can't communicate, these are not always obvious to the parent or caregiver. Examples include the following:

- abdominal discomfort or cramping (often includes crying, screaming or holding the abdomen)
- constipation or diarrhea
- indigestion, bloating and gas
- inadequate digestion (the evidence of which is often seen in stools)

- inflammation
- yeast or bacterial overgrowth
- serious food sensitivities

When gastrointestinal disorders are suspected, a thorough examination by a gastroenterologist is called for. That examination may include an endoscopy and/or colonoscopy. Based on this exam, the physician has many options to help support whatever conditions are present. These options may include:

- prescription antifungals, antibiotics, or other drugs
- over-the-counter pharmaceuticals
- special diets including gluten-free/casein-free (GF/CF) or Specific Carbohydrate Diet (SCD)
- probiotics to support good flora and crowd out undesirable organisms
- products that support tissue healing
- digestive enzymes to support proper food digestion

TRYING SPECIAL DIETS

Hidden sensitivities are often a contributing factor to GI problems. During a GI evaluation, the health professional may suspect a sensitivity to casein, gluten, soy, or complex carbohydrates as is the case with a majority of autistic individuals. If that is the case, a special diet would become an obvious intervention to try. Special diets can be very useful in alleviating GI symptoms as well as eliminating the cascade of other behavioral, neurological, and immunological symptoms. The most popular diet with the greatest success rate is undoubtedly the GF/CF diet. After following a strict GF/CF diet for a sufficient period of time (up to 6 months), if the desired results have not been seen, some practitioners recommend SCD. Please refer to the chapters in this book that explain these diets.

Therapy #2—Improving Nutritional Status

Following gastrointestinal evaluation and utilizing special diets if appropriate, improving nutritional status should become the next focus. This should be done by combining the proper healthful, nutritious foods with nutritional intervention using dietary supplements. Poor nutrition is very prevalent in autistic individuals for numerous reasons. A balanced diet is usually not the rule. This can happen for any (or all) of several reasons: (1) special diets such as GF/CF or SCD may be in place; (2) a person's tastes and attitudes can be such that their diet is very deficient in vitamins, minerals, or other necessary nutrients; or (3) a facet of biochemistry can be irregular, making the absorption of nutrients suboptimal.

The first step in improving nutritional status in an autistic patient is to do a thorough analysis of the patient's eating habits and supplement regimens. Physicians often turn this task over to a registered dietician or certified nutritionist who will lay out the person's typical diet and make recommendations for diet and supplementation.

Typical questions will include:

- What are the food groups consumed?
- How much in the way of protein sources, fruits, vegetables, carbohydrates, sugars, fiber, fats and oils are eaten daily?
- Are the foods consumed healthful?
- What nutrients do they provide?
- Are quantities consumed in the correct proportions?
- Is the method of cooking such that nutrients are not substantially depleted?
- What dietary supplements are also being taken?
- Given the food consumed and the additional supplements included, how does the regimen need to change to balance the person's nutritional status?

The diet must often change. But will it or can it? Often it is not possible because of the behavior or preferences of the individual. If the diet cannot improve sufficiently, then dietary supplements supplying vitamins, minerals, essential fatty acids, fiber, and antioxidants need to be added. An individualized diet plus the addition of the required supplements will greatly improve nutritional status, and results and rewards will generally be very obvious as signs of poor nutrition diminish.

Poor nutrition can often be recognized by:

- vision issues
- unhealthy skin tone
- extreme tiredness or lack of energy
- lethargy
- behavioral issues
- failure to thrive
- frequent illness because of immune dysfunction

For those on a casein-/dairy-free diet, calcium supplementation is essential to ensure proper bone development and growth. In addition, a comprehensive vitamin and mineral supplement is essential when the diet is unbalanced and nutrients deficient, which is often the case if all food groups including protein and carbohydrate sources and fruits and vegetables are not being consumed. Cod liver oil and omega-3 fatty acid supplements can help support good vision and healthy skin. Irregularities in biochemical pathways are often supported by B-6/magnesium supplements, folic or folinic acid, or sulfation aids (see below).

Certain nutrients are essential for proper support of the immune system. Zinc, vitamin A, vitamin C, vitamin D-3, vitamin E, and selenium are examples of nutrients that improve immune response. Suboptimal levels of these nutrients can sometimes lead to a weak immune system which can lead to frequent illnesses.

PROPER ABSORPTION OF NUTRIENTS AS ANOTHER FACTOR IN NUTRITIONAL STATUS

Often with autistic persons, even a balanced diet with the addition of the required dietary supplements fails to improve nutritional status to optimum levels because of a deficiency of pancreatic digestive enzymes or a lack of their proper secretion.

Digestive enzymes are those enzymes found in the body and secreted by the pancreas that function as biological catalysts to begin the breakdown of foods so that the important nutrients in the food can be properly absorbed and utilized. All food contains nutrients and potential nutritional value; however, until enzymes start the digestive process, the nutrients are "locked up" in the cellular structure and are not yet available to be absorbed by the body. For example, the fiber and vitamins in breakfast cereal provide no value until digestive enzymes start the digestion process and unlock the nutrients. Similarly, meat or fish do not deliver the protein necessary for growth and development until protease enzymes digest the protein.

When this type of enzyme insufficiency is taking place, adding oral digestive enzymes can make a dramatic, positive difference for an individual by improving digestion and absorption of nutrients. These enzymes can be administered as a prescription medication or as a dietary supplement. Some of the conditions that suggest digestive enzyme insufficiency include:

- malnutrition due to insufficient absorption of nutrients
- abnormal growth patterns
- vitamin and mineral deficiencies
- immune system impairment and frequent illness
- abnormal skin conditions
- gas, diarrhea, constipation, and/or foul smelling stools
- undigested food in the stool
- digestive tract discomfort (e.g., stomach, colon, or rectum)

Typically, a 3-to 4-week trial on a comprehensive multiple digestive enzyme will determine whether this intervention will be helpful.

Therapy #3—Use of Probiotics

Probiotics are defined scientifically as "living microorganisms that when ingested or locally applied in sufficient numbers can fill one or more specified, demonstrated functional or health benefits on the host." Probiotics have been called nature's "internal healers" because of their crucial role in the health and functioning of the intestinal tract. Probiotics are actually friendly (desirable and beneficial) bacteria that help keep the flora of the gastrointestinal tract within the correct balance of good and bad organisms.

One hundred trillion bacteria live in the human body, and of those, a healthy individual normally has a balance of about 85% good bacteria and 15% bad bacteria. When this ratio gets significantly out of balance, gastrointestinal problems arise. Individuals with autism are known to have imbalanced intestinal flora, with an excess of bad bacteria and a deficiency of good bacteria.

Supplementation of probiotics containing *Lactobacillus, Bifidobacterium* and other lactic acid bacteria strains are known to exert a profound positive influence in balancing intestinal flora. They are recognized to guard against intestinal inflammation, strengthening the immune barrier function of the intestines, and in helping to normalize intestinal permeability problems (aka "leaky gut"). They also produce antimicrobial substances, which are active against harmful bacteria, yeast, and viruses. By competing for intestinal nutrients and attachment sites, probiotic bacteria perform a crucial function in inhibiting the growth of harmful and potentially pathogenic bacteria.

Benefits of probiotics include:

- helping to regulate intestinal mobility, thereby normalizing bowel transit time
- producing lactic acid for reduction of colonic pH
- aiding digestion
- helping alleviate occasional diarrhea or constipation
- breaking down toxic byproducts of invading bad bacteria through a natural detoxification process
- increasing concentrations of healthy flora
- enhancing immune response
- decreasing infectious disease rates
- decreasing use of antibiotics
- decreasing serious allergic-type reactions

Results of using probiotics with individuals with autism having gastrointestinal and immune issues have been remarkably successful.

RESULTS OF THERAPIES 1, 2, AND 3

Gastrointestinal evaluation and support, a special diet (if required), and improving nutrition with use of digestive enzymes and probiotics should yield noticeable, favorable results for the person with autism within several weeks to several months. Once those improvements are noted and continuing support is established, there are other therapies that can be tried for numerous other symptoms the individual may exhibit.

Therapy #4—Improving Sleep Patterns

Individuals with autism suffer from sleep problems such as trouble falling asleep, periodic night waking, and nightmares. Parents of children on the autism spectrum have observed these problems to be more severe and/or frequent than those that occur in neurotypical children. These sleep problems can be all or in part due to underlying physiological conditions such as digestive discomforts; gastrointestinal pain from irritation, ulceration, reflux, or inflammation; or other causes of pain. Poor nutrition and metabolic issues can also contribute to poor sleep patterns.

Dietary supplements that have proven very useful in allowing autistic persons to maintain restful sleep include:

• melatonin
• magnesium
• L-Taurine
• 5-HTP
• GABA
• L-Threonine

All of these supplements are safe, usually without side effects, and should be tried one at a time for about a week in the order listed above. If one does not seem to help, stop and try the next one. Getting restful sleep can greatly improve other symptoms of autism because the body is rested and operating efficiently.

Therapy #5—Improving Behaviors, Cognition, and Social Skills

Behavioral, learning, and social challenges are very common in autistic individuals. Because each person displays different behavioral traits and ultimately has a unique biochemical profile, it is sometimes challenging to find the right interventions.

Common behavioral and social challenges involve the following:

• speech delay or absence of speech
• inability to put words or sentences together

- learning disabilities
- social skill/communication challenges
- lack of eye contact or unable to focus eyes on an object
- aggressive behavior
- passive behavior
- depression
- anxiety
- tics or abnormal nerve responses

The list of supplements and interventions that have been used in dealing with these behavioral, learning, and social issues is long. The supplements that qualify for the cutting-edge label based on their frequent success rate are high B-6/magnesium supplements, dimethylglycine (DMG) or trimethylglycine (TMG), L-Taurine, omega-3 fatty acids, and cod liver oil. The Autism Research Institute publishes a list of nutritional supplements and drug products, listing their success rate as reported by responding parents. These rank amongst the top performers.

Omega-3 fatty acids are somewhat of an exception because they are good for all individuals with autism and will, without a doubt, improve overall health status in the long run.

Therapy #6—Improving Immune Function

The immune system is a complex and dynamic network of many soluble components including specialized cells, membranes, and a mini circulatory system separate from blood vessels. These entities all work together to protect us from infection by opportunistic microbes, bacteria, viruses, fungi, and parasites. The immune system also constantly scans our bodies for any signs of abnormal cell growth and keeps our bodies in check with regard to recognizing the differences between antigens and allergens. This is why a compromised immune system often leads to a shift in T-cell types, which can lead to an individual developing more allergic-type reactions. Autistic individuals are almost always immunocompromised in some ways. Gastrointestinal issues often are immune related as are sensitivities to foods and allergens.

The signs of an immune problem are often quite easy to recognize over time. Persistence of the following conditions is key to suspecting immune deficiencies.

- frequent illness or illnesses of long duration
- continuous food allergies or an increased number of such allergies
- inadequate detoxification as indicated by laboratory testing
- low glutathione levels as indicated by laboratory testing
- impaired methylation pathway and inability to detoxify

Autistic individuals are especially prone to immune problems, and parents' observations conveyed to the physician are extremely important in helping the doctor recognize this problem because it is often hard to judge at an office visit.

There is a long list of nutritional supplements that support and strengthen the immune system. The most important of these include:

- zinc
- vitamin C
- vitamin D
- vitamin E
- selenium
- coenzyme Q-10
- reduced L-Glutathione (as prescribed by your physician)

You will recognize some of the above nutrients as being present in the multiple vitamin and mineral you may be using, but generally the multi will contain relatively low potencies. To better support a compromised immune system, additional supplementation of these immune-boosting nutrients is recommended. Increasing zinc to 50 mg. daily, vitamin C to 1000-3000 mg. daily, vitamin D-3 to 1000 IU or more daily, vitamin E to 200-400 IU daily, selenium up to 75 mcg. daily, and coenzyme Q-10 up to 100 mg. daily will be beneficial. As with the omega-3 supplements mentioned earlier, a regimen boosting immune response will be advantageous to all autistic individuals, so there is no reason not to use this proven therapy.

Therapy #7—Improving the Sulfation Pathway

The sulfation process is linked to an enzyme system known as phenol sulfotransferase (PST). Normally, PST is involved in a process called sulfoconjugation, whereby a group of potentially harmful chemicals known as phenols are attached to sulfate and thereby eliminated from the body. When there is a deficiency of sulfate in the bloodstream, phenolic compounds may build up in the body, and this in turn can interfere with neurotransmitter function. Sulfate deficiency and the resulting impairment of PST activity may explain some sensitivity reactions to a variety of phenol-containing foods, such as apples, grapes, chocolate, food colorings, and some herbs and spices.

Autistic individuals seem to have only about 20% of the normal level of sulfate in their bodies, the rest having been excreted excessively in the urine. In addition to the phenolic buildup described above, sulfate deficiency can contribute to other negative aspects of body chemistry including:

- preventing the detoxification of metals and other environmental toxins from the body

- inhibiting the release of pancreatic digestive enzymes, thereby hindering digestion
- limiting the activation of the hormone cholecystokinin (CCK), which plays a role in socialization
- contributing to a leaky gut because of an unhealthy ileum

Sulfation can often be regulated and improved by giving individuals Epsom salt baths once or twice daily. Dissolve some pharmaceutical grade Epsom salt (magnesium sulfate) in warm bath water. These baths have been remarkably helpful in autism. A topical Epsom salt preparation such as a cream or lotion can also be useful to improve sulfation, or a combination of the two may be convenient (such as using the cream in the morning and giving a bath at night). Oral sulfate such as glucosamine sulfate may be effective to some degree in certain individuals, but it is not purported to be as effective as the Epsom salt preparations or baths. Epsom salts are particularly helpful on days when an individual with autism has been swimming in a chlorinated pool.

Therapy #8—Improving the Methylation Pathway

Methylation is a series of very important biochemical reactions in the body that are responsible for overall good health. In individuals with autism, this process is very often lacking, making these individuals poor methylators. A properly functioning methylation pathway is necessary for the following:

- proper brain function
- healthy detoxification
- proper reproduction
- DNA protection
- a healthy, normal, non-premature aging process

There are many nutritional supplements that support proper methylation. Options should be discussed with the physician carefully because each autistic individual's needs are unique, and the protocol should be specifically tailored to their lab test results. Products used to support the methylation process include:

- methyl B-12 injections or other form of supplementation
- DMG or TMG
- folic or folinic acid
- vitamin B-6/magnesium
- SAMe (S-Adenosyl methionine)

- selenium
- zinc

Therapy #9—Detoxification

Substantial evidence is emerging linking a myriad of medical irregularities to negative environmental factors, including many conditions that are found in individuals diagnosed with autism. The frequency of many of these irregularities is increasing, which leads to further speculation that outside environmental factors are involved.

Included in the list of environmental insults that can affect disease states are toxic chemicals, heavy metals, PCBs, and pesticides present in the products we use, the air we breathe, and the water we utilize and drink. Preservatives may also contribute.

These environmental pollutants can affect the body in numerous ways. Natural body defense mechanisms such as immune response can be bombarded with the insults, thereby becoming less effective because of the toxic load.

The following conditions may be linked to continued exposure to environmental toxins:

- learning or speech difficulties
- social skills challenges
- aggressive behavior
- passive behavior
- poor immune response
- biochemical pathway issues

Certain nutrients are considered natural detoxifiers and can help mitigate exposures and enhance the body's natural detoxification process. Examples of such vitamins and minerals are zinc, vitamin C, vitamin E, vitamin D-3, and selenium. Other nutritional factors that can be helpful are L-Taurine, N-Acetyl Cysteine, and reduced L-Glutathione.

In addition to the nutritional detoxifiers mentioned above, chelation using approved drugs can be very effective in detoxifying certain heavy metal contaminants such as lead, mercury, arsenic, cadmium, antimony, and others deemed to be a health risk. On the Autism Research Institute's chart of effective therapies, chelation actually heads the list in its success rate. This would be a topic to discuss with the individual's physician, and regular medical monitoring and laboratory testing are recommended when chelating agents are used. Your physician trained and experienced in the physiological conditions underlying an autism diagnosis should also advise you on nutritional supplementation with minerals and the scheduling thereof during a chelation protocol.

Conclusions

It is likely that some of these interventions will help all autistic individuals to some degree. The challenge to parents after receiving an autism diagnosis is finding out which of the specific therapies will help their child. A doctor trained and experienced in the physiological conditions underlying an autism diagnosis may help, especially in conjunction with a certified nutritionist. Many children, parents, and families have found positive rewards at the end of the process.

48

OCCUPATIONAL THERAPY AND SENSORY INTEGRATION

BY MARKUS JARROW

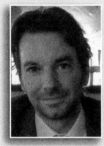

Markus Jarrow, OTR/L, C/NDT

Clinical Director
The SMILE Center | The Sensory Motor Integration + Language
Enrichment Center
171 Madison Avenue 5th Floor
New York, NY 10016
(212) 400-0383
markus@smileny.org
www.smileny.org

Markus Jarrow received his BA in Occupational Therapy from Sargent College of Boston University in 1997. Markus has more than twelve years of experience in pediatrics, specializing in the evaluation and treatment of children with autism spectrum disorders, sensory integration dysfunction, and neuromuscular disorders. Markus has extensive training in Sensory Integration, Neuro-Developmental Treatment, and DIR/Floortime methodologies. His approach to treatment draws from the fundamentals of these three models in a comprehensive style that addresses the whole child. Markus co-founded The SMILE Center | The Sensory Motor Integration and Language Enrichment Center in 2009, a state-of-the-art pediatric treatment facility in New York City.

Why does my child spin? Why does my child refuse so many foods? Why does my son scream every time I try to put a coat or hat on him? Why does my daughter always hum and look out of the corner of her eyes?

Occupational therapists can provide valuable insight, both practical and neurological, to help families better understand many of the questions they struggle with when raising a child with an autism spectrum disorder. Occupational therapy and sensory integration (SI) can be very effective treatment approaches for children with ASD. In order to understand how sensory integrative treatment can be effective, it is important to understand the basics of sensory integration theory and dysfunction. This chapter will provide you with a brief overview.

What is Occupational Therapy?

Occupational Therapy is a broad profession that shares a common goal of utilizing functional and purposeful activities, or occupations, to increase an individual's functional independence. In the scope of treatment of children with autism spectrum disorders, occupational therapy can be very effective in improving functional fine and gross motor skills, postural control and movement patterns, motor planning, self-help skills, hand-eye coordination, and visual perceptual and spatial skills. However, perhaps most significant is the impact that a sensory integration treatment approach can have on a child's sensory processing skills. After all, if a child cannot maintain an optimal level of arousal and appropriately integrate sensory information, his or her ability to learn and acquire new skills will be greatly comprised. A child who relies of self-stimulatory or self-regulatory behaviors to control their arousal level, or tune out adverse stimuli, is a child less available for engagement, learning, and skill acquisition. Therefore, with this population in particular, sensory integration is one of the primary frames of reference utilized by occupational therapists.

History of Sensory Integration

Sensory integration is a theory and treatment approach originally developed by the late occupational therapist, Dr. A. Jean Ayres, Ph.D., OTR in the 1960s. She defined sensory integration as the ability to organize sensory information for use by the many parts of the nervous system, in order to work together to promote effective interactions with the environment. Sensory integration had evolved over the years, but much of the original theory remains. It is a dynamic and child-directed treatment approach based on specific principles, treatment techniques, and equipment. It is a problem-solving and individualized approach that requires ongoing analysis and assessment in order to monitor changes in the child and adapt the treatment accordingly. A trained occupational therapist utilizes a wide range of techniques and strategies in order to help a child achieve and maintain an optimal level of arousal. It is in this state that adaptive responses can be made to incoming sensory information. This in turn, enables them to become more confident, successful, and interactive explorers of their worlds.

While Dr. Ayers's treatment and research pertained primarily to the vestibular, proprioceptive, and tactile systems, toward the end of her life, she began to look much more closely at the important roles of the auditory and visual systems. Unfortunately for all of us, she was unable to conclude her work as she lost her life to cancer. More recently, several occupational therapists have made great strides in further identifying the important roles of the auditory and visual systems. Two therapists in particular turned their research and experience into very effective and practical treatment modalities and protocols: Therapeutic Listening and Astronaut Training.

What to Expect From Sensory Integration Therapy

Typically a child will first be evaluated by an occupational therapist trained in sensory integration. This process may include a variety questionnaires and evaluation tools including the Sensory Integration and Praxis Test (SIPT). The evaluation will also consist of interviewing with the caregivers as well as further clinical observations of the child in order to obtain insight into their sensory profile and needs. The entire process may take anywhere from a few hours to a few lengthy visits over the span of several sessions. Following a thorough assessment, a treatment plan will be formulated and a recommendation will be made regarding the frequency and duration of the child's treatment.

Sensory integrative treatment is best implemented in a therapy gym outfitted with a wide variety of specific equipment and adaptable environments. These treatment facilities are referred to as sensory gyms. Therapists, however, have found creative solutions to providing treatment with limited space and materials, such as in schools and in the home. Treatment should only be carried out by a clinician trained in sensory integration and should involve the parents/caregivers, as carryover into the home is critical. No matter how effective the clinician is, he or she may only have an hour or two a week with the child. It is therefore essential that a home program be implemented. This may include simple modifications to the home, adaptations to the child's routines, toys, clothing, etc. as well as specific, scheduled treatment strategies to be carried out in the home and/or school. This is referred to as a sensory diet. This piece is critical in ensuring optimal progress.

In treatment, you may see your child flying and spinning through space on suspended equipment. You may see her climbing over or under enormous padded obstacles, up rope ladders, or through suspended tunnels. She may zip by you on a scooter board with headphones on, holding tight to a bungee cord, or jump from a platform into a crash mat or ball pit. She may be laying on her side, rhythmically spinning to the sounds of outer space.

Treatment with another child may appear completely different . . . at least initially. You may see him sitting with the clinician in a dimly lit room, wearing a weighted vest, covered in heavy blankets, attending to an activity. You may see him gently rocking on a swing with the clinician cradling him from behind, or slowly rolling over a soft surface to a rhythmical hum of the therapist. SI treatment can appear very different from one child to the next, as it is individualized to each child's unique sensory needs. While an experienced clinician can make treatment simply look fun and playful, rest assured, careful clinical reasoning is behind every move.

The cost of an evaluation can range from a few hundred dollars to a couple thousand dollars. Private treatment ranges greatly from less than one hundred to two hundred dollars or more per one-hour session. Sessions can be as short as thirty minutes; however, the nature of the treatment tends to lend itself to longer sessions. Occupational therapy evaluations and treatment are typically covered, to some extent, by local school systems as well as Early Intervention programs for children less than three years of age.

Occupational therapists can work with children with ASD in a variety of settings. In schools, treatment often carries over to the classroom as the primary focus is improving function in school related tasks and environments. In a private practice, sensory gym, or outpatient setting, the OT typically has access to more therapy equipment and can address issues related more to the home and community, as the parents are generally more present.

What is Sensory Integration and Sensory Integration Dysfunction?

In order for a child to appropriately move through space and interact with their world in an alert, regulated, and effective manner, they must take in an extraordinary amount of sensory information, unconsciously interpret it, and then make appropriate adaptive responses on a rapid and continuous basis. This is an incredibly complex process that relies on an intricate network of sensory systems functioning appropriately and simultaneously. It is called sensory integration. It's an amazing process that most of us take for granted; it just happens and we never think twice about it. However, for many of the children with ASD, this is not the case.

For a child with sensory integration dysfunction, the seemingly simple task of walking across a classroom, putting on a T-shirt, finding a toy in a closet, listening to mom on a busy street corner, walking barefoot on a beach, skipping down the sidewalk, or playing in a swing in the park may be perceived as overly challenging, seemingly impossible or even terrifying. Sensory integration dysfunction can impact every aspect of development including: social-emotional, behavioral, attention and regulation, gross and fine motor, postural, adaptive and self-help, visual motor, visual spatial/perceptual, speech and language, and academic. Our ability to appropriately meet the many challenges faced in our daily lives is a result of the integration and proper "wiring" of five major sensory systems: vestibular, proprioceptive, tactile, auditory, and visual.

The vestibular system is located in the inner ear and is the integral system that responds to gravitational forces and changes in the head's position in space. It is the sense that tells you when you're right side up or upside down, and is responsible for helping with balance and spatial orientation. The vestibular system is also responsible for proving a stable basis for visual function, even when the head is moving through space. Also, for example, when an object is getting larger in your visual field, your vestibular confirms that you are not moving, thus indicating that the object is coming toward you. The appropriate response can then be made, whether it's to move out of the way, catch it, etc.

Movement is a component of almost everything that we do; so vestibular function applies to almost every interaction we have with the world. It's the sense that, when overstimulated, makes one feel seasick and carsick. It's the sense that thrill seekers try to satiate with roller coasters, bungee jumping, and skydiving. Because of its role in movement and space, it works hand in hand with the auditory and visual systems in order to provide us with a sense of our three-dimensional spatial envelope, compelling us to move, explore, and understand. This collaborative system is referred to as the vestibular-visual-auditory triad.

Without this functioning triad, it would be impossible to appropriately process movement, space, time, and sequencing. When we enter a new restaurant for the first time, we immediately take in a sense of the room's size, relative shape, and arrangement of its contents. After navigating the delicate environment and casually taking a seat, we understand the quiet clinging of pots is coming from the open kitchen behind us and to the left; the gentle humming sound is coming from overhead ceiling fans; and the waitress walking slowly from across the room will be within a respectful distance in seven or eight seconds; the necessity to kindly request a glass of water in a suitable volume level for the environment. None of these seemingly simple processes that we take for granted would have been possible without appropriate integration of the vestibular-visual-auditory triad. This same analysis can be reapplied to countless scenarios, in countless environments, on countless different levels.

"Without a properly functioning vestibular system, sights and sounds in the environment do not make sense—they are only isolated pieces of information disconnected from the meaningful whole. It is the integration of the sensory information that holds the key to finding the meaning in the world. Because movement is part of everything we do in life, it could be said that the vestibular system supports all behavior and acquisition of skills, as well as helping to balance the stream of sensory information that constantly bombards the system." (Astronaut Training: A Sound Activated Vestibular-Visual Protocol for Moving, Looking and Listening; Kawar, Frick & Frick, 2005)

The proprioceptive system is a network of sensors throughout our muscles and joints that work together to create an internal body map. It is through proprioceptive awareness that we know the position of our body, even when we cannot see it. It is through intact proprioception that we can navigate a dark, familiar environment, or reach and grab something behind us without looking. It is also the sense that grades our pressure, allowing us to use the appropriate force when picking up a brick, versus a thin paper cup of water.

Input to the proprioceptive system through deep pressure, and much more significantly, resistive muscle activation, or "heavy work," enhances serotonin release and can be very grounding and organizing. This is why some people stomp their feet or clench their fists when they are angry or overwhelmed. This is why others chew on hard plastic pen caps when their attention wanes in a lecture. It is difficult to feel secure in oneself or in one's environment without a secure sense of body scheme. The proprioceptive system collaborates extensively with the closely associated tactile system. Together, they provide us with the critical sense of body awareness.

The tactile system is made up of the largest organ of our body, the skin. It is the system that provides us with the sense of touch for pleasure, pain, discrimination, and protection. Being that the tactile system is our exterior boundary, it is critical that it appropriately processes the wide variety of elements and touch sensations that surround us. If dysfunctional, pleasurable touch can instead be misinterpreted as noxious, or potentially dangerous sensations can go unregistered and become damaging.

Each of these systems must function properly and collaboratively in order to support appropriate sensory integration. A typical sensory system processes a wide variety and range of intensity of information, and makes the necessary filtrations in order for a person to function comfortably and without conscious effort. However, with many children with autism spectrum disorders, we find that one or more of these systems does not function properly. Any of the sensory systems can be hyper-responsive (sensory avoiding) or hypo-responsive (sensory seeking) to incoming information.

This can be easily demonstrated with an example of the tactile system. A hyper-responsive tactile system (sensory avoiding) is generally associated with a high level of arousal. This child is typically in varying states of fight or flight and is therefore less available for engagement and learning. She may avoid messy play and unfamiliar textures at all cost, may hold objects in her finger tips, avoiding contact with palms, may need to remove tags from shirts and only wear soft old clothes, may avoid standing close to peers and other people, may resist cuddling and affection even from parents and family members, may present with poor body awareness, stiff movement patterns, delayed motor planning, and difficulty with fine motor skills. This girl may tend to be inflexible and rigid in her ways, in an effort to attempt to control a world that she perceives as threatening.

A hypo-responsive tactile system (sensory seeking) is generally associated with a low level of arousal. This child may typically appear "tuned out" and is therefore also less available. In order to obtain input to raise his arousal, he may gravitate to messy and unfamiliar textures in an effort to better process his body and the things around them, may not seem to notice or mind when socks or clothing are twisted in uncomfortable ways or when sticky food is on his hands or face, may frequently bump into others or play excessively rough without ill intentions, and may present with poor body awareness and poorly graded, ballistic movement patterns, delayed motor planning, and difficulty with fine motor skills. This boy may tend to be disorganized in his ways, as he has difficulty making sense of his world.

Sensory issues can often be mistaken for behavioral problems. If a child has vestibular and visual issues, which impact his perception of his position in space, he may have great difficulty sitting upright in a chair without falling from time to time. To avoid falls or embarrassment, he may fidget to better process his body, or get out of his seat often. He, in turn, will present as a child who "won't" stay seated. Another child with severe tactile defensiveness may be terrified to stand in line next to his peers due to the fear of being touched. To protect himself, he stands away from the group with his back against the wall or casually wanders out of reach. He again, will present like a child who "won't" stay in line. With children with sensory integration dysfunction, it is important to remember that these behaviors may be nothing more than effective coping mechanisms. When the underlying sensory issues are addressed, the behavior may disappear all together.

What is Sensory Integration Therapy?

Sensory integration is a complex treatment approach. A breakdown of a few of the basic principles can help to provide a general understanding. We, as humans, need a wide variety of sensory and motor experiences to develop and sustain typical nervous system function. Much like plants need a full spectrum of light to grow and flower to their potential, we respond strongly to sensory information. Consider the devastating effects of prolonged sensory deprivation. Consider the positive effects of gently rocking a baby or tightly hugging a friend in need. Within the range of typically functioning systems, we find some variance. One "typical" adult may ride roller coasters every Saturday afternoon. Another may gasp at the sight of one. With a little encouragement, perhaps, she hops on and keeps her eyes closed. These two people are quite different, yet fall within a range where they experience a variety of rich sensory movement experiences. Children with ASD sometimes present with a much greater range. For whatever reasons, their nervous systems are wired differently.

Children inherently attempt to provide themselves with what they need and avoid what they are frightened by. They constantly listen to their bodies and try to regulate themselves. By listening to what their bodies tell us, we can help them to make a great deal of positive change. A therapist can provide them with calculated input that is stronger and more effective in reaching the threshold of the system the child is trying to stimulate. In turn, the child may begin to process the input more appropriately and therefore need less of it over time, demonstrating fewer sensory seeking or self-stimulatory behaviors. Children demonstrate self-stimulating behaviors for a reason. It is our responsibility to determine why.

The child who avoids sensory input faces another challenge. They develop compensatory strategies to protect themselves, and seldom subject themselves to the sensory information. Therapists utilize various strategies to help desensitize the child. This is never done through repeated exposure of the noxious experience. It often involves looking carefully at the stimuli and the relationships of the supporting sensory system. The clinician can then systematically address them in order to support sensory integration. For example, a defensive tactile system may better process touch following appropriate input to the proprioceptive system. A vestibular system may better process movement following appropriate input to the auditory or proprioceptive system.

Consider This Example:

One young girl may spin around for hours and never get dizzy. Another young boy may fearfully cling to his mother when she tries to put him in a swing at the park, or even just picks him up. These ranges pose a problem. The first child appears hypo-responsive (sensory seeking) and unable to provide herself with strong enough movement input to satiate her vestibular system. This compels her to spin, climb, run, jump, and crash. After all, if you were hungry, wouldn't you eat something? The second child, on the other hand, appears hyper-responsive (sensory avoiding) and avoids movement at all cost. If you had arachnophobia would you pet a tarantula? His vestibular system, however, still requires and craves input despite his interpreted fear. So almost instinctually, he has discovered that by looking out of the far corners of his eyes, by looking at spinning objects, or by closely following long linear edges visually, he can stimulate his vestibular system.

These two children are significantly impacted by this relatively simple sensory dysfunction and have developed effective coping mechanisms. However, the vestibular system works closely together with other systems to support many functions, so the ramifications may increase and broaden over time if left unaddressed. Both of these children are less available for engagement and learning.

The first child can only provide herself with so much movement input, due to human limitations. A trained therapist on the other hand, can make informed clinical decisions after assessment, and assist the child in obtaining calculated rotation and movement experiences in all planes that provide strong and organizing input to every receptor of the vestibular system. This may be followed with further resistive activities that activate her core muscles to provide additional grounding and organizing information. The movements can provide the vestibular system with its threshold of input, allowing it to better process movement and support more refined motor skills. It can also result in a substantial period of time to follow in which she seeks less movement and is more available to the world around her. Due to the plasticity of our nervous systems, this input can decrease over time as the system becomes rewired, or integrated.

Based on the profile of the second child, he likely presents with poor tactile and proprioceptive processing. This is commonly associated with low muscle tone and poor postural control. This typically results in decreased body awareness and motor planning, with one of the end functional outcomes being a fear of moving through space. If this child does not perceive his body properly when seated or walking, he most certainly will not feel safe when placed in a swing and pushed three feet off of the ground. A trained therapist will identify these patterns and recognize the need to address his tactile and proprioceptive systems, despite the fact that the initial red flag went off when mom reported an issue that appear to be related to his vestibular system. All involved systems will be addressed in treatment.

Specific brushing /deep pressure strategies and resistive activities that connect him to the support surface can be very effective in improving body awareness. A child needs to feel connected to the ground before they can feel free in space. Core muscle activation can improve alignment and postural control and help lay the foundation for the introduction of new, controlled movement experiences. A careful sequence of movement may now be explored, paired with continued body awareness work. All activities are paired with his passions and interests. He ideally gains ownership of his body in space and begins to freely explore on his own. The timid, fearful child can now become a confident explorer.

This example provides a little insight into the SI treatment approach. These principles can be applied to a variety of issues involving all of the sensory systems. Sensory integrative treatment can effectively help to change a child's "wiring." It is the clinician's goal to provide the child with the tools necessary to create their own ideas and develop more naturally and spontaneously in a world that they can make sense of and feel safe in.

PARENT SUPPORT

BY DR. LAUREN TOBING-PUENTE

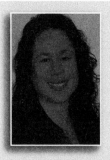

Lauren Tobing-Puente, Ph.D.

361 East 19th Street
New York, NY 10003
(917) 838-9274
services@drtobingpuente.com
www.drtobingpuente.com

Dr. Lauren Tobing-Puente is a NYS Licensed Psychologist with many years of clinical experience with children and families, specializing in autism-spectrum disorders (ASDs). She received her Ph.D. in Clinical Psychology from Fordham University, with a specialization in child and family therapy. As a Developmental Individual Differences and Relationship-based (DIR) model Certificate Candidate (Level II), Dr. Tobing-Puente uses the DIR approach both in her private practice and as the Clinical Coordinator of the Rebecca School, one of the largest DIR schools worldwide. Dr. Tobing-Puente has expertise in the assessment and treatment of children, and in providing support groups for siblings and parents. She has worked with parents of children with special needs in a variety of school, home, community-based, and hospital settings, and has used a variety of psychotherapeutic, developmental, and behavioral treatment approaches. Her research studies on the experiences of parents of children with ASDs have been presented at national conferences and have been published by reputable scientific journals.

The following is a brief overview of the role of parent support in the treatment of children with autism spectrum disorders (ASD). This chapter provides an understanding of the need for parent support, focuses on the impact on caregivers raising children with ASDs, and the various supports available to them, so that they can be most effective in their parenting, in their implementation of the child's treatment program, and in other aspects of their lives. This overview is based on both the research literature and on the author's wealth of clinical experience in this area.

Impact of Parenting a Child with an Autism Spectrum Disorder

Parents of children with ASDs are impacted by their children's challenges in many ways, including emotionally, financially, with respect to their marriages and partnerships, and their everyday routines. Regarding the emotional impact, much research has shown that mothers of children with ASDs consistently report very high levels of child-related parenting stress (parenting stress related to the child), with parenting stress scores ranging from the 95th to 98th percentiles.[1] Parenting stress has been found at greater levels for parents of children with ASDs than for parents of children with normal development[2] and parents of children with other special needs.[3] Parents of children with ASDs also have reported more general psychological distress than parents of children with other special needs, including depression[4] and anxiety. Likewise, parents with higher levels of parenting stress have reported higher levels of psychological distress.[5]

Many parents of these children report high levels of guilt and/or self-blame regarding their children's diagnoses, despite no evidence in the scientific literature that parents' behaviors play a role. Years of clinical work with parents have indicated that without the identification of the exact cause(s) of ASDs, many parents reflect on things they did or did not do during pregnancy or infancy, resulting in blaming themselves and experiencing guilt related to their child's diagnosis.

Parenting satisfaction (how satisfied one is in the parenting role) and parenting efficacy (how competent one feels as a parent) are impacted for parents of children with ASDs. Mothers of children with ASDs have reported lower parenting satisfaction and parenting efficacy than parents of children with normal development.[6] Parents' sense of their child's attachment to them is also often impacted, due to the difficulties children with ASDs have forming relationships. Such is often the case for parents of children who look at their parents less often, who initiate affection with them with less frequency (or do not accept affection), and/or show significant difficulties being soothed by their parents when they are upset. This results in the self perception by parents that they are less effective in the role of a nurturing parent and a decrease in satisfaction in the caregiver role. Lower levels of parenting satisfaction are associated with higher levels of psychological distress for mothers of children with ASDs.[5]

Raising a child with an ASD impacts family's everyday routines in many ways. Any family dynamic is disrupted when a crisis is introduced particularly in the form of illness, or developmental challenges. Parents of children with ASDs consistently report much less "free time" available, related to the amount of time necessary to participate in their children's therapies at home and after school hours. As a result, there is often limited time and/or energy for parents to spend on themselves, for both necessary tasks (e.g., trips to the supermarket) and leisure activities (e.g., going out for dinner; exercise). Parents of children with ASDs often report a significant impact on their relationships with friends and family members. Such parents often report isolation from those who have supported them in the past. This can occur both as a result of others spending less time with them due to their discomfort around or limited understanding of children with ASDs, or from parents having limited time to maintain their connections.

The impact of raising a child with ASD on parents' marriages and partnerships has been a focus in recent years. Lower relationship satisfaction scores have been found for couples raising children with ASD than for couples with children without developmental disorders.[2] For parents who do find occasional time for themselves or with their partner, child care is often an issue. Children with ASDs have specific needs that the average babysitter is not skilled to manage.

Support for Parents of Children with ASDs

Support for parents of children with ASDs is a critical component of their children's treatment. Just as is the case with any responsibility humans have, their ability to carry it out depends on their resources, and their physical and emotional states. For example, people are less likely to perform well on a test when they are more fatigued or feeling anxious or sad. Likewise, parents' ability to take part in their child's treatment is a function of how well they themselves are functioning. With the high levels of parenting stress and psychological symptoms that parents of children with ASD often experience, many parents find it difficult to fully take part in their children's treatment, especially in the context of typical family responsibilities (e.g., career, homework, housework, etc.). Support can help parents manage these challenges.

Parents of children with ASDs benefit from a range of supports that vary in terms of their focus and setting. The following are ways that parents of children with ASD can be supported in order to decrease symptoms of distress and, in turn, be increasingly available for involvement in their children's treatment. The supports described are not exhaustive, and their effectiveness may differ depending on how they are delivered and on the individual characteristics of the parent who receives them. Just as children's treatment protocols are individually tailored to meet their needs, so should the support provided to their parents. The quality of support may be more important than the quantity, as parents reporting higher satisfaction with their social supports, but not a greater number of social supports reported lower levels of psychological distress.[5]

Developing a Sense of Parental Mastery

One of the initial sources of support parents receive is often from the therapists who work with their children. Support is provided by enhancing the parents' understanding of the nature of their children's challenges and their progress, and teaching parents strategies that work best for their children. It is quite helpful having regular access to and communication with one or more professionals that clearly understand the child's challenges and the best ways of helping them succeed.

Parents' ability to take part in their children's treatment, including their sense of mastery over its components and carrying over strategies into their daily routine are critical factors for children's progress. From the Developmental Individual-Differences and Relationship-based (DIR) perspective,[7] parents are recommended to play a primary role in the development of children with ASDs. Support from the therapists working with one's child can significantly help parents in this way and can have a positive impact on parents' sense of competence and their satisfaction with parenting.

Parents often benefit from individual support that focuses on their own specific issues related to themselves and their child. Individual counseling with a mental health clinician allows opportunities for focusing on parents' own experiences and developing coping strategies that can help them manage their parenting stress and any symptoms of psychological distress. Here, they can specifically address their struggles in order to become more effective in their parenting role and feel increased contentment overall. Self-care is imperative for parents so that they are available to their child to help them develop the key components for social, emotional, and intellectual development, including the ability to focus and attend, engage, interact, and use ideas creatively and logically.[7] Marriage counseling with a mental health clinician who has a background in families of children with ASDs is often helpful for addressing issues within the marriage. Support for the siblings of children with ASDs is also important for addressing the impact on the entire family.

Enhancing Social Connections

Parents of children with ASDs also find support in settings in which they can interact with parents of children with similar challenges. Parent support groups, often led by a mental health clinician, are provided regularly by many schools and local organizations. Such groups provide opportunities for parents to share their experiences, discuss ways of helping their children (e.g., by sharing information on treatment protocols and behavioral strategies) and caring for themselves. With the guidance of mental health clinicians, parents can receive psychoeducation about the latest research on ASDs and treatment and strategies that can help their children and themselves. Education regarding what is known about the cause(s) of ASDs is often crucial for parents who experience guilt and self-blame. Listening to others who have had similar experiences helps parents feel a sense of community, contrasting their experience of isolation from others.

Modern technology has provided parents with other options for informal support. This is often helpful for parents who aren't able to attend support groups (e.g., due to scheduling or babysitting difficulties). Message boards and listservs for parents of children with ASDs have become very popular in recent years. Benefits of message boards and listservs include their convenience and accessibility, without the challenges of scheduling of face-to-face support groups. This can be especially helpful for parents who live in remote areas. However, online technology does not afford the personal contact of support groups or provide the same opportunity to develop true relationships with other parents. Another concern with online technology is how the content is monitored. Without consistent moderation by a clinician, it is difficult to ensure that the content is appropriate and factual.

Financial Support

Financial support is often a vital aspect of support for parents and their children, as parents often report stress related to financial strain. There is often an enormous financial toll of diagnostic second opinions, follow-up appointments, and additional therapies for their children as all of these services may not be provided by schools or covered by insurance companies. Parents are often unaware of the financial resources that may be available to them, such as the Medicaid waiver program or Supplemental Security Income (SSI) that can provide eligibility for certain therapies or services (e.g., respite care) or a monthly stipend to assist in their child's care. Parents can contact their child's service coordinator, social worker, or an agency that advocates on behalf of families confronting ASD, and provides information about entitlements and resources.

In summary, parents of children with ASDs experience high levels of parenting stress, psychological distress (e.g., depression, anxiety, guilt), marital strain, and social isolation. Parents should be as much the focus in treatment as the children themselves, as their well-being is critical to their ability to be a part of their children's therapy. The optimal functioning of the parents is essential if the treatment strategies are to be successfully implemented. These families require access to a variety of supports, including communication with children's treatment providers, individual and group counseling, and advice regarding financial management and entitlement benefits.

PHYSICAL THERAPY

BY MEGHAN COLLINS

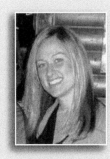

Meghan Collins, MPT

Rebecca School
40 E. 30th Street
New York, NY 10016
mcollins@rebeccaschool.org

Born and raised in New York. Graduated from the University of Scranton, 2005. Started working with children on the autism spectrum shortly after graduating. Currently, Physical Therapy Supervisor at Rebecca School. I want to thank my parents, Pat and Gene, for being a constant source of support and love.

Movement is a cornerstone for successfully functioning in one's environment and developing a sense of self. It is a sensation that a typically-developing individual becomes aware of and learns to modulate and control through various experiences. Multiple sensory systems, including the vestibular, proprioceptive, visual, and tactile, impact how a person perceives they are interacting with their environment. As babies, we practice interacting with our environment through both repetitive and spontaneous movement and a sense of where our bodies are in space develops. After we develop a sense of our bodies and where they are in space, movement is typically task-specific.

Motor development is an integrated experience between internal physiological development and the external environment. Richard Schmidt took Piaget's theory of scheme formation and related it to movement. Four things that impact the schema formation of motor learning, according to Schmidt, are the initial conditions of the movement, the response parameters for the motor program, sensory consequences of the movement, and the movement outcome. Motor learning is "a set of [internal] processes associated with practice or experience leading to relatively permanent changes in the capability for responding."

The World Confederation for Physical Therapy defines physical therapy as "a health care profession that provides treatment to individuals to develop, maintain and restore maximum movement and function throughout life. This includes providing treatment in circumstances where movement and function are threatened by aging, injury, disease or environmental factors."

Physical therapy with children on the autism spectrum may look very different from the physical therapy you or I may seek out. While we may have experienced some physical impairment that has impacted our ability to function successfully in our environment and need help in restoring, for those with autism, physical therapy can be used for a variety of developmental purposes. Children with autism typically have difficulties processing and integrating sensory information, including movement. For example, they may have low muscle tone, or have a tough time with coordination and sports. These issues can not only interfere with basic day-to-day functioning but can have an impact on social and physical development.

Younger children with autism often exhibit significant delays in reaching developmental milestones. Therefore the earliest forms of physical therapy may include working on skills such as sitting, rolling, crawling, standing, and walking. As the children get older, they may receive physical therapy to address concerns regarding muscle strength, endurance, balance, coordination, motor planning, ball skills, and various forms of locomotion.

Core muscle weakness and low muscle tone are common issues that need to be addressed during physical therapy with children on the autism spectrum. Core muscle strength and tone impact many aspects of movement and motor control such as postural control, balance, and coordination. Postural control is the ability to maintain the position required to perform other movements or tasks. When a person has poor core muscle strength and postural control, it makes it difficult to perform or participate in activities away from their body or outside their base of support such as throwing or kicking a ball. A common therapeutic intervention used is maintaining upright in various positions (sitting and lying on back, front, or side) and planes (frontal, sagittal, or transverse) on a therapy ball. The child may need support from the therapist to maintain a desired posture. They may also be able to perform another activity simultaneously increasing the difficulty of the task and challenging their ability to adapt or modify their posture accordingly. Core muscle strength and postural control are essential is general play, such as riding a tricycle or bicycle, or scooter.

Another common issue addressed during physical therapy is praxis or motor planning. This is an individual's ability to formulate a plan, organize their body appropriately, and execute the plan. The first step in praxis is ideation, formulating an idea or plan, and is the cognitive part of the process. Children with autism often have difficulty with ideation as it is thought to be largely related to integrate the sensory information they are receiving from their own body and environment. Next is the subconscious organization or development of a plan of how they are going to accomplish the task at hand. Lastly, the plan gets executed, which is the physical or motoric part of the process. The amount of thought and effort a typically-developing individual puts into learning a novel skill may be the same amount of thought and effort a child with autism has when learning how to run, skip, or hop. Creating, constructing, and executing an obstacle course play or negotiating playground equipment are common ways a child may work on their motor planning skills during a physical therapy session.

Overall muscle strength and endurance may be addressed during community walks or stair climbing. Limited range of motion or muscle flexibility may be addressed by traditional stretching or massage. Aerobic fitness may be a concern as weight-gain and lethargy are common side effects of various medications children on the autism spectrum may take. Traditional exercise may be performed during therapy sessions, such as push-ups, sit-ups, or jumping jacks, to improve aerobic capacity. Successfully moving through a classroom or hallway requires good body awareness, visual spatial ability, modulation and coordination. Balance activities may include negotiating stairs with and without support from the railing or wall, walking across a balance beam, standing one foot, hopping, moving onto, off of, or across uneven or moveable surfaces, and roller-skating.

Another very useful tool often used in physical therapy is ball play. Ball skills require knowing where one's limbs are in relation to the rest of their body and modulation of force. One should be able to orient one's body in order to send or receive a ball. Ball skills include overhand and underhand throwing, kicking, and catching. When evaluating child's ability to throw a ball, a physical therapy will typically evaluate the fluidity of movement, the ability of the child to hit the target (overshooting or undershooting), repeated misses of the target in the same direction, or stepping with the opposite foot. When kicking a ball, a physical therapists will typically evaluate the fluidity of movement, appropriate ball contact, coordinated knee bending, the ability of the child to hit the target (overshooting or undershooting), or repeated misses of the target in the same direction. When catching a ball or receiving it after a kick, a physical therapist may evaluate the ability of the child to follow the trajectory of the ball as it approaches them, correct orientation of the body with regard to the ball's height, direction, or force, and hand placement (e.g., are their hands open and ready, are they closing their hand too soon or too late, are their hands rigid or stiff.) If a child is having difficulty catching a medium-size ball, balloons serve as good substitutes until the child becomes more familiar with the task.

A child receiving physical therapy will improve their gross motor function which is an important aspect of socialization, allowing the child to participate in general play, physical education, or sports. The key to a successful physical therapy session is making the activities during the session motivating for the child. Ultimately kids just want to have fun!

PSYCHOTROPIC MEDICATIONS AND THEIR CAUTIOUS DISCONTINUATION

BY DR. GEORGIA A. DAVIS

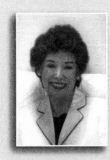

Georgia A. Davis, MD

Director
Genetic Consultants of Springfield, IL
1112 Rickard Rd # B
Springfield, IL 62704-1022

Dr. Davis is board certified as a Diplomat in the specialty of psychiatry by the American Board of Psychiatry and Neurology. She is also board certified in forensic psychiatry and forensic medicine and is a Diplomat of the American Board of Forensic Examiners.

Dr. Davis' private practice includes the diagnosis and treatment of children, adolescents and adults. She's a dedicated psychiatric intensivist and provides individualized care which is state of the art and quite comprehensive.

She is currently an adjunct faculty member of the University of Illinois at Chicago where she specializes in the use of nuclear brain imaging for the evaluation and treatment of mild to severe brain trauma, dementia and cognitive decline, seizure activity, atypical and refractory psychiatric disorders, aggressive/violent behavior, brain effects of substance abuse, exposure to toxic substances, suicidal behavior, temporal lobe dysfunction and forensic/legal evaluations.

I n this article, we'll discuss factors to consider when assessing a child's readiness or need to discontinue medications and how to do so safely, comfortably and successfully.

Reasons to Discontinue Medications:

Allergic Reactions: Due to the fact that children with autism spectrum disorders (ASD) usually have immune systems that are dysregulated, they may be prone to experiencing allergic reactions not only to foods and environmental triggers but also to medications and even supplements. Some of these medications or supplements may be critical to their recovery but, unfortunately they may be unable to tolerate them—even in small doses. If this is the case with your child, a pharmacist specializing in compounding medications can be very helpful. The pharmacist can compound a medication or supplement in a hypoallergenic form by using a different base, binding agent, or other components.. This may be all that is necessary to eliminate any "allergic" reaction. If this does not work, then the medication or supplement probably would need to be stopped. This needs to be done, however, in a manner which would allow a gradual, gentle tapering that minimizes withdrawal effects. Your pharmacist can compound a sustained-release form of the medication at the dosage your doctor has prescribed which would enable a gradual, gentle tapering and yet allow a faster taper than would ordinarily be possible with the usual form of the medication.

Unfortunately, it may become necessary to taper more quickly than either you or your doctor would prefer due to severe allergies or liver problems. You will be relying on your doctor's experience and expertise. He or she may suggest using additional medications or supplements for a short time to offset or minimize the withdrawal reaction. TAPS, Silymarin and Milk Thistle have proven very effective in supporting the liver and restoring its health and functionality. Ammonia levels are more sensitive indicators of liver problems than are routine liver function tests and most local hospitals can run these quickly if there is reason to be concerned. Follow your doctor's instructions to the letter, keep a log and don't hesitate to notify your doctor if you observe anything unusual. **Never worry alone.**

If at first you don't succeed, try again at a later time. Allow the elimination diet to have more time for healing of the gut and treat any dysbiosis, inflammation or oxidative stress with appropriate probiotics and/or supplements.

Intolerable Side Effects: ASD children may also have more intense side effects related to medications or supplements than their neurotypical peers. Parents will want to eliminate serious side effects quickly. Since most ASD children have a problem eliminating many toxic substances, e.g., heavy metals, pesticides, phthalates, they may develop a retention toxicity more easily than their peers. In the process of detoxification, which occurs in two phases in the liver, a *more toxic* substance is produced in Phase I. Phase II, in ASD children is compromised, making it more difficult for them to get rid of the more toxic substance and as a result side effects may be more pronounced.

Other Less Pressing Reasons: There are at least three other situations in which you might want to discontinue a medication, but would not have the time-pressure imposed on this endeavor by the situations described above.

1.) Should a *"Black Box"* warning be placed on a medication your child is currently taking, your doctor should notify you that a problem has been identified concerning the use of this medication. Your doctor will give you details regarding the issue that has come to light and you will then need to make a decision whether or not this "Black Box" warning identifies a serious risk for your child now or that there is a likelihood that it may become a problem in the future.

2.) If the medication is simply ineffective and you chose to discontinue it, you have the luxury of doing this at your convenience, perhaps replacing it with an alternative drug, supplement or therapy. (See recommendations below.)

3.) Of course, the most desirable reason for discontinuing a medication would be that the underlying problem has been identified and corrected, and the medication is no longer necessary.

Is Your Child Ready to Discontinue Medication?

1. This is difficult to address but is your doctor supportive of your wish to discontinue medication for your child or, if not, will you have to find another physician to guide you through the process and be available in the event that something unexpected happens? You will need a plan and help if you run into problems and a doctor you can work with to anticipate potential problems and to develop a plan to address them if it becomes necessary. Discontinuing medications is a challenge for both parent and child so a sympathetic caring physician will make the process somewhat easier.

2. Are the initial symptoms well controlled? Think back to why the medication was necessary in the first place. What were the target symptoms? Are they under good control now?

3. Have you identified the biochemical pathways that may have contributed to your child's symptoms? Become acquainted with the Citric Acid Cycle; the Serotonin, Epinephrine, Norepinephrine and Dopamine Pathways, Methylation Pathway, Transulfuration Pathway, and Cholesterol Pathway. Review your child's previous test results and re-test, if necessary, to make sure that nutritional and chemical deficiencies have been corrected, otherwise tapering may be premature and your child may regress precipitously.

4. Is the timing right? For school children, choosing summer vacation, Christmas break, Spring break or a time when a little extra help at home is available makes it easier to accomplish what might be difficult during times of busy family schedules. Always allow time for the unexpected.

5. Make Safety a priority! You and your child's doctor must work together to accomplish medication discontinuation. Discuss problems, no matter how small with your doctor and consider the pros and cons of discontinuation as well as what to expect in terms of withdrawal symptoms. Realize that the risk for withdrawal symptoms increases with younger age and female gender. Also remember that early adverse reactions when initiating a medication or supplement may predict withdrawal reactions.

6. Is your child in one of the high risk categories for discontinuing medications safely or easily? Children with a history of seizures, hypoxic or traumatic brain injuries, untreated infections, co-morbid conditions such as asthma, allergies, thyroid or adrenal problems, toxic markers, markers of inflammation or oxidative stress, problems with liver or kidney function may experience more difficulties when beginning medications or discontinuing them. Here again, work closely with your doctor to address these issues.

OK! If all of the above issues have been considered and discussed with your child's physician then you are ready to begin.

How to Discontinue Medications

1. Know what withdrawal symptoms to expect and how long they are expected to last. You may need to research how to minimize withdrawal symptoms or how to offset them. (See examples below).

2. Be prepared for *rebounding*. Withdrawal of some medications causes a rebound effect in which the symptoms for which the medication was given in the first place return in full force, that is, the symptom may be more severe. Sleep medications are infamous for this, causing children to have more difficulty sleeping that they had before the medication was given. Withdrawal symptoms and rebound symptoms are not the same thing.

3. Know the half-life of your child's medication that is, how long does it take for half of the drug to be eliminated from your child's system. A medication with a short half-life, e.g. 2-4 hours, usually carries a higher risk of withdrawal symptoms than one with a long half life, e.g., 24–36 hours. The shorter the half-life of a medication, the smaller should be the increment by which it is reduced and a longer time should be allowed between dosage reductions.

4. Find another medication in the same class but with a longer half-life and transition to that medication as a tapering strategy. There will be fewer and less intense withdrawal reactions using a medication with a longer half-life.

5. Reduce the dosage in very small increments. *Start low and go slow.* Remember that withdrawal symptoms may emerge even at the end of a slow taper. Therefore,

the lower the dose, the slower you go. Timing is important here too. Start on a week-end when your child will be with you most of the time. No one knows him like you do, so others are unlikely to spot something unusual as quickly as you will.

6.   Calculate the total daily dose of the medication to be tapered and plan to keep the same dosing schedule, but decrease each dose by a very small increment.

7.   Alternatively, start with the least necessary dose. If mornings are good now, but afternoons and evenings are still rough, the morning dose should be the first to go. If unsure, try giving the dose you plan to discontinue an hour or two later than usual. If problems develop, either choose a different dose to taper or decrease the amount by which you are reducing the dose. (Example: instead of lowering the dose in 25mg increments, lower it by 5-10mg increments only and reduce it more slowly.) If you have the luxury of time, slow tapering is the key to successful withdrawal.

Common Symptoms And What To Do About Them

Sleep Disturbances: Even a very slow and careful taper of most psychotropic medications can disrupt sleep in various ways. Tapering by too large an increment can cause sleep problems including difficulty falling asleep, staying asleep, early morning awakening, vivid dreams, nightmares, or night terrors.

1.   Is your child having trouble getting to sleep? Among the natural sleep aids, many parents find a small dose of regular Melatonin given an hour before bedtime to be quite helpful. GABA is a natural neuroinhibitory neurotransmitter that I have also found to be quite useful. For children with allergies who have dark circles under their eyes, have a nasal crease or awaken with nasal congestion, a small dose of Benadryl or Sudafed may be helpful.

2.   Is the problem staying asleep? Consider Melatonin Controlled Release (CR). It comes in chewable tablets making it easy for children to accept them.

3.   Does your child wake up early in the morning? This may be a sign of a biological depression due to a problem in the serotonin pathway. The main components of this is pathway can be examined through specialized urine tests that can pinpoint deficiencies in vitamins, minerals or amino acid precursors needed to synthesize serotonin, a neurotransmitter thought to be important in alleviating depression However, early morning awakenings may also occur due to adrenal fatigue. In this case, the early awakening is triggered by a drop in blood sugar because of the adrenal gland's inability to mobilize stored glycogen sufficiently to prevent hypoglycemia during an overnight fast.

Neuropsychiatric Symptoms: Discontinuance of psychotropic medications often results in the following neuropsychiatric symptoms.

1. Anxiety/panic

   Check out the adequacy of serotonin precursors,. Rule out magnesium deficiencies, hypercortisol states and eliminate glutamates from the diet. Provide nutritional support with L-Theanine and Taurine and increase B vitamins. Consider GABA , Xymogen's "RelaxMax" or a beta-blocker.

2. Compulsivity, Obsessionality, Aggression

   Inositol or IP-6, can be extremely helpful. It is available without a prescription and is very affordable, especially if purchased as a powder. It tastes sweet, so there should be no problems administering this one.

3. Depression or mood swings

   Again, review the test results looking for the functionality of the Serotonin and Epinephrine pathways, Copper/Zinc levels and adequacy of B-vitamins. Consider increasing or balancing omega-3 fatty acids with B-6's and B-9's. Rule out and correct Candida overgrowths, thyroid problems, adrenal insufficiency, anemias, pyroluria and abnormal histamine levels. Readjust as necessary and try again.

4. Irritability, impulsivity, confusion, paranoia, suicidal ideation, psychotic symptoms.

   Rule-out dietary infractions, especially gluten and sugar. Rule-out dysbiosis and overgrowth of pathogenic bacteria, especially certain species of Clostridia and Pseudomonas. Rule out other toxic exposures with tests for heavy metals, molds, pesticides, insecticides, phthalates etc. Check out acid/base balance and correct with alkalinizing foods, probiotics, biofilm protocols, enzymes, Omega 3 fatty acids and L-Glutamine. Eliminate as many glutamates as possible.

Flu-like Symptoms: These symptoms are very common on withdrawal of psychotropic medications.

1. Headache, muscle aches, fatigue, sweating, flushing, chills, temperature changes/intolerances, lethargy and lassitude are very common symptoms experienced when discontinuing psychotropic medications. Fortunately, these symptoms are generally benign although very uncomfortable for your child. They usually resolve within 1-2 weeks.

2. Treat flu-like symptoms with Epsom salts baths, correcting pH with alkalinizing foods, Alka-Seltzer Gold, Activated Charcoal and Trisalts.

3. Give a lot of fluids and go back to the previously well-tolerated dose of medication. Slow down the taper and decrease the dosage increment or switch to another medication in the same family, but with a longer half-life.

4.   If necessary, a teeny, tiny dose can be compounded and given at more frequent intervals to prevent these withdrawal symptoms.

Gastrointestinal Symptoms:

1.   Nausea, vomiting and loss of appetite; treat with Alka-Seltzer Gold, Activated Charcoal, or Tri-Salts and optimize hydration. In addition, discontinue solids and put your child on a clear liquid diet. Call your doctor's office if vomiting or diarrhea continues for more than 24 hrs.
2.   Diarrhea or loose stools , abdominal cramps, bloating; rule out dietary infractions, especially gluten, casein and soy. Eliminate all sugars, and fruits except berries (no strawberries though) and pears until stools normalize.
3.   Increase probiotics and enzymes and obtain a comprehensive stool analysis.
4.   If these measures fail to improve symptoms, discontinue solid foods and call your doctor for further instructions.

NeuroMotor Symptoms:

1.   Tremors, difficulty walking (ataxia), muscle jerks, restless legs, involuntary movement of the neck, tongue or eyes or difficulty with speech. Prevent these neuromotor symptoms by increasing magnesium and taurine. Treat with Cogentin, beta-blockers, Clonidine, Glutathione (NAC by nebulizer) or IV Glutathione.
2.   Hyperarousal, sense of inner restlessness, agitation, anxiety. Use magnesium, GABA, L-theanine, Benztropine, Clonidine, propranolol to ease these.

   Neuro-Sensory Disturbances: Numbness, tingling sensations, shock-like sensations, ringing in the ears, hypersensitivity to sound, tactile sensitivities, unusual visual disturbances—like visual trails, blurring of vision are not as common as flu-like symptoms and are generally short-lived if they are experienced, but they can be quite disconcerting. Generally all that is required is reassurance, but magnesium, taurine or a short course of very low-dose Valium (1mg in the morning and 1 mg in the evening) can help these symptoms resolve more quickly.

RELATIONSHIP DEVELOPMENT INTERVENTION

BY LAURA HYNES

Laura Hynes, LMSW; RDI Program Certified Consultant

Extraordinary Minds, Inc.
308 Forest Avenue
Staten Island, New York 10301
(347) 564-8451
L.Hynes@yahoo.com
www.extraordinaryminds.org
RDIconnect.com

Laura Hynes graduated from Stony Brook University with a Bachelor of Arts in Psychology and a minor in Child and Family Studies in 2001. She obtained a Masters in Social Work in 2005 from New York University and is a licensed social worker in the State of New York. In 2008, Laura became certified in Relationship Development Intervention She is the president and founder of Extraordinary Minds, Inc., where she currently provides RDI services to families.

Relationship Development Intervention is a unique approach to treating autism spectrum disorders. Developed by Dr. Steven Gutstein, RDI is based on the most recent research in autism spectrum disorders (ASD), neurology, and developmental psychology. The RDI theory is based on the premise that autism spectrum disorders prevent a child from providing their parent with adequate social-emotional feedback, thereby disrupting the typical parent-child relationship. RDI provides a second chance for parents and their child to reestablish that parent-child relationship. RDI's main objective is to provide individuals with ASD opportunities to attain a better quality of life than what is typically expected for them. It is a parent-based approach, whereby a trained consultant teaches parents how to change the way they are communicating and interacting with their child to reestablish the disrupted relationship thereby improving the child's dynamic intelligence.

"Give a man a fish and you feed him for a day. Teach a man to fish and you feed him for a lifetime."

—Chinese proverb

To best understand dynamic intelligence, one must understand static intelligence. Most individuals with ASD are quite proficient in static areas. Think of static intelligence as anything that has a right or wrong answer, that is unchanging and always produces the same outcome. Labeling, requesting, social scripts, academics, following directions, and memorization are all examples of static skills, and likely what a child with ASD is adept at.

Think about dynamic intelligence as the ability to manage situations that present themselves with elements of uncertainty. Examples of dynamic skills include the ability to problem solve, share experiences with others, curiosity, empathy, and taking another's perspective. All of these things are uncertain, in that there is no wrong or right answer, and no way to predict what specific outcome will occur. This type of intelligence is what is most often lacking in individuals with ASD.

There are other interventions for ASD that focus primarily on strengthening static skills; increasing language, teaching scripts to navigate social situations or following a schedule. Challenge yourself to think of these types of skills as compensatory for deficits in dynamic thinking.

- Is increasing one's vocabulary improving the ability to share experiences and communicate with other people?
- Is teaching a child a social script for the playground preparing them for what to do when they don't get the response they were taught to expect?
- Is creating a picture schedule teaching a person to be flexible and manage the real world, where unexpected things happen all the time?

"One can imagine training or therapies that are designed to teach the various parts of the brain to work together in a more coordinated way, to make them function as a team rather than individuals players."

—Marcel Just, MD

Years ago, the scientific community believed that the brain was unable to change. The only way we knew how to teach individuals with ASD was to give them the skills to compensate for their brain's difficulty managing uncertainty. We know now that the brain is an experience dependant organ; it changes and grows based on the types of learning experiences it is exposed to on a day to day basis. It is not only possible to but critical to begin addressing and remediating the deficits of ASD instead of merely working around them.

"Children's cognitive development is an apprenticeship–it occurs through guided participation in a social activity with companions who support and stretch children's learning."

—Barbara Rogoff

Neurotypical individuals begin thinking dynamically very early in life. The relationship between parent and child, called the guided participation relationship, is critical for the development of active thinkers and communicators. Guided participation is found cross-culturally, in every society, since the beginning of time. Children act as cognitive apprentices to more skilled and competent adults who provide them with ongoing challenges and the support necessary for them to be successful with life's challenges. Guides balance teaching various skills with a more important goal, providing the foundations for active thinking, learning, and cognitive growth.

Consider a young child raking leaves with his/her father. The father is not teaching his child to rake the leaves in a way that he would expect the child to go out and independently do this the following weekend. The father is teaching his child the child the goals beneath the goal; the foundations for learning. The child is learning how to collaborate with his father, how to flexibly manage problems and come up with solutions, and how to anticipate and communicate to one another about what they are doing.

Unfortunately, when ASD is added to the guided participation relationship, the child provides the parent with poor social and emotional feedback, leaving the parent with inadequate information to provide the child with opportunities to learn in a dynamic way. This is where RDI becomes so valuable.

"There is no greater reward than serving as a catalyst for another person's journey towards fulfilling their true potential."

—Dr. Steven Gutstein

Dr. Gutstein, developer of the RDI program looked closely at the guided participation relationship between typically developing children and their parents and how parents provide their children with opportunities for dynamic growth. He was able to identify where the breakdown in this relationship occurs with children with ASD. The RDI program is designed to reestablish the guided participation relationship, thereby improving the child's ability to function in a dynamic, ever-changing world.

Through his extensive research on autism and the guided participation relationship in autism, Dr. Gutstein identified several core areas of dynamic intelligence that are lacking in individuals with ASD. These elements of dynamic thinking are incorporated into guided participation objectives that make up the dynamic intelligence curriculum.

Parents often yearn for their child to develop peer relationships. Peer relationships, as all relationships, require the ability to collaborate, where partners are able to coordinate their actions, thoughts, and ideas to reach a common goal. Parents and professionals alike want nothing more than for the child with ASD to go out on the playground and make up a game with a peer. This type of collaborating requires a more basic understanding of social reciprocity called co-regulation that is also typically lacking in individuals with ASD.

Co-regulation is the most basic form of interaction and communication. It is simply, when one person takes an action in response to their partner's action. There is no end goal or task involved. It is purely about being in the moment with the other person. Oftentimes, individuals with ASD are either, passive and prompt dependant or controlling and rigid. To establish co-regulation with a passive partner, the parent must help the child to understand that he/she can bring something to the interaction without being told what to do. To establish co-regulation with a controlling child, the parent must provide the child with an authentic role that allows the child to provide suggestions for enhancement without the usual controlling features. Co-regulation can be established. As the individual with ASD understands and participates in basic social reciprocity, many new opportunities for interacting and communicating occur.

There are two types of communication, instrumental and experience sharing communication. Instrumental communication is used to obtain something and a specific response is expected. Examples of this would be requesting a toy, asking a question or providing a direction. Once the desired objective is received, the question answered, or the direction taken there is no longer a need to communicate with the other person.

Experience sharing communication, by nature, does not require a specific response. When you express what you like or dislike, what you are feeling or describing about your day, you will expect a relevant but not right or wrong response. Think about all the things that have to be considered in order to successfully have a conversation. We must interpret the other person's language, his or her non-verbal communication; gestures, facial expressions, intonation change, pauses and innuendo; and we decipher all of that simultaneously.

The value of language in the human experience is to communicate and share experiences with others. In an RDI program, parents look at what type of communication they are using with their child. Is it mostly instrumental; asking questions or providing directions or is it mostly experience sharing; commenting, sharing preferences and ideas? Parents are taught to strive for a balance of instrumental and experience sharing language that is found in conversational language among most people. To do this, parents increase their experience sharing language and decrease their instrumental language with their child with ASD. By providing the child with ASD language that does not require a specific response, parents are teaching a child the true value of language, to share with others. Parents find that by changing their own communication to become more experience sharing in nature, their child with ASD soon follows suit and begins commenting and sharing experiences spontaneously and independently.

The RDI program also teaches parents to create an environment conducive to the development of non-verbal communication. A great percentage of communication in the world is conducted non-verbally. Using and reading non verbal communication is inherently difficult for individuals with ASD. Often times, parents and professionals compensate for this deficit by using language as the primary and often only form of communication. Individuals with ASD do not naturally monitor their communication environment, resulting in parents and professionals prompting them to attend and/or make eye contact. Instead of trying to change their behavior, think about changing yours. If we are always providing individuals with ASD auditory information, they never have the need to look or monitor their environment. By reducing language, prompts for eye contact and incorporating more non verbal communication into everyday experiences, parents create a need for the child to look, monitor, and become a more active communicator.

By utilizing non verbal and broadband communication, parents are also increasing the child's opportunities to reference. Social referencing, the ability to seek out information from a parent or guide when wary or unsure, is in place by twelve months of age in typically developing children. A twelve month old, exploring child who is feeling uncertain will reference his mother to see her emotional reaction. If mom appears encouraging and calm, the child will continue in his exploration. If the mother appears distressed, the child will cease exploration and may seek comfort. Individuals with ASD have great difficulty using social referencing to manage uncertainty. When faced with a situation that is uncertain, they will often respond with fight or flight, meltdown or withdrawal. Referencing, often a deficit, is a better option. The goal is to allow the child to discover that there is value in looking to their more competent guides for information, to "borrow" their perspective when they are unsure as how to process the information. The RDI program teaches parents how to create moments of productive uncertainty that create just enough curiosity without being so uncertain that the child feels anxious. The productive part of productive uncertainty will vary for every individual. For example, parents can create productive uncertainty by merely stopping while walking together. Some individuals will however require a more deliberate or extreme approach to productive uncertainty such as pulling a hammer out of a washing machine while doing laundry together.

By teaching the value in looking to more competent guides for help processing information, we are actually teaching them how to become more effective problem solvers. True, independence begins with a healthy dependence on a parent or guide. No child is born into the world with the knowledge as to how to navigate it. Many individuals with ASD never develop a healthy dependence on their parent which results in great difficulty managing uncertainty, inability to appraise social situations and inadequate problem solving skills.

The RDI program teaches parents the value in helping their child to become more active thinkers and problem solvers. There are many ways to do this on a day to day basis, but the first is to look at areas where they may be overcompensating, perhaps doing things for their child that he or she is likely capable of doing. To create a feeling of competence in a child, the child needs opportunities to be successful at thinking, considering and problem solving. Take a simple everyday example of a child who wants a drink. Mom holds the juice and places the cup in front of the child, upside down. By just waiting and not providing the solution to "turn over your cup", mom has created a an uncertain moment where she is asking the child to monitor his/her environment, think about and consider the situation and take some kind of action to fix it. If the child is unable to figure out what it is that the mother is asking of him/her, mom can use a statement such as, "I don't think I can pour the juice yet", or "Your cup is upside down!" This type of statement is stating the problem instead of the solution, allowing the child the opportunity to think and problem solve on his/her own. The RDI program teaches parents how to identify opportunities and create dozens of moments such as these throughout the day.

> **"If there is anything that we wish to change in a child, we should first examine it and see whether it is not something that could better be changed in ourselves."**
>
> —C.G. Jung

Relationship Development Intervention is considered a developmental approach to treating autism spectrum disorders. This is because RDI, as other developmental approaches, is based on the concept that in autism, developmental milestones are missed yet can be revisited and addressed directly. Newer therapies and approaches are moving from traditional, behavioral based thinking that teach individuals with autism skills to compensate for these developmental deficits to addressing the deficits in development directly.

RDI is unique from other developmental approaches in that it is based on extensive research of the typical parent-child relationship; it is not a therapy that has been "created" to treat autism. It is a program that allows parents to go back and look at their child's development, learn where, exactly the gaps in development are and how to teach those missing milestones the way typically developing children learn them. Because an RDI program is based on typical development, it is an appropriate intervention for individuals with autism of all ages and levels of severity. All individuals with autism regardless of severity, co-occurring conditions or age will benefit from addressing deficits in dynamic intelligence and revisiting missed developmental milestones.

Critics of RDI and other developmental approaches often take the stance that individuals with autism learn a certain way and do not learn the way typically developing children learn. An RDI program will show you that this is actually untrue. When parents slow down and become more deliberate in their interactions, individuals with autism can learn what and how neurotypical children do. Anyone who tells a parent that this is untrue is not allowing individuals with autism reach their true potential.

The RDI program is broken down into systematic and workable objectives. Because it is a parent based intervention, parents work on their own objectives prior to the assignment of any objectives for the child. As parents move through their own objectives and as they change their behavior, many child objectives are inadvertently addressed. Thus early on, from the very beginning observable improvements in the child's dynamic abilities are often noticed early on.

RDI begins with an in depth look at the parent's readiness to begin the work of reestablishing the guided participation relationship. Parents work collaboratively with their consultants to develop long and short term goals for themselves, the child with ASD as well as siblings, they examine and modify current schedules to create more quality time for guided participation, and they work to improve their limit setting and identify and modify areas where they may be overcompensating for the child.

Once parents are demonstrating readiness to learn how to guide their child, a dynamic assessment is done. The Relationship Development Assessment looks at the state of the guided participation relationship and consists of parents and child engaging in predetermined activities provided by the consultant. Based on the information gathered during the RDA, objectives are assigned.

As parents adopt guided participation as their primary mode of parenting and become more competent guides, they begin using the dynamic intelligence curriculum for their child. They dynamic intelligence curriculum is comprised of over one thousand, dynamic, developmental objectives that follow the continuum of typical development. The RDI program thus provides parents, children and adults a second chance at getting back on developmental track with mastery of small manageable and observable objectives and goals.

Face to face meeting between parents, consultant and child occur regularly, several times per month. During these meetings, assignments are broken down, plans for work at home through role play and demonstrations occur. Parents leave their meetings with an assignment to complete at home with their child based on what particular parent or child objective is being addressed between sessions. They provide the consultant with videos, journals and other forms of communication demonstrating how they are working on their current assignment and how they are actively analyzing and evaluating the work they are doing with their child. From the very beginning of the RDI program, parents are taking the responsibility to think about and consider their success and breakdowns with their child and eventually to guide their child without the support of a consultant.

The RDI program is a unique and invaluable resource to families. It values parents as the most important influence in their child's life. Parents are provided the skills and direction to become successfully reconnected with their child. Knowing that their child's growth is due to their own guidance empowers parents to persevere through difficult times and look to the future with a great deal of hope.

SENSORY-BASED ANTECEDENT INTERVENTIONS

BY DR. GINNY VAN RIE AND DR. L. JUANE HEFLIN

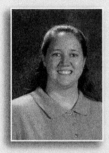

Georgia State University
Educational Psychology and Special Education
PO Box 3979
Atlanta, GA 30302-3970
(404) 413-8333

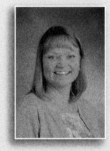

Ginny L. Van Rie, Ph.D.
ginny.vanrie@gcsu.edu

L. Juane Heflin, Ph.D.
jheflin@gsu.edu

Dr. Van Rie is an Assistant Professor of Special Education at Georgia College & State University. She is a certified special educator who taught children with ASD and extremely challenging behavior for over 9 years. She currently teaches behavior management courses to pre-service undergraduate and graduate-level teacher candidates to help them intervene positively and proactively to minimize maladaptive behavior and support student achievement. Her goal is to create environments to match the learning and behavioral needs of each student with ASD. She was honored as the "Outstanding Doctoral Student" in Special Education at Georgia State University in 2009. Dr. Heflin has over 25 years of experience learning about and advocating for individuals with ASD and coordinates the autism program at Georgia State University. She co-edits the journal, *Focus on Autism and Other Developmental Disabilities* and coauthored the book, *Students with Autism Spectrum Disorders: Effective Instructional Practices*, published by Prentice Hall in 2007. Both Dr. Van Rie and Dr. Heflin have been recognized "Heroes for Autism" by the Greater Georgia Chapter of the Autism Society of America.

Researchers have provided copious evidence that modifying antecedent events (those that occur prior to instruction) can have a strong positive effect on student engagement and success.

In some situations, the antecedent variables that occasion student resistance are predictable, such as giving the student a large amount of work to do (Sweeney & LeBlanc, 1995). For many of those with ASD, the antecedent conditions are uniquely individual, as was the case of a child who interacted willingly unless his shirt was wet or his toys had been moved, at which point he became aggressive (Napolitano, Tessing, McAdam, Dunleavy & Cifuni, 2006). Banda and Kubina (2006) discovered that asking two or three conversational questions that the adolescent answered willingly (e.g., "Did you watch football yesterday?"), prior to asking him to empty his backpack, arrange his daily schedule, and go to his locker resulted in quicker transitions and less resistance. Reinhartsen, Garfinkle, and Wolery (2002) documented that allowing children to choose the toy they wanted to play with resulted in higher levels of appropriate engagement as compared to when teachers gave children a preferred toy. Other antecedent interventions that have been used to increase adaptive behavior and reduce what others thought to be problem behaviors in individuals with ASD include the use of Power Cards (Keeling, Myles, Gagnon, & Simpson, 2003), alternative seating (Schilling & Schwartz, 2004), and self-operated auditory prompts (Taber, Seltzer, Heflin, & Alberto, 1999). The National Autism Center (2009a, p. 43) determined that sufficient empirical validation existed to identify antecedent interventions as "Established Treatments." However, none of the variations cited in the *National Standards Report* relate to sensory-based interventions.

It is well documented that individuals with ASD process sensory stimuli differently than individuals with typical development and those with other disabilities (e.g., Ben-Sasson et al., 2007; Crane, Goddard, & Pring, 2009; Ermer, & Dunn, 1998; Harrison, & Hare; 2004; Rogers, Hepburn & Wehner, 2003; Tomcheck & Dunn, 2007). These differences in sensory processing result in reduced availability for instruction that inhibits learning. Sensory-based antecedent interventions support the attainment of optimal levels of arousal to promote the acquisition of skills necessary for independent functioning.

Primary Developers

The theory of optimal arousal, introduced by Lueba (1955) and extended by Zentall and Zentall (1983) is based on the premise that all organisms have an optimal level of arousal and engage in behaviors either to increase or decrease stimulation in order reach those optimal levels. Dunn (1997) stated that individuals could be both hypo- and hyper-responsive to sensory stimuli and that an individual's response to the same sensory stimuli can change over time. She developed a conceptual model of sensory processing in which individuals respond to sensory stimuli based on their sensory receptor thresholds. Individual could have high thresholds and not register sensory input or need to seek additional sensory input to trigger their sensory thresholds. In contrast, individuals could have low sensory thresholds and be overly responsive to sensory stimuli or try to avoid sensory stimuli because the stimulation makes them uncomfortable (Dunn, 2001).

Success rate (including a "Best case" anecdote)

Van Rie and Heflin (2009) conducted a study to determine which form of sensory-based antecedent interventions would establish optimal levels of arousal as measured by correct responses on instructional tasks. Consistent with Dunn's (1997) premise, the type of sensory-based intervention needed to match the arousal level of the child in order to produce a level of arousal that facilitated learning. In the study, each child participated in five minutes of antecedent sensory-based activities prior to instructional tasks. The sensory-based interventions consisted of bouncing on an exercise ball and swinging in a suspended swing. Use of a rigorous research methodology, including analysis via an alternating treatment design with replication, resulted in the ability to draw conclusions about the effects of the interventions. The two students who were over-aroused in the classroom setting, Tony and Al, gave a greater number of correct responses after they spent five minutes swinging in a slow linear manner. Carl, who was under-aroused in the school environment, performed better on the instructional tasks after he spent five minutes bouncing on the exercise ball. These results can be interpreted not only to substantiate the variability of sensory processing difficulties present in the diverse population of individuals with ASD, but also to implicate the need to evaluate each individual's sensory processing patterns in order to select the most appropriate sensory interventions.

Risk and/or side-effects (including a "Worst case" anecdote)

Given the frequency with which sensory-based interventions are used (Heflin & Alaimo 2007; Hess, Morrier, Heflin, & Ivey, 2008; Schreibman, 2005) and a lack of reported adverse effects, there is little risk in using sensory-based antecedent interventions. As documented by Van Rie and Heflin (2009), the critical factor is choosing the appropriate sensory activity to facilitate rather than inhibit learning. The greatest risk manifests in using arousing activities (e.g., bouncing, jumping, running) for children who already are over-aroused or using calming activities (e.g., slow swinging, slow rocking, relaxation) for students who already are under-aroused. In these cases, the levels of arousal would deviate further from those which are needed for optimal arousal. A worst case anecdote is illustrated when Troy, who was over-stimulated in the classroom, was invited to bounce on the exercise ball prior to instruction. Using a Pairwise Data Overlap calculation (Parker & Vannest, in press) the effect size for bouncing was .52, indicating the intervention did not support Troy's learning. In contrast, the effect size was 0.97 for swinging, indicating that the intervention which modulated his level of arousal to optimal was highly effective for enabling Troy to respond correctly on his instructional tasks.

Contact Information for Developers/Practitioners/Clinics

Many practitioners and parents can intuitively determine if a child is over- or under-aroused. If a formal measure is needed, The Sensory Profile (Dunn, 1999), which includes the Short Sensory Profile (McIntosh, Miller, Shyu, & Dunn, 1999) can be used to identify sensory processing challenges. The measure is available from Pearson Assessments

A number of authors have described alerting and calming activities that can be used to affect levels of arousal. Readers are referred to the texts by Heflin and Alaimo (2007), Myles, Cook, Miller, Rinner, and Robbins (2000), and Yack, Aquilla, and Sutton (2002).

Documentation of the effects of an intervention is critical to determining whether or not an appropriate intervention is being used. Resources that describe the process of creating and analyzing graphed data to allow decisions to be made about continued use of an intervention include texts by Heflin and Alaimo (2007), Alberto and Troutman (2009b), and the guide entitled "Evidence-Based Practice: Autism in the Schools" created by the National Autism Center and available free online (www.nationalautism-center.org).

54

SENSORY GYMS, ACADEMICS, AND GROWING MINDS

BY AMANDA FRIEDMAN AND ALISON BERKLEY

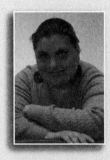

Amanda Friedman, MSEd
Amanda@emergeandsee.net

Alison Berkley, MS
Alison@emergeandsee.net

Emerge and See
www.emergeandsee.net
Twitter: EmergeandSeeEdu
Facebook: Emerge and See Education Center
and Social Groups
(917) 312-6600
(914) 494-9888
361 E 19th Street @ 1st Avenue, New York, NY

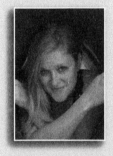

Emerge & See is excited to again be included in *Cutting-Edge Therapies for Autism*. Journeying into their second year of operation at Watch Me Grow (a sensory gym providing OT, PT, speech, and counseling services) E&S has begun preparing to reach beyond their education center, social groups, and workshops by applying to open a school. Amidst running programs, hosting community workshops on Medicaid, Embedded Educational Skills in Play, and events including Mommy Makeovers and Family Photo Shoots, Emerge & See owners, Amanda Friedman and Alison Berkley have submitted the initial application for NYC and Albany to open a non-for-profit private school for children and young adults with Autism and other developmental differences. The Atlas School intends to serve students between 7 and 21 years old and utilize a unique method of individualized components of TEACHH, ABA, and DIR/Floortime as well as a self-created FunQual (Functional Quality of Life) Curriculum to address activities of daily living (ADLs) and social/emotional skill sets. The Atlas School will carry on Emerge & See's philosophy of supporting the whole child with regards to academic growth (following NYS Standards), social awareness, and sensory integration. Emerge & See Education Center and Social Groups will continue to service children ages 3.5–21 in 1:1 tutoring sessions, after-school and holiday social groups, academic assessments and by hosting community workshops. Beginning January 2011 Emerge & See will be available to do trainings for families, schools, and community programs eager to understand Autism and how to support the ASD population. The company name serves to reflect our most highly valued philosophy: that we aim for our students to fully emerge into the world around them, but to also have the world see them for who they are. Hence, the name Emerge & See.

The Emerge & See Mission Statement: To incorporate love of learning, trust of self and the community, and respect into a fun and developmentally sound educational program for students with developmental and emotional differences.

Who Makes Up the Emerge & See Team?

The program is run by directors Amanda Friedman and Alison Berkley. Amanda Friedman is a special education teacher with over ten years experience within the educational field. She has completed the Administrative Certification Program from the College of Saint Rose/CITE and is awaiting approval of her SDL and SBL license. She has worked with students ranging in age from 3–25 years old with an array of differences including autism, mental retardation, emotional disturbances (PTSD, schizophrenia, oppositional defiant disorder, etc.). She has acted as the vice president for the Hudson Valley Autism Society, sat on several Walk for Autism Committees, and is a parent advocate for families at CSE and school meetings. Amanda has been through certified trainings in ABA, TEACCH, BART, and multiple trainings in DIR/Floortime. Alison Berkley is a special education teacher with four years experience in the classroom and worked for four years providing alternate-to-home schooling to students ranging in age and ability, and working as a SEIT (Special Ed Interim Teacher). She has had multiple trainings in DIR/Floortime and ABA and possesses strong ability in implementing assessments, curriculum adaptation and development, and research and data collection. Alison received her master of science in teaching degree (childhood education) at Pace University where she has been awarded a Dean's Scholarship. Alison graduated on the dean's honors list for her BS in psychology from NYU in 2006. In 2002 Alison traveled to Jordan on a medical mission to help provide 117 children with cleft palates/lips to receive reconstructive surgery via the Operation Smile Program. Her passion for progressive education utilizing the newest technologies and informed by the latest research is evident throughout the offerings of the Emerge & See Education Center.

Emerge & See is a proud employer of both part-time assistants and independent contractors who contribute a wealth of creativity, work ethic, and insight to the learning environment. While all Emerge & See staff and contractors are not required to hold degrees within the field of special education, they must have a minimum of two years experience in working with children and/or adults with developmental differences and fulfill a three-month probation period. They are also bound to follow our pledge:

- To inspire students to joyfully emerge into a world of love of learning, relationships, and to truly see their own abilities and potentials.

- To follow NYS Standards to support academic learning in our students.
- To support our students in being successful members of school, home, and community.
- To work collaboratively and respectfully with one another acting, always as role models for our students and families
- To be there for our students and families understanding the sensitivity surrounding their circumstances offering them every opportunity to feel a part of the education community and knowing there is always hope for a greater tomorrow!

What is the Emerge & See Advantage?

The goal of E & S is to foster within students an understanding of and ability to make gains in the following areas:

- Self-confidence
- Communication
- Academic Learning
- Sensory Regulation
- Imagination
- Emotional Growth
- Initiation
- Problem-Solving
- Independence
- Friendship

The layout of space within the sensory gym at Watch Me Grow and the office space naturally lends itself to work on transitions, group activities, and 1:1 interactions. Constant engagement with other students is readily available while highly motivating materials and sensory equipment aid in facilitating back and forth circles of communication both verbally and gesturally. All E&S staff provides respectful engagement with the expectation from EVERY child to communicate. The observation of students' behavior (facial, language, movement, etc.) is discussed regularly and opportunities are intentionally created within play and learning scenarios to expand communication skills. Most significant expectations are to:

- Give students a model of language with which to identify desired objects and places (including spoken words, written words, pictures, manipulatives, and gestures)
- Respect the child and work through anxiety, identifying emotions, and having clear expectations

- Ask questions and give fair time for students to process, think, and respond, remembering always that answers come in many forms (eye contacts, language, vocalizations, omissions, movements, etc.)
- Talk naturally (and not robotically or condescendingly by "baby talking") to a child who may have developmental delays but is chronologically older.
- Listen to students' nuances and expand on them, acknowledging all behavior as communication and aiding them to occur more appropriately.
- Offer help before a challenge becomes pure frustration.
- Become a partner, not just a boss, to the students maintaining a firm but loving demeanor.
- Remember there is no such thing as "nonfunctional behavior" (see chapter 13 on Breaking through Behavior)
- Maintain high and reasonable expectations
- Ensure critical thinking by students in an array of settings
- Support students fully and challenge them constantly to reach for new goals and opportunities

Emerge & See Services

Emerge & See provides an array of student services, each targeting different areas of need and which foster development of the whole child. Our services stand apart from other centers in their range and breadth. Our services include 1:1 tutoring sessions, social groups, holiday camps, summer day camps, sibling dyads, peer play-dates, after-school programs, academic evaluations and assessments, and consultations. Each service is never simply delivered in isolation, but rather integrates the individual student into a comprehensive and targeted program. The educational programs at E&S are aimed at propelling academic, social, and emotional growth as fast and as effectively as possible. E&S continually adapts programs so that they can best help students follow a positive and productive developmental trajectory.

Each student, upon entering our center is individually assessed in several areas of functioning and skill development. These assessments actively inform the creation of a truly individualized program uniquely fitting the needs of that particular student. E&S makes good on the claim that so many others falsely promise: to create fully individualized programs catered to the student and not vice versa. Many other programs remain rigid despite the need to adapt, and force students (and parents) to conform to and abide by their uniform methodology or approach. Childhood education should embrace the full diversity of development by fluidly adapting each service to meet the varying needs of each child. E&S is driven to overturn the current, inadequate status quo in special education by providing a variety of services where each and every session is adapted to the ongoing and ever-changing needs of the student.

There is a dire need for a new vision of education and a new form of engagement with those on the autism spectrum. The services E&S offers have expanded to meet the needs spoken of by so many parents and professionals in the community. A true embodiment of academic instruction balanced with structured movement-based activities and play therapy, E&S continually meets students' greatest capacity for learning without ceiling and nurtures strong developmental foundations. Inevitably, we cemented our own personal and professional belief that *every child can learn.*

1:1 TUTORING SESSIONS

Individual sessions typically run for 1–2 hours and incorporate a wide variety of activities, lessons, and movement-based activities. Prior to beginning individual sessions, each student is assessed developmentally, socially, and academically. These assessments actively inform the formation of that student's program. Combining formal and informal assessments, observations, and parent interviews this input provides insight and understanding of that particular student's areas of strengths and those of weakness, as well as their passions and aversions. From this informed starting point, the E&S team is able to leverage student interests to maintain motivation and engagement across contexts and emotions.

Goals are never blanketed across age groups or students. Every student that enters our office is welcomed and encouraged to express their individual personalities and to flourish in a structured learning environment. Many clients seek additional academic instruction at E&S to supplement school programs and to accelerate development across content areas. Other clients obtain our services in order to support their child emotionally. Amanda Friedman specializes in working with older children and young adults: she creates a supportive, loving and trusting relationship within which students can express any and all of their ideas and emotions while also teaching them how to be appropriate and effective in their social lives.

WEEKDAY AND AFTER-SCHOOL PROGRAMS

Weekday social groups and after-school programs are more academically focused relative to other social groups we hold, although peer interaction and effective communication are still strongly emphasized. The groups are structured in such a way that a balance is struck between social skills building among the whole group and 1:1 work to address individual academic goals. Each session entails work in content areas such as math or literacy, group games such as parachute play or basketball, and targeted movement activities such as obstacle courses or yoga. These activities and games are specially designed to elicit meaningful two-way interactions and to embed academic learning throughout each activity.

WEEKEND AND HOLIDAY GROUPS

Weekend and holiday groups run much longer, for 4–5 hours, which allows for a schedule that varies from movement-based activities to project-based learning. Again, each group strikes a balance by embedding academic learning into virtually every portion of the day, yet offering students a fun and playful reprieve from the high demands of their school programs. The extended time frame also allows for community outings and events. In the past, E&S groups have ventured out to restaurants, parks, and museums in the community. Last spring, E&S took nine of its students to see the Gazillion Bubble Show. The outing was tremendously successful and all students enjoyed the full seventy-minute show so much so, in fact, that many of the kids asked for "bubbles" again! This is but one example of E&S's dedication to community integration. We aim to help all of our students gain confidence and comfort within community situations, and outings to places like live theater help us support our students in doing just that. Yet, E&S prides itself on another kind of community integration: being an active and contributing member to the special needs and larger New York City community. Weekend and holiday groups pose numerous opportunities to expose our students to new places, people, and events. For E&S students to become productive citizens of the world, we must equip them with the knowledge and skills needed to navigate any social or physical landscape. Community integration, in this sense, promotes greater awareness, empathy and understanding of children with autism. The community (and companies like E&S) must work diligently in order to not simply accommodate special needs children, but to warmly welcome them as a member while embracing their unique differences.

ADDITIONAL SERVICES:

- Peer Playdates
- Sibling Dyads
- Assessments and Evaluations
- Consultations
- Workshops and Professional Development
- Events (Mommy Makeover, Family Photo Shoot, Medicaid Waiver Informational Evening, etc)

The Science of Emerge & See

Movement's positive impact on student learning is blatantly apparent. Codirector Alison Berkley has been fascinated with movement-based activities within the learning environment. For example, she has been an avid learner of yoga techniques and has become a huge proponent of its positive effects, particularly for those with Autism. Every Saturday, all of the students participate in 20–30 minute yoga sessions led by Mrs. Berkley. For this time, students are sharing attention, communicating with one another, and moving their bodies in new and challenging ways, all while calming their bodies and minds. These yoga sessions prompted Mrs. Berkley to pursue scientific research on movement's relationship to learning.

Mrs. Berkley created and carried out an extensive study on the ways in which academic performance scores were impacted by movement. The sample population was a neuro-typical class of first graders and the research was conducted in a New York City public school. The students were given access to 25 minutes of movement-based activity on certain days and then given a math assessment immediately following the period of movement in order to gauge student performance. These assessment scores were compared to baseline scores created from randomly selected student work samples. In this way, one could clearly see any and all increases or decreases in performance scores. Data collection spanned 25 days (duration was an unavoidable limitation of the experiment), the results of which were both conclusive and persuasive. All students, no matter their baseline academic performance level (high-, middle-, or low-performing) improved their scores significantly. (See graph on the next page)

When analyzing the graph, it is evident that movement-based activity directly preceding academic content produced impressive positive effects, especially in the low-performing students. These students improved drastically with performance scores jumping the equivalent of a full letter grade. Movement *never* detracted from academic performance and *always* improved it. All students benefitted significantly while struggling and at-risk students benefitted most.

The implications for this study are far-reaching. It would behoove schools and school districts to increase movement-based activity throughout each and every school day. Here at Emerge & See, we already incorporate movement into nearly everything we do, and this study can be adapted, replicated, and administered to our own students. A similar study (data collection is being piloted currently) using special needs students as the sample population will help us scientifically monitor and analyze specific ways in which movement facilitates, maximizes, and cements learning.

This research speaks to the ways in which Emerge & See grounds all that it does in science. Data and research inform the directors' knowledge, educational curricula,

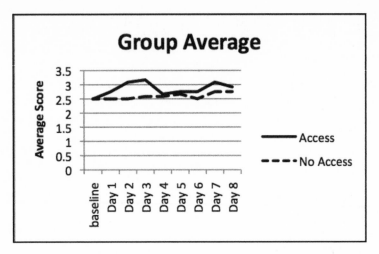

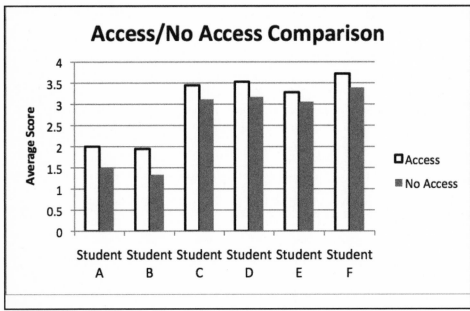

and interventions. All too often schools and programs fail to systematically track student progress. Solely using qualitative and informal documentation of student profiles places massive constraints on one's ability to adapt interventions appropriately and effectively. Data should be collected on new interventions and critically analyzed to inform the program. In this way there is a continuous feedback loop between student functioning, data collection, analysis, and the intervention.

For complete data sets and research, please contact Alison Berkley.

55

THE SENSORY LEARNING PROGRAM

BY MARY BOLLES

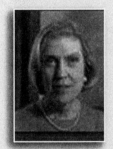

Mary Bolles

Sensory Learning Institute
P.O. Box 11047
Boulder, CO 80301
(888)720-5437
www.sensorylearning.com

Mary holds a liberal arts degree from Bowling Green State University in Ohio. When Mary looked at available therapies to help her son who was not speaking at three and was exhibiting behaviors consistent with children on the autism spectrum, she believed therapy could help him interact with his environment more successfully if it were multi-sensory. With the notion of combining aspects of vision therapy, auditory training, and occupational therapy, the Sensory Learning System uses visible light, modulated music, and vestibular stimulation. This program has a twenty year history of clinical success with children on the spectrum. She has trained many allied health professionals and doctors to be providers of the program nationwide and internationally.

I remember many years ago when I had a five year old daughter who never stopped talking and a three and a half year old son who wasn't talking at all. He had never said "mom" or "ball" or anything. We had just put the two children in their car seats for an hour long trip back home from shopping for school clothes. It was past their bedtime and the situation with my overtired son felt like a major meltdown brewing. His father was driving so I picked the screaming child up and held him, his left ear against my body. Jason had never wanted to be held, so it was quite a treat for me that he fell asleep in my arms. All the way home he slept quietly. All the way home his sister talked. She was trying to learn the rhyme that goes, "How much wood would a woodchuck chuck if a woodchuck could chuck wood?" She's getting it all tangled up and I'm feeding it back to her correctly over and over. When the car stopped in front of our house the most amazing thing happened, Jason woke up and clearly said the whole rhyme. I wondered over and over, "What was it that allowed him to speak for the first time?" As Jason grew older, I began connecting the experiences that were unique to him: laying chest-down in the warm soil after a hard day at kindergarten. Always being too loud, too fast, too strong except when he was sick and then it was magical as the intensity of his every sense and motor activity seemed to match the rest of family for a short while. It was these sensory experiences that led me to develop an intensive multi-sensory therapy as a way to help him.

Jason taught me that sensory messages can be a bridge or a barrier. The main goal of the Sensory Learning Program is to strengthen a natural sensory connection to the physical world. The three main sensory systems that help living organisms relate to the physical world are the visual, auditory and the vestibular or balance system. This intervention uses vibration in the form of visible light. This narrow band of frequencies in the electromagnetic (EM) spectrum is able to be detected by the human eye. The vibration of sound is detected by the cochlea in the middle ear. The position of the head in relationship to the geomagnetic force of gravity is detected by the vestibular system in the inner ear. When these three sensory messages are integrated and organized by the brain, successful interaction with the physical environment is achieved automatically.

A more specific focus of the Sensory Learning Program is to strengthen connections between the three major sensory systems to better handle sensory demands of the environment. Firing neurons with simultaneous stimulation can allow them to wire together more easily. Abnormal neural connectivity and under-connectivity are known to disrupt the way children on the spectrum process information. White matter long-range connections between neurons are needed for areas of the brain to interrelate in a healthy way. Complex behavior, such as language and social interaction, depend upon long-range connections between distant brain regions. Post-natal development is dependent on sensory experience to bring forth brain functions in the maturation process. Early emerging sensory skills are body awareness and attention to sensory input. Sensory systems do not work independently and complex perception depends on efficient integration. The vestibular system is closely tied to tactile messages coming from the skin and proprioceptive messages coming from the muscles, tendons and joints. The vestibular system is the frame of reference for all the visual messages and most of the auditory. Well organized connections between the vestibular and the visual system allow gross and fine motor skills. Connections between the vestibular and auditory are how the child can sequence sounds for receptive language and initiation and execution of speech. Connections between the auditory and visual are abstract and involve the left hemisphere thinking in words and the right hemisphere thinking in pictures.

A third intention of the Sensory Learning Program is to facilitate the orienting response to the external environment. A general spatial temporal orientation, knowing where your body is in space and time, is the result of integrating visual, auditory and vestibular input. This then allows the performance skills of reading and math and oral and written language to later emerge. Adapting to challenges imposed by the environment and making transitions to the sensory demands of different environments often cause much anxiety and overwhelm children on the spectrum. Sensory pathways related to the ability to accept comfort, think positively, have hope and form affective relationships with others are often limited. Severely affected autistic children alternate from one sensory input to another, from one modality to another, without integration of the experience as a whole. Theirs is a world of fragmented sensory inputs, unrelated to each other, without meaning. The brain is not talking to itself, integrating new stimuli with existing information and thus developing new perspectives, new ideas and the ability to see a "bigger picture."

A fourth therapeutic assist of the Sensory learning Program is to stimulate brain development through environmental signaling which is critical for the maturation process. After the neurons migrate to where they will live in the brain, environmental signaling plays a major role in how these neurons hook up through white matter. The brain is designed to filter and organize bits of sensory information into an integrated experience. The brainstem area develops first, then emotional centers, and then cognitive centers. As children proceed through the sensory integrative process in a normal and healthy way, they become able to respond to sensations with adaptive responses that are increasingly more mature and complex. Improved regulation of core physiological states have a broad positive impact on resolution of emotional dysregulation, dissociative symptoms, and social interaction. The Sensory Learning Program can provide for integration and processing of disruptive emotions and sensations as well as cognitive inhibition of these arousal states. The program is a "bottom up" approach to challenge development associated with gaining control over behavior that is organized at a lower level. Higher cortical brain areas can function effectively only if they are able to interrelate in a healthy way with lower brain levels. Upper cortical connections from the prefrontal areas provide the capacity for emotional regulation, gaining autonomy from sensory reactivity and the acquisition of cortical control over behavior.

During the Sensory Learning sessions, the participant lies on a trochoidal motion table that slowly rises and descends in a circular pattern, providing vestibular stimulation. At the same time, the participant's eyes follow a stationary light instrument that provides frequencies of colored light. Modulated music is introduced through headphones that are worn during the session. Children do two ½ hour sessions a day for twelve consecutive days and then have a light instrument at home for the balance of the month. The rhythm of the table entrains the cerebral spinal fluid flowing through the ventricles to the rate of flow when the body is in a 'resting' state. Use of colored light from developmental and behavioral optometry serves three purposes: (a) introduction of various frequencies of light along the energetic portion of the optic nerve pathway to add flexibility to the firing pattern of the hypothalamus; and (b) exercise of the extrinsic eye muscles to strengthen the parvo pathway for sustained vision in higher cortical activities and(c) to allow more light to travel along the optic nerve resolving constricted visual fields. The auditory stimulation with processed music introduces varying volume and random filtering of frequencies. The unique quality of the music challenges the participant's cognitive processes, allowing sensory integrative processes to progress unconsciously.

When a child adapts to the unique multi sensory environment of the Sensory Learning sessions, we see them adapting to typical environments more successfully. Improved sensory integration can allow a wide spectrum of benefits resolving or partially resolving toilet-training problems, disintegrated primitive reflexes, low muscle tone, motor planning problems, tactile defensiveness, self-stimming behaviors, restrictive and repetitive behaviors, language deficits, cognitive impairment, and unusual fears and anxiety.

I believe no mother, no father, no sibling, no child should have to go through the sensory struggles of autism. The Sensory Learning Program is a functional approach, allowing children to learn sensory skills, a necessary bridge to interact successfully with the environment. This multi-sensory approach matches the challenges of the real world. The program can strengthen a natural sensory connection to the physical world, strengthen neural connections between the three main sensory systems, help achieve spatial temporal orientation, and stimulate developmental milestones.

56

SOUND-BASED THERAPIES— DAVIS MODEL OF SOUND INTERVENTION

BY DORINNE DAVIS

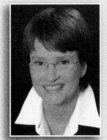

Dorinne S. Davis, MA, CCC-A, FAAA, RCTC, BARA

The Davis Center 19 State Route 10 East, Suite 25
Succasunna, NJ 07876.
(862) 251-4637
info@thedaviscenter.com
www.thedaviscenter.com
www.dorinnedavis.com

Ms. Davis is President/Founder of The Davis Center, the world's premier sound therapy center in Succasunna, NJ. She is the author of four books, including the primer on sound-based therapy, *Sound Bodies through Sound Therapy* and *Every Day A Miracle: Success Stories through Sound Therapy*. She established The Davis Addendum to the Tomatis Effect and designed The Tree of Sound Enhancement Therapy and The Diagnostic Evaluation for Therapy Protocol. She has a radio show on AutismOne.org radio once a month. She is recognized as THE expert on sound-based therapies.

Sound-based therapies use the vibrational energy of sound to make change with learning, development, and wellness challenges with special equipment, specific programs, modified music, and/or specific tones/beats, the need for which is identified with testing. Many sound-based therapies have been demonstrated as helpful to autistic individuals.

While there are many different sound-based therapies which have made change, identifying which methods can be most appropriately used is the foundation of *The Davis Model of Sound Intervention*. This model utilizes the analogy of a tree, *The Tree of Sound Enhancement Therapy,* for discussing how the many therapies make change for each person. *Root System* Therapies address one's sense of hearing. *Seed* Therapies address one's body rhythms. *Trunk* Therapies address the ability to process all basic sound stimulation. *Leaves and Branches* Therapies address auditory processing issues.

The *Head* surrounding the Tree portion addresses general wellness. All of the therapies use the vibrational energy of sound to make change for the specified processes.

The pieces of the Tree come together by understanding three key points: 1) There is a connection between the voice, the ear, and the brain supported by five laws known as The Tomatis Effect and The Davis Addendum to The Tomatis Effect; 2) Every cell in your body resonates sound; and 3) Your ear helps stimulate all of your senses by sound vibration, not just hearing.

The *Diagnostic Evaluation for Therapy Protocol (DETP)* evaluates each person's responses for the various levels of the Tree analogy and determines if, when, how long, and in what order any or all of the many different sound-based therapies should be appropriately applied. This battery of tests is key for determining how to best use any sound-based therapy. Assuming that each person starts with *The Root System* therapy is incorrect. Not everyone needs every therapy. The test battery takes the guesswork out of determining if a sound-based therapy is appropriate and provides the order for the correct administration of a sequence of therapies. Currently the assessment can only be obtained at www.thedaviscenter.com.

By using *The Tree of Sound Enhancement Therapy*, some of the various therapies are as follows:

1. The *Root System* therapies are called "Auditory Integration Training," The origi-nator of this type of therapy is Dr. Guy Berard, a French physician, who wanted to establish a program that would create a kind of physical therapy for the ear, which has been demonstrated with this author's research on the acoustic reflex muscle of the middle ear. His method is now known as Berard Auditory Integra-tion Training. The equipment used in his method is either an Audiokinetron or an Earducator. His method can only be applied in a practitioner's office. There are other applications within the generalized term "Auditory Integration Training" that can be used at home. The equipment applicable for home programs are FST, DAA, and BGC and all do a similar yet different type of physical retraining of the acoustic reflex muscle. Each of these programs is modeled after Dr. Berard's work. All "Auditory Integration Training" programs address the person's "sense of hearing." The programs last for ten days and the person listens for ½ hour in the morning and afternoon to specially chosen music played through the appropriate device. While listening, little or no sensory stimulation should occur because it is possible to negate the positive effects of retraining the acoustic reflex muscle.

    Symptoms helped: one type of hearing hypersensitivity, lack of sound aware-ness, inability to discriminate sound differences, sense of self, body move-ment/rhythm, eye contact, awareness of the world around them, motor skills and more.

Testimonials from parents of autistic children:

    a.   My child no longer covers his ears in uncomfortable listening situations.

    b.   My child no longer reacts to fluorescent lighting.

    c.   My child responds immediately when his name is called.

www.berardaitwebsite.com and www.AITinstitute.org

2.   The *Seed* therapies all make a change with body rhythmical patterns. Our body has many rhythms and patterns such as our heart rate and breath stream. Currently two therapies exist at this level: REI and Cymatherapy.

    a.   REI was developed by Jeff Strong and uses rhythmical drum patterns to stimulate and repair the nervous system. A pair of custom made CDs are created and used for a ten-week period.

        Symptoms helped: inability to "fit in" with the rhythms of those around them, significant sensory processing issues, self-stimulatory behaviors, attention span, sleep, aggression, and more.

        Testimonials from parents of autistic children:

        1. My child fell asleep faster and more calmly.

        2. My child became less aggressive.

        3. My child became less impulsive.

www.reiinstitute.com

    b.   Cymatherapy represents the work of Dr. Guy Peter Manners, who explored sound as a healing modality. This approach uses sound frequency stimulation on different parts of the body working to balance the body's energy patterns. The current device is called the Cyma1000.

        Symptoms helped: issues with attention, behavior, social connections, cognition, and much more.

        Testimonials from parents of autistic children:

        1. My child waited and listened for instructions.

        2. My child waited his turn better.

        3. My child wanted to be around his family more.

www.cymatechnologies.com

3.   The *Trunk* therapies are called "Listening Training Programs" and are modeled after the work of Dr. Alfred Tomatis, the founder of all sound-based therapies. The therapies at this level are "core" therapies because they incorporate one of the main points behind The Davis Model of Sound Intervention—the connection between the voice, the ear and the brain. Dr. Tomatis was the first to discover that the voice produces what the ear hears and when the distorted frequencies

are reintroduced to the ear, the voice regains coherence or stability. This became known as The Tomatis Effect and he incorporated this process into The Tomatis Method. He differentiated between hearing and listening. Hearing is the passive reception of sound and we hear without thinking about it. But listening involves mentally thinking about what is heard. We must tune into what is heard. By doing so, we cortically "recharge" the brain. When recharging the brain, the body's full response to sound must be stimulated. Every cell of the body must be stimulated. Every sense will be stimulated. Every way that the body responds to sound must be stimulated. Listening Training Programs must include air conduction vibration of sound, bone conduction vibration of sound, filtered and gated music, specific sound delays, and actively incorporating one's speaking and/or singing voice in the programming.

The programs are brain intensive, meaning that the program lasts for many days in order to make sufficient change at the cortical level. Practitioners should incorporate activities that address the person's whole body response to sound, not just one type of skill such as academics or sensory integration as the full ability to balance the person's skills will not be met. Basic programs last for sixty hours, often applied with a break after thirty hours. Listening occurs for two hours per day for fifteen days, then a three- to six-week break, followed by another fifteen days of two hours per day. Some centers administer the second set in eight and seven days with another break in between. For people with autism, this basic program is typically not enough stimulation to establish sufficient skills for communication, so additional sessions are encouraged depending upon each person's needs. Follow up sessions should be determined by a proprietary Listening Test which shows the levels of progress. Each person's voice should begin to show a change in its tonal quality as progress occurs.

a.   The Tomatis Method was established by Dr. Alfred Tomatis. He felt that a good listener was a good learner and by training a person to listen well provided them to opportunity to reach their full potential. He identified the benefit of a dominant right ear, supporting the most direct pathway to the language center in the brain. His method supports learning how to filter out irrelevant information and supports capturing the energizing frequencies of the speech sound spectrum. He uses all of the connections between the voice, the ear and the brain by stimulating the weaker body processes in order to advance overall skill levels resulting in improved listening and enhancement of body sensory needs and communication needs. When using this method at *The Trunk* level make sure it is a full individualized program and not a generic newer program.

Symptoms helped: some hypersensitivities to sound, hyposensitivity to sound, sensory processing issues, oral motor issues, social/emotional connectedness, expressive/receptive language skills, sense of self, inappropriate behaviors, fluency of speech, vestibular imbalances, movement and rhythm, fine/gross motor skills, posture, and more.

Testimonials from parents of autistic children:

1. Within two years following The Tomatis Method, my child was declassified.
2. My child began eating different foods and trying different textures of food.
3. My child's high pitched voice disappeared.
4. My child's reading skills jumped three years growth in six months time.
5. My child began using full sentences to express his thoughts.
6. My child's anxiety to large groups practically disappeared.

www.tomatis.com and www.tomatis-group.com

b. EnListen was developed by Drs. Billie and Kirk Thompson and modeled from the concepts established by Dr. Tomatis. Their proprietary software program provides stimulation with air conduction, bone conduction, sound delays and filters, and active voice work for developing targeted learning skills. This process stimulates growth of new and underutilized neural pathways.

Symptoms helped: weak receptive/expressive language skills, weak motor skills, poor communication skills, sense of self, poor social skills, disorganization, poor reading skills, singing abilities, phonics skills, and more.

Testimonials from parents of autistic children:

1. My child began trying to connect socially with other children around him.
2. My child began combining three or four words in utterances.
3. My child no longer craved spinning.
4. My child began tasting new and different foods.
5. I was able to leave my child playing independently for up to ½ hour at a time.
6. My child's stammer disappeared.

www.enlisten.com

3. Some sound-based therapies are modeled after the work of Dr. Tomatis but do not include ALL of the requirements for a Listening Training Program at The

Trunk level of *The Tree*. However, they can be inserted at the Upper Trunk/Lower Leaves and Branches of The Tree analogy because they offer more higher functioning changes. Some of these programs are:

a. The Listening Program was developed by Advanced Brain Technologies as a music-based sound stimulation program designed to enhance listening skills and remediate auditory perceptual skills. The basic program included eight CDs that incorporated music and nature sounds to create a balance of exercises for the middle ear muscles. A filtration system and a gating technique is also utilized supporting a full spectrum of sound frequencies. These CDs are listened to for a half hour per day, five days per week for eight weeks typically. Extended sessions are sometimes needed and the program has different levels now. A bone conduction segment has been added with practitioner supervision. The concept is for the brain to receive, process, store and retrieve the information from a person's surrounding sound environment.

> Symptoms helped: learning challenges, attention/focus weaknesses, reading challenges, sense of self, communication weaknesses, sensory processing issues, self-regulation, and more.
>
> Testimonials from parents of autistic children:
>
> 1. My child began to have an interest in socially interacting with his peers.
> 2. My child began drawing clearly and writing legibly.
> 3. My child began to verbally label his drawings.

www.advancedbrain.com

b. The Samonas Method was developed by Ingo Steinbach. Samonas stands for "spectrally activated music of optimum natural structure." By using his Sonas System, he was able to create a system for recording music where the therapeutic value of the music and the effectiveness of the musical recording could be maintained. This new system could only be produced on compact discs. He created CDs that emphasized high frequency listening, presented the sensation of being in the location of the music, created a calming effect on the body, while monitoring the overtone effects of most musical selections. The concept is to experience the energizing effects of sound through the expression of the overtones within the music. The Samonas CD's are generic in nature and no specific "therapy" regimen is currently established for any one type of challenge.

> Symptoms helped: vitality, stress, limited concentration, vestibular imbalances, lack of creativity, and more.
>
> Testimonials from parents of autistic children:
>
> 1. My child immediately began to notice everything going on around him.

2. My child could focus on an activity for a longer period of time.

3. My child decreased his need to spin constantly.

www.samonas.com

4. The *Leaves and Branches* of *The Tree of Sound Enhancement Therapy* reflects auditory processing skills like memory, discrimination and sequencing skills. These skills are higher functioning skills than basic sound awareness and utilization. These are skills inherent for our understanding of the communication process, including reading. However, these skills need the support of the more foundational skills established in *The Root System, The Seed,* and *The Trunk* of *The Tree* analogy in order for the reception, expression and interpretation of these skills to be well embedded for each person. Without the foundational skills well established, these skills simply become "splinter skills" and testing can show that these skills have improved; but skill testing doesn't show how the body is fully integrating the skills. The Davis Model of Sound Intervention encourages the full integration of all skills to maximize learning and developmental changes. A few of these therapies are:

a. Fast ForWord is a series of programs that use an interactive computer training system to retrain language, reading and learning skills. The initial program targeted receptive language skills and retrained the skill of temporal sequencing—a skill necessary for auditory discrimination, auditory figure ground, and auditory sequential memory. By retraining how the brain comprehends and uses speech information, the person is better able to distinguish the many different components of speech sounds. The basic program still retrains temporal sequencing although the Fast ForWord series of programs now heavily emphasizes skills for reading. The basic program averages between six to eight weeks for approximately 1½ to 2 hours per day.

Symptoms helped: two listening comprehension, phonological awareness, specific language structures, oral language skills, and more.

Testimonials from parents of autistic children:

1. My child wants to listen on the telephone now to his grand parents.

2. My child is able to go shopping with me at the mall now without covering his ears.

3. My child is understanding more of what is being said to him.

www.scilearn.com

b. Interactive Metronome was developed by James Cassily who thought that learning, cognition and social skills were influenced by the ability to plan and sequence motoric actions. These actions are processed through the sensation of vibration through the ear and are therefore at this level of *The Tree* analogy. Mr. Cassily's theory was that man's intelligence is connected with the ability to process rapid movements and developed a computer-based interactive version of the musical metronome. The purpose of the program is to develop precise control over basic mental functions through the use of body movements. The average program is composed of fifteen one-hour sessions over a period of three to five weeks.

Symptoms helped: attention, motor control, reading, language processing, regulation of behavior, and more.

Testimonials from parents of autistic children:

1. My child began to talk more and became more engaged with those she was communicating with.
2. My child's sleeping patterns improved.
3. My child became less tactilely defensive.

www.interactivemetronome.com

5. The *Head* surrounding *The Tree of Sound Enhancement Therapy* brings the connection between the voice, the ear and the brain full circle and demonstrates the laws within *The Davis Addendum to the Tomatis Effect* as making an important contribution to the full effect of how sound-based therapies make change in learning, development and wellness. Whereas The Tomatis Effect suggests that the voice produces what the ear hears, The Davis Addendum to the Tomatis Effect suggests that the ear also emits (yes, the ear gives out a sound) the same stressed frequencies as the voice and once the imbalanced frequencies are returned to the ear, the voice regains stability or coherence. *The Head* then represents the wellness piece of how sound impacts the entire body. Currently, the science of BioAcoustics is used to help identify how well the body is able to support the changes possible with the other portions of *The Tree* analogy.

Human BioAcoustics was developed Sharry Edwards and after many years of research, the idea of vocal profiling has supported the idea that the body is a mathematical matrix of predictable frequency relationships. Every cell is the body vibrates and emits its own sound frequency. These cellular frequencies must stay "in tune" in order for the body to maintain its wellness. For the autistic person, this piece is often the key for determining if the other many different sound-based therapies will make a change and more importantly maintain any changes.

Symptoms helped: anything related to the body and wellness

Testimonials from parents of autistic children:

1. My child's sound sensitivities decreased dramatically.
2. My child can maintain his focus so much better.
3. My doctor likes supporting my child's detoxing with BioAcoustics.

www.soundhealthinc.com

Overview

The Davis Model of Sound Intervention incorporates all of the many different sound-based therapies only after appropriately using The Diagnostic Evaluation for Therapy Protocol to determine if the therapies are needed, and if so, in the correct order. There are many stories of people using one or another of the therapies with limited or no success, or losing the effects after a period of time. Some people do need more than one therapy and some may need "tuneups" periodically if their body doesn't maintain the support well enough.

Any sound-based therapy can produce change but for some, the change may take place over an extended period of time as the body integrates the changes so that higher ordered skills can develop. To date, most research on these methods have measured skill changes but the responses of sound go further into the body at the cellular and brain level, and researchers are beginning to recognize this fact.

Can there be side effects to this approach? Sound-based therapies can produce skill changes, but the main change goes more deeply to core body needs. Picture the peeling of an onion—each layer represents a layer of development. For some children, many layers need to be removed to get to the heart of their issues and these main issues need to be repatterned so that movement forward can occur. Some people consider this as regression but in reality this repatterning is movement forward—a positive change. It is important not to get "stuck" at this lower functioning level, though, so for many, movement up *The Tree* is necessary to help the person move toward higher progressive levels.

The Davis Model of Sound Intervention offers an alternative approach for addressing the learning, developmental, and wellness challenges associated with autism from a holistic paradigm.

SPEECH-LANGUAGE THERAPY

BY LAVINIA PEREIRA AND MICHELLE SOLOMON

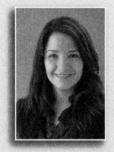

Lavinia Pereira, MA, CCC-SLP

lavinia@firstsoundseries.com

Lavinia Pereira, MA, CCC-SLP is a speech-language pathologist in private practice on Manhattan's Upper East Side. She specializes in the evaluation and treatment of children diagnosed with moderate to severe developmental disorders, including autism spectrum disorders and childhood apraxia of speech.

Lavinia's experience in the field of speech language pathology is multifaceted; she has supervised graduate students at New York University and has guest lectured on the topics of therapeutic planning and treatment techniques at both New York University and Columbia University. She is trained in ABA, Floortime, Oral Motor Therapy, and is a PROMPT trained clinician.

Lavinia earned her Master's degree in Speech-Language Pathology from New York University and holds the Certificate of Clinical Competence from ASHA. She is a licensed speech-language pathologist in New York State.

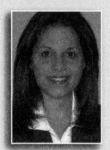

Michelle Solomon, MA, CCC-SLP, PC

michelle@firstsoundseries.com

Michelle Solomon, MA, CCC-SLP, PC graduated from New York University with a Master's degree in Speech-Language Pathology. She holds the Certificate of Clinical Competence from ASHA, has New York licensure in Speech-Language Pathology and earned her degree as a Teacher of the Speech and Hearing Handicapped.

Michelle is currently in private practice in New York City. She specializes in the assessment and treatment of children diagnosed with autism spectrum disorders, childhood apraxia of speech, dysarthria, and other motor speech disorders. In addition, she works with children diagnosed with central auditory processing disorder and language delays/disorders.

Michelle is trained in a variety of techniques including ABA, Floortime, Oral Motor Therapy, Beckman Oral Motor, and is a PROMPT Certified Clinician and PROMPT Instructor.

Together, Lavinia and Michelle develop and present workshops in speech and language development as part of their commitment to educating parents. In addition, they founded *First Sound Series,* a series of interactive, repetitive books developed for children with speech and language delays and motor planning disorders.
www.firstsoundseries.com

It can be an overwhelming process to find a Speech-Language Pathologist (SLP) and once you have, what can you expect during the assessment process? How will he or she teach your child to communicate? Will he or she be trained in the most "cutting-edge" techniques and have enough knowledge about the dynamic disorder of autism? Will the communication skills your child learns in session generalize to your home, school and community? What role will the therapist play outside of the therapy sessions and will this therapy be helpful in teaching your child to communicate effectively?

What is a Speech-Language Pathologist?

A Certified Speech-Language pathologist may also be referred to as an *SLP* or *speech therapist*. This title infers that the individual has completed a master's, doctoral, or other recognized post-baccalaureate degree. In addition, the individual has passed a national examination and successfully completed a supervised, clinical fellowship post graduation. The SLP will then be recognized by ASHA (American Speech-Language-Hearing Association) and earn their Certificate of Clinical Competence (CCC).

An SLP is a "professional who engages in clinical services, prevention, advocacy, education, administration, and research in the areas of communication and swallowing across the life span from infancy through geriatrics" (www.asha.org). SLP's work in a variety of settings including public and private schools, in a client's home, hospitals, rehabilitation clinics, universities, and nursing homes. SLP's work on remediation of feeding and swallowing (Dysphasia) disorders as well as a variety of communication disorders.

SLP's can provide remediation for the following communication disorders:

- **Language disorder:** impairment of receptive (comprehension), expressive (use of spoken), written, and/or other symbol systems;
- **Speech disorder:** impairment of the articulation of speech sounds, fluency or voice;
- **Pragmatic disorder:** impairment of the ability to use and understand social language (verbal and nonverbal);
- **Hearing disorder:** impairment of the auditory system;
- **Central auditory processing disorder:** impairment of the ability to process, retrieve, and/or organize information through the peripheral and central nervous systems;
- **Prosody disorder:** impairment of the suprasegmentals of speech (intonation, stress).

Where Can You Find an SLP?

Children ages zero to three and school-age children may be eligible for speech and language services through the state in which they reside. Government agencies within your state will be able to provide contact information to begin the assessment process, which will determine eligibility for services. School age children may be evaluated to determine the need for speech-language therapy within the school setting. In addition, licensed therapists in your area can be located by visiting the ASHA website (www.asha.org), asking your child's doctor, or by contacting local support groups and agencies.

What Can You Expect From the Assessment Process?

An SLP may be performing the assessment individually or as part of a comprehensive assessment. The following information may be asked of you at the time of your child's assessment (Hegde, 1999):

Case History:

- Prenatal and birth history (complications, C- section)
- Medical (surgeries, illnesses, ear infections)
- Family makeup (siblings, ages)
- Home environment (parent's occupations, single parent household)
- Developmental Milestones (crawling, walking, first words)
- Allergies/ Medications (food, environmental/name, dose)
- Diet Restrictions (gluten free, casein free, picky eater)
- Languages spoken in the home (primary language, additional languages)
- Schooling (name, days/hours per week, contact information)
- Previous and current therapies received (types, length of time, contact information)
- Current ability to communicate (expressive, gestures, signing)
- Receptive language skills (follow directions, understand labels and actions)
- Play Skills (interests, peer interaction, participation in games)
- Behaviors (stereotypical, aggressive, injurious)
- Family history of communication disorders or other relevant disorders/delays
- Copies of additional reports (neurological, psychological)

Informal Observation:

The clinician will spend time with your child and assess a variety of areas through play, observation, and interactions that elicit the skills in question. The following is a condensed list of several of the areas assessed in an informal observation:

- Expressive and receptive language (gestures, pointing, following directions, comprehension of a variety of concepts, length of utterance, vocabulary, use of questions words, echolalia)
- Play skills (child-directed, symbolic play, narrative play, expanding on ideas)

- Pragmatic language (eye contact, joint attention, turn taking, body in space awareness, reading of facial cues, topic maintenance, conversational exchanges)
- Intelligibility of speech sounds in isolation, words, phrases
- Orofacial assessment (range of motion of articulators—jaw, lips, tongue, dentition)
- Muscle tone (body and face, control of oral secretions, posture, grip)
- Sensitivity to touch (hyper- or hyposensitive)
- Rate and volume of speech appropriate for age
- Feeding skills (manipulation of a variety of textures, tastes, temperatures)
- Behavior (compliance, attention, willingness to try new materials)
- Stereotypical body movements
- Pre-academic/ academic skills (literacy)

Formal Assessment:

The clinician may want to administer standardized tests to further assess speech and language development. Standardized tests yield several different scores (standard score, percentile rank, age equivalency, etc.) and may compare your child's development to that of a typically developing child of the same age. There are a variety of standardized tests that may be appropriate for your child. The SLP will choose tests based on your child's age, development, language abilities and capability of sitting through formal testing procedures.

Once your SLP has completed the assessment he or she will likely write a detailed report of the findings which will be carefully reviewed. Based on the findings, an SLP may recommend further assessments be conducted by other disciplines (Occupational Therapist, Neurologist, Audiologist, Developmental Pediatrician, etc.), may provide an additional diagnosis (Childhood Apraxia of Speech, Dysarthria), or include short and long term goals that are appropriate for your child. It is important that the assessment results and goals are shared with other therapists and teachers working with your child to ensure collaboration and carry-over. The assessment itself can be very overwhelming however, with this information comes the knowledge and power to seek the most appropriate treatment.

What are Some of the "Cutting Edge" Treatments Being Used Today?

There are several techniques that are in current use with individuals diagnosed on the Autism Spectrum. Each technique is unique and may or may not be right for your child. The experienced SLP will not only be trained in a variety of techniques, but will know which techniques will be most beneficial and at what point in your child's development each will yield the best results. Below is a list of several highly recognized techniques and a brief description. Additional information can be obtained by visiting their respective websites.

- **PROMPT**: "Prompts for Restructuring Oral Muscular Phonetic Targets," was developed in the 1970s by Deborah Hayden. It has continued to evolve and today is taught and used worldwide by licensed SLP's. PROMPT incorporates the use of organized and systematic tactile (touch) input to the oral musculature to facilitate and/or improve speech production. Seven stages or subsystems (tone, phonatory control, mandibular (jaw) control, labial-facial (lip) control, lingual (tongue) control, sequenced movements (co-articulation), prosody (suprasegmentals) are assessed to determine the child's weaknesses and strengths within a stage and develop core vocabulary that is functional across settings. PROMPT is a dynamic and holistic approach that emphasizes the importance of assessing and targeting the development of the whole client (cognitive-linguistic, social-emotional, physical-sensory) through the use of functional activities and meaningful interactions for communication. Minimally, a licensed SLP must participate in two three-day courses (Introduction to PROMPT and Bridging PROMPT Technique to Intervention), a PROMPT Technique Practicum and complete a four-month self-study in order to become PROMPT Certified. Visit www.promptinstitute.com to learn more about PROMPT, read research articles, or find an experienced PROMPT therapist in your area.

- **Oral Motor (TalkTools Therapy)**: Sara Rosenfeld-Johnson, the founder of Innovative Therapists Int'l, Inc. and TalkTools Therapy tm, is known worldwide for providing educational courses and developing tools designed to assist in implementing oral-motor therapy. Oral motor therapy focuses on assessment and remediation of oral motor deficits (jaw instability, poor lip rounding, poor tongue control, etc.) through the use of specific tools (e.g., horns, bubbles, straws, chewy tubes). In addition, techniques and tools for feeding therapy are utilized to improve strength and coordination. *The Homework Book* is available for clinicians to select exercises for the caregiver to carryover at home. A licensed SLP may participate in a two-day workshop for either treatment planning for oral motor therapy or feeding therapy to become trained in the respective area. Visit www.talktools.net to learn more about oral motor therapy, read articles, find a local therapist who is experienced with oral motor techniques or join a parent group.

- **The Hanen Approach**: The Hanen Approach encourages SLP's to work closely with parents and family members to develop a child's language skills and ultimately increase communication. It is a child-centered approach that can be utilized in a variety of settings and promotes intervention in a naturalistic setting. The program stresses the importance of the family's involvement in a child's success and strives to empower parents to help their child learn to communicate. There are a number of programs available specifically designed for children on the autism spectrum (*More Than Words, TalkAbility*). Workshops are three days in length. Visit www.Hanen.org to learn more about the programs available, purchase materials, find a trained *Hanen* therapist in your area, and read helpful parenting tips.

- **Beckman Oral Motor:** Developed in 1975 by Debra Beckman for individuals with poor oral motor skills who may not have the cognitive ability to follow directives such as "stick out your tongue." The technique focuses on "increas[ing] functional response to pressure and movement, range, strength, variety and control of movement for the lips, cheeks, jaw and tongue." Beckman recommends multidisciplinary involvement in improving an individual's oral motor skills with the speech-language pathologist assessing and planning the treatment protocol. There are two courses available; Beckman Oral Motor Assessment and Intervention and Beckman Oral Motor Oro-Facial Deep Tissue Release. Visit www.beckmanoralmotor.com to locate a therapist in your area, find information on workshops and or learn how to become involved in research.

- **Augmentative and Alternative Communication (AAC):** is defined as any form of communication (other than oral speech) that is used to express thoughts, needs, wants, and ideas (www.asha.org). AAC is a broad term that encompasses both unaided and aided systems. Unaided communication is the use of signs and gestures without supportive equipment. Aided systems include external devices such as pictures, letters, words, communication books such as PECS (Picture Exchange Communication System), and VOCAs (Voice Output Communication Aids). Children on the autism spectrum are often good candidates for AAC devices as a way to either expand their verbal output or as an alternative to verbal communication. Choosing which type of AAC is most appropriate will be based on your child's communication and motor strengths and weaknesses as well as what is best for your family and the educational setting. Although there is controversy as to which method is most effective with those on the Autism Spectrum, many will use and benefit from a combination of aided and unaided systems (PECS and signing). One commonly used aided system with individuals on the spectrum is PECS.

- **PECS:** Picture Exchange Communication System is an augmentative alternative communication system developed in 1985, by Andrew S. Bondy, Ph.D. and Lori Frost, MS,CCC/SLP. It was specifically developed for children and adults with Autism and related developmental disabilities. The primary goal is functional spontaneous communication via the exchange of pictures. It is considered a visual method and recommended for those with motor impairments due to the ease of retrieving and exchanging a picture with a communication partner. The PECS system consists of six phases: how to communicate; distance and persistence; picture discrimination; sentence structure; answering questions; and commenting. Although certification in the method is not required, it is recommended that any professional or parent using the method consider attending a training session as it is essential to follow the correct protocol. Visit www.pecs.com to learn more about the PECS system, how to become trained or certified, to join PECS user groups, and to purchase products.

How Will Understanding Autism Shape Your Child's Speech-Language Sessions?

SLP's play a critical role in facilitating the social communication skills of individuals on the autism spectrum (Schwartz & Drager, 2008). Social communication, also known as pragmatics, requires social as well as linguistic skills, which are areas of weakness for this population (Siegel, 1996). Pragmatic skills include eye contact, turn taking, joint attention, topic initiation, maintenance and elaboration. These skills are compromised by the difficulty those with ASD have in imitating others, maintaining attention, generating new ideas, and finding social experiences inherently rewarding. An experienced SLP will treat your child holistically and dynamically, frequently re-assessing and treating all areas of development (cognitive, linguistic, social, physical, sensory, behavior) while maintaining focus on the development of social language skills. For example, your SLP may engage your child in games that encourage turn taking while reinforcing the development of related expressive and receptive language skills and appropriate behaviors.

In addition to significant social language delays, individuals on the autism spectrum often present with challenges (e.g., behaviors, sensory regulation difficulties) that can interfere with learning. Furthermore, different learning styles, limitations, and needs will result in the development of treatment plans that are specifically designed for each individual. One of the biggest challenges your SLP will face will be determining what additional modifications and support strategies should be implemented to facilitate learning. It is the SLP's observations and interactions with your child that will assist in deciding what environmental modifications, behavioral management plans, supporting materials and activities will promote an optimal and motivating setting to learn and support communication.

Environmental modifications: When working with a child on the autism spectrum it is vital that the surroundings are modified to lessen distractions and provide support for additional needs such as sensory and attention deficits.

- Decrease visual distractions (little or no decorations)
- Supportive seating

- Facing away from the window
- Good lighting
- Established work area and sensory or "break" area
- Awareness of noises that might be distracting to the child (buzzing of light, air conditioner/heat)
- Toys and materials out of reach and in enclosed cabinets

Behavior management/regulation: Children with ASD may have behavioral difficulties resulting from frustration, sensory regulation difficulties, self stimulatory behaviors, and/or an inability to communicate their needs and wants effectively. Your SLP will evaluate what behavior management strategies need to be utilized to facilitate a successful session and to develop and maintain a trusting relationship with your child. Just as Autism is a dynamic disorder, a behavioral plan will be a work in progress and continuously altered to meet your child's needs. There are many behavioral modification techniques that can be implemented.

- Use of preferred activities
- Choice boards
- Consistency and following through
- Establishing clear and realistic expectations
- Use of reinforcers (tangible, social, auditory, visual)
- Token system
- Verbal praise
- Replacing negative behaviors with more appropriate behaviors
- Prevention of negative behaviors
- Use of timers to indicate the initiation/completion of a task or transition
- Structured and predictable sessions
- Sensory breaks (physioball, vibration, massage, wheel-barrel walking)

Supporting materials: To maximize learning and your child's ability to communicate the SLP will often use additional supporting materials. These materials enhance nonverbal and verbal communication and provide the structure that children on the autism spectrum often benefit from. In addition, many of these activities foster the development of early sight reading and literacy.

- Use of pictures/words to create a daily schedule
- Use of pictures/words to create an activity schedule for one session to assist in transitioning from one activity to the next
- Written words on objects around room
- Choice board with pictures/words

- Use start-to-finish activities that have a clear beginning and end facilitate
- **Supporting activities**: Children on the autism spectrum often require the use of unique activities to learn various language skills; particularly social language skills. These activities support and encourage communication and interaction.
- Use of routines (daily living activities - dressing, snack time, bedtime routine)
- Use of scripts to learn and practice social scenarios (inviting a peer to play)
- Social stories (address problematic situations by reading stories)
- Repetition of material to foster learning (books, songs, carrier phrases such as "I want__")
- Use of cloze sentences ("Birds fly in the (sky)") and fill-ins ("Ready set (go)")
- "Sabotaging" of materials and environment (desired toy out of reach, piece of a toy missing)
- Group therapy (sessions with typical peers to provide modeling of appropriate social behavior)
- Sessions in a natural setting to promote carryover
- Use of technology (computers, hand held game systems) to encourage independent learning and visual feedback
- Establishing a routine to the sessions
- Keep pace of sessions relative to attention span

How Will Your SLP Facilitate Carryover and Generalization?

Individuals on the autism spectrum often have difficulty generalizing skills learned in a therapy setting to the "real world." Therefore, working in a naturalistic setting is strongly recommended. A naturalistic setting promotes inclusion in "normal" everyday situations, teaches the individual how to interact with others, and allows for more "teachable" moments. Furthermore, when therapy is provided in a natural setting activities are more purposeful and meaningful which will increase your child's motivation and desire to participate. For example, an SLP would make learning the labels of food more salient if it is taught and experienced in a kitchen with real food items and engaging activities (cooking, cutting, tasting) versus through the use of pictures and pretend play food in an office or bedroom setting.

Speech-language pathologists who work with children on the autism spectrum realize the importance and necessity of carryover and generalization of skills to a variety of settings and across different people. Your SLP will collaborate with other team members (multi-disciplinary approach) to share current goals, strategies, and concerns. For example, your SLP may ask others on the team to encourage a verbal request for a desired toy during their respective sessions. Your SLP in turn may incorporate other team member's goals into their sessions (gripping a writing utensil appropriately, providing scheduled sensory breaks). Communication between the service providers (Occupational therapist, Physical therapists, home-based therapists, Psychologist, Play therapist, etc.) educational providers (teachers, special education itinerant teachers, small class instructors, etc.) and family members/caregivers is essential to your child's ability to transfer what is learned in a speech- language session to other environments and people in their life. Your SLP can promote carryover and generalization in a variety of settings.

Educational Settings (Outside Of the Home):

- Your SLP may:
- Observe the classroom and make suggestions
- Spend time with your child in school to demonstrate strategies used in sessions to foster communication
- Train teachers to use PECS, signs, or other aided/unaided AAC
- Collaborate with school therapists
- Keep a shared notebook to communicate successes, goals, concerns on a session to session basis

Home Environment:

- Your SLP may:
- Work with parents, extended family members, babysitters
- Provide homework for parents to do each week
- Facilitate sibling interactions
- Suggest appropriate toys, games, and other materials
- Collaborate with home-based therapists
- Participate in team meetings

In the Community:

- Your SLP may:
- Teach about the community
- Visit local stores
- Prepare your child for difficult outings/activities (getting a haircut, going to the dentist)
- Teach appropriate behavior and social language for various settings/events in the community

What Other Roles May the SLP Play in Your Life?

Your SLP will not only work with your child but will also be someone you, the parent, can turn to for suggestions, advice, and to gain knowledge on the constantly changing world of Autism. For example, your SLP may act as an advocate for your child by attending school meetings or writing letters to recommend an increase in services. He or she will share their knowledge on various treatments, local school programs, support groups and therapies available. In addition, your SLP can provide you with resources such as recent books and articles published as well as connect you with other families who are going through similar experience.

Is Speech and Language Therapy Helpful for Your Child?

Yes! "Clinical evidence indicates that children and adults with ASD benefit from assessment and intervention services provided by speech-language pathologists." (Perlock, www.asha.org) Speech-language Pathologists have significantly more training and experience working with children on the autism spectrum than ever before. As the prevalence of Autism continues to rise, SLP's are seeing an increase in the number of children with ASD on their caseload (Schwartz & Drager, 2008). As a result, Speech-language Pathologists now receive training, certification or become familiar with techniques such as applied behavioral analysis (ABA) and relationship development intervention (RDI). Your speech-language pathologist plays a crucial role in your child's development and will aid in the maintenance and generalization of life changing communication skills.

Although speech-language pathologists today have more experience with those individuals on the Autism Spectrum, not every professional will be a "good fit" for your child. There is no exact recipe to working with a child on the spectrum and therefore what works for one child may or may not work for another. An experienced SLP will have training in multiple techniques and find what works for your child. If you are not seeing progress or have doubts about the services your child is receiving please seek out additional resources and recommendations.

As speech-language pathologists who have many years of experience with children on the autism spectrum, we are familiar with the questions and concerns parents may have. The purpose of this chapter was to give you an overview of speech-language pathology and what to expect when your child has been diagnosed with ASD. Our goal was to provide you with the knowledge you need to be an informed parent; which is an empowered parent. You are your child's biggest advocate and the more information you have, the more your child will benefit from speech-language services.

THE STRUGGLE TO SPEAK: IMPLEMENTATION OF THE KAUFMAN SPEECH TO LANGUAGE PROTOCOL (K-SLP)

BY NANCY R. KAUFMAN

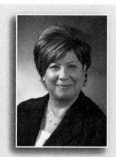

Nancy R. Kaufman, M.A., CCC/SLP

Kaufman Children's Center for Speech, Language, Sensory-Motor and Social Connections, Inc.
6625 Daly Road
West Bloomfield, MI 48322
(248)737-3430
Kidspeech.com

Since 1979, Nancy Kaufman has dedicated herself to establishing a treatment approach, the Kaufman Speech to Language Protocol (K-SLP), to help children become effective vocal communicators. She is the author of many materials related to the K-SLP method, most recently the Kaufman Speech to Language Protocol Instructional DVD Set. Families from around the globe visit the Kaufman Children's Center for Speech, Language, Sensory-Motor, & Social Connections, Inc. in Michigan to benefit from Nancy's expertise in the area of childhood apraxia of speech and other speech sound disorders. She lectures locally, nationally, and internationally and serves on the professional advisory board of the Childhood Apraxia of Speech Association of North America. Nancy is the recipient of the 2010 Michigan State University College of Communication Arts & Sciences Outstanding Alumni Award and the 2011 Distinguished Service Award from the Michigan Speech-Language-Hearing Association.

Children with autism spectrum disorders (ASD) often struggle to speak. There are many reasons why speaking may be especially difficult for the ASD population. One of them is that children with ASD often have difficulty processing and comprehending spoken language. A good analogy about this is to think of oneself in a foreign country without knowing the language. Conversational language sounds like "gibberish" as it is difficult to perceive where each word begins and ends. As a result, the speech of a child who is trying to mimic the language that is heard but not comprehended also sounds like gibberish.

However, once the child understands the meaning of a word, they also have a better idea of the acoustic properties of the word (hearing where it begins and ends) and are better able to produce it. For children who struggle to speak for the reason that they don't easily process and comprehend spoken language, we would want to focus our efforts upon helping them to understand language, but also to physically produce the words that are important to them. We would be working on auditory recognition, comprehension, retention and integration skills (such as through an ABA verbal behavior program) but would also work on the pronunciation of favorite foods, drinks, toys, activities and significant people in their environment. We are thus focusing on the input system (auditory linguistic processing or receptive language) and the output system (motor-speech and expressive language).

Another reason that children with ASD may struggle to speak is because they may have weak oral musculature. Very often in the ASD population we find difficulty with upper body strength or low muscle tone. One can also have low tone of the oral musculature, resulting in weak, garbled and imprecise speech. If this same child has difficulty with quality sucking, chewing and swallowing different textures of foods, they would benefit from therapy that will directly help with quality feeding, while also working on the oral postures or placements needed for increased accuracy of vowels and consonants. `Sara Rosenfeld Johnson's Talktools would be ideal for this challenge, though oral placement therapy must be paired with the vowel or consonant oral motor movements themselves to increase the vowel and consonant repertoire, and to help in the oral muscle tone and strength to maintain accuracy in connected speech.

A third reason that children with ASD may struggle to speak may be due to Childhood Apraxia of Speech (CAS). These are children who may be able to produce vowels and consonants accurately in isolation, but struggle to combine these motor movements into different syllable shapes or gestures at will (on volitional muscle control). They may even struggle to produce isolated vowels and consonants, though not because of oral motor weakness or some type of dysarthria (usually flaccid). It is difficult to determine if children with ASD actually have Childhood Apraxia of Speech (CAS) as there is usually not enough vocal/verbal output to examine. However, best practices for CAS are often successful for children with this profile.

One of the challenges we face as speech-language pathologists is that often, children with ASD who are not vocal/verbal communicators also struggle to imitate vowels and consonants. They may not understand the task of vocal imitation and may also struggle to imitate gross motor movements in general. For these children we like to begin with sign language as a bridge to vocal/verbal communication. This is an ABA verbal behavior method that requires very specific teaching methods.

In general, we observe the child and determine what items and activities are motivating to them. Once the child shows motivation for a specific item (reaches for a cookie) or activity (attempts to get on the trampoline) we take their hands and shape them to make the single sign for that item or activity (cookie or jump). However, just as important, we must say the word *cookie* or *jump*, three times, in a natural voice, while shaping the child's hands for the sign and then deliver a small piece of cookie or the opportunity to jump (just once) on the trampoline. We want to do this for possibly hundreds of trials until we can simply move our hands toward the child's hands but not touch them, and perhaps the child will make the sign without help. In this case we would still say the name of the item or activity a few times, and deliver more of the item or activity. Since the sign has always been paired with the item or activity, the production of the sign by the child themselves may trigger the word vocally as a reflex, in which case we would offer the full cookie or many opportunities to jump on the trampoline with much excitement. If speaking the word is never triggered as a reflex, we would wait until the child makes some sort of vocalization with the sign before we reinforce.

Eventually we would work on their favorites through echoics or vocal imitation tasks to help them to at least produce an approximation of that word. The two most important aspects in using sign language as a bridge to vocal communication are that we only choose words that are motivating to the child while the child is actually showing motivation for it, and we first work on them as a "mand" or a request rather than working on them as a "tact" or a label. There is a complete manual and kit about this type of approach entitled the *K&K Sign to Talk-Nouns* and *K&K Sign to Talk-Verbs* (Kasper, Kaufman). It is a helpful resource in explaining this ABA verbal behavior approach to shaping signs toward vocal/verbal skills. Once the child is vocalizing more and getting reinforced for this behavior, we can start working on refining their motor-speech coordination.

The Kaufman Speech to Language Protocol (K-SLP) is designed to work on simple to complex motor-speech patterns to increase motor-speech coordination. We also work on the child's list of favorites by shaping vowels and consonants toward best approximations. We can then move into helping the children with two–and three-word combinations to progress toward expressive language development. There is a complete manual for the K-SLP within the *Kaufman Speech Praxis Treatment Kits 1 and 2*. Also available is the *K-SLP Instructional DVD* that details the K-SLP approach, offered through www.kaufmandvdcom. The K-SLP Instructional DVD is not specifically detailed for children with ASD but showcases close to 50 children who all struggle to speak with various communicative profiles, to include those with ASD.

When working on a child's list of favorites, having them attempt to produce the full word would be difficult and frustrating. We would want to probe through successive approximations to determine their closest approximation of these important words on a simplified (motor) level and by using cues, help them to say these best approximations when requesting their favorite items or activities. SLPs are familiar with phonological process terminology, which is the way children simplify spoken words based on the principle of the least physiological effort. We would thus simplify difficult words for the children by employing phonological processes and by using cues, fading cues and using powerful motivation (toys and items of interest to the child).

We might have to delete a final consonant to help them with the basic consonant and vowel of the word so that *ball* might first be produced as *baw*. We may have to reduce a cluster of consonants so that a word such as *blue* might have to be first produced as *boo* or *stop* may have to be produced as *top*. We might have to allow the children to use "fronting" for the sounds of /k/ or /g/ that may not yet be in their repertoire, such as producing *cookie* as *tootie* until they do have the appropriate consonant, /k/. Children's names are also usually quite difficult to produce. We would examine the motor complexity of each word that is important in the child's world, and help them to produce their best approximations so that they can use them functionally. We would then extinguish lower patterns of words and replace them with higher approximations which have been taught in our therapy sessions. So, for example, as soon as the child is successfully able to produce a /k/, we would extinguish the /t/ and replace it with the /k/ for *cookie*.

These are some of the main issues that occur in children with ASD who also struggle to speak. Some children have a combination of these issues and we will need to work on each with the appropriate techniques. Repetition, providing cues and fading cues as well as utilizing powerful reinforcement are the keys to a successful program. Though many children are not motivated by typical toys, it is our responsibility to find the items and activities that are motivating, giving them freely at first, gaining their trust, and gradually helping them to perform the tasks we are asking of them with a strong promise of wonderful things to come. Eventually, the ability to speak will be the motivation as well as the reward!

TECHNOLOGICAL-BASED INTERVENTIONS FOR AUTISM—THERE'S AN APP FOR THAT!

One exciting tool/therapy that has really come on in the last twelve months since we published the first edition of *Cutting-Edge Therapies* is the iPad. As you may be aware there are dozens of apps currently available for the iPad and similar devices that have a basis in helping kids with autism communicate, organize their day, and even help parents keep track of therapy schedules. In addition, many other computer-based therapies have recently upgraded their offerings and it seems each month there are more programs/apps being launched. In light of this we have created this special technology section to provide a brief look at what is available.

The section leads off with Valerie Herskowitz returning to provide an overview of "Computer-Based Interventions: What's It All About?" Patti Murphy follows, writing on ACC: Augmentative and Alternative Communication. Robert Tedesco is next with HandHoldAdaptive, creator of such apps as iPrompts, and we close with Rachel Coppin introducing us to Proloquo2Go.

COMPUTER-BASED INTERVENTION—WHAT'S IT ALL ABOUT?

BY VALERIE HERSKOWITZ

Excerpt from the book, *Autism & Computers: Maximizing Independence Through Technology.*

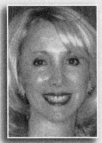

Valerie Herskowitz, MA, CCC-SLP

info@valerieherskowitz.com
www.valerieherskowitz.com

One of the world's foremost speakers on the subject of computer-based intervention (CBI) with autism, Valerie Herskowitz was the founder of Dimensions Therapy Center. She has expanded her computer-based intervention for families on an international scale by establishing a "global autism support village" through podcasts, webcasts, and other cyber tools. Ms. Herskowitz's career as a speech pathologist spans the past thirty-two years, and she was the recipient of the Stevie Lifetime Achievement Award in 2004 for her work with individuals with autism. Her youngest son, Blake, was diagnosed in 1993 with autism. Her professional journey as a therapist and as a parent of a child with autism have combined to give Ms. Herskowitz the unique insights to help families cope with problems they face in parenting a child with autism. She is the author of the book, *Autism & Computers: Maximizing Independence Through Technology* (2009). For more information about computers and autism, or to buy her book, log onto: www.valerieherskowitz.com.

It is important to start on the road to technology literacy early. The reason is based on the science and research that supports early training of any sort. It deals with early intervention and neuroplasticity, which revolves around the brain's ability to reorganize itself by forming new neural connections throughout life (Medicine.net). The brain is an organ that changes from response to experience.

There are several studies that support early intensive behavioral intervention (e.g., Anderson et al., 1987; Fenske et al., 1985; Lovaas, 1987; Smith et al., 2000) Though the types of therapy models have varied in the studies, they have certain things in common. They all incorporated curriculums in the areas of attention and focusing, language, and social skills, and they all used a behavioral approach. Each model utilized twenty-five hours per week of structured stimulation, and they promoted the inclusion of parents and families into the intervention process. When these factors occur together, there is evidence that many children show significant increases in communication, IQ, and educational placement.

Computer-based intervention or CBI incorporates all of the above features. There are software programs that teach skills in the areas of attention, language, and social interaction, and they are taught using effective behavioral methods. I don't recommend that CBI be implemented twenty-five hours a week, but I do feel that it needs to be an integral part of a home-based intervention program. And I highly recommend that family members become active in the process.

From a physiological perspective, let's look at the reasons why early intervention is successful in utilizing the concept of neuroplasticity. According to the website Neuroscience for Kids, neuroplasticity consists of several different processes that occur throughout a person's life. There are certain periods of one's life, however, where plasticity occurs more frequently. During the first two years of life, the synaptic connections of each neuron increase until there are twice as many synaptic connections as in an adult's brain. As time continues, there is a degenerative process called pruning which continues until the cell dies. This pruning process can be affected by the activity of cell interaction, however. Therefore, cells that are activated are strengthened, and those that are not activated are pruned. The pruning process continues until approximately age sixteen, so as you can see, early stimulation has a huge impact on brain development.

From a cellular and molecular level, researchers have demonstrated how sensory, perceptual, and language functions are influenced by our experiences. They have surmised that the brain is most susceptible to modifications for language acquisition within the first six years of life. The brain still retains the ability to acquire language skills in a slower manner up until the age of twelve. After that, there is a significant slowdown. It doesn't come to a complete halt by any means, but it may be more difficult to accomplish.

Helping Older Children and Adults

What if your child or student is older? Is all hope lost? Certainly not! As previously mentioned, brain plasticity does not stop for the entire lifetime of a person. Dr. Merzenich, the neuroscientist often referred to as the "father of neuroplasticity," has been involved in some interesting work regarding older individuals. He and his colleagues have recently created a computer-based program called Brain Fitness, which is designed to strengthen the brain in order to increase speech and agility. Dr. Merzenich's early work involved the research design of a similar computer-based training program called Fast ForWord. This program was designed for children and adolescents who demonstrate significant language impairments.

Think about the last time you tried to learn a new skill. Perhaps you and your spouse decided to take dance lessons, you decided to try to learn a little Italian before your trip to Italy, or you needed to learn a new computer application at work. There may have been a little bit of a learning curve, but you probably were able to gain some skill in these areas. Granted, it wasn't easy, and you probably won't be on *Dancing With the Stars* in the near future. But I'm sure you were able to learn enough to add enjoyment to your life.

Taking on technology in later years is much the same way, even for a person with developmental disabilities. I have a student that is actually my age. (If you have done the math, you may have figured out that I'm in my early fifties.) We started working together approximately seven years ago. Bobby lives with his brother, who referred Bobby to me. At the time, Bobby's language consisted of one- to two-word sentences, and he was difficult to understand. He had no reading skills and was unable to tell time. He was high functioning in other areas and held a job in the food court at the local mall, but he had virtually no experience using computers or any other technological application.

Initially, I felt that Bobby should focus on developing his language skills. I wanted to increase his ability to produce longer sentences, so I introduced him to a program called Sentence Developer, which I created for the students in my office. It's a visual system designed to teach sentence structure. From a technological prospective, it's fairly easy to use. Bobby was able to learn how to use a mouse very quickly, so the touchscreen wasn't necessary.

This program was Bobby's first introduction into the world of computers. Though the technological learning curve was short, the impact of these exercises on his language development was significant. This experience also gave him the confidence to move on to more sophisticated computer usage.

We moved on to programs designed to improve his speech production. These applications, which are a little bit more involved from a technological perspective, allowed Bobby to record his own voice. We also incorporated a reading program, as well as an application to teach Bobby some time-telling skills. Through the last few years, Bobby has become quite skilled in computer technology. Aside from the skills he has acquired through the training, he feels that he's part of the world that he lives in and feels pride in his accomplishments.

Bobby loves the fact that he is computer literate at this time of his life. His brother purchased the reading program, and Bobby enjoys practicing the exercises at home. Bobby's story shows that we are never too old to acquire computer or technology skills.

Had Bobby been given the opportunity to obtain computer training when he was young, would he have been more able to utilize technology than he is today? My experience tells me that the answer to this question is yes, but this type of instruction simply wasn't available to him until seven years ago. Still, what he has accomplished in that span of time is quite remarkable and compelling. So, if anyone ever tries to convince you of the old adage, "You can't teach an old dog new tricks," please disregard it as an untruth.

Why CBI is Successful

I have identified several factors that CBI offers which explain its success with individuals on the autism spectrum.

Predictability. Every parent, teacher, or therapist of a child with autism will agree that, for the most part, our children have issues with new people, new foods, and new experiences—just about "new" anything. Conversely, they seem to handle familiar situations well. They thrive in a ritualistic environment and deteriorate when something is strange to them. Computer-based intervention offers a mode of treatment that can provide familiarity and predictability. Certainly, this isn't the case the first time the individual begins the process, but as time goes on, the training takes on a *sameness* even when the actual exercise changes. The program starts up the same each time, and/or the animation is the same. The format of the exercises is the same, and if you use multiple programs from a particular software manufacturer, the format of other programs is similar, if not identical, to the programs the child is already using.

As therapists, teachers, or parents, we will have a shorter learning curve as well, since the software designers often create a series of programs that present different exercises in the same format.

Animation. I feel that animation is a make-it or break-it situation. Some children need the animation that is provided by many of these programs, and others find it a major distraction, may be afraid of it, or become overstimulated by it. This is why many of the manufacturers of these programs have included the ability to turn the animation feature on or off. You don't have this ability, however, with off-the-shelf software or programs that you purchase in a store rather than from a vendor who sells software specifically for the special needs population.

The animation can be used for several purposes: First, it's used as a reinforcer, so that when the child performs the task correctly, an animated character comes out and congratulates the child for a job well done. Another function of the characters is as a prompt device. Often, they will appear above the correct answer when the child has demonstrated the need for cuing. Then, as the child progresses, the animation will not appear. Lastly, there are several programs that utilize animation as the actual characters in the program. In this case, the intention is to increase attention and focus on the task.

If you take a look at off-the-shelf software, you often find that animation is used for other purposes as well as the above. There may be several animations on the screen at a time, and this can be quite distracting to many of the kids. The last thing we need is for our children to be *more* distracted than they already are.

Looking forward instead of down. When I started working with children on the computer, there was one thing that I noticed immediately. It seemed that they had a much easier time focusing on what they saw on the computer versus what I presented on a table when I worked with them off the computer. I initially concluded that it was the computer program alone that caused them to be more focused and attentive. But after a while, I began to realize that it was because they looked forward when working on a computer rather than down. When they looked straight ahead, I was able to maintain their attention for a much longer period of time.

I have done my own quasi-experiment and have often utilized this vertical plane presentation when working off the computer with the children as well. Sure enough, I have found that children do seem to be able to sustain attention more appropriately this way. It makes sense. It's more natural if you think about it. When you watch TV or talk to someone, what direction are your eyes looking? You may sometimes look slightly down or slightly up if you're talking to someone who is shorter or taller. But most often, we are looking forward. It's not only a better way to teach our kids, but it's also more pragmatically appropriate. Do we really want to teach our children to focus down? No, we want them to focus forward as they will need to do when conversing with another person or watching the teacher at school.

From a therapeutic and educational sense, it's important to always try to maximize learning for all students. One way that therapists and teachers accomplish this is by recognizing different learning styles in their students. Some obvious ones are auditory learners versus visual learners. Delving into the entire subject of various learning styles is beyond the scope of this book, but software manufacturers of these types of programs have taken into account that individuals will vary greatly in terms of which sense they learn from. Therefore, they have made considerable efforts to include a great deal of auditory and visual approaches. For example, pictures are one stimulus, as well as the voice of the narrator who gives the directive. The only time that this varies is when the task requires the individual to just respond to a visual *or* auditory directive. Then, of course, both the visual and the auditory are not given. We call this a multimodality approach.

The term "modalities" refers to the way information is processed. If it is processed by seeing the information, it's obviously visual. If it's processed by hearing the information, it's auditory. Even though every individual learns through one channel better than the other, in most cases, presenting information in both an auditory and visual format is the best way to maximize learning. So, the child sees the picture, hears the words, maybe sees the written words, and sometimes gets visual cuing, etc. This multi-stimulation is often how we can make sure that the student has had the best opportunity for learning.

AAC: AUGMENTATIVE
AND ALTERNATIVE
COMMUNICATION

BY PATTI MURPHY

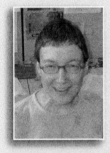

Patti Murphy

Patti Murphy writes for DynaVox Mayer-Johnson in Pittsburgh, Pennsylvania. She has written on disability issues for more than 15 years, specializing in augmentative and alternative communication (AAC) for the past decade. Her work has also appeared in ADVANCE for Speech-Language Pathologists, Closing the Gap, Exceptional Parent Magazine and the Pittsburgh Post-Gazette. She thanks the speech-language pathologists on staff at DynaVox Mayer-Johnson for the expertise and insight they shared for this chapter and the direction they provided. Thanks also to the many young people who use AAC, their parents, siblings, teachers and therapists who over time have graciously shared their experiences for their inspiration. Though each has taken a distinctive path on their communication journeys, collectively they speak with one voice.

DynaVox Mayer-Johnson (www.dynavoxtech.com) is the leading provider of speech-generating devices and symbol-adapted special education software used to assist individuals in overcoming speech, language and learning challenges.

The ebb and flow of everyday communication can be cloudy when autism is part of the equation. It is important to remember that with proper tools and support every individual with autism, even those with significant challenges, is capable of improving their communication skills. A good mix of human and technological elements, some of which you may already be utilizing, may clear a path to more meaningful communication.

Since the early 1980s, ACC interventions have increasingly gained recognition in consumer and clinical circles as a viable way to support communication among those with autism spectrum disorders, their families, friends and others they meet throughout their lives.

In the introduction to the 2009 book *Autism Spectrum Disorders and AAC*, Pat Mirenda discusses scientific roots of AAC for this population that date back more than 40 years, and involve studies conducted with chimpanzees then replicated with children. The studies included teaching a male chimp to use American Sign Language (Gardner & Gardner, 1969); teaching a female chimp to associate plastic chips with more than 130 words categorized by parts of speech based on the colors and shapes of the chips (Premack & Premack, 1974) and teaching a group of chimps to communicate with the aid of abstract lexigrams comprised of 9 geometric forms. The chimps accessed the lexigrams through computer-linked, touch-sensitive display panels. In the project's early phases, the panels produced illuminated symbols and later, synthetic speech. (Rumbaugh, 1977; Savage-Rumbaugh, Rumbaugh & Boysen, 1978).

Mirenda writes of the unsettling nature of the research. "The sad and distasteful logic inherent in these early AAC experiments was that if chimps could learn to communicate, perhaps people with autism also could."

The visual-graphic emphasis that shaped AAC strategies and technologies near the end of the 20th century opened new roads for those with autism and their communication partners. In 1985, Andy Bondy and Lori Frost introduced the Picture Exchange Communication System (PECS), commonly used to teach children to request preferred items or activities. Symbols used on AAC devices, were less abstract than in the past. Devices with static visual displays and limited vocabulary, the most advanced available in the early 1980s and still frequently used for beginners, gave way to dynamic-display technology by the end of the decade. Dynamic displays, based on natural language formation, changed according to the vocabulary selections of person using the device, offering better command of expressive language and understanding of context, bolstered by the concreteness of the symbols, their written labels and the corresponding speech output.

Soon the debut of Boardmaker and similar page creation software tweaked the communication process for everyone involved. Parents and teachers no longer needed to spend hours creating paper overlays for a child's device. The software also provided an alternate means of communication (page printouts that the child could point at in the absence of the device) and helpful tools for schoolwork.

AAC devices were also becoming consumer friendlier from a hardware standpoint, smaller, less industrial in appearance and smaller. With nearly each new generation, the devices were lighter in weight, had exponentially greater memory and synthesized speech sounding more like a human voice.

AAC use does not deter and may encourage speech development (Silverman, 1980; Berry, 1987 and Daniels, 1994). For those with autism, "enhanced speech production is usually viewed as a 'bonus' side effect of AAC rather than as a primary goal"

(Millar, 2009.) Diane Millar also writes, "Some have estimated that as many as one half of individuals with autism never develop speech to the level that they are functionally able to use it as an adequate means of communication," reflecting research published in the 1990s. (Peeters & Gillberg, 1999; Light, Roberts, DiMarco, & Greiner, 1998 and Mesibov, Adams, & Klinger, 1997).

Historically, AAC interventions have been somewhat slower to catch on for people with autism spectrum disorders than for those with complex communication needs primarily associated with physical impairment from conditions such as cerebral palsy or traumatic brain injury. One reason, Mirenda writes, is that those with autism were considered too "something: (e.g. too young, too old; too cognitively, behaviorally or linguistically impaired) to qualify for AAC services" or prospects for speech development seemed too good. Recommendation of advanced technologies despite such challenges is becoming more acceptable. A lot depends on the person's desire to communicate and implementation strategies, issues covered later in this chapter.

Lack of awareness is another issue. It is believed that just 5 percent of the estimated 1 in 8 Americans who cannot speak due to a variety of health conditions use AAC technology. The rest know little, if anything, about it.

In the new millennium, AAC is virtually synonymous with technology that may be called a speech communication, speech-output, or voice-output or speech-generating device. Device use, sometimes referred to as aided AAC, is often one facet of an eclectic approach to communication that also combines lighter technologies and technology-free (or unaided) strategies we all use—including natural speech. From stories of communication success that parents, colleagues and professionals in clinical and educational settings from across the country have shared with me in the past decade, AAC is clearly an embraceable approach.

AAC means more than talking or technology alone, for it encompasses unaided strategies that we all use naturally to convey a message, such as facial expressions, body language or clearing our throats for attention. It includes a variety of simple tools—alphabet or word boards accessed by pointing and picture books like Mary Claire's binder, for example. These modes of communication work in concert to promote effective communication. As a staple of a comprehensive communication system, AAC device use is meant to complement, not replace other effective methods of communication.

The How and Why of AAC Success

Parents and other significant adults in the life of a child with autism attribute positive outcomes of AAC device use to its capacity for drawing on strengths while mediating challenges inherent to the child. In some respects, the opportunity to use the technology may be more motivating than actual opportunities for communication. Some children are naturally more comfortable with things than people, and tend to think more literally than figuratively. They find the technology's audio-visual format attractive and appreciate the often sequential arrangement of content (letters, words, symbols or images) on a device. Its structure and predictability, elements often missing in complex verbal exchanges, make information tangible and the sequence of communication easier to follow. Children benefit from seeing concrete images of what they hear, as Michael does while using his counting pages to manage stress, and Casey while consulting pages on his device to manage his routine.

It is important to introduce AAC gradually and sensitively, taking into account a child's comfort level with various communication modalities and settings. A picture symbol book or photo album may be more practical than an AAC device in a loud, crowded restaurant. An older child with good literacy and typing skills may do well with a keyboard-based device, using rate enhancement features such as word and phrase prediction to keep communication moving at a steady pace.

Communication is very complex and filled with behavioral expectations. The mere expectation of interaction with another individual, perhaps the most basic requirement of communication, can unduly overwhelm some individuals with autism, shutting down their auditory processing and word retrieval abilities while triggering anxiety, aggression or withdrawal. Lacking a reliable means of articulating needs and desires, the person may utilize less socially appropriate behavior such as yelling or grabbing in an attempt to convey their message. At times, the aberrant behavior becomes the equivalent of communication for the person. It may also be the surest way to get attention, which is reinforcing even when it is negative attention. AAC, well-known as an effective behavior management tool, presents a more acceptable option.

Joanne Cafiero (2007) writes: "Sadly, these challenging behaviors become the rationale for NOT providing an AAC intervention. Practitioners reason that behaviors must be brought under control before AAC is introduced. Or that it is not safe for an aggressive person to have an AAC device. These belief systems set in motion a cycle of despair for both the practitioner and the student."[5]

Cafiero (2004) has also written that "AAC tools can be both a buffer and a bridge between the communication partners." High–and low-tech visual supports are a prime example of tools that promote language comprehension as well as successful AAC use. The goals are often equally important. Many people with autism, including some with extensive vocabularies, experience deficits in receptive as well as expressive language. Visual supports used to reinforce or enhance both include illustrated calendars, rules and instructions for the classroom or workplace. Variations on token reward systems used with small children may be helpful during school-to-work transitions. By viewing a series of digital images on an AAC device, a student training for a restaurant job learned that it was OK to drink pop after cleaning three tables. Photos on an AAC device (Figure 1) visually reminded the student of tasks to be completed on the work shift.

Scripting and social narratives are visual supports offering tools for self-regulation and communication in new or difficult circumstances. Each can help individuals make sense of confusing situations, understand expectations and deal with transitions, aspects of daily life that may be taxing without a concrete frame of reference. Scripting guides individuals through the beginning, middle and end of a specific social exchange—introducing oneself or accepting a compliment, for instance. It provides language and cues needed to get a communication partner's attention, maintain and close a conversation, and for transitions such as changing the conversation topic. Social narratives similarly integrate vocabulary with visual cues, and help children respond appropriately in unfamiliar situations. Effective in addressing behavioral problems, teaching social skills and promoting good communication from early childhood through middle school, narratives are generally short, and may be tailored to individual learners.

Figure 2 shows a behavioral support page that a speech therapist created on the spot using a template on a child's AAC device. The child, frightened by a power outage that had occurred at school, used narrative language on the page to clarify feelings about the situation. Within minutes, the child calmed down and navigated to another page on the device to ask the therapist if they could resume the task at hand.

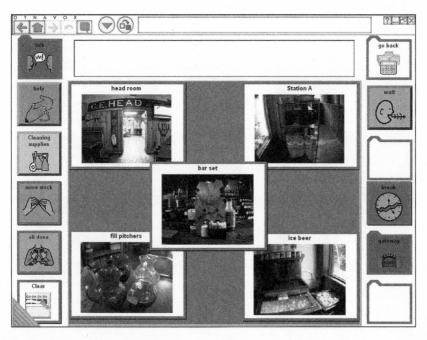

Figure 1. Photos and audio messages on an AAC device help a young restaurant worker in training keep focused on the job.

Behavioral support pages may be customized to help children better understand the consequences of their choices and actions through meaningful contingencies. A good-better-best hierarchy of choices works well in some cases. Consider these two mealtime vocabulary selections that parents gave their child: "If I finish half my dinner, then I can have pretzels" or "If I clean my plate, then I can have a cookie," which the child deemed a more desirable treat. Parents may also find that positively reinforcing messages ("If I walk home from the playground, we will stop for ice cream" or "If I set the table, then I can do puzzles") are more effective than messages with negative overtones—"If I don't eat this meal, then I can't have a snack later," or "If I don't do my chores, then I can't play outside," for instance.

Device content reflecting what matters to your child similarly encourages meaningful communication. Freedom to avoid a situation or activity may be more motivating than permission to have a treat or to do something fun. They can convey that with cognitively and age-appropriate messages, like those that Mary Claire and Casey use when they want to be left alone. Ready-to-use vocabulary common in today's devices keeps the words at your child's fingertips.

Helping children with autism progress beyond communication primarily for fulfillment of wants and needs presents unique challenges because conversation for its own sake may not be as motivating. Children may show interest in a topic (as Michael

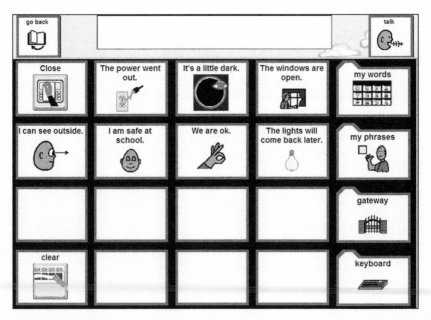

Figure 2. This behavioral support page helped a child communicate and cope with fear experienced during a power outage at school.

does when prompted to talk about horses, and Mary Claire through her enthusiasm when sharing pictures), but struggle with unfamiliar people and nuances of social interaction—interruptions, turn-taking, and changes in the tone of a partner's voice, for instance. They can learn social skills through use of an AAC device (or low-tech tools), modeling, practice and reinforcing items. Instead of having a child ask a peer for a desired toy, the child may be prompted to ask "Can I play with you?" Through repetition of the scenario, the child sees that there is a relationship between interacting with the peer and playing with the toy.

With consistent support, effective instruction, realistic expectations from family and care team members, and AAC as a catalyst, young people with autism can cultivate social communication opportunities and skills needed for success in life. Personal observations and successes shared with me include:

A child independently asked a school aide for help and ordered a drink on a lunchtime field trip to a neighborhood restaurant using an AAC device. Previously, the child typically made repetitive sounds or exhibited frustration to voice desires.

Another child stayed actively engaged in an after-school music program with the aid of visual cues from an AAC device.

Teachers designate periods for social interaction between a student using an AAC device and typically speaking peers. The students exchange brief pleasantries ("Hi, how are you?", "Have a great day!) before class. Or they play board games, allowing the student to initiate communication with vocabulary such as "Your turn," "My turn" or "Next" on the device.

Small steps leave a lasting imprint. The pride and joy that parents experience upon first hearing a child's voice through technology often stems from watching the seeds of self-esteem take root because the child is sure of being heard and understood by others. Whether the child speaks his name, asks to be excused from the dinner table or says that she wants to play, the message is clear.

"What If...?"

Adopting AAC solutions is an ongoing, fluid process driven by the goal of developing skills and supports children need to communicate throughout their life. Questions that may arise along the way, and some short answers, are:

What If My Child is Too Young or Old?

When in doubt, trust that now is the best time to explore AAC options. Some experts consider ages 1 to 5 a prime time to introduce AAC. AAC will lead children to greater skill development, self-sufficiency and social acceptance in years to come. Millar writes that "hesitation about introducing AAC out of fear that AAC will impede speech development is understandable; however, there are serious clinical implications in adopting such as 'wait and see' approach, especially with regard to problem behavior and language development."

It may be argued that the later the initial intervention occurs, the more effort it requires. Early intervention is ideal. However, intervention at any age can bring good results. As children grow up, their behavior patterns, strengths and preferences may become clearer, allowing parents and care team members to make better informed AAC decisions. While discussing the fear that challenging behavior may preclude successful device use, Cafiero (2007) also notes that past failure with AAC technology is not a valid reason to forego it in the present.

Where Do We Begin?

AAC interventions typically begin with traditional speech therapy focusing on language development, particularly for younger children Speech Language Therapy is a related service provided within the educational environment. A referral can be made to the speech-language pathologist (SLP) for children enrolled within educational system. The SLP may conduct a comprehensive assessment to determine the appropriateness of the use of AAC and which technologies are most compatible with the child's language, cognitive and physical abilities. Therapists working within the autism population find it crucial to keep assessments flexible and motivating. Some recommend performing the evaluation in short increments, each followed by a short break, to help children stay relaxed and focused. Awareness of factors that may overload the child, such as device volume, is also important.

How Can I Be Sure That Recommended AAC Tools Are a Good Match for My Child?

Recommendation of a particular device is based primarily on whether, and how, it will make functional communication possible. Technology improves every year and each generation of devices brings advancements. These advancements are usually secondary matters as functional communication is the goal and many devices are available to address children's needs.

It is important to start with the person, not the technology, when recommending AAC solutions. For people with autism, AAC technology is most helpful by providing language in a form they readily understand, and for many, that is a visual form.

"If a child truly doesn't understand the give and take of communication, **and** they don't understand symbolic language, you have to teach these things concurrently, using very powerful and motivating messages," says Vicki Clarke, M.A., CCC-SLP, of Dynamic Therapy Associates, her Kennesaw, Georgia-based practice.

Some children are comfortable with multiple forms of language including visual scenes or text that they type. Others may favor text–over symbol-based vocabulary.

Motor planning or sensory issues may be a consideration. The assessment typically includes a trial period of device use in a variety of settings, which helps to ensure that the device gives the child efficient access to language he or she can use effectively.

What About Device Funding?

The odds of receiving an approval for coverage from most device funding sources increase substantially when an SLP holding a Certificate of Clinical Competence from the American Speech-Language-Hearing Association completes and provides documentation of the assessment. Video of the assessment or device trial period may also be requested. Third-party sources that fund the purchase of devices include Medicaid (regulations vary from state to state), Medicare, the Veterans Administration (coverage is available for beneficiaries of veterans), Vocational Rehabilitation and private insurers. Many device manufacturers employ specialists to assist families and individuals with the funding process. Some manufacturers also offer training and technical support when the device is obtained.

What If There Are Gaps Between School and Home in Device Implementation?

Though a child's academic ability may become apparent or improve through his or her use of a device and other modalities, functional communication must take precedence in AAC use. "There has to be some type of communication goal in mind," says Tina Murphy, M.S, CCC-SLP, an AAC specialist with Florida's Palm Beach County Schools. "Unfortunately, not everyone thinks that way. Some of it stems from lack of understanding as to what AAC is for."

Educators may also use the device to assist with learning. A teacher may, for example, hold up objects for the student to identify or count objects using single-word vocabulary programmed on the device for the lesson, as a recall task. For the student to learn to use the device optimally, communication goals must be incorporated into academics. In a math lesson on counting, for example, the student may be expected to respond in a detailed manner, such as "There are 5 books in the picture you showed me."

Communication is about people making connections, not testing, Cafiero wrote in 2007. "Beware of using a device for drills or practice ...There have been reports of students rejecting their devices because they have been used for "work" rather than communicative interactions. The tool or device then becomes an aversive. If, and only if, the device is viewed by the student as his voice, it may be used for academic tests, but only with extreme caution and respect."[8]

Parents and school teams stress the importance of using consistent symbol sets and word-based vocabulary for greetings, meals, telling jokes and other situations occurring at home and school. Device content is often a tool for maintaining open lines of communication. Teachers, therapists or paraprofessionals may assist children in creating and updating news pages for sharing daily school happenings at home. Parents or siblings can help with a "Weekend" or "Last Night" page that a child may use to tell classmates or teachers about life at home. Figure 3 shows a visual scene and pop-ups with related vocabulary (3A and 3B) that a child uses at bedtime to tell family members about the day at school and plan for tomorrow.

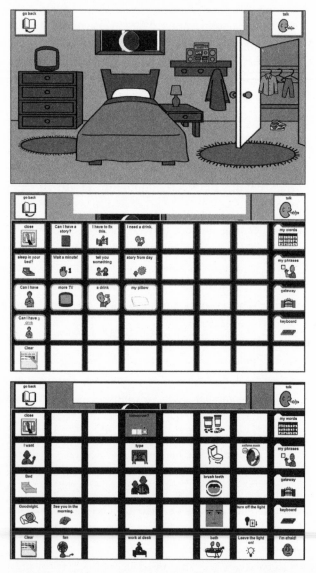

Figures 3, 3A, and 3B. A child uses this visual scene on an AAC device and two pop-ups containing relevant vocabulary as a tool for sharing information about the school day, carrying out bedtime tasks and discussing plans for tomorrow with family members.

HANDHOLD ADAPTIVE

by Robert Tedesco

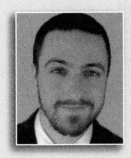

Robert C. Tedesco

Robert C. Tedesco is Co-Founder and Senior Vice President of Research and Development at HandHold Adaptive (makers of iPrompts and AutismTrack), where he has led the company's research, product and business development efforts since 2009. Prior to HandHold Adaptive, Rob developed, managed, and supported the licensing of a $700 million-valued portfolio of technology patents while at Stamford, Connecticut's Walker Digital Gaming from 2003 through 2008. He is named as an inventor on 193 pending and issued U.S. patents, and also worked as Director of Software Development at Yappr.com, a language-learning Web site with more than 7 million users. Rob holds an MBA from the Stern School of Business at New York University.

HandHold Adaptive, LLC produces applications designed for use by caregivers of those with special needs, including those with autism. Whereas many applications for the iPhone, iPod Touch and iPad are designed for direct use by individuals with autism, HandHold Adaptive has focused on creating software controlled by parents and professionals.

One such application is iPrompts®, a picture-prompting tool introduced in May of 2009. iPrompts allows caregivers to create and present several different types of visual prompts. These prompts are designed to help those with autism transition between activities, understand upcoming events, make choices, focus on tasks, and learn socially appropriate behaviors. When using iPrompts, parents and professionals hold the hand-held device, and present the screen to the individual with autism after configuring the desired visual prompt.

Three different types of visual prompts are available (see Figure X). A "Schedules" template allows users to create and save and unlimited number of visual schedules—for example, different sets of pictures for different activities, sequences, days of the week, or individuals. A "Timer" template displays an image of the caregiver's choice along

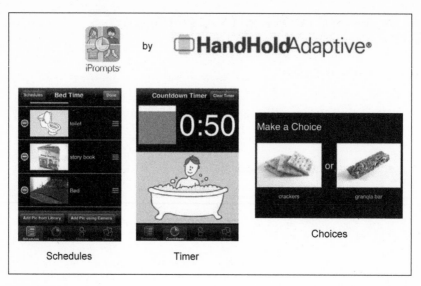

Figure X

with a graphical countdown timer (set to any duration), and is useful for demonstrating how much time is left until a current activity ends, or before the next pictured activity begins. A "Choices" template enables caregivers to select any two images and offer them as a choice, empowering those who cannot vocalize their preferences. When rotated horizontally, the Choices and Schedules features enlarge and orient images for display to individuals needing visual support.

To populate these three templates with pictures, caregivers use an expandable Library of images. The Library includes several hundred "stock" illustrations and digital pictures across numerous categories. Additional pictures may be incorporated by users in a variety of ways, including (1) transferring pictures from a personal computer, (2) taking pictures "on the fly" using the built-in camera of the iPhone or iPod Touch, and (3) searching the Internet and adding pictures from directly within the application's Library.

One of the first autism-specific "apps" on the market, iPrompts is consistently one of the highest-grossing titles in the Medical category on the Apple iTunes Store, and is the focus of U.S. Department of Education research initiative exploring handheld technology in classrooms for students with autism. According to Dan Tedesco, the company's Founder and himself parent of a young boy with autism, "Our goal with iPrompts was to create a portable, flexible, easy-to-use, stigma-free and eco-friendly alternative to using Velcro-backed and laminated cards or magnet boards. We hope iPrompts is especially helpful in reducing the frustrations of everyday life when traveling or on the go."

AutismTrack™, the second application released by HandHold Adaptive, is a data-tracking tool for the iPhone, iPod Touch and iPad. Caregivers use AutismTrack on a daily basis to record information about any medications, diets, supplements or therapies administered, and also to track behaviors and symptoms. This information may then be reviewed, analyzed, and shared among family, friends, and professionals. Over time, AutismTrack may help caregivers to discover and better understand the behavioral trends of individuals with autism, and how therapeutic interventions may seem to influence these trends.

Caregivers begin by setting up a profile, and then track interventions and behaviors on a regular basis, periodically creating trend analysis reports and reviewing progress (see Figure Y). The "Person & Day" tab allows caregivers to establish profiles for an unlimited number of individuals with autism. After providing basic information like age and diagnosis, caregivers then track any medicines, diets, supplements or therapies administered on a daily basis, using checkboxes accessed through the "Interventions" tab (e.g., if a Vitamin B12 supplement was taken today, the checkbox is marked). The default set of interventions is customizable, such that caregivers may tailor their data collection to any specific therapies undertaken with regard to a given individual (e.g., a customized entry of "Massage Therapy" may be tracked). The "Behaviors" tab then allows caregivers to track behaviors on a daily basis, using touch-sensitive sliding scales. If a behavior such as "Eye Contact" was desirable on a particular day, the slider may be moved to the right (the rightmost position is 100% or "Most Desirable"). If another

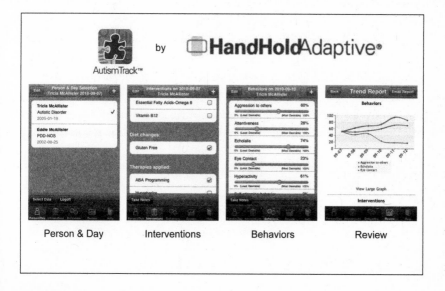

| Person & Day | Interventions | Behaviors | Review |

Figure Y

behavior, such as "Echolalia," was poor on a particular day, the slider may be dragged to the left. All interventions and behaviors may be customized, and optionally supplemented with detailed notes typed by the caregiver.

The "Review" tab then allows for three specific types of data analysis: (1) Daily Logs, which provide a snapshot of the data collected for any one selected day; (2) Trend Reports, which allow caregivers to graph any desired behaviors over time, showing compliance with different interventions during that period (e.g., during a given two-week period, "Aggression" trended downward, while compliance with "ABA Programming" was 50%); and (3) Raw Metrics, which may be exported into a spreadsheet format. Daily Logs and Trend Reports may also be emailed (in PDF format), so that caregivers may share information on their search to discover the unique patterns and trends experienced by individuals with autism.

All collected data are stored in a secure, account-based, password-protected online server (a Wi-Fi or cellular Internet connection is required to use the application). The server-based architecture provides several benefits. One, multiple caregivers may use separate devices to track a single individual with autism, which may be useful in achieving consensus around the individual's current level of performance, or in simply confirming whether or not medications were already administered for the day. Two, caregivers who register to use AutismTrack may rest assured that if their device is misplaced or breaks, data are recoverable through HandHold Adaptive's secure server.

Users of AutismTrack are required to agree to a standard User Agreement that, among other things, requires a HIPAA waiver and an acknowledgment that Hand-Hold Adaptive does not recommend any medications or treatments, and does not provide any medically diagnostic information. In the future, HandHold Adaptive hopes that AutismTrack can help improve autism research, as aggregate data from households may one day be provided to researchers looking to better understand causes and treatment options.

Each of HandHold Adaptive's applications may be downloaded for a one-time fee of $49.99 from the iTunes Store online. For more information, visit: www.handhold-adaptive.com.

INTRODUCING PROLOQUO2GO

by Rachel Coppin

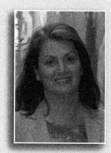

Rachel Coppin MS,CCC-SLP

Anne Carlsen Center
701 3rd St. NW
Jamestown, ND 58401
rachel.coppin@annecenter.org

Rachel Coppin is a Speech Language Pathologist whose caseload is predominantly focused on individuals on the Autism Spectrum. She has a Master's degree and has been working in the field for twenty-five years.

Proloquo2Go is a symbol and text based Augmentative and Alternative Communication application that will run on iPhone, iPad and iPod touch. The name Proloquo is latin for "speak out loud" and 2Go alludes to it being an extremely mobile system.

Proloquo2Go is a product by AssistiveWare that was originally created by David Niemeijer and Samuel Sennott.

Proloquo2Go was designed for use on iPhone, iPod touch and iPad devices in order to provide an easy to use, portable and affordable communication option for people who are nonverbal or have difficulty speaking. The portability of these devices allows the user to have them at home, work, school and during recreational activities. The list just goes on and on. These devices are also extremely popular among individuals of all ages, so carrying them around doesn't make you stand out or look different from other people in any way. These devices are multi-purposed so they can be used for other things than just communication.

One of the best features about Proloquo2Go is its price. This application, which can be purchased through iTunes, currently costs $189.99. Proloquo2Go, along with whichever of the above devices you choose, is just a fraction of the cost of most other augmentative devices. It has a vocabulary of over seven thousand items and close to eight thousand built-in symbols from SymbolStix. It has natural sounding text-to-speech voices from Acapela Group.

Proloquo2Go can be set up in either a list or a grid view. Vocabulary is set up in categories, which are color coded for parts of speech. It has text-to-speech and allows for the automatic conjugation of verbs and plurals and possessives for nouns using grammatical technology from Ultralingua. It is easy to customize and has basic tutorials that walk you through how different features of the application can be used or changed in order to fit the individual user's needs. This allows you to get started immediately without a complete understanding of the software and allows you to go back and make changes as you learn.

When you open the Proloquo2Go application you immediately come to the Home page screen. It is set up with folder-style items that contain information of different types. Items such as basic information you might need to tell people about yourself, greetings, basic starter phrases, questions, comments, a keyboard and a folder that brings you to all the categories of vocabulary that are available for your use. Tap on any item to make Proloquo2Go speak that item. To navigate to other categories simply press one of the folder-style items. At the top of the display is a Message Window. This will speak the currently displayed message. At the bottom of the page you will see the toolbar. This allows you to change between grid and list views, gives you access to punctuation, allows you to edit the page and will get you back to the home page. You can adjust what is available to match the needs and abilities of the user. You can allow them full capability of editing their own system down to locking them out completely to keep items from being changed or deleted by accident. To access the Proloquo2Go settings you need to exit Proloquo2Go and go to the iPhone/iPod/iPad home screen. At that point you tap on the icon of the Settings application and make any changes you feel appropriate for the current user.

Proloquo2Go can be used for a single user or multiple users depending on whether it belongs to a particular person or is being used for evaluation purposes. As the application is being customized the changes can be backed up to a computer in order to save the customized vocabulary in case of accidental deletions or changes to the work. As an evaluation tool, different set-ups can be backed-up and downloaded depending on who you are going to be working with.

Proloquo2Go also has six available settings: Appearance, Interaction, Restrictions, Speech, Grammar, and Demo Mode. These give you numerous options to allow for maximum customization for individual users.

Proloquo2Go allows you to choose whether or not there is a message displayed on the device or whether it is just spoken. You can choose how many items you have displayed on each page. You can start with one and move all the way to sixty-four if you are using an iPad. You can also change the color of the screen, text, text background and the item background. You also have the option of turning the color-coding off if desired. You can have the text appear above or below the images or have two lines of text.

Proloquo2Go allows you to customize how to access vocabulary not immediately visible on a single screen. You can choose to use the flicking motion to scroll line by line or a screen at a time.

In Restriction Settings you can restrict or allow as much access to the Edit mode as your user is capable of handling. This allows you to manage how much control you want the user to have in modifying what you have set up for them. This will help keep items from being accidentally deleted and changes being made to the vocabulary that you don't want.

Speech Settings allows you to determine when Proloquo2Go will speak. When users are in a classroom setting you may only want it to speak when a sentence is built and the Message Window is tapped. This is the "Speak message only" setting. If the user needs everything spoken in order to confirm their item choice then "Speak all items" should be used.

Grammar Settings allows you to keep the automatic conjugation and pluralization feature on or off. You can turn it off by turning off Grammar support. Whether or not you use this is determined by the user's capabilities.

Demo Mode allows you to restore Proloquo2Go to the default vocabulary, options and settings. You can choose to let it reset itself after quitting the application or after midnight (i.e. once a day). This might be something you would choose to leave on if you are evaluating or demonstrating to several individuals each day.

Adding new vocabulary items and editing existing ones is easy and can be done right on the iPhone, iPod touch or iPad. Proloquo2Go records all utterances created by the user and allows you to create unique vocabulary based on those utterances. For example, if a user generates unique vocabulary based on a specific activity, Proloquo2Go allows you to capture those utterances for future use.

Proloquo2Go also allows you to edit items in several ways. It allows you to use symbols from an existing library or you can import photos into the app. These allow for a high level of customization that is meaningful to each individual.

Proloquo2Go gives you an option of starting vocabulary sizes from very small to very large. You can choose which is most appropriate for the user's capabilities. This allows them to learn at the level they are currently at but can grow with them as they mature and become comfortable with the app.

Proloquo2Go will allow you to easily customize or create activity specific vocabulary. You can copy already created items and paste them from various locations within the app to a specific location. This allows you to quickly create vocabulary for an activity the user is going to participate in. For example, if you are going out to eat you can quickly copy vocabulary items that will allow the user to do his or her own ordering and/or interacting while in the restaurant.

This has been an excellent tool to use in helping people on the Autism Spectrum find a means of communication that is versatile and mobile. The inexpensiveness of the application with the iPod touch and iPad has made it feasible when expensive dedicated devices were not found to be the right fit. These devices are accepted socially by their peers and are yet another way to help them fit in.

Proloquo2Go is a versatile, mobile, inexpensive alternative to dedicated communication systems. It fills a much-needed niche in the array of communication choices for people who are nonverbal or have difficulty speaking.

TRADITIONAL AND INDIGENOUS HEALING

BY DR. LEWIS MEHL-MADRONA

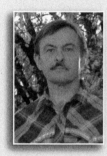

Lewis Mehl-Madrona, MD, Ph.D., MPhil

Education and Training Director
Coyote Institute for Studies of Change and Transformation
Burlington, VT and Honolulu, HI

Department of Family Medicine
University of Hawaii School of Medicine,Honolulu, HI

PO Box 9309, South Burlington, VT 05407.
mehlmadrona@gmail.com
(808) 772-1099

Dr. Lewis Mehl-Madrona graduated from Stanford University School of Medicine and completed his family medicine and his psychiatry training at the University of Vermont College of Medicine. He earned a Ph.D. in clinical psychology at the Psychological Studies Institute in Palo Alto and also became a licensed psychologist in California. He took a Master's in Philosophy degree from Massey University in New Zealand in Narrative Studies in Psychology. He is American Board certified in family medicine, geriatric medicine, and psychiatry. He is the author of *Coyote Medicine*, *Coyote Healing*, *Coyote Wisdom*, *Narrative Medicine*, and most recently, *Healing the Mind through the Power of Story: The Promise of Narrative Psychiatry*. He is the Education and Training Director for Coyote Institute for Studies of Change and Transformation, based in Burlington, Vermont and in Honolulu, Hawaii, and is Clinical Assistant Professor of Family Medicine at the University of Hawaii in Honolulu.

Recently, traditional cultural healings have become more widely discussed in the area of autism thanks to Rupert Isaacson's recent book and film about taking his son to African and then to Mongolian healers. Significant improvement occurred through this journey/interaction, though not cure. Parents are ever vigilant for new sources of miracles, and, thanks to the book, several parents of my patients are making the journey to Mongolia this next summer.

Isaacson noticed immediate improvement in his son's language skills when he started riding horses. He had previously trained horses for a living, but had never seen a horse and a child bond so spontaneously. Rowan's tantrums were nearly driving Isaacson and his wife, Kristin Neff, to divorce. All the while, his son was withdrawing more and more. Isaacson began riding Betsy, a neighbor's horse, with his son.

According to preliminary analysis of an ongoing study by Dismuke-Blakely, hippotherapy has been shown to increase verbal communication skills in some autistic children in as little as eighteen to twenty-five minutes of riding once a week for eight weeks. "We see their arousal and affect change. They become more responsive to cues. If they are at a point where they are using verbal cues, you get more words," Dismuke-Blakely said. "It's almost like it opens them up. It gives us access."

After about three weeks, Isaacson says, Rowan's improved behavior was translating into the home and outside world as well. But not consistently. In late 2004, Isaacson brought a delegation of African Bushmen from Botswana to the United Nations. The traditional healers of the group offered to work with Rowan. "For the four days while they were with him, he started to lose some of his symptoms. He started to point, which was a milestone he hadn't achieved," Isaacson said. When the tribal healers left, Rowan regressed.

Isaacson decided to visit healers in Mongolia, the oldest horseback culture on Earth. Just trekking across the Mongolian prairie on horseback changed his son's behavior dramatically.

"Rowan came back without three key dysfunctions that he had. He went out to Mongolia incontinent and still suffering from these neurological firestorms—so tantruming all the time and cut off from his peers, unable to make friends—and he came back with those three dysfunctions having gone. He's . . . becoming a very functional autistic person," Isaacson said (Bonifield, 2009).

Traditional healers abound here in North America, though the journey to reach them is less far, and probably less exotic. Traditional healing in North America includes elements of ceremony, manual medicine, energy medicine, storytelling, hypnosis, and psychotherapy. Indeed, traditional medicine could be the standard from which we evaluate more modern forms of psychotherapy, medicine, or healing. Traditional healers have been assisting children and adults diagnosed with autism for as long as this label has existed. Traditional healers use their gifts to assist the individual and the family to transform to the extent that the spirits who assist the healers can facilitate. Traditional healers do their work throughout the world, as evidenced by a brief mention of them in a South African medical article about autism (Mubaiwa, 2008).

Elsewhere (Mainguy & Mehl-Madrona, 2009), we have written about how traditional healers in North America go about doing this, and have compared the methods of traditional healers to those of contemporary creative arts therapists in terms of their use of art, music, and drama. For example, the Bonny Method of Guided Imagery and Music therapy integrates visual and auditory experience into a unified journey, similar to what traditional healers do

While considering traditional healers, we must not underestimate the use of the horse as a means to improve balance, strength, and motor coordination. As responsive, moving, and exciting living beings, horses can motivate and stimulate the child with autism in unique ways. Being on a horse may provide strong sensory stimulation to muscles and joints, impact the balance and movement sense detected by sensory receptors in the inner ear, and provide varied tactile experiences as the rider hugs or pats the horse. The therapist addresses communication goals by asking the rider to follow simple or multistep directions, such as "turn to face backwards and give me high five." The rider is encouraged to communicate directions to the horse to "go" or "whoa," by using words, sign language, or pointing to pictures. In addition, pulling on the reins indicates stop, and a kick tells the horse to get going. Clients are taught to relate appropriately to the horse with gentle pats. The consequences of inappropriate behaviors are easy to implement. The horse stops. Good behavior is rewarded with short trots.

Within the indigenous worldview, all healing is fundamentally "spiritual healing." Spirits are the source of all inspiration for healing. Spirits are everywhere. Spirits guide the treatment. Healers are adept at narratives without words. The sacred songs of ceremonies convey rich cultural messages through music. Elders teach people diagnosed with autism to participate in their specific socio-cultural context, through whole body communication. Rather than teaching a set of behaviors, the elders encourage increased self-awareness/self-other awareness, leading to more overt social interactions.

Music therapy principles can link to what elders do with children diagnosed with autism, and can play an important role for parents of children with autism by fostering relationships and developing positive interactions. Most approaches to music therapy rely on spontaneous musical improvisation just as elders do. Drumming has its impact in both traditional healing and musical therapy. Dance movement therapy and drama therapy are used with autistic children, just as traditional healers incorporate people diagnosed with autism into ongoing dance ceremonies. Body-centered therapies can bring important comfort to individuals struggling with autism, and parallel the spontaneous cultural therapies into which elders introduce autistic individuals.

Bernard Williams (1993) has proposed that all cultures share a "belief-desire-intent" psychology. Boyd (2009:257) notes that animals other than humans understand the concepts of desire and intention. Human children understand intention in their first year and desire by their second year. Belief-desire-intention represents a fundamental cross cultural psychology (Saxe, 2004; Premack & Premack, 2003). Autistic individuals lack the capacity to understand others' beliefs, desires, and intentions. Through stories and ceremony, traditional healers attempt to provide them with a better sense of others' beliefs, desires, and intentions.

Indigenous healers conceptualize illness very differently from conventional medicine.[2] Contemporary medicine bases its diagnoses on structural changes in tissues, while indigenous cultures are more concerned with disharmony and imbalances in social relationships (Mehl-Madrona, 2003). Medicine is noun based, while indigenous thought is verb based. While biomedicine traces the sources of structural tissue changes, indigenous healers contemplate the source for disturbances in the harmony of individuals within their communities and in all their relationships. When the harmony within relationships is disturbed, imbalances result that lead to illness and therefore to suffering. The two views are not necessarily contradictory. They can be linked, though not within the restricted perspective of contemporary biomedicine. The linkage occurs from our observation that sufficient degrees of disharmony and imbalance lead to tissue damage. It is associated with suffering. For example, different cytokines (messenger molecules of inflammation) are out of balance for a variety of disease (arthritis, asthma, diabetes). Different imbalances are seen for each disease; what is consistent is the presence of imbalance.

Most people spontaneously experience mental images while listening to music (Goldberg,1995). The musicality of traditional healers may be an important aspect of their ability to provide assistance to people with a diagnosis of autism.

The "natural history of disease" concept of biomedicine compares and contrasts to one of disharmony and imbalance, in which larger levels of disharmony are associated with greater strength for those forces that oppose health. To accept this, we must accept the idea that how we live and the stories we enact relate to the health of our bodies, and that our psychological resilience parallels, in some manner, our physical resilience. Biomedicine has difficulty traveling here, though the concept is becoming more commonly discussed in narrative medicine circles (Mehl-Madrona, 2007).

Storytelling seems to evoke a response from children with autism. They lack the usual intense interest in monitoring other people, and lack a well-developed theory of mind. They are relatively unable to tell a good story. Through the telling of stories in an inherent musicality, the elders help children to develop an interest in others, especially since so many of the characters in the stories are animals.

Ceremony

Here is a ceremony I watched an elder do with a person diagnosed with autism: The mother brought the son to the elder's home and we sat in the living room. We chatted while normal household activity transpired and then the elder took us into a small bedroom that he reserved for his healing activities. He took an iron pot and put sage into it. He lit that sage, and waved the smoke all around the child. He sang a song that I recognized as a spirit calling song. Then he talked to Hank, the child, about new beginnings, about letting everyone go and starting over. Then he drummed and sang with the child and prayed more. He waved his eagle feather over Hank and blessed him. He sang another prayer song and began a long chant with Hank. When it was over, Hank told him about six white geese feathers he found. He talked about and orange and gold sunset with geese and some buffalo horns he found.

Elsewhere, we (Mainguy & Mehl-Madrona, 2009) published three case stories of children who worked with elders:

Case 1. Regina was a twenty-four-year-old adult who had been diagnosed with moderately severe autism. She had lived most of her life in Pittsburgh, but had recently been brought back to her home reserve in upstate New York because her mother feared for her own health and wanted Regina to develop relationships with other relatives to sustain her, in the event that her mother became too ill to care for her or died.

When Regina first arrived, she showed minimal interest in any social relationships. Her interest instead was in cemeteries, which she visited for hours, as well as standing in what appeared to be strange postures for hours, or massaging herself. She also talked incessantly about the internal organs of the abdomen. When the traditional healer met her, the healer sat in the cemetery with her, speculated about which internal organ might be trying to speak, and gifted her with a new toy pickup truck. The healer also brought a drum. While they were doing other activities, the healer began to drum . . . and drum . . . and drum. Eventually Regina was engrossed in the drumming, nodding her head in rhythm. Finally the healer handed Regina the drum and invited her to play. Almost magically, another drum appeared and they banged away together.

I know that Regina's mother had given the healer tobacco in request for his help with Regina, but could afford little else. She had barely enough money to stay stocked with cigarettes. The healer clearly cared about Regina, as did others in the community. He kept coming to visit her. Slowly but surely they developed a relationship focused upon the drums. Subtly, the elder began to add singing and chanting to the drumming. Regina began humming along. Over time she began to learn the words. The elder sat with her periodically. The elder also gave Regina a can of paint and let her paint anything she wished on the elder's house. Michael spent hours on this project in which the elder, joined him occasionally, painting along with him or chatting away.

Eventually Regina began attending ceremonies. She appeared proud to be within the sweat lodge ceremony *(inipi)*, drumming. The elder gave her a special sweat drum to bring to ceremony. Regina was beginning to form social awareness. Over the course of the next two years, Regina became progressively more oriented into the healer's *hoc-okah*, or circle of people who relied upon him. Then her mother died. Regina cried, but virtually the entire community came out for him. The funeral lasted four days, as was customary. Regina was seamlessly integrated into the community. She danced at pow-wows. Over four years, she had developed a social self.

Case 2. Brad was a three-year-old child diagnosed with autism. Consistent with contemporary health care, Brad had waited eighteen months from recognition to diagnosis. No services were available to him once diagnosed. Donald lived on a reserve about two hours from any major urban area. Friends of Brad's mother encouraged her to connect with me. My first response, despite whatever else could be done, was to introduce Brad and his mother to one of the local healers. I encouraged Mary Jane, Brad's mother, to start coming to ceremony and bringing Brad, who was initially relatively new to human contact. This example convinced me that community could overcome great obstacles. We watched Brad make great strides to catch up with his age-mates. More than just the drumming and singing and dancing, Brad became a most adorable powwow dancer, even when he was clueless about how to dance. His mom learned to make elaborate costumes, which made up for his missed steps and puzzled expressions on his face.

More than the support for Brad, was the support for his single mother. People often underestimate the support that a community can provide, despite poverty and adverse conditions. Faye had previously run in a hard group—drugs, heavy drinking, and gangsters. The shock of Brad's diagnosis opened a door in her heart to embrace the traditional stories of her Cree origins. She sat for long talks with elders. She began learning traditional ways. Three years later, Brad was dramatically improved.

Case 3. Ralph was eight years old, and insisted on dressing like a rabbit. He wouldn't go outside without his bunny ears. He liked wearing bunny shoes as well. Ralph liked to watch fire. He lit matches whenever possible and stared at the flame until the fire burned his fingers. His parents lived in fear that he would burn down the house. He communicated very little, except through lighting fires.

Ralph couldn't sit unless he was wearing his bunny ears and his bunny shoes. Otherwise, he would pace incessantly. If enough time elapsed without his bunny slippers, he would begin to bang his head against the wall.

When Ralph's family moved back to the reserve (because a house opened in which they could live), Ralph was slowly adopted by the community. At first people were scared of him. With time, he grew on everyone. The elder began to invite him to light the fire to heat the stones for the sweat lodge ceremony. Others let him burn their garbage. Others protected him when he ventured into dangerous places on the reserve, and kept him from hurting himself. Eventually Ralph had free run of the entire reserve, because everyone took care of him.

Over time, Ralph became interested in the pipe. I suppose it was because it kept being lit on fire. Here is a story the elder told this autistic boy about his sacred pipe:

Ralph seemed to listen to the elder's stories indirectly. He slowed his play, attending longer to a particular object, and returned to his former speed and easy distractibility only after the story ended. Over time, Ralph began to act as if he were more aware of the elder. He slowly developed a sense of social relatedness, though it took four years for him to have a conversation with the elder. By eight years, Ralph was interacting almost normally. He seemed to respond to the containment by the community, to the persistent efforts of the elder to engage him, to the music, the rhythm, the consistency of humans in his life, and to the presence of his family.

Explanation

In each of my stories, the elders relied heavily upon drumming and singing to integrate the diagnosed with autism individuals into their circles of concern. In keeping with their general approach, they were completely permissive and non-judgmental, refusing to accept the autism diagnosis. Rather, as one elder said, "That's just how Michael is. He's okay. When he wants to be different, he will be. Until then, let him be." Within this permissive and accepting approach, Michael was encouraged to attend all ceremonies and powwows. The protection of the elder assured a minimum of teasing. Michael was encouraged to dance, regardless of how clumsy he looked. "We dance," the elder said, "because that is our nature."

Drama therapy is also used with autistic children, and relates directly to what elders do. Drama includes physical exercises that emphasize embodiment, discovery of the way we present ourselves in roles, and encourages a gently paced exploration of the self in the context of others (Landy, 1996). Drama therapy uses mirroring, a technique that encourages two people to mirror the movements of each other without words, which promotes understanding. Adding vocalization and then emotions can happen through mimicking correspondent facial and body tension. Therapists use a "back to back" game, which can be used to work with physical contact without eye contact. This gives the patient some indication of the impact of his strength on another body. Emotions, as different social attitudes can be sculpted on the other body, varying from a low to a high amount of physical contact, and playing on the repertoire of different social attitudes.

Thus, a traditional healing approach to autism uses elements of what conventional medicine calls spiritual healing, energy medicine, drama therapy, music therapy, and relationship to call forth a healing response. I suspect these approaches have evolved over thousands of years of trial and error with the affected person and have a stronger degree of success (based upon their sustainability) than we have yet appreciated.

TRANSCRANIAL DIRECT CURRENT STIMULATION, IMPLICIT TEACHING, AND SYNTAX ACQUISITION IN MINIMALLY VERBAL CHILDREN WITH AUTISM: GETTING KIDS TO SPEAK

BY DR. HARRY SCHNEIDER

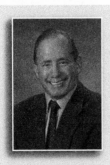

Harry D. Schneider, MD

146A Manetto Hill Road, Suite 207
Plainview, NY 11803
(516) 470-1930

491 North Indiana Avenue
Sellersburg, IN 47172
(516) 477-7682
hds7@columbia.edu or debra@harrydschneidermd.com
www.harrydschneidermd.com

- Advanced degrees in language and linguistics. Upcoming doctorate in Speech-Language Pathology.
- World Health Organization, Pan American Studies and Research
- A neuroscientist at Columbia University Medical Center, where he has specialized in understanding the language circuits of the brain, having sent his research on these topics for publication to eminent peer-reviewed journals (www.fmri.org)
- A research fellowship in Neuroimaging at the Program for Imaging and Cognitive Sciences, Columbia University Medical Center, New York, New York
- Specialized training in diagnosing and managing autism at the Neurologic and Psychiatric Institute in New York, New York
- Investigational studies and clinical trials using novel forms of language therapy combined with investigational use of music, cerebellar-based physical activities, and neuromodulation (transcranial electromagnetic stimulation) to restore language function in minimally verbal ASD children

Editor's Note: We preface Dr. Schneider's update with a selection from last year's chapter which serves to introduce the reader to the therapy elaborated on within:

After my linguistics lecture, the parents were still waiting for an answer to their original question: "How are you going to help my child?" I told them that the (functional MRI) fMRI neuroimaging study was the first part of my journey. The Columbia research work I had co-investigated led me to develop a treatment plan for autism, which I currently employ in my private practice on Long Island. I explained that this treatment protocol applies cutting-edge technology called transcranial direct-current stimulation (tDCS). It is the application of weak electrical currents (1–2 mA) to modulate the activity of neurons in the brain. When the electrode sponges are placed on the scalp, the amount of electricity produced in the brain is exceedingly small, changing the activity of the nerve cells minimally. In 1998, it was demonstrated that even a weak direct current delivered over the scalp can influence the excitability of the underlying cerebral cortex. These effects were reported to last for an appreciable amount of time after exposure.

TDCS is not "stimulation" in the same sense as conventional electric shock treatment for depression (it is 1/1,000—one millionth of that dose). It does not appear to cause nerve cell firing on its own and does not produce discrete effects such as the muscle twitches associated with classical stimulation. If a part of an existing speech network is not functional, we try to make it become functional, or create a different neural network to do the job; neurons are plastic and can take over the functions of other neurons, and it is possible to stimulate a brain's white matter and cause it to rewire. Currently tDCS is being studied for the treatment of a number of conditions, including major depression, brain injury affecting muscle movement, and memory. tDCS has been used to enhance associative verbal learning, a process by which a word is learned through association with a separate, pre-occurring word (king-queen). This is an implicit skill, crucial for both acquiring new languages in healthy individuals and for language reacquisition after neurological damage. Therapeutic cortical stimulation in general has become applicable to many conditions, from motor disorders (e.g., Parkinson's disease) to depression. In this study, we are attempting to restore function to those areas of the brain that deal with the acquisition of grammar. These sites of action can be distant from the site of stimulation with tDCS, because axons with remote projections are more prone to be activated than local cell bodies. We have also noted that functional and clinical effects occur both during and beyond the time of stimulation, which relates to processes of synaptic plasticity induced by the stimulation. The cortical stimulation we use may activate, various cortico-subcortical networks (the grammar machine), depending on what part of the brain we attempt to stimulate.

It is said that when a dog bites a man, that is not news, but when a man bites a dog, that is news. In this simple sentence, the order of the nouns placed in the subject and object positions were simply reversed, thereby rendering it newsworthy. Every language has rules of word order: where do the subject, verb and object go in the sentence? In the English sentence above, "The man bites the dog," the word order is Subject-Verb-Object (SVO); this is the standard word order in English. In German, however, if we want to learn German, we have to say, "Ich möchte Deutsch lernen," or literally "I want German to learn." Here the sentence has a Subject-Object-Verb (SOV) construction. These linguistic rules are referred to as syntax, which consists of the principles of word order for constructing sentences to properly convey intention and which may impart meaning. For those of you reading this article who speak more than one language, see which order your native language uses. For example, the SVO construction is used in English, Spanish, French, Italian, Bulgarian and Chinese. The SOV order is used in Japanese, Turkish, Korean, and many of the Indian dialects, such as Hindi, Tamil and Telugo to name a few.

Most people reading this article know the core features of autism: difficulty with social interactions, stereotypical behaviors and deficits in language function and communication. This is a very short version of the core features, to be sure. Many parents want to know why minimally verbal children can understand much more than they can speak and why children who have more verbal language cannot initialize or maintain a conversation. When typical children, or those of who have mastered a second language begin to speak fluently, the use of syntax becomes automatic, unconscious and systematic. To get a little technical here, we linguists say that such fluent use of the grammar and syntax has achieved "linguistic competence." This type of knowledge is actually *implicit* and is referred to as *knowing how*. It is information we recall unconsciously in order to do things like tie our shoes, ride a bicycle, or drive a car. Implicit memory is a type of memory in which previous experiences help us in things we do on a daily basis without conscious awareness of them. When we speak our native language, we really don't have to think before we talk (which often gets us into trouble), unless we are trying to think of a particular way to say what we want to convey to others.

There is a actually a brain network dedicated to implicit memory, which in neuroscience terms is called the "procedural memory network." The ability to perform skills and procedures without thinking (knowing how) is part of this specialized brain network and is responsible for linguistic competence. On the other hand, learning words, such as "book" or "juice" is a different story. Our ability to learn words is *explicit and conscious* and is referred to as *knowing that*. This type of knowledge is stored in the brain in separate areas and pathways from those used for grammar. It is part of a system we call the "declarative memory netork." These two neural networks, one implicit for grammar and one explicit for vocabulary, are responsible for learning language. And to make things even more complicated, we all must learn a part of language we call *pragmatics,* or we will never become fluent! Pragmatics is involved with how we convey the meaning of what we say. It depends not only on grammar and vocabulary, but also how we think people will understand our statement and what we intend to say often without even saying it. Some examples of pragmatics are: "I am sure you are all taking notes on this technical stuff"; "Flying planes can be dangerous"; and "I love your tie. Did you get it at a garage sale?" I will not get into pragmatics in this paper except to say that we finally have children who have mastered enough grammar to become conversational and now these children need to know that, "Really? Get outta here!" really means "that's hard to believe," not that they actually have to leave my office.

Language abnormalities are often the first symptoms of autism alerting parents to a possible communication delay. Standardized diagnostic testing such as the Autism Diagnostic Observation Schedule-Generic (ADOS-G) and the Autism Diagnostic Interview-Revised (ADI-R) employ standardized behavioural evaluations. Neuroimaging techniques such as functional magnetic resonance imaging (fMRI) and diffusion tensor imaging (DTI) are being used to complement the findings of behavioural testing. There is currently an investigation at Columbia University addressing the issue of diagnostic testing for children with autism in which fMRI is used as a potential indicator of autism and attempts to demonstrate that language disability due to autism can be detected by objective imaging techniques. While children are listening to recordings of their parents, fMRI activation within language-sensitive brain areas can distinguish between minimally-verbal children and normal controls (not often seen on regular MRI). The application of fMRI to determine physiological differences between autism and other developmental disorders may provide an objective biomarker to distinguish among other disorders. There are subtle differences in neuroanatomical features between autistic, specific language impairment(SLI)and attention-deficit-hyperactivity disorder (ADHD) subjects and fMRI may help in the diagnosis. Other neuroimaging studies have demonstrated both dysfunctional brain areas and aberrant connectivity patterns in patients with autism . The structural anatomy of the basal ganglia (BG), deep brain structures often referred to as being part of the primitive or reptilian brain are deformed and the cortical areas to which their axons projects (such as Broca's speech area) are pathologically distributed. These studies suggest that during the period of first language acquisition in infancy in children with autism, neurotypical pathways used for implicit (procedural) grammar acquisition became dysfunctional and inhibited normative implicit language. To state it more directly, grammar pathways in the brain did not develop normally and most kids with autism did not get their grammar!

Parents continue to seek treatment modalities to restore functional language. Treatment methods including behavioural interventions, traditional pharmacotherapy and complementary/alternative therapies have not shown significant success in increasing functional language. I have mentioned before that scientific research has demonstrated the success of neuromodulation techniques such as transcranial direct current stimulation (TDCS) will soon become a new, mainstream treatment modality for general cognitive dysfunctions. It is already being used in universities all around the world for language treatments , short-term memory loss language recovery from post-stroke aphasia and other language acquisition difficulties. It was shown to be successful in the facilitation of language acquisition for children with developmental disabilities. It demonstrated an increase in general sound and speech production in children age 3 to 6 with developmental delays without noticeable side effects.

As mentioned in my previous article in Cutting Edge Therapies for Autism, we have been evaluating children with autism at Columbia University and our Center for Medical and Brain Sciences (CMBS) in Long Island. We have been clinically assessing and treating children with autism with TDCS to modulate different features of language. In addition to traditional explicit language therapies (conscious learning) we must use implicit (unconscious) learning strategies to facilitate the acquisition of the rules of language . Our techniques are based on affective-humanistic activities to activate imagination, problem-solving activities, and interactive games. An overview of our children's language deficits, specifically those whose syntax was immature, demonstrated a need for us to formalize an appropriate protocol to assess and treat these deficits in syntax. We began conducting pilot studies to examine the strengths and weaknesses of our existing methodology to find the best platform for combining evaluations with treatments. The purpose of this was to publish an institutional review board (IRB) approved, peer-reviewed research investigation that would validate the clinical work we have been doing for years. We have finally completed this study of minimally verbal children with autism and it has been accepted for publication by a peer-reviewed journal. I shall notify all those who are interested when the paper becomes available.

For this particular paper, we elected to evaluate syntax acquisition in a population of children who had not yet developed this important skill, one that leads to fluency in language. Remember, as boring as it may sound, language proficiency is all about grammar! That said, I strongly emphasize that for children to be able to progress to the critical phase of acquiring grammar and syntax, they must first successfully go through some linguistic 'milestones': a prelinguistic communication period. It has long been known that, prior to attaining grammar and syntax, typically developing (TD) children demonstrate increasing abilities in conveying meaning to interactive part-ners. The children use intentional communication behaviors that have been shown to be *predictive* of normal language functioning. These behaviours, such as vocalizations and appropriate gestures need to have a particular function or meaning . They might take the form of communicative requests, comments, or even protests that a child intends to convey. The best outcomes for successful language development is that all these pre-linguistic behaviors display dome degree of joint attention. We have shown that in children with autism, achieving these same prelinguistic 'milestones' found in typical children are equally necessary before grammar can be acquired. Displaying these types of intentional communication are also very predictive of better language outcomes.

A rationale for our study was to see whether tDCS would bring about syntax acquisition in children with autism who had achieved these prelinguistic milestones, had all received both intensive speech and ABA therapies, but had still not yet acquired basic syntax. We had not witnessed *novel* verbal utterances in these children; rather we had been hearing their use of explicitly memorized phrases and simple repetitions of basic sentences—all this being indications of *not* having acquired syntax. Children with autism are often trained to respond to questions ('what is this'?) with scripted answers ('this is a book'), but are not able to generalize the notion of word order to novel sen-tences. We noted that these children also had reading comprehension difficulties at an entry level of academic complexity. We know that this lack of reading comprehension is consistent with an immature and underdeveloped level of syntax.

The study we have done will show that syntax acquisition in minimally verbal chil-dren with autism can be achieved with the use of Tdcs. Simply put, this study demon-strated a large difference in syntax scores before and after the use of tDCS. Not all of the children achieved 100 percent syntax accuracy even after brain stimulation. We should remember that acquisition of syntax is a slower process than learning vocabulary, as we have seen in typical infant development. The significant improvement seen in these children on the test most likely represent a rapid, but incomplete early phase of syntax learning that usually generalizes over time to other syntactic tasks. This is consistent with how the basal ganglia in our brains slowly process these grammatical, procedural rules. Infants start with slowly absorbing basic word order over years and eventually progress to more complex sentences. They do get there and they become quite chatty. We expect in time that many children on the spectrum will go through this same pro-cess—for the first time perhaps—and with careful guidance and continued stimulation of brain areas that are not yet completely functional, they will make it!

We noted during the vocabulary portion of this study that there were some chil-dren who obtained who had perfect scores on a vocabulary test, even before stimu-lation with tDCS. We were curious about the significance of this finding. We used statistical analyses to investigate any relationship between their scores on the vocabulary test and the syntax test. What we found was quite interesting and we think of importance to educators. Those children who had perfect scores on the vocabulary test performed worse on the syntax test! We admit that this should not be interpreted to mean that high vocabulary scores predict low syntax scores or that a great knowledge of vocabulary can adversely affect a child's ability to acquire grammar and syntax. One the one hand, this finding demonstrates simply that in minimally verbal children with autism, there may not be a strong relationship between vocabulary size and the ability to acquire syntax. On the other hand, it seems to confirm the linguistic theory that we have been postulating over the years and certainly in the previous Cutting Edge article: children with autism with particularly weak implicit, unconscious memory systems (due to the damage to these brain areas from autism) must rely to a greater extent on their conscious, explicit memory. We have all seen some children do well with vocabulary learning. We have scientifically shown that this is not something they can apply to learning grammar and syntax. In other words, the unconscious acquisition of grammar and syntax is not related to memorized vocabulary. The better their declarative memory for the use of consciously memorized words, the more children seem to rely on this same learning system to solve other tasks (as do normal second-language learners after the age of 6 or 7). This is a difficult concept to grasp and the explanation is described within the framework of the declarative/procedural model we cited in previous studies. The declarative (conscious) memory system is not related to nor does it transfer information to the procedural (unconscious) memory systems.

Let's return again to this idea of two memory systems: the declarative and procedural systems. This is a crucial element of language learning that can no longer be ignored, especially when thought is given to how we are going to rehabilitate and restore language function in minimally-verbal children with autism. We have seen that when people speak fluently, the way in which they use the rules of their grammar is methodical and systematic, not deviating from a certain norm that we all accept as correct language. This is what happens in typical children who are *not* taught how language works. Infants acquire this 'linguistic competence' incidentally (for example, they may consciously focus on the meaning of a sentence while at the same time they are unconsciously internalizing its syntactic structure!). Implicit memory is evolutionarily very old and considered the norm in many animal species in our world, while explicit memory appears in only the most evolved species. During the first year of life, an infant possess only implicit memory while explicit memory emerges later. Three year old children still display an unconscious implicit memory system that is better than their conscious explicit memory.

When you turn on a light switch at home, how do you know where it is without thinking, and how do you know which way to get hot water as opposed to cold when you turn on the faucet? Just as typical adults do, the infant's mind absorbs subtle patterns and learns about the world indirectly. The study of implicit learning is a relatively new frontier in psychology, but it has the potential to not only revolutionize how we understand our experiences, but to allow us to optimize approaches to learning new information, such as the learning of grammar rules in children with autism. This is the kind of learning that happens when minimally verbal children are playing, listening to music, or jumping on a trampoline—that is when they are focused on enjoying themselves—they are unconsciously and incidentally picking up rules of grammar by a sort of 'osmosis'. As they unconsciously learn new motor skills such as skipping or walking down the stairs, they also unconsciously acquiring the 'skills' of the rules or their language– as long as they are listening to someone speak in full sentences to them at the same time. Children will inadvertently pick up new cognitive skills and unconsciously develop intuitions about how other people will act. We think that for children with autism it is much more important for them to adapt to new places and people than to devote more time to conscious forms of learning, such as memorizing words. Implicit learning is outside of awareness and educators do not often realize how important it is. Despite new and important studies showing that implicit learning is essential for learning about many properties of our world and the people in it, declarative learning and memory (our ability to memorize facts) has received much more attention than implicit learning. This has occurred in part because implicit learning is a less obvious phenomenon and is difficult to observe and measure. This style of learning is subtle, and occurs without intention or conscious awareness that the learning is taking place. It is also not easy to explain. Often people can't fully articulate what they've learned, even though they may have absorbed and retained significant amounts of information.

We must remember that our imaging studies have shown that these autistic children have brain areas and conections that are not functional for all aspects of language: the grammar pathways are simply 'broken'. We have shown that tDCS, together with both explicit and implicit language learning, is capable of restoring language to minimally children with autism. I personally want to appeal to parents, speech therapists , ABA interventionists and all health-care professionals involved in treating autism that children will not be able to speak fluently and functionally unless all these types of language teaching are incorporated into one language program. To the wonderful supermoms and dads of children on the spectrum I say that you must continue to ensure that your child has these services available, that all efforts are made to ensure that children are at their behavioral best—not an easy task to be sure—and that you never give up hope that your child, at any age, can manage to converse with you one day.

TRANSCRANIAL MAGNETIC STIMULATION

BY DR. JOSHUA BARUTH, DR. JOSHUA M. BARUTH, DR. ESTATE SOKHADZE, DR. AYMAN EL-BAZ, DR. GRACE MATHAI, DR. LONNIE SEARS, AND DR. MANUEL F. CASANOVA

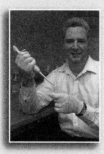

Joshua M. Baruth, PhD[1,2]
Estate Sokhadze PhD,[2]
Ayman El-Baz, PhD[3]
Grace Mathai, PhD[4]
Lonnie Sears, PhD [4]
Manuel F. Casanova, PhD [1,2]

Affiliations:

[1] Department of Anatomical Sciences and Neurobiology, University of Louisville School of Medicine, Louisville, KY 40202,
[2] Department of Psychiatry and Behavioral Sciences, University of Louisville School of Medicine, Louisville, KY 40202,
[3] Department of Bioengineering, University of Louisville J.B. Speed School of Engineering, Louisville, KY 40208,
[4] Department of Pediatrics, University of Louisville School of Medicine, Louisville, KY 40202

Dr. Manuel Casanova did his basic training at the University of Puerto Rico and continued his specialty training at the Johns Hopkins University and the National Institutes of Mental Health. He is a Board Certified Neurologist with specialty training in both Neuropathology and Psychiatry. At present Dr. Casanova serves as the Vice Chair for Research within the Department of Psychiatry at the University of Louisville. He is also the Gottfried and Gisela Kolb Endowed Chair in Psychiatry for the same institution. Dr. Casanova was a founding member of the National Alliance for Autism Research (now merged with Autism Speaks) and the Autism Tissue Program. He chaired for several years the Developmental Brain Disorders Study section of the National Institute of Health. He serves as an editor for five different journals. Among his many recognitions Dr. Casanova is the recipient of an EUREKA award from the NIMH for innovative research in regards to autism. In 2010 he was a plenary speaker at the World Organization of Autism Congress in Monterrey Mexico. His CV shows 191 refereed articles, 49 books chapters, 3 edited books, and close to 300 congress presentations.

Transcranial magnetic stimulation (TMS) allows scientists to stimulate the brain noninvasively in alert, awake patients. The first TMS device that could stimulate focal regions of the brain was developed in Sheffield, England by A.T. Barker and colleagues in 1985 (Barker et al., 1985). TMS operates based on Faraday's law of electromagnetic induction (1831) which describes the process by which electrical energy is converted into magnetic fields and vice versa. The TMS apparatus achieves the induction of a magnetic field by using a power supply to charge capacitors which are then discharged through the TMS coil and this creates a magnetic field pulse. The principle of electromagnetic induction proposes that a changing magnetic field induces the flow of electric current in a nearby conductor--in this case the neurons below the stimulation site. Typically TMS coils are designed to produce magnetic fields in the range of 1 tesla (T) which is powerful enough to cause neuronal depolarization. The focal point of stimulation is about 1 cm^2 in area, and maximal induction is proposed at 90 degrees to the magnetic field (see George & Belmaker, 2007).

TMS can be administered in a single-pulse manner where single or paired pulses are delivered non-rhythmically and not more than once every few seconds or repetitively (rTMS) where pulses are delivered at specific frequencies in trains with precise inter-train intervals (ITI). Generally, single-pulse TMS is used for physiological research or diagnostic purposes while rTMS is used to alter the excitability and function of targeted areas of cortex. rTMS can be divided into low-frequency rTMS (≤1Hz) and high-frequency rTMS (>1Hz), which categorically affect cortical excitability in different ways. Studies have shown that low-frequency or 'slow' rTMS (≤1Hz) increases inhibition of stimulated cortex (e.g., Maeda et al., 2000), whereas high-frequency rTMS (>1Hz) increases excitability of stimulated cortex (e.g., Pascual-Leone et al., 1994). It has been proposed that the effect of 'slow' rTMS arises from increases in the activation of inhibitory circuits (Pascual-Leone et al., 2000). Long-term potentiation may be a model for understanding the mechanisms of high frequency rTMS, whereas long-term depotentiation (whereby synaptic weights are "reset" to baseline levels) may be proposed as the most relevant model for understanding the inhibitory effect of low-frequency rTMS (Hoffmann & Cavus, 2002). (see Hoffman & Cavus, 2002 for review).

rTMS is a simple outpatient procedure lasting approximately 20 minutes. Patients are seated in comfortable, reclining chair and are fitted with a swim cap to outline the TMS coil position and aid in its placement for each session. Before the procedure begins the 'motor threshold' is determined in each patient. 'Motor threshold' is the intensity of the pulse delivered over the motor cortex that produces a noticeable motor response. Sensors are applied to the hand muscle (i.e., the first dorsal interosseous) opposite the site of stimulation and motor responses are monitored with physiological monitoring tools on a PC computer. The output of the machine is gradually increased by 5% until a 50μV deflection on the monitor (i.e., electromyograph) or a visible twitch of the muscle is observed. Once the patient's 'motor threshold' is determined the coil is moved to the site of stimulation (e.g., the prefrontal cortex) and the pulse intensity is adjusted relative to the patient's 'motor threshold'. Common dosing schedules include one to two visits per week, and typically patients are welcome to read a book or magazine during the procedure (Fig. 1).

TMS is generally regarded as safe without lasting side effects. Reported side effects include a mild, transient tension-type headache on the day of stimulation and mild discomfort due to the sound of the pulses; earplugs are recommended especially at higher frequencies of stimulation. Given the modulatory effect of rTMS on cortical excitability, there is a very small risk of inducing a seizure with rTMS (see Wasserman et al., 1996). Given this risk, participants with epilepsy or a family history of epilepsy are generally excluded of rTMS studies, and as a safety precaution, most rTMS studies adjust the stimulation intensity below the participants 'motor threshold' (e.g., 90% of motor threshold). rTMS is generally considered safe for use in pediatric populations, as no significant adverse effects or seizures have been reported (see Quintana, 2005 for review)

rTMS has been applied to a wide variety of psychiatric (e.g. ADHD, depression) and neurological disorders (e.g. Parkinson's Disease). A number of studies report an improvement in mood after repeated frontal lobe stimulation in depression (e.g. George et al., 1995), and it has been found that rTMS may improve certain symptoms associated with anxiety disorders, like Post Traumatic Stress Disorder (PTSD) and Obsessive-Compulsive Disorder (OCD) (see George & Belmaker, 2007). In Attention Deficit Hyperactivity Disorder (ADHD) TMS has proven to be a useful tool for investigating neurophysiological mechanisms underlying ADHD symptomatology. In Parkinson's disease (PD) most studies to date have shown beneficial effects of rTMS on clinical symptoms (Wu et al., 2008).

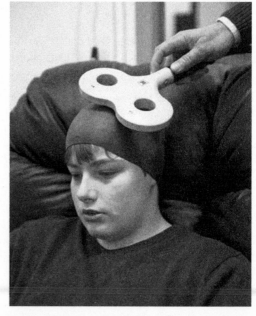

Within the context of autism spectrum disorders (ASD) rTMS has unique applications as a treatment modality. ASD is associated with disturbances in social interaction and communication, restricted and stereotyped behavioral patterns, and frequently abnormal reactions to the sensory environment (American Psychiatric Association, 2000; Charman, 2008). It has been suggested that a

Figure 1. Patient receiving Transcranial Magnetic Stimulation treatment.

wide range of deficits in autism might be understood by an increase in the ratio of cortical excitation to cortical inhibition (Casanova et al., 2003; Rubenstein & Merzenich, 2003) and increases in local cortical connectivity accompanied by deficiencies in long-range connectivity (Casanova et al., 2006b; Rippon et al., 2007). Locally overconnected neural networks may explain the superior ability of autistic children in isolated tasks (e.g., visual discrimination), while, at the same time, deficiencies in long-range connectivity may explain other features of the disorder (e.g., lack of social reciprocity). An increased ratio of cortical excitation to inhibition and higher-than-normal cortical 'noise' may explain the strong aversive reactions to auditory, tactile, and visual stimuli frequently recorded in autistic individuals as well as a higher incidence of epilepsy (Gillberg & Billstedt, 2000).

One possible explanation for higher-than-normal cortical noise and abnormal neural connectivity in ASD is the recent finding of minicolumnar abnormalities. Minicolumns are considered the basic anatomical and physiological unit of the cerebral cortex (Mountcastle, 2003), and contain pyramidal cells that extend the cortical width surrounded by a neuropil space consisting of several species of GABAergic, inhibitory interneurons (i.e. double-bouquet, basket, and chandelier cells) (Casanova, 2007). The double-bouquet cells impose a strong vertically directed stream of inhibition (Mountcastle, 2003) surrounding the minicolumnar core. The narrow vertical distribution of the double bouquet cells is so specific and restricted that it creates a narrow vertical cylinder of inhibition running geometrically perpendicular to the surface of the brain (Mountcastle, 1997; Douglas & Martin, 2004). Our preliminary studies indicate that minicolumns are reduced in size and increased in number in the brain of autistic individuals, especially the prefrontal cortex (Casanova et al., 2002ab, 2006ab). More specifically minicolumns in the brains of autistic patients are narrower and contain less peripheral, neuropil space (Casanova, 2006ab). The lack of a 'buffer zone' normally afforded by lateral inhibition and appropriate neuropil space may adversely affect the functional distinctiveness of minicolumnar activation and could result in isolated islands of coordinated excitatory activity (i.e., possible seizure foci); this autonomous cortical activity may hinder the binding of associated cortical areas, arguably promoting focus on particulars as opposed to general features. In addition the effect of loss of surround inhibition may result in an increase in the ratio of cortical excitation to inhibition and signal/sensory amplification which may impair functioning, raise physiological stress, and adversely affect social interaction in patients with ASD.

We hypothesize that contrary to other inhibitory cells (i.e., basket and chandelier), whose projections keep no constant relation to the surface of the cortex, the geometrically exact orientation of double-bouquet cells and their location at the periphery of the minicolumn (inhibitory surround) makes them the appropriate candidate for induction by a magnetic field applied parallel to cortex (Fig 2). Over a course of treatment 'slow' rTMS may restore the balance between cortical excitation and cortical inhibition and lead to improved long-range cortical connectivity.

Thus far our laboratory has focused on clinical, behavioral, and neuroimaging outcome measures, in order to access the effectiveness of rTMS treatment in ASD. One neuroimaging modality that has unique applications to ASD research is electro-encephalography (EEG). EEG is the non-invasive measurement of the summation of postsynaptic currents via scalp electrodes; the oscillatory frequency ranges of the post-synaptic currents can be divided into delta (0-4Hz), theta (4-8Hz), alpha (8-12Hz), beta (12-30Hz) and gamma (30-80Hz) frequencies. It is well known that the generation of normal gamma oscillations directly depends on the integrity of networks of inhibi-tory interneurons within cortical minicolumns (Whittington et al., 2000). Addition-ally the synchronization of cortical activity over wide-ranging cortical regions in the gamma range as been linked to the connectivity or 'coherence' of assemblies of neurons working on the same object (percept, idea, cognition) (Brown et al., 2005).

In one of our recent investigations (Sokhadze et al., 2009b) we measured the EEG gamma band in 12 children with ASD and 12 controls during a visual attention task and then measured the EEG gamma band in the ASD group after 6 sessions of 'slow' rTMS to the prefrontal cortex. We hypothesized that the ASD group would have excess gamma band activity due a lack of cortical inhibition and treatment with 'slow' rTMS would help restore inhibitory tone (i.e., reduce excess gamma band activity). We also ana-

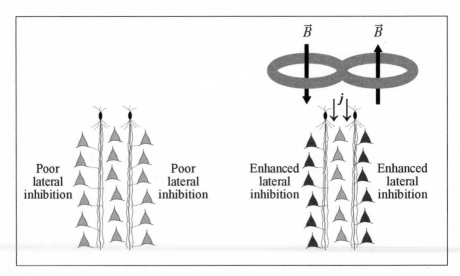

Figure 2. Magnetic field applied parallel to the cortex enhances surround inhibition on the periphery of the minicolumn.

lyzed clinical and behavioral questionnaires assessing changes in symptoms associated with ASD after rTMS treatment. The visual attention task employed Kanizsa, illusory figures which have been shown to readily produce gamma oscillations during visual tasks (Fig. 3). Subjects are instructed to press a button when they see the target Kanizsa square and ignore all other stimuli: Kanizsa stimuli consist of inducer disks of a shape feature and either constitute an illusory figure (square, triangle) or not (colinearity feature); in non-impaired individuals gamma activity has been found to increase during the presentation of target visual stimuli compared to non-target stimuli.

We found that the power of gamma oscillations was higher in the ASD group and had an earlier onset compared to controls--especially in response to non-target illusory figures over the prefrontal cortex (Fig. 4). Additionally there was less of a difference in gamma power between target and non-target stimuli in the ASD group particularly over lateral frontal and parietal recording sites. After 6 sessions of 'slow' rTMS applied to the left prefrontal cortex the power of gamma oscillations to non-target Kanizsa figures dramatically decreased at frontal and parietal sites on the same side of stimulation, and there was more of a difference between gamma responses to target and non-target stimuli. According to clinical and behavioral evaluations the ASD group showed a significant improvement on the repetitive behavior scale (RBS) which assesses repetitive and restricted behavior patterns associated with ASD (e.g., stereotyped, self-injurious, compulsive, and restricted range) (Bodfish et al., 1999).

In a more recent investigation with more participants (Baruth et al., 2010a) we investigated gamma band activity in 25 subjects with ASD and 20 age-matched controls using Kanizsa illusory figures and assessed the effects of 12 sessions of bilateral 'slow' rTMS applied to the prefrontal cortices in 16 of the ASD participants. In individuals

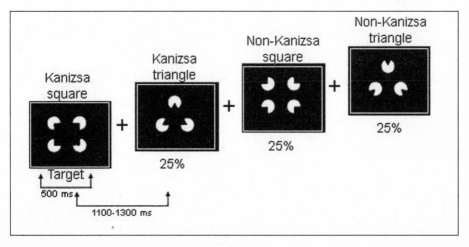

Figure 3. Target and Non-target Kanizsa illusory figures.

with ASD gamma activity was not discriminative of stimulus type, whereas in controls early gamma power differences between target and nontarget stimuli were highly significant. Following rTMS individuals with ASD showed significant improvement in discriminatory gamma activity between relevant and irrelevant visual stimuli, and there was also a significant reduction in irritability and repetitive (Fig 5 & 6).

In another investigation our laboratory analyzed gamma coherence before and after 12 sessions of 'slow' rTMS in 14 subjects with ASD. Analysis at 4 sites of EEG over frontal and parietal sites revealed significantly lower coherence in the ASD group before rTMS while after rTMS there was a significant improvement pointing to an increase in global cortical connectivity.

We have also been interested in investigating event-related potentials (ERP) abnormalities in ASD: ERPs provide a neurobiological measure of perceptual and cognitive processing and represent scalp-recorded, transient changes in the electrical activity of the brain in relation to the onset of a stimulus. In a previous paper (Sokhadze, et al. 2009a) we investigated ERPs in a three-stimuli, visual task of selective attention in 11 high-functioning children and young adults with autism spectrum disorder (ASD) and 11 age-matched, typically developing control subjects. Patients with ASD showed significantly amplified and prolonged cortical responses to irrelevant, visual stimuli compared to controls; these results were recently confirmed in a following study assessing ERP responses in 15 subjects with ASD and 15 controls in a similar task using illusory figures (Baruth et al., 2010b).

In a follow-up investigation (Sokhadze, et al. 2009c) we assessed the effects of 6 sessions of 'slow' rTMS stimulation applied to the left prefrontal cortex on performance in a three-stimuli, visual task of selective attention, as well as clinical and behavioral questionnaires in 13 individuals with ASD. Low-frequency rTMS minimized early cortical responses to

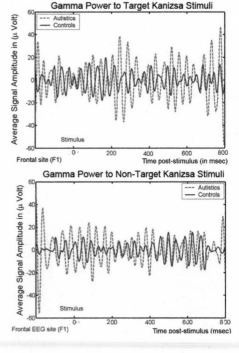

Figure 4. Gamma power is higher in ASD group as compared to controls, especially to non-target stimuli.

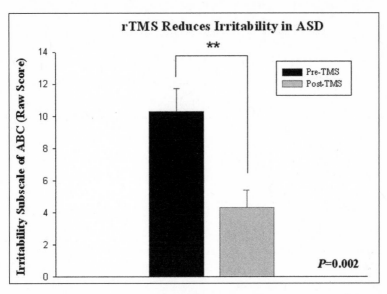

Figure 5. rTMS treatment resulted in a significant reduction in irritability in ASD (Baruth et al., 2010a).

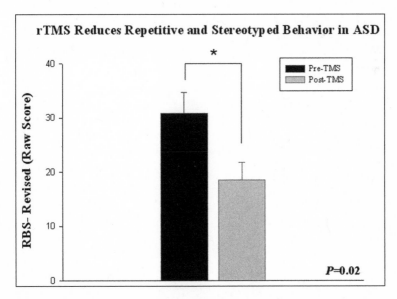

Figure 6. rTMS treatment resulted in a significant reduction in repetitive and stereotyped behavior in ASD (Baruth et al., 2010a).

irrelevant stimuli in this task and increased responses to relevant stimuli indicating improved selectivity and better stimulus differentiation. Additionally, there was a significant reduction in the percentage of errors in motor responses to target stimuli and in agreement with our previous results (Baruth et al., 2010a; Sokhadze et al., 2009b) we found a significant reduction in repetitive behavior according to the RBS. Furthermore, these results were recently confirmed in 24 subjects with ASD by finding significantly improved ERP indices of attention and executive functioning after 12 sessions of bilateral 'slow' rTMS applied to the prefrontal cortices. (Fig. 7).

Our findings of excessive gamma oscillations and ERP responses in visual tasks are in agreement with other studies noting that neural systems in the brains of autistic patients are often inappropriately activated (e.g., Belmonte & Yurgelin-Todd, 2003); this may be due to a disruption in the ratio between cortical excitation and inhibition (Casanova et al., 2002ab; Casanova, 2006ab; Rubenstein and Merzenich, 2003). In autism, increased cortical activity made evident by gamma and ERP responses indicate that activity induced by perceptual processes starts earlier and continues longer, because the neural networks subserving cognitive processes involved in combining information processing are not functioning normally. A reduction in the ability to decrease these cortical responses may reflect inhibitory deficits, and may result in the brain of autistic patients being over-activated. Abnormally large cortical responses to sensory stimuli (i.e. signal/sensory amplification) may play an important role in the manifesta-

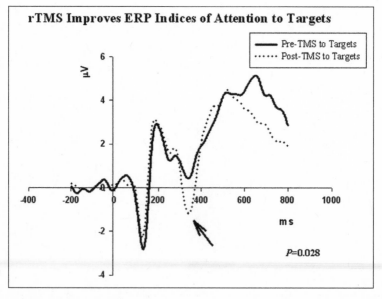

Figure 7. ERP indices of attention and executive functioning were significantly improved as a result of rTMS treatment.

tion of symptoms of ASD (e.g. sensory hypersensitivity, impaired social interaction). Enhanced and weakly differentiated responses to both target and non-target stimuli in sensory specific cortical areas (e.g., visual cortex at occipital EEG sites) and low functional connectivity supports the hypothesis of abnormal regional activation patterns (local over-processing vs. global under-processing).

Overall, our preliminary results show promising results for TMS as a treatment modality targeting core symptoms of ASD. Treatment with 'slow' rTMS decreased excess gamma activity and amplified ERP responses in ASD patients during visual tasks and improved the signal differentiation between processing relevant and irrelevant stimuli (Baruth et al., 2010a; Sokhadze et al., 2009bc). Treatment also provided a significant reduction in the percentage of errors in motor responses to target stimuli (Sokhadze, et al. 2009c). Additionally 'slow' rTMS dramatically improved the coordinated activity or coherence between different regions of the brain and significantly improved repetitive and restricted behavior patterns associated with ASD (Baruth et al., 2010a; Sokhadze et al., 2009bc). Our results suggest that low-frequency rTMS may improve the inhibitory tone and decrease the ratio of cortical excitation to inhibition in ASD, and this may lead to improved long-range connectivity. TMS has the potential to become an important therapeutic tool in ASD treatment and may play an important role in improving the quality of life of many with the disorder.

VISION THERAPY

by Dr. Jeffrey Becker

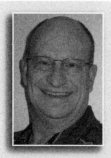

Jeffrey Becker, OD

NeuroSensory Center of Eastern Pennsylvania
250 Pierce Street, Suite 317
Kingston, Pennsylvania 18704
(570) 763-0054
Jbecker@Keystonensc.com
www. Keystonensc.com

Dr. Becker is a neurodevelopmental/behavioral optometrist with board certification and specialty training in neurosensory disorders. Dr. Becker is a Defeat Autism Now! (DAN!)-certified clinician. He is the director of Vision Rehabilitation Services for the Neurosensory Center of Eastern Pennsylvania. He has participated in multiple research projects involving neurologically impaired individuals. He has spoken about vision and learning at national and international autism conferences. He most recently published an article in *Autism File* is titled "Vision Therapy Can Help Children with Spectrum Disorders." Dr. Becker is also an adjunct faculty member of Misercordia University, Dallas, Pennsylvania, where he teaches vision rehabilitation courses to master's-level occupational and physical therapy students. In more than twenty-seven years of clinical and research experience, Dr. Becker has examined and treated over 3,000 patients who are neurologically impaired with neurosensory disorders.

"Vision" refers to how the visual system coordinates function between the two eyes and the brain. (Cohen, et al., 1988) We ask questions like: Do both eyes perceive the same image at the same time? Do both eyes move in unison? Do both eyes have equal focusing power? Do both eyes do all these visual requirements easily, fluidly, and for an extended length of time? If the answer to any of these questions is "No," then vision therapy may be indicated. Vision therapy is done in a sequential manner that mirrors normal developmental processes. This allows the child to most readily relearn the visual skills that were lost, or to learn those that were never developed. It is therefore necessary to start with very easy tasks and work toward more difficult tasks. The Piagetian approach to development indicates that this is the best way to remediate vision-related problems.

The therapy has been used by optometrists for years in the general population in those who have visual functioning disorders and now it can be adapted to autistic spectrum disorder (ASD) individuals by developmental/behavioral optometrists. (Trachman et al. 2008) It is important that these clinicians have specific training with these disorders through DAN! and other agencies such as Autism Research Institute (ARI).

Fifty-three percent of children who are poor readers have some form of visual functioning disorder, and it has been estimated that up to 80 percent of children with special needs have significant visual functioning disorders that affect the learning and developmental process. (Cohen, et al., 1988)

Success is based on visual, subjective, and functional findings. Success rates vary depending on the initial functional loss. Studies indicate that success rates range from 63 percent to as high as 89 percent. This depends on the frequency and number of sessions completed. (Cohen, et al. 1988)

DG, an eight-year-old boy, sat in my examination chair after his mother had completed all the appropriate intake forms as recommended by the Defeat Autism Now! protocol. She tried to control her son as he attempted to touch the bright instruments in my examination room. The paperwork indicated that DG had been diagnosed with ASD at two years of age. He was in and out of different programs and, at one time, was labeled as dyslexic. The interview proceeded typically, but his mother was not quite sure why she was here with her son, even though an observant occupational therapist had suggested she make an appointment with me. She said, "I've had my son's eyes checked before every school year, and he has always had 20/20 vision." My comprehensive neurosensory examination, along with the functional and developmental vision examination, indicated that the other eye care specialists were correct. DG did have 20/20 visual acuity in both eyes. But they had apparently not assessed another aspect of vision, which is very important. (Holmes, et al., 2008) DG had significant eye tracking and eye focusing problems, reduced convergence difficulty with depth perception, and vestibular inaccuracies.

At this point, I explained to DG's mother the difference between sight (acuity) and vision. Sight is the ability to see a certain size object at a certain distance. The standard means to assess acuity was conceived by Herman Snellen in 1862, and since that time we have referred to normal sight as 20/20. The top number indicates the distance of the observer from the acuity chart, and the bottom number is the size of the letter being viewed. All this really means is that a person can see a certain size letter at a certain distance. This terminology is, of course, important for many aspects of our lives. However, even more important to our children with ASD, like DG, is functional/behavioral vision. Deficits with their visual systems can be very disabling.

Children with ASD, like DG, appear more likely to have visual functioning disorders than the general population. (Taub, 2007) When doing the intake form for DG, it was noted that he disliked doing any near point tasks. He preferred to run randomly around the room, picking up items along the way. He would briefly look at them and then put them down quickly when he saw another item to view, examining the new item for a very short period of time. This behavior was repeated consistently. His mother noted that she felt DG was very smart because he could easily memorize songs and verses. (My experience has been that ASD children are very smart but are unable to utilize their intelligence in the positive and productive manner that we all expect.) He would not engage in eye contact and would attend to objects out of the corner of his eyes. Instead of moving his eyes, he turned his head to see objects.

DG's evaluation, which took over two hours, indicated visual functional deficits that needed to be remediated in order for DG to be able to function visually in the world. This two-hour evaluation included tests with the Sensory View diagnostic system. (NeuroSensory Centers of America, 2009) This system assists in the evaluation of myelin health, eye movements, balance, proprioception, and dynamic visual acuity. After these tests are done, an additional evaluation is done to assess depth perception, visual suppressions, visual focusing, ocular health, and the ability of the eyes to work together. These tests, which are done by an eye care specialist trained in these procedures, need to be done without the use of the phoroptor, an instrument normally utilized in routine eye examinations.

Vision therapy can be done in an office by a trained therapist, in an outpatient rehabilitation center, or at home. Vision rehabilitation to correct most oculomotor, eye focusing, and eye deviation deficits typically continues for six to eight months when done two or three times per week. Treatment also requires home participation for thirty to forty-five minutes per day for five days per week on an outpatient basis. This does not mean that the rehabilitation cannot be concluded earlier (or later) than this prescribed time. Program length is dependent on the child's participation level and attendance.

Due to DG's particular needs, I began his therapy program in my office. The eye movement exercises I prescribed consisted of computer-based therapy, as well as hand-held therapy techniques. Both techniques have the same end result, but I have found that the computer techniques seem to work more quickly, and the results are more consistent in nature than those using the handheld therapies. The disadvantage of the computer therapies is that many children with ASD have difficulties sitting at the computer for any length of time, thus making the sessions more frustrating for them. Therefore, we incorporated both therapy techniques into DG's treatment program.

The computer programs we have had success with come from a company in Gold Canyon, Arizona. (HTS, 2009) The programs can be tailored for each child and his or her skill level. We can incorporate therapies for all visual deficits, including gross motor, fine motor, vestibular, and focusing issues, into this program. The computer programs allow easy progression for each child and can be modified when a child has difficulty with certain tasks. I review progress at least two times per month but usually more frequently, making sure that the child is meeting the proper goals.

Case Example

DG's mother was completely amazed at her son's progress. His eye contact improved, his visual stimming significantly decreased, and his school performance accelerated. His teachers wanted to know what his mother had done to get him this far. He was a more pleasant child, according to what others told DG's mother. Most importantly, DG now knows that he can do these tasks and has improved self-esteem.

What is Visual Stimming?

Many parents ask, "Why does my child do this?"

There are many theories about the function of visual stimming and peripheral viewing, and the reasons for its increased incidence in those on the autism spectrum. The Bio-medical approach states that visual stimming can be a result of yeast over growth. For hyposensitive people, it may provide needed nervous system arousal, releasing beta-endorphins. For hypersensitive people, it may provide a "norming" effect, allowing the person to control a specific sense, and is thus a soothing behavior. Visual stimming can be demonstrated as flapping hands, blinking and / or moving fingers in front of eyes, and staring repetitively at a light. (http://autism.wikia.com/wiki/Stimming)

Besides yeast over growth, there are many other reasons why visual stimming and peripheral viewing occur. If a person has visual misalignment, then visual stimming can be the product of this visual condition and the person feels better by performing this activity. Another reason is that these individuals have either an intermittent and/or alternating visual suppression. The brain only sees images out of alternating eyes and the person then visually stims, trying to understand and/or perceive images out of the other eye. When a child visually stims under stress or under new environmental conditions, this should be considered a visual breakdown due to the stress of the new environment. Again, the brain is not simultaneously processing images from each eye.

Visual stimming first needs to be evaluated by a qualified doctor who understands these conditions. The best form of treatment is visual therapy procedures to correct this disorder and sometimes, specialized prisms may be used with the therapy and with other therapies to improve the ability of the eyes to work together. My experience has been that in most cases, the therapy works better than using prisms alone, although many times, using both systems of treatment jointly may be indicated.

Once the in-office rehabilitation program is completed, a reduction in rehabilitation time is given to the child, and a phase-out program is begun for several months. This is done to monitor and maintain all visual skills that are learned and to make sure the child has adapted adequately to the new visual functioning environment.

As a final step, DG was given a home maintenance program to follow and is checked every three months in the office to confirm that he has not regressed. The home maintenance program can be a computer-based program (HTS) or the procedures that are outlined in the next section. It is very important to do this program with the understanding that these visual skills have been learned and can easily be unlearned, if not reinforced on a routine basis at home. (Becker et al., 2009)

Checklist for possible developmental visual deficits related to ASD. If you can answer yes to two or more of these signs, your child should engage in a complete neurosensory and developmental vision evaluation:

1.   Child likes to look out of the corners if his/her eyes when doing either near point or distance viewing.
2.   Child only does near tasks for short periods of time, then goes back to task after a few short minutes.
3.   Child turns head to the left or right to view distant or near objects.
4.   Child bends head to either shoulder when viewing distant or near objects.
5.   Child covers or closes an eye when looking at near point tasks.
6.   Child likes to visually stim with his hands in front of one eye or another.
7.   Child moves closer and closer to near point tasks over a short period of time.
8.   Child rubs eyes frequently.
9.   Child's eyes tend to water when doing near point tasks.
10. Child likes to turn head up or down and moves head in strange positions to do near point tasks.

How to Find a Qualified Eye Care Specialist

To locate a neurodevelopmental optometrist in your area, log onto www.nora.cc (Neuro-Optometric Rehabilitation Association). When making an appointment, ask the following questions:

1.   How frequently does the doctor examine children with autism spectrum disorders?
2.   Does the doctor do functional vision testing, not just acuity testing?
3.   Does the doctor prescribe vision therapy, and who carries out the therapy?
4.   How long is the examination process with the doctor? (It should last at least sixty to ninety minutes to get a good understanding of the child's deficits.)
5.   Will the doctor write and correspond with the school and/or other professionals?

THE ROLE OF THE MICROBIOME/BIOME AND CYSTEINE DEFICIENCY IN AUTISM SPECTRUM DISORDER: THE IMPLICATIONS FOR GLUTATHIONE AND DEFENSINS IN THE GUT-BRAIN CONNECTION

BY DR. JEFF BRADSTREET

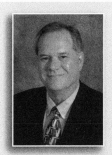

James Jeffrey Bradstreet MD, MD(H), FAAFP

International Child Development Resource Center
3800 West Eau Gallie Blvd
Melbourne FL 32934
321-259-7111
DrBradstreet@aol.com

Jeff Bradstreet, MD, MD(H), FAAFP, graduated from the University of South Florida College of Medicine and received his residency training from Wilford Hall USAF Medical Center. As a flight surgeon, he was involved in aerospace medicine research, and he has extensive experience and training in environmental medicine, hyperbarics, and toxicology. He is extensively published in autism research and outcome studies and serves as an adjunct professor of pediatrics at Southwest College of Naturopathic Medicine in Tempe, Arizona. Dr. Bradstreet is the founder and director of the International Child Development Resource Center (www.icdrc.org), which is located in Melbourne, Florida, with a satellite office in Irvine, California. His son, Matthew, is recovering from autism with the combined help of biomedical and behavioral interventions.

Autism spectrum disorders (ASD) are complex developmental abnormalities defined on the basis of the severity of symptoms in three domains: language, socialization and stereotypical behaviors. Although it is recognized that various chromosomal, mitochondrial and metabolic disorders can present with autistic features, the biological aspects of this disorder are not generally considered in the evaluation and diagnosis of the condition. Over the last 3 decades we have seen accumulating evidence of immune dysregulation in ASD. Although the nature of the immune aberrations is somewhat elusive and inconsistent, the general pattern indicates an imbalance resulting in proinflammatory and autoimmune conditions. This was recently reviewed by Careaga, et al.[1] as well as Gupta, et al.[2] These effects are present in the gut and the brain of a significant subset of ASD affected individuals.[3] As early as 1982, Weizman, et al., found abnormal cell-mediated immune responses to brain proteins in 13 of 17 ASD children tested.[4] Chez and colleagues noted extremely high cerebral spinal fluid to plasma ratios of TNF-alpha (a powerful inflammatory mediator), even in immunologically treated cases of ASD.[5] Researchers at Johns Hopkins also found persistent neuroinflammatory changes at the time of autopsy even into the 4th decade of life.[6] The implication of these inflammatory changes persisting despite either steroids or intravenous immunoglobulin therapies cannot be understated. Some force is driving the ongoing central inflammatory response in ASD. It is tempting to speculate that a persistent neurotropic pathogen (e.g., virus, atypical bacteria, etc.) is present in the central nervous system (CNS), but after several decades none has been identified with any consistency. However, in 2004, working with molecular virologists at Coombs Women's Hospital in Dublin, Ireland, Bradstreet, et al., reported the first three cases of measles virus F gene in the spinal fluid of ASD children with concurrent gastrointestinal inflammation.[7] That same year they reported MV F-gene was present in the cerebral spinal fluid (CSF) from 19 of 28 (68%) cases and in only one of 37 (3%) controls (RR = 25.12; 3.57-176.48, p<0.00001).[8] The three original cases are part of this cohort as well, so to date only 19 cases have been positively identified and reported. Even with the detection of the MV gene in the CSF, the actual cause and effect relationship between viral genome and autistic symptoms is hotly debated.[9]

In the absence of consensus on a central nervous system pathogen, others have focused on the role of the gut's complex ecosystem, the intestinal microbiome, as a potential source for immune activation and toxins capable of influencing the brain's development. This is an appealing theory that fits at least some of the clinical and laboratory observations. In 2000, Sandler et al., observed that 8 of 10 (80%) of children with ASD, regardless of intestinal symptoms, significantly improved after treatment with vancomycin.[10] The speculation was that this was related to *Clostridia* colonization, overgrowth or infection in the intestinal tract of these children. However, in this study, the researchers did not attempt to identify specific organisms that may be responding to the vancomycin. Dr. Sydney Finegold (who was a part of the vancomycin study) and colleagues recently applied pyrosequencing DNA detection techniques to evaluate the bacteria present in the feces of children with ASD.[11] This is a highly specific and sensitive method, and the results support the potential explanations why vancomycin could have been effective. At the same time, this study points us away from clostridial species to other anaerobic bacteria. One of the predominate organisms vastly overrepresented in the ASD group (as well as in their siblings) is the *Desulfovibrio* species. This becomes intriguing because of its potential relationship to the observations of cysteine deficiency in ASD. *Desulfovibrio* will compete with the host organism (a child with autism) for cysteine. So this provides at least one potential mechanism for the observed deficiency of cysteine in ASD.[12]

While it is easy to see how brain inflammation could lead to autistic features, it is more challenging to comprehend the microbiome-gut-brain connection in both creating and maintaining this ongoing CNS inflammatory response.

In the late 1990s, I had observed cysteine deficiency on amino acid testing of children with ASD. The availability of cysteine is considered to be the rate limiting step in the body's ability to manufacture intracellular glutathione. It would be hard to overemphasize the role of glutathione to human health. It is the main intracellular antioxidant and has been known for decades to protect neurons from oxidative stress.[13] In addition to more recent observations in autism, glutathione deficiency has long been known to be associated with a variety of disorders, including Parkinsonism,[14] schizophrenia,[15] ADHD,[16] HIV,[17] inflammatory bowel disease[18] and premature aging.[19] While working on research with Professor S. Jill James from the University of Arkansas for Medical Sciences, I observed dramatically lower cysteine and glutathione, as well as corresponding increases in oxidative markers in the ASD population.[20] With that study, we also found increased frequencies of genetic vulnerabilities to oxidation and glutathione metabolism.

Let's examine another critical part of this intestinal-immune puzzle. This part also relates to the vital role of cysteine. Defensins are produced by Paneth cells and are an inducible, yet nonspecific, antimicrobial defense mechanism, regulating the gut microbiome.[21] Thus defensins might be considered the extracellular counterpart of glutathione. They, too, are cysteine-dependent peptides critical to host immune function and protection.[22] It's likely, although at this time still speculative, that the type and magnitude of cysteine deficiency observed in ASD creates a relative defensin deficiency just as it creates a glutathione deficiency. This would be especially relevant to the local intestinal mucosal environment where *Desulfovibrio*, as a dominate organism, would be most locally competing for cysteine resources. In ulcerative colitis we see sulfur-reducing bacteria implicated in causation.[23]

So far we have the following overlapping observations: CNS inflammation, an abnormally skewed microbiome capable of competing with the body for valuable cysteine resources, low cysteine in the blood of ASD children, evidence of oxidative stress, potential responses to antibiotics capable of reducing anaerobic bacteria like *Desulfovibrio*, and suspected defensin deficiency. But is this enough to explain the catastrophic developmental changes we label "autism"?

Over the past several decades, both children and their mothers have been exposed to increasingly powerful broad-spectrum antibiotics. This is an unprecedented factor in human development since there is growing acceptance that humans coevolved with their microbiome.[24] Undoubtedly, this has radically altered the gut microbiome in a way that predisposes to inflammatory bowel disease.[25] At the same time, cultural changes as humans left the farm and gathered in cities have resulted in what is now referred to by Dr. William Parker of Duke University as "biome depletion."[26] Simply stated, biome depletion recognizes the regulatory roll of helminthic species (worms). Rather than being the yucky and the presumed evil bloodsuckers envisioned by most of us, there is abundant evidence that certain helminths are mutualistic symbionts. In an excellent review on this subject, McKay states the following:

> There is unequivocal evidence that parasites influence the immune activity of their hosts, and many of the classical examples of this are drawn from assessment of helminth infections of their mammalian hosts. Thus, helminth infections can impact on the induction or course of other diseases that the host might be subjected to. Epidemiological studies demonstrate that world regions with high rates of helminth infections consistently have reduced incidences of autoimmune and other allergic/inflammatory-type conditions.[27]

Elliott and colleagues at the University of Iowa had this to say about our dependent relationship with worms:

> Immune-mediated diseases (e.g., inflammatory bowel disease, asthma, multiple sclerosis, and autoimmune diabetes) are increasing in prevalence and emerge as populations adopt meticulously hygienic lifestyles. This change in lifestyles precludes exposure to helminths (parasitic worms). Loss of natural helminth exposure removes a previously universal Th2 and regulatory immune biasing imparted by these organisms. Helminths protect animals from developing immune-mediated diseases (colitis, reactive airway disease, encephalitis, and diabetes). Clinical trials show that exposure to helminths can reduce disease activity in patients with ulcerative colitis or Crohn's disease.[28]

Mount Sinai School of Medicine has an ongoing trial of helminthic therapy for autism. No results are available at this time. The study is investigating *Tricuris suis* ova (TSO: pig whipworm eggs). As with any monotherapy for a complex disorder like autism, it is doubtful it will produce dramatic results in language and stereotypical symptoms over a short course. TSO does show impressive results in refractory inflammatory bowel disease,[29] but there we are not dealing with complex CNS/developmental abnormalities. When applied to existing respiratory allergies, TSO had no measurable benefit on nasal allergy symptoms in a recent controlled study.[30] It has been observed that there is a mutually exclusive relationship between *Schistosoma* infection and multiple sclerosis, implying a protective effective of helminthic colonization.[31] And while helminths have been shown to have a protective effect by preventing the induction of experimental encephalomyelitis,[32] it is unknown if it can reverse the course of established brain inflammation as observed in ASD.

It is reasonable—even likely—that the regulatory role of both the biome and the microbiome needs to be first established in the maternal environment prior to pregnancy.[33,34] These data point to very early immune programming of the brain's future developmental response. They also establish a link between maternal immune dysregulation and ASD. It may also be that the same microbiome/biome effects that disrupt the maternal immune system are passed along environmentally to her offspring. As will be described in detail later, the ecosystem of the gut is set very early in life.

This brings up the issue of artificially changing the intestinal ecosystem. The logic seems to follow that if the nature of the gut flora is the problem, why not just change them with different—presumably healthier—bacteria (probiotics)? This was discussed briefly by Garvey,[35] but no systematic investigation has been published. Despite this, numerous clinicians and parents undertake the use of bacteria supplementation.[36] My experience provides a mixture of results from the use of probiotic supplements. Some children are immediately benefitted by probiotics: demonstrating improved bowel function, decreased hyperactivity, increased eye contact, and better attention. The dose and type of probiotic tolerated seems highly variable. Some children do well, but only with small doses (in bacterial terms this is 1-10 billion bacteria per day). Other children are helped, but only by massive doses (upwards of 450 billion per day). There is support in the pediatric literature for high-dose *Lactobacillus* in ulcerative colitis (UC).[37,38] VSL-3® has been tested in adults with proven efficacy for UC in this older population as well.[39] However, evidence is lacking for VSL-3® efficacy in Crohn's disease, which is a different type of inflammatory bowel disease.[40]

The nature of the inflammatory bowel disease in autism is immunologically distinct from both UC and Crohn's disease.[41] So, this creates the need for specifically testing the ASD population for the efficacy of any proposed probiotic. At this point, any large scale scientifically rigorous study of probiotics in ASD is unlikely to be financially feasible. Despite this obstacle, clinicians can reasonably try probiotics in population on an N of 1 study model. In essence, each child's baseline serves as his or her own control point for observations. The probiotic can be started initially at low doses and subsequently increased to tolerance. It is especially helpful to use biomarkers of gut inflammation wherever possible. For a review of these biomarkers and the clinical application of them to autism interventions, please see Bradstreet, et al.[42]

Recently, another form of microbiome modification has been proposed for autism: fecal transfer or transplantation (Finegold, et al. ibid 11). This presents some daunting challenges. There is growing evidence the immune system programs itself to accept a specific microbiome very early in life.[43] Within days of birth, the gut of all infants is colonized by the child's mother and specific environment and diet. Various factors, including the route of delivery, formula versus breast and in various combinations, influence the composition of the child's gut microbiome.[44] Once established, the microbiome drives nutrient digestion and absorption, further determining the composition of the intestinal ecosystem.[45] There is evidence this ecosystem becomes stable by 1 year of life, and even after antibiotics it tends to return to the immunologically programmed microbiome within a few months.[46]

When and how this microbiome became disrupted in autism is poorly understood. As mentioned earlier, vancomycin resulted in temporary improvement of autistic symptoms, but after a few months the children relapsed, implying a return to the old microbiome. In some cases, microbiome disruption caused by antibiotics is potentially life-threatening, as with *Clostridium difficile* colitis. Some cases are refractory to treatment with *C. difficile* specific antibiotics. In these cases the new harmful microbiome becomes established and the host lacks the ability to revert to the earlier ecosystem. Various factors contribute to this: 1) the chronic form of colitis is debilitating and creates nutritional deficiencies; 2) the inflammatory response alters local bacterial regulatory factors; and 3) the *C. difficle* biochemically defend their ecological niche.

In these entrenched, chronic cases, doctors have resorted successfully to fecal bacteriotherapy (FB), also known as fecal transfer or transplantation.[47] This has been successful in pediatric cases as well.[48] Naturally, there is going to be significant consumer resistance to this therapy for many obvious reasons. I have had the pleasure of discussing the early use of fecal bacteriotherapy with Professor Emeritus Tore Midtvedt, MD, PhD, from Karolinska University in Sweden. In the early 1950s, he was asked to help a Norwegian community plagued with chronic infectious diarrhea that had resisted all efforts of the local physicians to eradicate the infections. With a great deal of effort, they identified an ideal donor and were able to instill the feces into the infected individuals using enemas. This early experience was complicated by the challenges of finding a suitable donor. The difficulty of donor screening and identification has escalated in an age of antibiotics and occult viruses like HIV and the newly discovered retrovirus, XMRV (xenotropic murine leukemia virus-related virus). Despite these challenges, FB research continues at several institutions.

Fecal bacteriotherapy can be accomplished in a variety of ways.[49] The simplest technique would be swallowing oral time-delayed capsules. This is envisioned but to my knowledge not available to consumers at this time. The high-end recent research has used colonoscopies to deliver the fecal transplant to the cecum (first portion of the large bowel). Both nasogastric tubes and retention enemas have also been used to deliver the new microbiome. Most of the protocols involve pretreating the gut with some antibiotic (like vancomycin) or antibiotic combinations. Since there have been few clinical trials published, the best methods are not yet established, and no one has yet to publish the application of this therapy to treat the microbiome of ASD. Given the link between bowel flora and at least some of the behaviors observed in autism as well as its potential benefit on the immune dysregulation observed in ASD I suspect we will see more discussions and potential clinical trials with FB and ASD.

Now we face the challenge of linking these observations into a logical disease model to guide both our diagnostic evaluations and therapeutic efforts. The data points out the following potential problems leading to and then likely maintaining the autistic state.

1. Disruption of the maternal ecosystem.
2. Altered microbiome with flora which tend to disrupt her immune balance and that of her offspring, including antibodies directed against the fetal brain.
3. Further complicated by biome (helminthic) depletion such that the pregnant woman is unable to counter the autoimmune/proinflammatory influences of her microbiome.
4. The early-life establishment of an undesirable microbiome for her offspring.
5. Cysteine depletion created at least in part by sulfur-reducing intestinal bacteria overgrowth.
6. Cysteine-dependent defensin deficiency that alters the microbiome and permits greater numbers of potentially pathogenic organisms (presumed).
7. Glutathione deficiency and increased intracellular oxidative stress in all organs. The brain is especially sensitive to glutathione deficiency.
8. This combination of antecedents opens the door to brain inflammation and altered development (perhaps as early as intrauterine development).

Intervening in this process must start early in life—ideally prior to conception—with properly conditioning the maternal biome/microbiome. That will be no small challenge in its own right—given the resistance to change noted in the gut ecosystem. For existing cases of autism, early and appropriate restoration of the gut flora could offer significant benefits. In clinical observations, we have seen efforts to benefit the microbiome proving successful—if only temporarily so. Improved diagnostic methods of detecting microbiome disruption (e.g., pyrosequencing) may become clinically available soon and assist the clinician in therapeutic interventions. Multiple means are available in our efforts to alter the intestinal ecosystem. Although not previously discussed, dietary changes may offer significant advantages during the attempts to alter the gut environment. Anecdotal observations support interventions ranging from gluten and casein elimination to even more restrictive and challenging diets, such as the Specific Carbohydrate Diet™. All of these dietary changes would be expected to modify the immune and microbiome responses of the child. Novel microbiome therapies like fecal bacteriotherapy loom in the future even as biome therapy with TSO is being investigated. Probiotics are readily available, but dosing and strain selection is still incompletely understood. Methods to address brain inflammation are being discussed, and some have proposed nature provided anti-inflammatories to address this need.[50]

In conclusion, the complex interactions of maternal and child immune and intestinal environments seem to play a major role in the development of ASD and, therefore, are important targets for therapeutic interventions.

RESEARCH AT THE UNIVERSITY OF LOUISVILLE AUTISM CENTER

DR. MANUEL F. CASANOVA, DR. ESTATE SOKHADZE, DR. AYMAN EL-BAZ, DR. JOSHUA BARUTH, DR. GRACE MATHAI, DR. LONNIE SEARS.

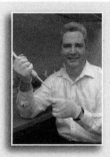

Manuel F. Casanova, MD[1,2]
Estate Sokhadze, PhD[1]
Ayman El-Baz, PhD[3]
Joshua M. Baruth, PhD[2]
Grace Mathai, PhD[4]
Lonnie Sears, PhD[4]

[1] Department of Psychiatry and Behavioral Sciences
[2] Department of Anatomical Sciences and Neurobiology
[3] Department of Bioengineering
[4] Department of Pediatrics

University of Louisville Health Sciences Center
500 South Preston Street, Building 55A Room 217
Louisville, KY 40202

Dr. Manuel Casanova did his basic training at the University of Puerto Rico and continued his specialty training at the Johns Hopkins University and the National Institutes of Mental Health. He is a Board Certified Neurologist with specialty training in both Neuropathology and Psychiatry. At present Dr. Casanova serves as the Vice Chair for Research within the Department of Psychiatry at the University of Louisville. He is also the Gottfried and Gisela Kolb Endowed Chair in Psychiatry for the same institution. Dr. Casanova was a founding member of the National Alliance for Autism Research (now merged with Autism Speaks) and the Autism Tissue Program. He chaired for several years the Developmental Brain Disorders Study section of the National Institute of Health. He serves as an editor for five different journals. Among his many recognitions Dr. Casanova is the recipient of an EUREKA award from the NIMH for innovative research in regards to autism. In 2010 he was a plenary speaker at the World Organization of Autism Congress in Monterrey Mexico. His CV shows 191 refereed articles, 49 books chapters, 3 edited books, and close to 300 congress presentations.

From a traditional neurological perspective, the clinical syndrome of autism is characterized by abnormalities in higher order cognitive abilities, complex behavior, and the presence of seizures in a significant number of patients. In autism these symptoms occur in the absence of long tract signs, blindness or deafness. This constellation of symptoms is associated in neurology with dysfunction of the outer grey matter of the brain or neocortex. Research studies support the suggested localization as studies of eye tracking movements have documented generalized abnormalities in the integrative circuitry of neocortex. Functional MRI studies have similarly revealed abnormalities in neocortical activation to different tasks (e.g., theory of mind, face recognition, executive, and language) suggesting underdevelopment of higher order integrating connections of the neocortex in autism. The reported increase in volumes of gray and white matter confirms the presence of neocortical abnormalities and in its connections through the white matter.

The above characteristics of cognition in autism suggest problems with information processing that are expressed in different ways in different tasks. Across characteristics, it appears that as tasks get more demanding or require reliance on global versus local information, performance fails; emergent skills normally present are absent, thus making it impossible to assume the processing load as demands increase. The question many researchers would like to answer is what is the underlying mechanistic framework for these cognitive abnormalities or is there a unifying framework at all? One possibility is that disturbance of global precedence and possibly even hypersensitivity to complexity may arise from the use of sharply tuned, narrowly focused receptive fields in cortical connections. This may result from an abnormality in the internal structure of neocortical minicolumns which may be amenable to therapeutical interventions.

A comprehensive program of basic, applied, and outcomes research has been created at the University of Louisville with the goal of increasing our understanding of autism. The Autism Center aims to study how the brain analyzes information, what the underlying deficits might be, explore possible clinical interventions, and determine the efficacy and quality of those interventions. The center unites areas of the University of Louisville that already focus on autism: the Department of Psychiatry, the Department of Pediatrics, and the Kentucky Autism Training Center (KATC) in the College of Education and Human Development. The research director of the University of Louisville Autism Center is Dr. Manuel Casanova, Associate Chair for Research and the Gottfried and Gisela Kolb Chair in Psychiatry.

Research at the Autism Center of the University of Louisville presently focuses on how the brain processes signals. Information processing is viewed as a common characteristic of the behavioral and cognitive abnormalities in autism, and thus an organizational framework for hypothesis testing. Initial research has looked at the anatomy of the cell minicolumn, the smallest cortical unit capable of information processing. Previous studies have found this anatomical and functional unit of the brain to be altered in patients with autism. More specifically, minicolumns in the brains of autistic patients were described as being narrower and more numerous per linear length of tissue section examined as compared to controls. Since the minicolumn re-iterates itself millions of times throughout the brain, variations in the total number and width of minicolumns can result in macroscopic changes of the brain's surface area and/or gyrification. In this regard, our Autism Center is currently trying to establish a correlation between autopsy and neuroimaging (postmortem MRIs) findings in autism. The intent is to develop markers of the condition that can be detected while the patient is alive. Another innovative aspect of the research is an attempt to validate current diagnostic screening techniques against autopsy findings.

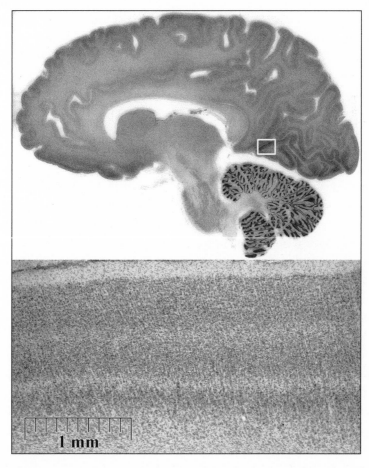

Figure 1. Above, a postmortem section of a human brain has been stained for cell bodies, so that the gray matter comprising the cerebral cortex appears dark. Below, a portion of the primary visual cortex, falling within the outlined area in the top image, was photographed at 40× magnification. Minicolumns, arrays of pyramidal cells running from top to bottom in this image, give the cortex a characteristic streaky texture.

Basic research within the Autism Center includes the study of functional circuitry associated with the impact of stimulus saliency, novelty and typicality on information processing from the visual perceptual or local level processing to the conceptual level processing. Topographical studies of the cell minicolumn indicate a gradient of severity spanning idiotypic (least affected) brain regions to heteromodal regions (most affected). Our results thus suggest that lower level of visual processing performed by idiotypic (e.g., calcarine) cortex will be sparred or even enhanced. How this normal function translates into higher level processing deficits (e.g., working memory, executive functions, complex figure recognition tasks) and abnormalities typical of autism is a major aim of our Autism Center.

At the Autism Center diffusion tensor imaging (DTI) is being used to investigate microstructural abnormalities in white matter pathways between brain structures related to the signs and symptoms of autism and the molecular mechanisms involved in cell-cell interaction in the cortex of autistic patients and controls. Computer programs and algorithms have been created that help define morphometric measures of cortical circuitry. Findings from these minicolumnar studies are being modeled as simulations of cell migration during brain development to define a time window of vulnerability for the condition.

Applied research focuses on investigating the human side of the disorder through studies of lifespan, treatment, social, and vocational activities. Case definition strategies are being explored by measuring variables on cases and controls and interview data on spouses and other relatives to allow the investigation of the impact of autism on the family. Future studies will include an attempt to define autism as a spectrum based on how far from the mean persons score on the Social Responsiveness Scale and clinical trials to study the impact of possible therapeutic interventions on automatic information processes.

Outcomes research seeks to understand the end results of medical, psychosocial, behavioral, and educational interventions. For individuals with chronic conditions, end results include those personal experiences that influence quality of life, morbidity, and mortality. Outcome research also helps in predicting the impact of various influences. As part of the diagnostic endeavors, the clinical core of the Autism Center explores case definition and risk factors for autism. As an immediate benefit, these studies provide patients and their relative's evidence about benefits, risks, and results of treatments so they can make more informed decisions.

Clinical colleagues in the Systematic Treatment of Autism and Related Disorders program (STAR) at the University of Louisville pursue applied and outcomes research initiatives, which also include translational research on the effectiveness of clinic-based and community-based interventions for autism. Particular attention to outcomes of

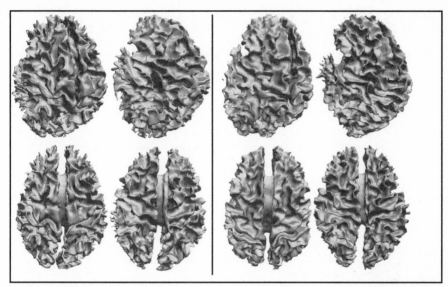

Figure 2. The white matter surface, i.e. the boundary between the grey matter of the cerebral cortex and the underlying white matter, was reconstructed from MRI data. White matter surfaces for two people with autism (left) and two neurotypical comparison clients (right) are shown. Our research has found that the gyri (ridges) in these surfaces are narrower in autism.

teacher training in autism, effectiveness of social skills interventions, parent training and outcomes, and services research are highlighted.

Educators at the Kentucky Autism training Center serve as a resource for families and teachers in bridging the research to practice gap by instituting evidence-based practice for families, teachers and schools. The KATC tests and evaluates services for patients within the autism spectrum of disorders and facilitates data collection at all levels of operation.

THREE DRUGS THAT COULD CHANGE AUTISM

BY MEGHAN THOMPSON

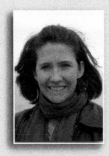

Meghan Thompson

mthompson.writer@gmail.com

Meghan Thompson is a freelance writer, researcher and editor and has just finished her first novel, *Resurrected*. A contributor for the websites *The Examiner* and *Rebel Mom*, Meghan's features focus on ways to live a more fulfilling life. Meghan also works for Consilium Global Research, a financial firm helping companies increase their exposure to the investment community. Her interests include politics, exotic travel, education, and good pizza.

Introduction

While there may never be a silver bullet to eradicate autism—the causes and manifestations are too complex and individual to hope for one cure—biotech and pharmaceutical companies are finding ways to use recent discoveries in autism research to create exciting new drugs that may be able to treat or even perhaps, cure some forms of autism. Recent disclosures by Novartis and Pfizer that they have teams dedicated to autism research shows the progress being made for a condition once thought to have little chance for a pharmaceutical treatment. While there is skepticism about the drugs currently in development, several are showing promise and offering hope to the autism community. Three, in particular, are showing great potential for treating the underlying causes of autism, not just the symptoms: Cellceutix's KM 391, Curemark LLC's CM–AT and Seaside Therapeutics' STX209.[1]

CELLCEUTIX KM-391

Overview: KM-391 is a novel compound in the early stages of research and development, which shows promise for increasing brain serotonin and plasticity. In studies with rats that have been chemically-induced to present specific characteristics of an autistic brain and the behavioral symptoms that result, treatment with KM-391 has produced significant improvements to repetitive behavior, self-induced injury, sensitivity to touch, positioning correction, group dynamics and curiosity. Cellceutrix believes that by focusing on normalizing brain serotonin levels, they have found a key to the treatment of autism.

How it works: Building on the studies that show individuals with autism often have decreased brain serotonin and plasticity, Cellceutix developed sophisticated animal models that mimicked these characteristics. KM-391 has been administered orally to rats over a period of 90 days. After treatment, the rats were found to have normalized levels of brain serotonin, increased brain plasticity and improved behavior. In other words, the "autistic" rats seemed to improve significantly.

Who could benefit: As its studies show that KM-391 will change the brain's plasticity and serotonin, Cellceutix hopes that it will be effective throughout the whole spectrum of autism.

Possible side effects: Thus far, there have been no apparent side effects in the rats who were treated with the KM-391 compound; however, further specific toxicology evaluations are needed. Until tests are done with humans, it is impossible to say with certainty what the side effects might be. But from the present findings, Cellceutix is projecting that the compound will be safe.

Clinical trial stage: Cellceutix's objective is to start clinical evaluations in 2012. Prior to submitting an Investigational New Drug application, the company must complete specific preclinical studies, including pharmacokinetic-pharmacodynamic (pk/pd modeling helps determine the appropriate dosage regimen for testing.), toxicology, chemistry and formulation.

Issues to consider: Cellcuetix is in the very early stages of developing the KM-391 compound and many more studies must be completed before they can even begin human testing. This means, of course, that KM-391 will not be available for years, if at all. Cellcuetix has a number of promising treatments in its pipeline—most notably, Kevitron, which treats drug-resistant cancers—but it is in need of capital to continue funding its research and studies.

From the company: "We have made significant advancements in the development of KM-391 as a treatment for autism. Animal studies support our contention that Cellceutix has created a novel compound for treating and healing a core cause of autism, not simply for treating the symptoms. With our innovative approach, we are attempting to keep hope alive for all who suffer from autism."

For more information: visit http://www.cellceutix.com/

CUREMARK LLC CM-AT

Overview: Curemark's enzyme replacement therapy, CM-AT, treats another possible underlying cause of autism: an enzyme deficiency that results in an inability to digest protein. Dr. Joan Fallon, Curemark's CEO, discovered this unexpected connection between autism and protein deficiency after observing that many autistic children choose a diet of carbohydrates and avoid proteins. She hypothesized that they were simply unable to digest the proteins and that correcting this problem could address core autism issues like communication, social awareness and repetitive behavior.[2] From this hypothesis, she developed CM-AT, an ingestible powder.

How it works: From Curemark's website: "The inability to digest protein affects the production of amino acids, the building blocks of chemicals essential for brain function," such as the areas of the brain that control the behaviors most often affected by autism: communication and social interaction. Curemark has identified a series of biomarkers that can determine which children have underlying digestive deficiencies. CM-AT is sprinkled on children's food three times a day to help them digest proteins and ingest amino acids, thereby producing key brain signaling molecules.

Who could benefit: CM-At could help autistic children who exhibit low levels of the biomarker chymotrypsin, indicating they suffer from enzyme deficiency. Curemark's research shows that between 50 and 70% of children with autism may benefit. However, in Virginia Hughes' article on the Simons Foundation Autism Research Initiative website, she quotes Christopher Smith, the head of the Southwest Autism Research and Resource Center in Phoenix, who is leading a trial. Smith said that four of the first seven children recruited for the study "were screened out because their levels of chymotrypsin were too high."

Possible side effects: According to Hughes' article, Fallon says, "Curemark has unpublished preliminary data from more than 350 children that show CM-AT's efficacy, with no observed adverse effects."

Clinical trial stage: CM-AT is in Phase III clinical trials, or the "final hurdle" before a company can submit an application for drug approval from the Food and Drug Administration. At 19 sites across the country, approximately 170 children, ages 3 to 8, will be testing CM-AT. Several centers were recruiting candidates as of February 2011.

Curemark received good news in February of 2010, when it learned CM-AT had been designated as a Fast Track drug by the F.D.A. This means the enzyme will receive an expedited review for its drug approval process.

Issues to consider: Curemark appears to be well funded. In October, 2009, an article in the *Westchester County Business Journal* reported that Curemark had closed a $6.5 million round of private funding and it had just opened a $20 million funding round to build its pipeline of drug applications.[3] And according to Hughes' article, the company is in talks with "several large pharmaceutical companies about licensing or other shared arrangements."

While there is a lot of hope for Curemark's research, some experts remain skeptical. In Hughes' article, she writes about Mel Heyman, chief of pediatric gastroenterology, hepatology and nutrition at University of California, San Francisco Children's Hospital, who describes two flaws in the reasoning. First, a pancreatic enzyme deficiency should also affect the breakdown of fats and carbohydrates, not just proteins; and second, malnourishment will affect all aspects of bodily function, not just the brain. But, the clinical trials are progressing, so if there are flaws in the logic, they will soon be exposed. Thus far, however, the progress seems positive for CM-AT.

For more information: visit http://www.curemark.com/ or http://www.clinical-trials.gov/ct2/results?term=curemark

SEASIDE THERAPEUTICS STX209

Overview: Fragile X is the most common known single gene cause of autism.[4] It refers to a mutation of the FMR-1 gene, which causes the gene to shut down and cease production of an important protein called FMRP. STX209, also known as arbaclofen, is a novel compound that has been shown to correct protein synthesis in the brain and improve the related characteristics of fragile X syndrome and autism, including agitation, tantrums and social withdrawal. In their open label study, they saw significant improvement in a number of measures including social responsiveness and communication. Subjects have been more engaged and interactive with their families, their peers, and with teachers and therapists.

How it works: The National Institute for Mental Health says "scientists theorize that, without FMRP, brain cells produce too much of certain other proteins, and that the mGluR5 receptor plays a key role in this process." MarkBaer, PhD Picower Professor of Neuroscience, Picower Institute for Learning and Memory, Massachusetts Institute of Technology Scientific Founder of Seaside Therapeutics, and his colleagues suggest that excess production of these other proteins contributes to the weakened connections between brain cells seen in people with fragile X syndrome. The compound STX209 is a selective gamma-amino butyric acid type B (GABA-B) receptor agonist that partially blocks mGluR5 receptors. In studies, reducing mGluR5 receptors has led to improvements in the functioning of individuals with FXS and ADS. "Recent studies in animals suggest that targeting mGluR5 receptors could prevent or treat fragile X syndrome."[5]

Who could benefit: Seaside Therapeutics has not reached a conclusion yet on the question of who could benefit from arbaclofen; but they are evaluating a number of patient characteristics to see if there is a subset of patients who respond to treatment.

Possible side effects: In its research to date, the company states that arbaclofen has been well tolerated by study participants and no metabolic side effects have been observed. Infrequent side effects possibly include headache and lethargy of short duration that goes away without any change in dose. Due to the study participants' use of other medications, though, it is difficult for Seaside to determine exactly which effects were caused by arbaclofen, if any.

Clinical trial stage: Arbaclofen began Phase II clinical trials with adolescents and adults in March 2009. Seaside Therapeutics included thirty-two patients with autism spectrum disorders, though 28 patients completed the study. The patients ranged in age from 6-17 years. Assuming safety and efficacy, Seaside Therapeutics hopes to expand the trial to include younger children.

In September 2010, the company announced positive results from its open label Phase II study. "We observed marked improvement in the majority of patients treated in the STX209 autism spectrum disorders study, including reductions in agitation and tantrums," said Craig A. Erickson, M.D., Assistant Professor of Psychiatry, chief of the Christian Sarkine Autism Treatment Center, chief of the Fragile X Research Treatment Center at the Indiana University School of Medicine and an investigator in the study.

Randall L. Carpenter, M.D., president and chief executive officer of Seaside Therapeutics said, "We have now observed significant improvement in social interaction across two studies. We believe the reduction in social withdrawal is important as it suggests that STX209 is demonstrating efficacy for a core symptom of both fragile X syndrome and autism. We look forward to initiating later stage clinical studies of STX209 in both fragile X syndrome and autism spectrum disorders."

Issues to consider: In September 2009, Seaside Therapeutics received a $30 million grant from an anonymous private, family investment firm and are well funded as they move forward with their clinical trials.

With continued positive results, Seaside is hopeful it can work the FDA to get the therapy to patients as soon as possible, perhaps in 2 to 3 years.

From the company: Seaside Therapeutics is creating new drug treatments to correct or improve the course of Fragile X Syndrome, autism and other disorders of brain development. We are dedicated to translating breakthrough discoveries in neurobiology into therapeutics that improve the lives of patients and their families.

For more information: visit http://www.seasidetherapeutics.com/index.html or http://www.clinicaltrials.gov/ct2/results?term=stx209

AFTERWORD

RESTORATION AND RESPECT

BY TERI ARRANGA

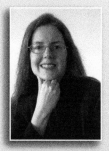

Teri Arranga

(714) 680-0792
tarranga@autismone.org
www.autismone.org
www.autismsciencedigest.com

Teri Arranga is the director of AutismOne, the vice president of the Global Autism Collaboration, and the secretary of the Strategic Autism Initiative. She is the editor in chief of *Autism Science Digest*. Teri is the editor of Dr. Andrew Wakefield's book *Callous Disregard: Autism and Vaccines—The Truth Behind a Tragedy*, which was published by Skyhorse Publishing. She is the co-host of the weekly program *Autism One: A Conversation of Hope* on the VoiceAmerica Health and Wellness Channel, and she has been involved with a number of media projects, including consulting for medical documentaries such as by award-winning filmmaker Lina Moreco of Canada. She received the National Autism Association's Believe Award for 2008. Teri has been an active advocate in the autism community for many years, including attending and broadcasting events in Washington, D.C. Ed and Teri Arranga have two boys on the spectrum, Jarad and Ian.

Autism is a whole-body condition affecting multiple physiological systems such as the immune, gastrointestinal, and endocrine systems and involving intestinal inflammation, metabolic abnormalities, immune dysregulation and detoxification impairment.

"Autism" has been a label used in ways that have impeded the children, in general, from getting the help that they need from mainstream medicine—specifically, addressing the roots/underlying conditions. "Autism" tells us nothing about what is going on internally. It follows the outdated paradigm of behaviors isolated from the rest of an individual's physiology. That is medically-medieval thinking because the brain is not separate from the body. This type of thinking can never respect the whole person. I feel that we need to continue to try to turn thinking around to recognize the underlying conditions (e.g., gastrointestinal pathology). Children are turned away by some gastroenterologists when the "autism" label is mentioned; "neurotypical" individuals with the same symptoms would be seen and treated. Our children deserve the same respect.

"Autism" is an "ism" that has engendered disrespect, like sexism and racism. Often when "autism" is mentioned, the listener ceases to view the whole person and focuses on one aspect—an aspect that society has wrongly devalued or marginalized.

There are people who, from a philosophical standpoint, heatedly argue against the verbiage of "curing" autism or "curing" a child who has autism. What we really want to "cure" are things such as gastrointestinal pathology and agonizing, debilitating, behavior- and toxin-producing associated symptoms. We want to "cure" immune dysregulation and anything else that causes distress to the child and threatens cognition and their having as safe, healthy, and functional a future as possible. We love, appreciate, and respect our children and their shining personalities. We don't want to change our children's spirits. We want to remedy the underlying disease—the same as any doctor or parent is expected to responsibly and compassionately do for any child, individual, or patient. People often do not make the distinction between more-able individuals and severely affected/severely ill children who are in pain and who will not be able to independently keep themselves safe and healthy and meet their basic human needs without intervention.

By viewing the child diagnosed with autism as a whole person, we respect that whole person—far from disrespecting the person and their personality, dignifying their real physical needs gives them respect.

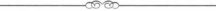

I join in spirit with the staff of Skyhorse Publishing in extending my best wishes for the future to you, your family, and your children. We are a team with our children: Together we will find the answers. Together we will have a voice.

Take joy in your child today.

With love, hope, and great respect,

— **Teri Arranga**

REFERENCES

THERAPIES

Chapter 1. Allergy Desensitization: An Effective Alternative Treatment for Autism, by Dr. Darin Ingels

1. Heuer L, Ashwood P, Schauer J, et al. Reduced levels of immunoglobulin in children with autism correlates with behavioral symptoms. *Autism Res.* 2008 Oct;1(5):275-83.
2. Careaga M, Van de Water J, Ashwood P. Immune dysfunction in autism: a pathway to treatment. *Neurotherapeutics.* 2010 Jul;7(3):283-92.
3. Trottier G, Srivastava L, Walker CD. Etiology of infantile autism: a review of recent advances in genetic and neurobiological research. *J Psychiatry Neurosci.* 1999;24(2):103-15.
4. Jyonouchi H. Autism spectrum disorders and allergy: observation from a pediatric allergy/immunology clinic. *Expert Rev Clin Immunol.* 2010 May;6(3):397-411.
5. Incorvaia C, Masieri S, Berto P, et al. Specific immunotherapy by the sublingual route for respiratory allergy. *Allergy Asthma Clin Immunol.* 2010 Nov 9;6(1):29.
6. Frati F, Scurati S, Puccinelli P, et al. Development of a sublingual allergy vaccine for grass pollinosis. *Drug Des Devel Ther.* 2010 Jul 21;4:99-105.
7. Scala G, Di Rienzo Businco A, Ciccarelli A, Tripodi S. An evidence based overview of sublingual immunotherapy in children. *Int J Immunopathol Pharmacol.* 2009 Oct-Dec;22(4 Suppl):23-6.
8. Pham-Thi N, de Blic J, Scheinmann P. Sublingual immunotherapy in the treatment of children. *Allergy.* 2006;61 Suppl 81:7-10.
9. Akdis CA, Barlan IB, Bahceciler N, Akdis M. Immunological mechanisms of sublingual immunotherapy. *Allergy.* 2006;61 Suppl 81:11-4.
10. O'Hehir RE, Sandrini A, Anderson GP, Rolland JM. Sublingual allergen immunotherapy: immunological mechanisms and prospects for refined vaccine preparation. *Curr Med Chem.* 2007;14(21):2235-44.

Chapter 2. Allergic-Like Symptoms, Blood-Brain Barrier Disruption, and Brain Inflammation by Dr. Theo Theoharides

1. Theoharides TC, Doyle R, Francis K, Conti P, Kalogeromitros D. Novel therapeutic targets for autism. Trends Pharmacol Sci 2008; 29(8):375-382.
2. Angelidou A, Alysandratos KD, Asadi S, Zhang B, Francis K, Vasiadi M, Kalogeromitros D, Theoharides TC. Brief Report: "Allergic Symptoms" in Children with Autism Spectrum Disorders. More than Meets the Eye? J Autism Dev Disord 2011.
3. Theoharides TC, Angelidou A, Alysandratos KD, Zhang B, Asadi S, Francis K, Toniato E, Kalogeromitros D. Mast cell activation and autism. Biochim Biophys Acta 2011.
4. Theoharides TC, Kempuraj D, Redwood L. Autism: an emerging 'neuroimmune disorder' in search of therapy. Exp Opinion on Pharmacotherapy 2009; 10(13):2127-2143.
5. Theoharides TC. Autism spectrum disorders and mastocytosis. Int J Immunopathol Pharmacol 2009; 22(4):859-865.

6. Theoharides TC, Doyle R. Autism, gut-blood-brain barrier and mast cells. J Clin Psychopharmacol 2008; 28(5):479-483.

7. Goines P, Van de Water J. The immune system's role in the biology of autism. Curr Opin Neurol 2010; 23(2):111-117.

8. Li Z, Okamoto K, Hayashi Y, Sheng M. The importance of dendritic mitochondria in the morphogenesis and plasticity of spines and synapses. Cell 2004; 119(6):873-887.

9. Theoharides TC, Spanos CP, Pang X, Alferes L, Ligris K, Letourneau R, Rozniecki JJ, Webster E, Chrousos G. Stress-induced intracranial mast cell degranulation. A corticotropin releasing hormone-mediated effect. Endocrinology 1995; 136:5745-5750.

10. Esposito P, Gheorghe D, Kandere K, Pang X, Conally R, Jacobson S, Theoharides TC. Acute stress increases permeability of the blood-brain-barrier through activation of brain mast cells. Brain Res 2001; 888:117-127.

11. Theoharides TC, Konstantinidou A. Corticotropin-releasing hormone and the blood-brain-barrier. Front Biosci 2007; 12:1615-1628.

12. Angelidou A, Francis K, Vasiadi M, Alysandratos K-D, Zhang B, Theoharides A., Lykouras L, Kalogeromitros D, Theoharides TC. Neurotensin is increased in serum of young children with autistic disorder. J Neuroinflammation 2010; 7:48.

13. Kempuraj D, Asadi S, Zhang B, Manola A, Hogan J, Peterson E, Theoharides TC. Mercury induces inflammatory mediator release from human mast cells. J Neuroinflammation 2010; 7(1):-20.

14. Romagnani P, de PA, Beltrame C, Annunziato F, Dente V, Maggi E, Romagnani S, Marone G. Tryptase-chymase double-positive human mast cells express the eotaxin receptor CCR3 and are attracted by CCR3-binding chemokines. Am J Pathol 1999; 155(4):1195-1204.

15. Theoharides TC, Kempuraj D, Tagen M, Conti P, Kalogeromitros D. Differential release of mast cell mediators and the pathogenesis of inflammation. Immunol Rev 2007; 217:65-78.

16. Middleton E, Jr., Kandaswami C, Theoharides TC. The effects of plant flavonoids on mammalian cells: implications for inflammation, heart disease and cancer. Pharmacol Rev 2000; 52:673-751.

17. Kempuraj D, Madhappan B, Christodoulou S, Boucher W, Cao J, Papadopoulou N, Cetrulo CL, Theoharides TC. Flavonols inhibit proinflammatory mediator release, intracellular calcium ion levels and protein kinase C theta phosphorylation in human mast cells. Br J Pharmacol 2005; 145:934-944.

18. Woodcock EA. Ucn-II and Ucn-III are cardioprotective against ischemia reperfusion injury: an essential endogenous cardioprotective role for CRFR2 in the murine heart. Endocrinology 2004; 145:21-23.

19. Kempuraj D, Tagen M, Iliopoulou BP, Clemons A, Vasiadi M, Boucher W, House M, Wolferg A, Theoharides TC. Luteolin inhibits myelin basic protein-induced human mast cell activation and mast cell dependent stimulation of Jurkat T cells. Br J Pharmacol 2008; 155:1076-1084.

20. Parker-Athill E, Luo D, Bailey A, Giunta B, Tian J, Shytle RD, Murphy T, Legradi G, Tan J. Flavonoids, a prenatal prophylaxis via targeting JAK2/STAT3 signaling to oppose IL-6/MIA associated autism. J Neuroimmunol 2009; 217(1-2):20-27.

21. Theoharides TC, Sieghart W, Greengard P, Douglas WW. Antiallergic drug cromolyn may inhibit histamine secretion by regulating phosphorylation of a mast cell protein. Science 1980; 207:80-82.

22. Klooker TK, Braak B, Koopman KE, Welting O, Wouters MM, Van Der HS, Schemann M, Bischoff SC, van den Wijngaard RM, Boeckxstaens GE. The mast cell stabiliser keto-

tifen decreases visceral hypersensitivity and improves intestinal symptoms in patients with irritable bowel syndrome. Gut 2010; 59(9):1213-1221.

23. Dimitriadou V, Pang X, Theoharides TC. Hydroxyzine inhibits experimental allergic encephalomyelitis (EAE) and associated brain mast cell activation. Int J Immunopharmacol 2000; 22:673-684.

24. Vasiadi M, Kalogeromitros K, Kempuraj D, Clemons A, Zhang B, Chliva C, Makris M, Wolferg A, House M, Theoharides TC. Rupatadine inhibits pro-inflammatory mediator secretion from human mast cells triggered by different stimuli. Clin Exp Allergy 2010; 151(1):38-45.

Chapter 3. Animals in the Lives of Persons with Autism Spectrum Disorder by Dr. Aubrey Fine

1. American Pet Products Association. (2009). *Industry statistics & trends*. Retrieved August 16, 2009 from: http://www.americanpetproducts.org/press_industrytrends.asp

2. Barol, J. (2006) *The Effects of AAT on a child*. Unpublished Thesis. New Mexico Highland University.

3. Dayton, L. (2010, January 23). Pets are a natural remedy for owners' health. *The Australian (Sydney, Australia)*.

4. Delta Society. (1996). *Standards of practice in animal-assisted activities and therapy*. Bellevue, WA: Delta Society

5. Fine, A.H. (2010) (Ed.), *Handbook on animal-assisted therapy: Theoretical foundations and guidelines for practice*. USA: Academic Press.

6. Fine, A.H., & Eisen, C. (2008). *Afternoons with Puppy: Inspirations from a therapist and his therapy animals*. West Lafayette, Indiana: Purdue University Press.

7. Foxall, E. L. (2002). The use of horses as a means of improving communication abilities of those with autism spectrum disorders: An investigation into the use and effectiveness of the horse as a therapy tool for improving communication in those with autism. Unpublished manuscript, Coventry, UK: Conventry University.

8. Friedmann, E., Locker, B. Z., & Lockwood, R. (1990). Perception of animals and cardiovascular responses during verbalization with an animal present. *Anthrozoos, 6*(2), 115-134.

9. Frewin, K. & Gardiner, B. (2005). New age or old sage? A review of equine assisted psychotherapy. In *The Australian Journal of Counseling Psychology, 6*, pp. 13-17.

10. Grandin, T. (2011). The roles that animals can play with individuals with autism. In P McCardle, S McCune, J. Griffin, L Esposito, & L Freund, *Human–Animal Interaction in Family, Community, and Therapeutic Settings*. **Baltimore, MD: Brookes Publishing, 183-195.**

11. Grandin, T., Fine, A., & Bowers, C. (2010). The use of therapy animals with individuals with autism. In A. Fine (Ed.) *The Handbook on Animal-Assisted Therapy: Theoretical Foundations and Guidelines for Practice (3rd Edition)*. New York: Elsevier Science Press.

12. Grandin, T., & Johnson, C. (2005). *Animals in translation*. New York, NY: Scribner.

13. Journal of the American Veterinary Medical Association. (1998). Statement from the committee on the human-animal bond. *Journal of the American veterinary medical association, 212*(11), 1675.

14. Levinson, B. (1969). *Pet oriented child psychotherapy*. Springfield, IL: Charles C. Thomas Publisher.

15. Martin, F. & Farnum, J. (2002). Animal assisted therapy for children with pervasive developmental disorders. *Western Journal of Nursing Research, 24*, 657-670.

16. Mason, M. A. (2004). Effects of therapeutic riding in children with autism. Unpublished dissertation. Minneapolis, MN: Capella University.

17. The North American Riding for the Handicapped Association (NARHA) (2010). Equine-facilitated psychotherapy and equine-facilitated learning FAQ. [Online]. Available: http://www.narha.org/faq#efp.

18. McNicholas, J. & Collis, G. M. (2000). Dogs as catalysts for social interactions: robustness of the effect. *British Journal of Psychology, 91,* 61-70.

19. McNicholas, J., & Collis, G. (2006). Animals as supports. Insights for understanding animal assisted therapy. In A. Fine (Ed.) *Handbook on animal assisted therapy (2nd Edition*, pp. 49-71). San Diego, CA: Academic Press.

20. Ming Lee Yeh, A. (2008). Canine AAT model for autistic children. At Tawian International Association of Human-Animal Interaction International Conference, Tokyo Japan, 10/5-8/2008.

21. Odenthal, J., & Meintjes, R. (2003). Neurophysiological correlates of affiliative behavior between humans and dogs. *Veterinary Journal,165,* 296-301.

22. Olmert, M. D. (2009). *Made for each other*. Philadelphia: De Capo Press.

23. Wells, D. L. (2009). The effects of animals on human health and well-being. *Journal of social issues, 65*(3), 523-543.

Chapter 5. Antifungal Treatment, by Dr. Lewis Mehl-Madrona

Ashwood P, Van de Water J. (2004). Is autism an autoimmune disease? *Autoimmunology Review, 3*(7-8):557–562.

Ashwood, P., Anthony, A., Torrente, F., & Wakefield, A. J. (2004). Spontaneous mucosal lymphocyte cytokine profiles in children with autism and gastrointestinal symptoms: mucosal immune activation and reduced counter regulatory interleukin-10. *Journal of Clinical Immunology, 24*(6):664–673.

Azcarate-Peril, M. A., Bruno-Barcena, J. M., Hassan, H. M., Klaenhammer, T. R. (2006). Transcriptional and functional analysis of oxalyl-coenzyme A (CoA) decarboxylase and formyl-CoA transferase genes from Lactobacillus acidophilus. *Applied Environmental Microbiology, Mar, 72*(3): 1891–1899.

Baggio, B., Gambaro, G., Zambon, S., Marchini, F., Bassi, A., Bordin, L., Clari, G., Manzato, E. (1996). Anomalous phospholipid in n-6 polyunsaturated fatty acid composition in idiopathic calcium nephrolithiasis. *Journal of the American Society of Nephrology, Apr, 7*(4): 613–620.

Chetyrkin, S. V., Kim, D., Belmont, J. M., Scheinman, J. I., Hudson, B. G., Voziyan, P. A. (2005). Pyridoxamine lowers kidney crystals in experimental hyperoxaluria: a potential therapy for primary hyperoxaluria. *Kidney International, 67,* 53–60.

Crook W. (1999). *The Yeast Connection.* Newton, MA: Professional Books.

Edelson (2006).The Autism Yeast Connection. At www.ei-resource.org/articles/autism-articles/the-candida-yeast%11autism-connection/. Last Accessed 09 Feb 2010.

Fomina, M., Hiller, S., Charnock, J. M., Melville, K., Alexander, I. J., Gadd, G. M. (2005). Role of oxalic acid oversecretion in transformations of toxic metal minerals by Beauveria caledonica. *Applied Environmental Microbiology, Jan 71*(1): 371–381.

Ghio, A. J., Roggli, V. L., Kennedy, T. P., Piantadosi, C.A. (2000). Calcium oxalate and iron accumulation in sarcoidosis. *Sarcoidosis Vasc Diffuse Lung Dis, Jun, 17*(2): 140–150.

Great Plains Laboratory. (2008). OXALATES CONTROL IS A MAJOR NEW FACTOR IN AUTISM THERAPY. July 2008 Newsletter.

Hornig, M., Lipkin, W. I. (2001). Infectious and immune factors in the pathogenesis of neurodevelopmental disorders: epidemiology, hypotheses, and animal models. *Ment Retard Dev Disabil Res Rev* 7(3): 200–210.

Jepson, B., Johnson, J. (2007) *Changing the Course of Autism: A Scientific Approach for Parents and Physicians.* New York: Sentient Publications.

Kumar, R., Mukherjee, M., Bhandari, M., Kumar, A., Sidhu, H., Mittal, R. D. (2002). Role of Oxalobacter formigenes in calcium oxalate stone disease: a study from North India. *Eur Urol Mar, 41*(3): 318–322.

Rimland, B. (1988). Candida caused Autism? *Autism Research Review International, 2*(2): 3.

Money, J., Bobrow, N. A., Clarke, F. C. (1971). Autism and autoimmune disease: A family study, *J Autism Child Schizophr, 1*:146.

Pardo, C. A., Eberhart, C. G. (2007). The neurobiology of autism. *Brain Pathology, 17*(4):434–447.

Rosseneu, S. *Aerobic gut flora in children with autism spectrum disorder and gastrointestinal symptoms.* Presented at Defeat Autism Now! Conference. San Diego, CA, October 3, 2003.

Ruijter, G. J. G., van de Vondervoort, P. J. I., Visser, J. (1999). Oxalic acid production by Aspergillus niger: an oxalate non-producing mutant produces citric acid at pH 5 and in the presence of manganese. *Microbiology* 145: 2569–2576.

Kornblum, Lori, *Feast Without Yeast: Four Stages to Better Health*, Madison, WI: Institute of Nutrition.

Shaw, W., Kassen, E., Chaves, E. (1995). Increased urinary excretion of analogs of Krebs cycle metabolites and arabinose in two brothers with autistic features. *Clinical Chemistry 41,* 1094–1104.

Shi, L., Fatemi, S. H., Sidwell, R. W., Shirane, Y., Kurokawa, Y., Miyashita, S,, Komatsu, H., Kagawa, S. (1988). Study of inhibition mechanisms of glycosaminoglycans on calcium oxalate monohydrate crystals by atomic force microscopy. *Urol Res, 27*(6): 426–431.

Stubbs, E. G. (1976). Autistic children exhibit undetectable hemagglutination-inhibition antibody titers despite previous rubella vaccination. *J Autism Child Schizophr., 6*(3):269–274.

Stubbs, E. G., Crawford, M. L. (1977). Depressed lymphocyte responsiveness in autistic children. *Autism Child Schizophr, 7*(1):49–55.

Takeuchi, H., Konishi, T., Tomoyoshi, T. (1987). Observation on fungi within urinary stones. *Hinyokika Kiyo May; 33*(5):658–661.

Vargas, D. L., Nascimbene, C., Krishnan, C., Zimmerman, A. W., Pardo, C. A. (2005). Neuroglial activation and neuroinflammation in the brain of patients with autism. *Ann Neurol, 57*: 67–81.

Vulvar Pain Foundation. Reducing Oxalate. http://vulvarpainfoundation.org/Low_ oxalate?treatment.htm Last accessed 8 February 2010.

Wakefield, A. J., Anthony, A., Murch, S. H., et al. (2000). Enterocolitis in children with developmental disorders. *Am J Gastroenterol, 95*: 2285–2295.

Chapter 6. Applied Behavior Analysis: What Makes a Great ABA Program? Sorting Through the Science, the Brands, and the Acronyms by Jonathan Tarbox and Doreen Granpeesheh

Cohen, H., Amerine-Dickens, M., Smith, T. (2006). Early Intensive Behavioral Treatment: Replication of the UCLA Model in a Community Setting. *Developmental and Behavioral Pediatrics, 2,* 145-157.

Eikeseth, S. (2009). Outcome of comprehensive psycho-educational interventions for young children with autism, *Research in Developmental Disabilities, 30,* 158-178.

Granpeesheh, D., Tarbox, J., & Dixon, D. (2009). Applied behavior analytic interventions for children with autism: A description and review of treatment research. *Annals of Clinical Psychiatry, 21,* 162-173.

Howard, J. S., Sparkman, C. R., Cohen, H. G., Green, G., Stanislaw, H. (2005). A comparison of behavior analytic and eclectic treatments for children with autism. *Research in Developmental Disabilities, 26,* 359-383.

Lovaas, I. O. (1987). Behavioral treatment and normal educational and intellectual functioning in young autistic children. *Journal of Consulting and Clinical Psychology, 55,* 3-9.

Sallows, G. O. & Graupner, T. D. (2005). Intensive behavioral treatment for children with autism: Four-year outcome and predictors. *American Journal on Mental Retardation, 110,* 417-438.

Zachor, D. A., Ben-Itzchak, E. L., Rabinovich, A. L., & Lahat, E. (2007). Change in autism core symptoms with intervention. *Research in Autism Spectrum Disorders, 1,* 304-317.

Chapter 7. Aquatic Therapy, by Andrea Salzman

1. Salzman, A. (2009). *Aquatic Therapy Boot Camp: Aquatic Therapy University.* Plymouth, MN. For more information: (800) 680-8624. www.aquatic-university.com

2. Salzman, A. New therapy pool especially for children with autism. Aquatic Therapist Blog. Plymouth, MN. July 08, 2008. www.aquatictherapist.com/index/2008/07/new-therapy-pool-especially-for-children-with-autism.html.

3. Bloorview Kids Rehab. Programs & Services: Community Programs: Snoezelen. January 19, 2010. www.bloorview.ca/programsandservices/communityprograms/snoezelen.php.

4. Aquatic Therapy University. 2010 Pediatric Certification Track. Aquatic Sensory Integration for the Pediatric Client: Using Water to Modulate Vestibular, Tactile, Proprioceptive, Visual & Auditory Input. Minneapolis, MN campus. For more information: (800) 680-8624. www.aquatic-university.com

5. Aquatic Resources Network. Aquatic Sensory Integration for the Pediatric Client (Distance learning DVD and manual). Plymouth, MN. For more information: (800) 680-8624. www.aquaticnet.com.

6. AquaticNet Social Network. Autism work group. Aquatic Resources Network. Plymouth, MN. To join discussion group: www.aquatictherapist.ning.com.

7. Vonder Hulls, D. S.; Walker, L. K., Powell, J. M. (2006). Clinicians' perceptions of the benefits of aquatic therapy for young children with autism: a preliminary study. *Phys Occup Ther Pediatr*, 26(1-2):13–22.

8. Huettig, C.; Darden-Melton, B. (2004). Acquisition of aquatic skills by children with autism. *Palaestra, 20*(2):20–46.

9. Bumin, G., Uyanik, M., Yilmaz, I., Kayihan, H., Topcu, M. (2003). Hydrotherapy for Rett syndrome. *J Rehabil Med, 35*(1): 44–45.

10. Yilmaz, I., Yanardag, M., Birkan, B., Bumin, G. (2004). Effects of swimming training on physical fitness and water orientation in autism. *Pediatrics International, 46*(5):624–626.

11. Aetna. Clinical Policy Bulletin: Pool Therapy, Aquatic Therapy or Hydrotherapy (Number: 0174). Revised April 3, 2009. www.aetna.com/cpb/medical/data/100_199/0174.html.

12. Salzman, A. Coding Confusion. Advance for Physical Therapy & Rehab Medicine. Merion Publications. King of Prussia, PA. November 8, 2004. http://physical-therapy.advanceweb.com/Article/Coding-Confusion.aspx.

13. Salzman, A. A Poolside Practicum: Part I. PTs can use aquatic therapy to teach transitions in children with autism. Advance for Physical Therapy & Rehab Medicine. Merion Publications. King of Prussia, PA. October 20, 2008. http://physical-therapy.advanceweb.com/Article/A-Poolside-Practicum-Part-I.aspx.

14. Salzman, A. A Poolside Practicum: Part II: PTs can use aquatic therapy to teach transitions in children with autism. Advance for Physical Therapy & Rehab Medicine. Merion Publications. King of Prussia, PA. November 18, 2009. http://physical-therapy.advanceweb.com/Article/A-Poolside-Practicum-Part-II.aspx.

15. Salzman, A. A Poolside Practicum: Part III: PTs can use aquatic therapy to enhance body awareness and kinesthesia. Advance for Physical Therapy & Rehab Medicine. Merion Publications. King of Prussia, PA. December 1, 2008. http://physical-therapy.advanceweb.com/Article/A-Poolside-Practicum-Part-III.aspx.

16. Salzman, A. A Poolside Practicum: Part IV: PTs can use aquatic therapy to alter tactile processing.Advance for Physical Therapy & Rehab Medicine. Merion Publications. King of Prussia, PA. December 29, 2008. http://physical-therapy.advanceweb.com/Article/A-Poolside-Practicum-Part-IV.aspx.

17. Salzman, A. A Poolside Practicum: Part V: PTs can use aquatic therapy to enhance vestibular input. Advance for Physical Therapy & Rehab Medicine. Merion Publications. King of Prussia, PA. January 27, 2009. http://physical-therapy.advanceweb.com/Article/A-Poolside-Practicum-Part-V.aspx.

18. Salzman, A. Poolside Practicum: Part VI: PTs can use aquatic therapy to offer visual challenges. Advance for Physical Therapy & Rehab Medicine. Merion Publications. King of Prussia, PA. February 24, 2009. http://physical-therapy.advanceweb.com/Article/A-Poolside-Practicum-Part-VI.aspx.

Chapter 9. Art Therapy Approaches to Treating Autism, by Nicole Martin and Dr. Donna Betts

American Art Therapy Association (2009a). *About art therapy.* Retrieved January 6, 2010 from www.arttherapy.org/aboutart.htm.

American Art Therapy Association (2009b). *How did art therapy begin?* Retrieved January 6, 2010 from www.arttherapy.org/faq.htm#howbegin.

Betts, D. J. (2003). Developing a projective drawing test: Experiences with the Face Stimulus Assessment (FSA). *Art Therapy: Journal of the American Art Therapy Association*, 20(2), 77–82.

Betts, D. J. (2009). Introduction to the Face Stimulus Assessment (FSA). In E. Horovitz & S. Eksten (Eds.), *Art Therapy Handbook: Assessment, Diagnosis, and Counseling.* Springfield, IL: Charles C. Thomas.

Evans, K., Dubowski, J. (2001). *Art Therapy with Children on the Autistic Spectrum: Beyond Words.* London: Jessica Kingsley.

Gilroy, A. (2006). *Art therapy: Research and Evidence-Based Practice.* London, UK: Sage Publications. (Reviews research on ASD from pages 144–146.)

Kramer, E. (1979). *Childhood and Art Therapy: Notes on Theory and Application.* New York: Schocken Books.

Martin, N. (2008). Assessing portrait drawings created by children and adolescents with autism spectrum disorder. *Art Therapy: Journal of the American Art Therapy Association*, 25(1), 15–23.

Martin, N. (2009a). *Art as an Early Intervention Tool for Children with Autism.* London: Jessica Kingsley.

Martin, N. (2009b). Art therapy and autism: Overview and recommendations. *Art Therapy: Journal of the American Art Therapy Association*, 26(4), 187–190.

Stack, M. (1998). Humpty Dumpty's shell: Working with autistic defense mechanisms in art Therapy. In M. Rees (Ed.), (1998), *Drawing on Difference: Art Therapy with People Who Have Learning Difficulties.* London: Routledge.

Chapter 14. CARD eLearning and Skills: Web-Based Training, Assessment, Curriculum and Progress Tracking for Children with Autism, by Dr. Doreen Granpeesheh and Dr. Adel C. Najdowski

Dixon, D.R., Tarbox, J., Najdowski, A.C., Wilke, A.E. & Granpeesheh, D. (2011). A comprehensive evaluation of language for early behavioral intervention programs: the reliability of the SKILLS language index. *Journal of Research in Autism Spectrum Disorders, 5*, 506-511.

Granpeesheh, D. (2008). Recovery from autism: learning why and how to make it happen more. *Autism Advocate, 50*, 54-58.

Granpeesheh, D., Tarbox, J., Dixon, D.R., Carr, E., & Herbert, M. (2009). Retrospective analysis of clinical records in 38 cases of recovery from autism. *Annals of Clinical Pyschiatry, 21(4)*, 195-204.

Granpeesheh, D., Tarbox, J., Dixon, D.R., Peters, C.A., Thompson, K., & Kenzer, A. (2010). Evaluation of a learning tool for training behavioral therapists in academic knowledge of applied behavior analysis. *Journal of Research in Autism Spectrum Disorders, 4*, 11-17.

Chapter 16. Chelation: Removal of Toxic Metals, by Dr. James B Adams

J. B. Adams, M. Baral, E. Geis, J. Mitchell, J. Ingram, A. Hensley, I. Zappia, S. Newmark, E. Gehn, R.A. Rubin, K. Mitchell, J. Bradstreet, J.M. El-Dahr, "The Severity of Autism Is Associated with Toxic Metal Body Burden and Red Blood Cell Glutathione Levels," *Journal of Toxicology*, vol. 2009, Article ID 532640, 7 pages, 2009. www.hindawi.com/journals/jt/contents.html

J. B. Adams, M. Baral, E. Geis, J. Mitchell, J. Ingram, A. Hensley, I. Zappia, S. Newmark, E. Gehn, R.A. Rubin, K. Mitchell, J. Bradstreet, J.M. El-Dahr Safety and Efficacy of Oral DMSA Therapy for Children with Autism Spectrum Disorders: Part A - Medical Results BMC Clinical Pharmacology 2009, 9:16 www.biomedcentral.com/1472-6904/9/16

J. B. Adams, M. Baral, E. Geis, J. Mitchell, J. Ingram, A. Hensley, I. Zappia, S. Newmark, E. Gehn, R.A. Rubin, K. Mitchell, J. Bradstreet, J.M. El-Dahr Safety and Efficacy of Oral DMSA Therapy for Children with Autism Spectrum Disorders: Part B - Behavioral Results BMC Clinical Pharmacology 2009, 9:17 www.biomedcentral.com/1472-6904/9/17

Bernard S et al, Autism: a novel form of mercury poisoning. *Med Hypotheses.* 2001 Apr;56(4):462–71.

James et al, Metabolic endophenotype and related genotypes are associated with oxidative stress in children with autism. *Am J Med Genet B Neuropsychiatr Genet.* 2006 Dec 5;141(8):947–56.

Nataf R et al., Porphyrinuria in childhood autistic disorder: implications for environmental toxicity. *Toxicol Appl Pharmacol.* 2006 Jul 15;214(2):99–108

Bradstreet J., Geier DA, Kartzinel JJ, Adams JB, Geier MR, A Case-Control Study of Mercury Burden in Children with Autistic Spectrum Disorders, *J. Am. Phys. Surg* 8(3) 2003 76–79.

Holmes AS, Blaxill MF, Haley BE. Reduced levels of mercury in first baby haircuts of autistic children. *Int J Toxicol.* 2003 Jul-Aug;22(4):277–85.

Windham et al, Autism spectrum disorders in relation to distribution of hazardous air pollutants in the San Francisco bay area. Environ Health Perspect. 2006 Sep;114(9):1438-44. Palmer RF et al., Environmental mercury release, special education rates, and autism disorder: an ecological study of Texas. Health Place. 2006 Jun;12(2):203–9.

Chapter 17. Craniosacral and Chiropractic Therapy: A New Biomedical Approach to ASD, by Dr. Charles Chapple

Goddard, Sally. (2005). *Reflexes, Learning and Behavior, a Window into the Child's Mind.* Eugene, OR: Fern Ridge Press.

Chapple, Charles W., D.C., F.I.C.P.A. (2007). Making the Connection Between . . . Primitive Reflexes, Sensory Processing Disorders and Chiropractic Solutions. *SI Focus Magazine Winter 2007,* 8–9.

Chapple, Charles W.D.C., F.I.C.P.A. (2005). A Biomechanical Approach for the Improvement of...Sensory, Motor and Neurological Function with Individuals with Autistic Spectrum Disorder (ASD), Pervasive Developmental Delay (PDD), and Sensory Processing Disorder (SPD). *SI Focus Magazine Autumn 2005,* 6–9.

Dodd, Susan B. A. (2005). *Understanding Autism.* Elsevier Australia.

Koester, Cecilia, M.Ed. (2006). *Movement Based Learning...For Children of All Abilities,* Reno, NV: Movement Based Learning Inc.

Kranowitz, Carol Stock, M.A. (2005). *The Out of Sync Child...Recognizing and coping with Sensory Processing Disorder,* New York: Penguin Group.

Melillo, Robert, DC. (2009). *Disconnected Kids*, New York: Perigee.

Upledger, John E., D.O., F.A.A.O. and Jon D. Vredevoogd, M.F.A. (1983). *Craniosacral Therapy*, Seattle: Eastland Press.

Williams, Stephen D.C., F.C.C. (paed), F.C.C. (2005). *Pregnancy and Paediatrics: A Chiropractic Approach*. Southampton, UK: Stephen P. Williams.

Chapter 18. Dance/Movement Therapy, by Mariah Meyer LeFeber

Adler, J. (2003). From autism to the discipline of authentic movement. *American Journal of Dance Therapy, 25*(1), 5–16.

American Dance Therapy Association. (2008). Retrieved October 28, 2008 from www.adta.org/about/factsheet.cfm.

Berrol, C. (2006). Neuroscience meets dance/movement therapy: Mirror neurons, the therapeutic process and empathy. *The Arts in Psychotherapy, 33*, 302–315.

Canner, N. (1968). *And a Time to Dance.* Boston: Beacon Press.

Erfer, T. (1995). Treating children with autism in a public school system. In F. J. Levy, J. P. Fried, & F. Leventhal (Eds.), *Dance and Other Expressive Arts therapies* (pp. 191–211). New York: Routledge.

Hartshorn, K., Olds, L., Field, T., Delage, J., Cullen, C., & Escalona, A. (2001). Creative movement therapy benefits children with autism. *Early Child Development & Care, 166*, 1–5.

Kestenberg, J. A., Loman, S., Lewis, P., & Sossin, K. M. (1999). *The meaning of movement: Developmental and clinical perspectives of the Kestenberg Movement Profile.* New York: Brunner-Routledge.

Levy, F. (2005). *Dance Movement Therapy: A Healing Art.* Reston, VA: National Dance Association.

Loman, S. (1995). The case of Warren: A KMP approach to autism. In F. J. Levy, J. P. Fried, & F. Leventhal (Eds.), *Dance and Other Expressive Arts Therapies: When Words Are Not Enough* (pp. 213–224). New York: Routledge.

Meekums, B. (2002). *Dance Movement Therapy: A Creative Psychotherapeutic Approach.* London: Sage Publications.

Wolf-Schein, E., Fisch, G., & Cohen, I. (1985). A study of the use of nonverbal systems in the differential diagnosis of autistic, mentally retarded and fragile x individuals. *American Journal of Dance Therapy, 8*(1985), 67–80.

Chapter 19. Dietary Interventions for Autism: Different Approaches, by Karyn Seroussi and Lisa Lewis, Ph.D.

1.   According to the Food Allergy & Anaphylaxis Network, eight foods account for 90% of all food allergies. These include milk, egg, peanut, tree nuts (walnuts, cashews, etc.), fish, shellfish, soy and wheat.

2.   Oski, Frank A., MD1996 *Don't Drink Your Milk*. Teacher Services, Inc.

3.   Iacono G, Cavataio F, Montalto G, Soresi M, Notarbartolo A, Carroccio A. Persistent cow's milk protein intolerance in infants: the changing faces of the same disease. *Clin Exp Allergy* 1998 Jul;28(7):817–23.

Chapter 20. Dietary Interventions for Autism: Specific Carbohydrate Diet, by Judith Chinitz

1   Yap, I.K.S, Angley, M., Veselkov, K.A., Holmes, E., Lindon, J.C., Nicholson, J.K. (2010). Urinary metabolic phenotyping differentiates children with autism, from their unaffected siblings and age-matched controls. *Journal of Proteome Research* .

2   Gomez-Llorente, C., Munoz, S., Gil, A. (2010). Role of Toll-like receptors in the development of the immunotolerance mediated by probiotics. Proceedings of the Nutrition Society, 69(3): 381-9.

3   Heijtz, R.D., Wang, S., Anuar, F., Qian, Y., Bjorkholm, B., Samuelsson, A., Hibberd, M.L., Forssberg, H., Pettersson, S. (2011). Normal gut microbiota modulates brain development and behavior. *Proceedings of the National Academy of Science*, as yet unpublished.

4   Riazi, K., Galic, M.A., Kuzmiski, J.B., Ho, W., Sharkey, K.A., Pittman, Q.J. (2008). Microglial activation and TNFalpha production mediate alterned CNS excitability following perifpheral inflammation. Proceedings of the National Academy of Science, 105(44): 17151-6.

5   Vargas, D.L., Nascimbene, C., Krishnan, C., Zimmerman, A.W., Pardo, C.A. (2005). Neuroglial activation and neuroinflammation in the brain of patients with autism. *Annals of Neurology*, 57(1):67-81.

6   Parracho, H.M.R.T., Bingham, M.O., Gibson, G.R., McCartney, A.L. (2005). Differences between the gut microflora of children with autistic spectrum disorders and that of healthy children. *Journal of Medical Microbiology*, 54, 987-991.

7   Goldstein, R., Braverman, D., Stankiewicz, H. (2000). Carbohydrate malabsorption and the effect of dietary restriction on irritable bowel syndrome and functional bowel complaints. *Israeli Medical Association Journal*, Aug,2(8):683-7.

8   Reif, S., Klein, I., Lubin, F., Farbstein, M., Hallak, A., Gilat, T. (1997). Pre-illness dietary factors in inflammatory bowel disease. *Gut*, June;40(6):754-60.

9   Gibson, P.R., Barrett, J.S. (2010). The concept of small intestine bacterial overgrowth in relation to functional gastrointestinal disorders. *Nutrition* 11-12: 1-38-43.

10   Gottschall, E. (2000). *Breaking the Vicious Cycle*. Ontario: Kirkton Press Ltd.

11   Chinitz, J. (2007). *We Band of Mothers: Autism, My Son and The Specific Carbohydrate Diet*. San Diego: Autism Research Institute.

Chapter 21. Drama Therapy, by Sally Bailey

Attwood, T. (1998). *Asperger's syndrome: A guide for parents and professionals*. London: Jessica Kingsley.

Bailey, S. (2009a). Performance in drama therapy. In D. R. Johnson & R. Emunah (Eds.), *Current Approaches in Drama Therapy,* 2 ed. (pp. 374–392) Springfield, IL: Charles C. Thomas Publisher.

Bailey, S. (2009b). Theoretical reasons and practical applications of drama therapy with clients on the autism spectrum. In S.L. Brooke (Ed.), *The Use of the Creative Therapies with Autism Spectrum Disorders* (pp. 303–318). Springfield, IL: Charles C. Thomas Publisher.

Bailey, S. (2006). Ancient and modern roots of drama therapy. In S. L. Brooke (Ed.), *Creative Arts Therapies Manual: A Guide to the History, Theoretical Approaches, Assessment, and Work with Special Populations of Art, Play, Dance, Music, Drama, and Poetry Therapy* (pp. 214–222). Springfield, IL: Charles C. Thomas Publisher.

Bolding, G. (2007, November 9) Student overcomes autism with acting. *The Kansas State Collegian,* p. 3.

Blair, R. (2008). *The Actor, Image, and Action: Acting and Cognitive Neuroscience.* London: Routledge.

Grandin, T. (2002). Teaching tips for children and adults with autism. [Electronic Version]. *Center for the Study of Autism.* Retrieved on August 2, 2005 from www.autism.org/temple/tips.html.

Iacoboni, M. & Dapretto, M. (2006, December 7). The mirror neuron system and the consequences of its dysfunction. *Nature Reviews: Neuroscience, 942–951,* Retrieved July 27, 2008 from www.csulb.edu/~cwallis/cscenter/mnc/abstracts/nn2024.pdf.

Iacoboni, M., Molnar-Szacks, I., Gallese, V., Buccino, G., Mazziotta, J.C., & Rizzolatti, G. (2005). Grasping the intentions of others with one's own mirror neuron system. *PLoS Biology, 3*(3) 79e. Retrieved January 23, 2006 from www.plosbiology.org.

Jensen, E. with Dabney, M. (2000). *Learning Smarter: The New Science of Teaching.* San Diego: The Brain Store.

McConachie, B. (2008). *Engaging Audiences: A Cognitive Approach to Spectating in the Theatre.* New York: Palgrave Macmillan. North Shore ARC brochure: *The Spotlight Program: Innovative drama-based social pragmatics for students ages 6–22.* Retrieved January 11, 2009 from http://spotlightprogram.com/Documents/Spotlight%20Brochure.pdf.

Posner, M., Rothbart, M. K., Sheese, B. E., & Kieras, J. (2008). How arts training influences cognition. In C. Ashbury & B. Rich (Eds.), *Learning, Arts, and the Brain* (pp. 1–10). New York: Dana Press.

Oberman, L. M. & Ramachandran, V. S. (2007). The simulating social mind: The role of the mirror neuron system and simulation in the social and communicative deficits of autism spectrum disorders. *Psychological Bulletin, 133*(2), 310–327.

Ramachandran, V. S. & Oberman, L. M. (2006, November). Broken mirrors: A theory of autism. *Scientific American,* 63–69.

Regan, T. (Director). (2007). *Autism: The Musical.* [Motion picture]. United States: Bunim-Murray Productions.

Chapter 22. Early Start Denver Model, by Dr. Sally Rogers et al.

1. Rogers, S.J., & Dawson, G. (2009). *Play and engagement in early autism: The Early Start Denver Model.* NY: Guilford.

2. Rogers, S. J., Herbison, J., Lewis, H., Pantone, J., & Reis, K. (1986). An approach for enhancing the symbolic, communicative, and interpersonal functioning of young children with autism and severe emotional handicaps. *Journal of the Division of Early Childhood, 10(2),* 135–148.

3. Rogers, S. J., & Lewis, H. (1989). An effective day treatment model for young children with pervasive developmental disorders. *Journal of the American Academy of Child and Adolescent Psychiatry, 28,* 207–214.

4. Stern, D. (1985). *The interpersonal world of the human infant.* New York: Basic Books.

5. Koegel, R.L., O'Dell, M., & Dunlap, G. (1988). Producing speech use in nonverbal autistic children by reinforcing attempts. *Journal of Autism and Developmental Disorders, 18(4)*, 525–538.

6. Schreibman, L., & Pierce, K. (1993). Achieving greater generalization of treatment effects in children with autism: Pivotal response training and self-management. *Clinical Psychologist, 46*, 184–191.

7. Dawson, G., Webb, S. J., Wijsman, E., Schellenberg, G. D., Estes, A., Munson, J. et al. (2005). Neurocognitive and electrophysiological evidence of altered face processing in parents of children with autism: Implications for a model of abnormal development of social brain circuitry in autism. *Development and Psychopathology, 17*, 679–697.

8. Rogers, S. J., & DiLalla, D. L. (1991). A comparative study of the effects of a developmentally based preschool curriculum on young children with autism and young children with other disorders of behavior and development. *Topics in Early Childhood Special Education, 11(2)*, 29–47.

9. Rogers, S. J., Lewis, H. C., & Reis, K. (1987). An effective procedure for training early special education teams to implement a model program. *Journal of the Division of Early Childhood, 11(2)*, 180–188.

10. Rogers, S. J., Hayden, D., Hepburn, S., Charlifue-Smith, R., Hall, T., & Hayes, A. (2006). Teaching young nonverbal children with autism useful speech: A pilot study of the Denver Model and PROMPT interventions. *Journal of Autism and Developmental Disorders, 36(8)*, 1007–1024.

11. Vismara, L.A., Colombi, C., & Rogers, S.J. (2009). Can one hour per week of therapy lead to lasting changes in young children with autism. *Autism, 13(1)*, 93–115.

12. Dawson, G., Rogers, S., Munson, J., Smith, M., Jamie, W., Greenson, J., et al. (2009). Randomized controlled trial of the Early Start Denver Model: A developmental behavioral intervention for toddlers with autism: Effects on IQ, adaptive behavior, and autism diagnosis. *Pediatrics, doi/10.1542/peds.2009–0958.*

13. Koegel, R.L., Koegel, L.K., & Surratt, A. (1992). Language intervention and disruptive behavior in preschool children with autism. *Journal of Autism and Developmental Disorders, 22(2)*, 141–153.

14. Koegel, L.K., Koegel, R.L., Hurley, C., & Frey, W.D. (1992). Improving social skills and disruptive behavior in children with autism through self-management. *Journal of Applied Behavior Analysis, 25(2)*, 341–353.

15. Ratner, N., & Bruner, J. (1978). Games, social exchange, and the acquisition of language. *Journal of Child Language, 5*, 391–402.

16. Rogers, S.J., Dawson, G., & Vismara, L.A. (in preparation). *The Early Start Denver Model Parent Curriculum*. New York, NY: Guilford Press.

17. Lord, C., & McGee, J. (Eds.), (2001). *Educating children with autism*. Washington, DC: National Academy Press.

18. McGee, G. G., Morrier, M. J., & Daly T. (1999). An incidental teaching approach to early intervention for toddlers with autism. *Journal of the Association for Persons with Severe Handicaps, 24*, 133–146.

19. National Research Council (2001). *Educating children with autism*.Washington, DC: National Academy Press.

20. Wetherby, A.M., & Woods, J.J. (2006). Early social interaction project for children with autism spectrum disorders beginning in the second year of life: A preliminary study. *Topics in Early Childhood Special Education, 26*, 67-82.

21. Kogan, M.D., Strickland, B.B., Blumberg, S.J., Sing, G.K., Perrin, J.M., & van Dyck, P.C. (2008). A national profile of the health care experiences and family impact of Autism Spectrum Disorder among children in the United States, 2005-2006. *Pediatrics, 122,* 1149-1158.

22. Kraus, M.W., Gulley, S., Sciegaj, M. & Wells, N. (2003). Access to specialty medical care for children with mental retardation, autism, and other special health care needs. *Mental Retardation, 41,* 329-339.

23. Ruble, L.A., Heflinger, C.A., Renfrew, J.W., & Saunders, R.C. (2005). Access and service use by children with autism spectrum disorders in Medicaid Managed Care. *Journal of Autism & Developmental Disorders, 35,* 3-13.

24. Oberleitner, R., Elison-Bowers, P., Reischl, U., & Ball, J. (2007). Optimizing the personal health record with special video capture for the treatment of autism. *Journal of Developmental Physical Disabilities, 19,* 513-518.

25. Stahmer, A.C., & Mandell, D.S. (2007). State infant/toddler program policies for eligibility and service provision for young children with autism. *Administration and Policy in Mental Health and Mental Health Services Research, 34,* 29-37.

26. Feil, E.G., Glasgow, R.E., Boles, S., & McKay, H.G. (2000). Who participates in Internet-based self-management programs? A study among novice computer users in a primary care setting. *The Diabetes Educator, 26,* 806-811.

27. Mackenzie, E.P., & Hilgedick, J.M. (1999). The Computer-Assisted Parenting Program (CAPP): The use of a computerized behavioral parenting training program as an educational tool. *Child and Family Behavior Therapy, 21,* 23-43.

28. Dudding, C.C. (2009). Digital videoconferencing applications across the disciplines. *Communication Disorders Quarterly, 30,* 178-182.

29. Baggett, K.M., Davis, B., Feil, E.G., Sheeber, L.L., Landry, S.H., Carta, J.J., et al. (2010). Technologies for expanding the reach of evidence-based interventions: Preliminary results for promoting social-emotional development in early childhood. *Topics in Early Childhood Special Education, 29,* 226-238.

Chapter 23. The Role and Treatment of Elevated Male Hormones in Autism Spectrum Disorders, by David A. Geier, Lisa Sykes, and Dr. Mark R. Geier

1. Auyeung B, Barson-Cohen S, Ashwin E, Knickmeyer R, Taylor K, Hackett G. Fetal testosterone and autistic traits. *British Journal of Psychology.* 2009;100:1-22.

2. Baron-Cohen S. The extreme male brain theory of autism. *Trends in Cognitive Sciences.* 2002;6:248-54.

3. Bryan KJ, Mudd JC, Richardson SL, Chang J, Lee HG, Zhu X, Smith MA, Casadesus G. Down-regulation of serum gonadotropins is as effective as estrogen replacement at improving menopause-associated cognitive deficits. *Journal of Neurochemistry.* 2010;112:870-81.

4. Dorn LD, Hitt SF, Rotenstein D. Biopsychological and cognitive differences in children with premature vs on-time adrenarche. *Archives of Pediatrics and Adolescent Medicine.* 1999;153:137-46.

5. Eaton GG, Worlein JM, Kelley ST, Vijayaraghavan S, Hess DL, Axthelm MK, Bethea CL. Self-injurious behavior is decreased by cyproterone acetate in adult male rhesus (Macaca mulatta). *Hormones and Behavior.* 1999;35:195-203.

6. Eriksson T. Anti-androgenic treatment of obsessive-compulsive disorder: an open-label clinical trial of the long-acting gonadotropin-release hormone analogue triptorelin. *International Clinical Psychopharmacology.* 2007;22:57-61.

7. Gaikwad U, Parle M, Kumar A, Kaikwad D. Effect of ritanserin and leuprolide alone and combined on marble-burying behavior of mice. *Acta Poloniae Pharmaceutica*. 2010;67:523-7.

8. Geier DA, Geier MR. A clinical trial of combined anti-androgen and anti-heavy metal therapy in autistic disorders. *Neuro-endocrinology Letters*. 2006;27:833-8.

9. Geier DA, Geier MR. A prospective assessment of androgen levels in patients with autistic spectrum disorders: biochemical underpinnings and suggested therapies. *Neuro-endocinology Letters*. 2007;28:565-73.

10. Geier DA, Young HA, Geier MR. Thimerosal exposure and increasing trends in premature puberty in the vaccine safety datalink. *Indian Journal of Medical Research*. 2010;131:500-7.

11. Geier MR, Geier DA. The potential importance of steroids in the treatment of autistic spectrum disorders and other disorders involving mercury toxicity. *Medical Hypotheses*. 2005;64:946-54.

12. Ingudomnukul E, Baron-Cohen S, Wheelwright S, Knickmeyer R. Elevated rates of testosterone-related disorders in women with autism spectrum conditions. *Hormones and Behavior*. 2007;51:597-604.

13. Knickmeyer R, Baron-Cohen S, Fane BA, Whellwright S, Mathews GA, Conway GS, Brook CG, Hines M. Autistic traits in people with congenital adrenal hyperplasia: a test of the fetal testosterone theory of autism. *Hormones and Behavior*. 2006;50:148-53.

14. Knickmeyer RC, Whellwright S, Hoekstra R, Baron-Cohen S. Age of menarche in females with autism spectrum conditions. *Developmental Medicine and Child Neurology*. 2006;48:1006-11.

15. Loosen PT, Purson SE, Pavlous SN. Effects on behavior of modulation of gonadal function in men with gonadotropin-releasing hormone antagonists. *American Journal of Psychiatry*. 1994;151:271-73.

16. Majewska MD, Hill M, Urbanowicz E, Rok-Bojko P, Namyslowska I, Mierzejewski P. Different levels of salivary steroids in autistic and health children. *European Neuropsychopharmacology*. 2010;20(Suppl 3):S615-6.

17. Manning JT, Barson-Cohen S, Wheelwright S, Sanders G. The 2nd to 4th digit ratio and autism. *Developmental Medicine and Child Neurology*. 2001;43:160-4.

18. Schwarz E, Guest PC, Rahmoune H, Wang L, Levin Y, Ingudomnukul E, Ruta L, Kent L, Spain M, Baron-Cohen S, Bahn S. Sex-specific serum biomarker patterns in adults with Asperger's syndrome. *Molecular Psychiatry*. 2010 Sep 28 [Epub ahead of print].

19. Tanaka T, Niimi H, Matsuo N, Fujieda K, Tachibana K, Ohyama K, Satoh M, Kugu K. Results of long-term follow-up after treatment of central precocious puberty with leuprorelin acetate: evaluation of effectiveness of treatment and recovery of gonadal function. The TAP-144-SR Japanese Study Group on Central Precocious Puberty. *Journal of Clinical Endocrinology and Metabolism*. 2005;90:1371-6.

20. Tordjman S, Ferrari P, Sulmont V, Duyme M, Roubertoux P. Androgenic activity in autism. *American Journal of Psychiatry*. 1997;154:1626-7.

21. Uday G, Pravinkumar B, Manish W, Sudhir U. LHRH antagonist attenuates the effect of fluoxetine on marble-burying behavior in mice. *European Journal of Pharmacology*. 2007;563:155-9.

22. Umathe S, Bhutada P, Dixit P, Shende V. Increased marble burying behavior in ethanol-withdrawal state: modulation by gonadotropin-releasing hormone agonist. *European Journal of Pharmacology*. 2008a;587-175-80.

23. Umathe SN, Bhutada PS, Dixit PV, Jain NS. Leuprolide: a luteinizing hormone releasing hormone agonist attenuates ethanol withdrawal syndrome and ethanol-induced locomotor sensitization in mice. *Neuropeptides*. 2008b;42:345-53.

24. Umathe SN, Bhutada PS, Jain NS, Dixit PV, Wanjari MM. Effects of central administration of gonadotropin-releasing hormone agonists and antagonist on elevated plus-maze social interaction behavior in rats. *Behavioral Pharmacology*. 2008c;19:308-16.

25. Umathe SN, Bhutada PS, Jain, Shukla NR, Mundhada YR, Dixit PV. Gonadotropin-releasing hormone agonist blocks anxiogenic-like and depressant-like effect of corticotrophin-releaseing hormone in mice. *Neuropeptides*. 2008d;42:399-410.

26. Umathe SN, Wanjari MM, Manna SS, Jain NS. A possible participating of gonadotropin-releasing hormone in the neuroleptic and cataleptic effect of haloperidol. *Neuropeptides*. 2009;43:251-7.

Chapter 24. Enzymes for Digestive Support in Autism, by Dr. Devin Houston

1. Ehren, J., Moron, B., Martin, E., Bethune, M. T., Gray, G. M., Khosla, C. (2009). A food-grade enzyme preparation with modest gluten detoxification properties. *PLos ONE 4*(7): e6313.

2. Scalbert, A., Johnson, I. T., Saltmarsh, M. (2005). Polyphenols: antioxidants and beyond. *Am. J. Clin. Nutr, 81*(S1): 21.

3. Scalbert, A., Williamson. G. (2000). Dietary intake and bioavailability of polyphenols. *J. Nutr. 130*: 2073S.

Chapter 27. Food Selectivity and Other Feeding Disorders in Autism (2), by Dr. Petula Vaz and Dr. Cathleen Piazza

Bachmeyer, M. H., Piazza, C. C., Fredrick, L. D., Reed, G. K., Rivas, K. D., & Kadey, H. J. (2009). Functional analysis and treatment of multiply controlled inappropriate mealtime behavior. *J Appl Behav Anal, 42*(3): 641–658.

Cohen, S. A., Piazza, C. C., & Navathe, A. Feeding and nutrition. In: Crocker ILRAC (Ed.). (2006). *Medical Care for Children and Adults with Developmental Disabilities*. Baltimore: Paul H. Brooks Publishing Co.

Freeman, K. A., Piazza, C. C. (1998). Combining stimulus fading, reinforcement, and extinction to treat food refusal. *J Appl Behav Anal, 31*:691–694.

Gulotta, C. S., Piazza, C. C., Patel, M. R., Layer, S. A. (2005). Using food redistribution to reduce packing in children with severe food refusal. *J Appl Behav Anal, 38*:39–50.

Keen, D. V. (2008). Childhood autism, feeding problems and failure to thrive in early infancy. *Eur Child Adolesc Psychiatry, 17*: 209–216.

Kelley, M. E., Piazza, C.C., Fisher, W. W., Oberdorff, A. J. (2003). Acquisition of cup drinking using previously refused foods as positive and negative reinforcement. *J Appl Behav Anal, 36*: 89–93.

Kerwin, M. E. (1999). Empirically supported treatments in pediatric psychology: severe feeding problems. *J Pediatr Psychol, 24*: 193–214; discussion 215–216.

Kodak, T., Piazza, C. C. (2008). Assessment and behavioral treatment of feeding and sleeping disorders in children with autism spectrum disorders. *Child and Adolescent Psychiatric Clinics of North America, 17*: 887–905.

Laud, R. B., Girolami, P.A. , Boscoe, J. H., Gulotta, C. S. (2009). Treatment outcomes for severe feeding problems in children with autism spectrum disorder. *Behavior Modification, 33*: 520–536.

Mueller, M. M., Piazza, C. C., Moore, J. W., et al. (2003). Training parents to implement pediatric feeding protocols. *J Appl Behav Anal, 36*: 545–562.

Mueller, M. M., Piazza, C. C., Patel, M. R., Kelley, M. E., Pruett, A. (2004). Increasing variety of foods consumed by blending nonpreferred foods into preferred foods. *J Appl Behav Anal, 37*: 159–170.

Munk, D. D., Repp, A.C. (1994). Behavioral assessment of feeding problems of individuals with severe disabilities. *J Appl Behav Anal, 27*: 241–250.

Najdowski, A. C., Wallace, M. D., Doney, J. K., Ghezzi, P. M. (2003). Parental assessment and treatment of food selectivity in natural settings. *J Appl Behav Anal, 36*: 383–386.

Patel, M. R., Piazza, C. C., Kelly, L., Ochsner, C. A., Santana, C. M. (2001). Using a fading procedure to increase fluid consumption in a child with feeding problems. *J Appl Behav Anal, 34*: 357–360.

Patel, M. R., Piazza, C. C., Layer, S. A., Coleman, R., Swartzwelder, D. M. (2005). A systematic evaluation of food textures to decrease packing and increase oral intake in children with pediatric feeding disorders. *J Appl Behav Anal, 38*: 89–100.

Patel, M. R., Piazza, C. C., Santana, C. M., Volkert, V. M. (2002). An evaluation of food type and texture in the treatment of a feeding problem. *J Appl Behav Anal, 35*: 183–186.

Patel, M. R., Reed, G. K., Piazza, C. C., Bachmeyer, M. H., Layer, S, A., Pabico, R. S. (2006). An evaluation of a high-probability instructional sequence to increase acceptance of food and decrease inappropriate behavior in children with pediatric feeding disorders. *Res Dev Disabil, 27*: 430–442.

Piazza, C. C., Fisher, W. W., Brown, K.A., et al. (2003). Functional analysis of inappropriate mealtime behaviors. *J Appl Behav Anal, 36*:187–204.

Piazza, C. C., Patel, M. R., Gulotta, C. S., Sevin, B. M., Layer, S. A. On the relative contributions of positive reinforcement and escape extinction in the treatment of food refusal. *J Appl Behav Anal, 36*: 309–324.

Piazza, C. C., Patel, M. R., Santana, C. M., Goh, H. L., Delia, M. D., Lancaster, B. M. (2002). An evaluation of simultaneous and sequential presentation of preferred and nonpreferred food to treat food selectivity. *J Appl Behav Anal, 35*: 259–270.

Reed, G. K., Piazza, C. C., Patel, M. R., et al. (2004). On the relative contributions of noncontingent reinforcement and escape extinction in the treatment of food refusal. *J Appl Behav Anal, 37*:27–42.

Rommel, N., De Meyer, A. M., Feenstra, L., & Veereman-Wauters, G. (2003). The complexity of feeding problems in 700 infants and young children presenting to a tertiary care institution. *Journal of Pediatric Gastroenterology and Nutrition, 37*: 75–82.

Sevin, B.M., Gulotta, C.S., Sierp, B. J., Rosica, L. A., Miller, L. J. (2002). Analysis of response covariation among multiple topographies of food refusal. *J Appl Behav Anal, 35*: 65–68.

Twachtman-Reilly, J., Amaral, S. C., Zebrowski, P. P. (2008). Addressing feeding disorders in children on the autism spectrum in school-based settings: Physiological and behavioral issues. *Language, Speech, and Hearing Services in Schools, 39*: 261–272.

Volkert, V. M., Piazza, C. C. (in press). Empirically supported treatments for pediatric feeding disorders. In P. Sturmey and M. Herson (Eds.), *Handbook of Evidence-Based Practice in Clinical Psychology*. Honoken, NJ: Wiley.

Werle, M. A., Murphy, T.B., Budd, K. S. (2002). Treating chronic food refusal in young children: Home-based parent training. *J Appl Behav Anal, 26*: 421–433.

Chapter 28. Gastrointestinal Disease: Emerging Concensus, by Dr. Arthur Krigsman

Afzal N, Murch S, Thirrupathy K, Berger L, Fagbemi A, Heuschkel R. Constipation with acquired megarectum in children with autism. Pediatrics. 2003 Oct;112(4):939–42.

Ashwood P, Wakefield AJ. Immune activation of peripheral blood and mucosal CD3+ lymphocyte cytokine profiles in children with autism and gastrointestinal symptoms. J Neuroimmunol. 2006 Apr;173(1-2):126–34.

Balzola F, Barbon V, Repici A, Rizzetto M. Panenteric IBD-like disease in a patient with regressive autism shown for the first time by the wireless capsule enteroscopy: another piece in the jigsaw of this gut-brain syndrome? Am J Gastro. 2005; 979–981.

Balzola F, Daniela C, Repici A, Barbon V, Sapino A, Barbera C, Calvo PL, Gandione M, Rigardetto R, Rizzetto M. Autistic enterocolitis: confirmation of a new inflammatory bowel disease in an Italian cohort of patients. Gastroenterology. 2005;128:Suppl.2;A–303.

Bolte ER. Autism and Clostridium tetani. Med Hypotheses. 1998 Aug;51(2):133–44.

Buie T, Campbell D, Fuchs G, Furuta G, Levy J, VandeWater J, Whitaker A, Atkins D, Bauman M, Beaudet A, Carr E, Gershon M, Hyman S, Jirapinyo P, Jyonouchi H, Kooros K, Kushak R, Levitt P, Levy S, Lewis J, Murray K, Natowicz M, Sabra A, Wershil B, Weston S, Zeltzer L, Winter H. Evaluation, Diagnosis, and Treatment of Gastrointestinal Disorders in Individuals With ASDs: A Consensus Report Pediatrics, Jan 2010; 125: S1 - S18.

Buie T, Fuchs G, Furuta G, Kooros K, Levy J, Lewis J, Wershil B, Winter H. Recommendations for Evaluation and Treatment of Common Gastrointestinal Problems in Children With ASDs Pediatrics, Jan 2010; 125: S19 - S29.

D'Eufemia P, Celli M, Finocchiaro R, Pacifico L, Viozzi L, Zaccagnini M, Cardi E, Giardini O. Abnormal intestinal permeability in children with autism. Acta Paediatr. 1996 Sep;85(9):1076–9.

Finegold SM, Molitoris D, Song Y, Liu C, Vaisanen ML, Bolte E, McTeague M, Sandler R, Wexler H, Marlowe EM, Collins MD, Lawson PA, Summanen P, Baysallar M, Tomzynski TJ, Read E, Johnson E, Rolfe R, Nasir P, Shah H, Haake DA, Manning P, Kaul A. Gastrointestinal microflora studies in late onset autism. Clin Infect Dis. 2002 Sep 1;35(Suppl 1):S6–S16.

Furlano RI, Anthony A, Day R, Brown A, McGavery L, Thomson MA, Davies SE, Berelowitz M, Forbes A, Wakefield AJ, Walker-Smith JA, Murch SH. Colonic CD8 and gamma delta T-cell infiltration with epithelial damage in children with autism. Pediatrics 2001;138:366–72.

Gonzalez L, Lopez K, Navarro D, Negron L, Flores L, Rodriguez R, Martinez M, Sabra A. Endoscopic and Histological Characteristics of the digestive mucosa in autistic children with gastrointestinal symptoms. Arch Venez Pueric Pediatr 69;1:19–25.

Horvath K, Papadimitriou JC, Rabazlan A. Gastrointestinal abnormalities in children with autistic disorder. J Pediatr 1999, 135:559–563.

Horvath K, Perman JA. Autistic disorder and gastrointestinal disease. Curr Opin Pediatr. 2002 Oct;14(5):583–7.

Jyonouchi, H, Geng, L, Ruby, A and Zimmerman-Bier, B. Dysregulated innate immune responses in young children with autism spectrum disorders: their relationship to gastrointestinal symptoms and dietary intervention. Neuropsychobiology, 2005;51(2):77-85.

Jyonouchi, H, Sun, S and Le, H. Proinflammatory and regulatory cytokine production associated with innate and adaptive immune responses in children with autism spectrum disorders and developmental regression. Journal of Neuroimmunology, 2001;120(1-2):170-179.

Knivsberg AM, Reichelt KL, Hoien T, Nodland M. A randomised, controlled study of dietary intervention in autistic syndromes. Nutr Neurosci. 2002 Sep;5(4): 251–61.

Knivsberg AM, Reichelt KL, Nodland M, Hoein T: Autistic Syndromes and Diet: a follow-up study. Scandinavian Journal of Educational Research 1995; 39: 223–236.

Knivsberg AM, Reichelt KL, Nodland M. Reports on dietary intervention in autistic disorders. Nutr Neurosci. 2001;4(1): 25–37.

Krigsman A, Boris M, Goldblatt A, Stott C. Clinical Presentation and Histologic Findings at Ileocolonoscopy in Children with Autistic Spectrum Disorder and Chronic gastrointestinal Symptoms. Autism Insights 2010:2 1–11.

Kuddo T, Nelson KB. How common are gastrointestinal disorders in children with autism. Curr Opin Pediatr 2003: 15(3); 339–343.

Kushak R, Winter H, Farber N, Buie T. Gastrointestinal symptoms and intestinal disaccharidase activities in children with autism. Abstract of presentation to the North American Society of Pediatric Gastroenterology, Hepatology, and Nutrition, Annual Meeting, October 20-22, 2005, Salt Lake City, Utah.

Melmed RD, Schneider CK, Fabes RA. Metabolic markers and gastrointestinal symptoms in children with autism and related disorders. J Pediatr Gastroenterol Nutr 2000:31(suppl 2) S31–32.

Parracho HM, Bingham MO, Gibson GR, McCartney AL. Differences between the gut microflora of children with autistic spectrum disorders and that of healthy children. J Med Microbiol. 2005 Oct;54(Pt 10):987–91.

Sandler RH, Finegold SM, Bolte ER, Buchanan CP, Maxwell AP, Vaisanen ML, Nelson MN, Wexler HM. Short-term benefit from oral vancomycin treatment of regressive-onset autism. J Child Neurol. 2000 Jul;15(7):429–35.

Song Y, Liu C, Finegold SM. Real-time PCR quantitation of clostridia in feces of autistic children. Appl Environ Microbiol. 2004 Nov;70(11):6459–65.

Torrente F, Machado N, Perez-Machado M, Furlano R, Thomson M, Davies S, Wakefield AJ, Walker-Smith JA, Murch SH. Enteropathy with T cell infiltration and epithelial IgG deposition in autism. Mol Psychiatry. 2002;7:375–382.

Torrente F, Anthony A. Heuschkel, RB, Thomson, M, Ashwood, P, Murch S. Focal-enhanced gastritis in regressive autism with features distinct from Crohn's disease and helicobacter Pylori gastritis. Am J Gastroenterol 2004 Apr;99(4):598–605.

Valicenti-McDermott M, McVicar K, Rapin I, Wershil BK, Cohen H, Shinnar S. Frequency of gastrointestinal symptoms in children with autistic spectrum disorders and association with family history of autoimmune disease. J Dev Behav Pediatr. 2006 Apr;27(2 Suppl):S128–36.

Wakefield AJ, Murch SH, Anthony A et al. Ileal-lymphoid nodular hyperplasia non-specific colitis and pervasive developmental disorder in children. Lancet. 1998;351:637–41.

Wakefield, AJ, Anthony, A, Murch, S, et al. Enterocolitis in Children with Developmental Disorders. American Journal of Gastroenterology, 2000;95(9):2285-2295.

Chapter 29. Helminthic Therapy by Judith Chinitz

Ashwood, P., Anthony, A., Torrente, F., Wakefield, A. J. (2004). Spontaneous mucosal lymphocyte cytokine profiles in children with autism and gastrointestinal symptoms: mucosal immune activation and reduced counter regulatory interleukin-10. *Journal of Clinical Immunology, 24*(6): 664–673.

Ashwood, P., Wakefield, A. J. (2006). Immune activation of peripheral blood and mucosal CD3+ lymphocyte cytokine profiles in children with autism and gastrointestinal symptoms. *Journal of Neuroimmunology, 173*(1-2):126–134.

Bashir, M. E. H., Andersen, P., Fuss, I., Shi, H. N., Nagler-Anderson, C. (2002). An enteric helminth infection protects against an allergic response to dietary antigen. *The Journal of Immunlogy, 169*: 3284–3292.

Becker, K. (2007). Autism, asthma, inflammation, and the hygiene hypothesis. *Medical Hypothesis,* doi:10.1016/j.mehy.2007.02.019.

Careaga, M., Van de Water, J., Ashwood, P. (2010). Immune dysfunction in autism: a pathway to treatment. *Neurotherapeutics*, Jul;7(3):283-92.

Correale, J., Farez, M. (2007). Association between parasite infection and immune responses in multiple sclerosis. *Annals of Neurology, 61*: 97–108.

Croonenberghs, J., Bosmans, E., Deboutte, D., Kenis, G., Maes, M. (2002). Activation of the inflammatory response system in autism. *Neuropsychobiology, 45*(1):1–6.

Croese, J., O'Neil, J., Masson, J., Cooke, S., Melrose, W., Pritchard, D. Speare, R., (2006). A proof of concept study establishing Necator americanus in Crohn's patients and reservoir donors. *Gut, 55*: 136–137.

Diaz Heijtz, R., Wang, S., Anuar, F., Qian, Y., Bjork, B., Samuelsson, A., Hibberd, M.L., Forssberg, H., Pettersson, S. (2011). Normal gut microbiota modulates brain development and behavior. *Proceedings of the National Academy of Science*, [Epub ahead of print—retrieved February 12, 2011 from http://www.pnas.org/content/early/2011/01/26/1010529108.long].

Elliott, D. E., Summers, R. W., Weinstock, J. V. (2007). Helminths as governors of immune-mediated inflammation. *International Journal of Parasitology, 37*(5): 457–464.

Elliott, D. E., Summers, R. W., Weinstock, J. V. (2005). Helminths and the modulation of mucosal inflammation. *Current Opinion in Gastroenterology, 21*: 51–58.

Feillet, H., Bach, J.F. (2004). Increased incidence of inflammatory bowel disease: the price of the decline of infectious burden? Current Opinion in Gastroenterology:20(6):560–4.

Fumagalli, M., Pozzoli, U., Cagliani, R., Comi, G.P., Stefania, R., Clerici, M., Bresolin, N., Sironi, M. (2009). Parasites represent a major selective force for interleukin genes and shape the genetic predisposition to autoimmune conditions. *Journal of Experimental Medicine, 206*(6): 1395–1408.

Gupta, S., Aggarwal, S., Rashanravan, B., Lee, T. (1998). Th1–and Th2-like cytokines in CD4+ and CD8+ cells in autism. *Journal of Neuroimmunlogy, 85*(1): 106–109.

Hamilton, G. (2008). Why we need germs. The Ecologist Report. Retrieved August 4, 2008 from www.mindfullly.org/Health/We-Need-Germs.htm.

Hayes, K.S., Bancroft, A.J., Goldrick, M., Portsmouth, C., Roberts, I.S., Grencis, R.K. (2010). Explitation of the intestinal microflora by the parasitic nematode Trichuris muris. *Science,* June 11;328(5984):1391-4.

Jyonouchi, H., Sun, S., Le H. (2001). Proinflammatory and regulatory cytokine production associated with innate and adaptive immune responses in children with autism spectrum disorders and developmental regression. *Journal of Neuroimmunology: 120*(1-2):170–179.

Li, X., Chauhan, A., Sheikh, A.M., Patil, S., Chauhan, V., Li, X.M., Ji L., Brown, T., Malik, M. (2009). Elevated immune response in the brain of autistic patients. *Journal of Neuroimmunology, 207*(1-2):111–116.

Maizels, R. M., Yazdanbakhsh, M. (2003). Immune regulation by helminth parasites: cellular and molecular mechanisms. *Nature Reviews/Immunlogy,* volume 3.

Mangan, N.E., Fallon, R.E., Smith, P., van Rooijen, N., McKenzie, A.N., Fallon, P.G. (2004). Helminth infection protects mice from anaphylaxis via IL-10-producing B cells. *Journal of Immunology, 173*: 6346–6356.

Molloy, C. A., Morrow, A. L., Meinzen-Derr, J., Schleifer, K., Dienger, K., Manning-Courtney, P., Altaye, M., Wills-Karp, M. (2006). Elevated cytokine levels in ch ildren with autism spectrum disorders. *Journal of Neuroimmunlogy, 172*(1-2):198–205.

Newman, A.(1999). In pursuit of autoimmune worm cure. *The New York Times* on the Web. Retrieved March, 25, 2008 from http://query.nytimes.com/gst/fullpage.html?res=9A0DE 6DB113BF932A0575BC0A96F958260&scp=1&sq=in%20pursuit%20of%20an%20autoim-mune%20cure&st=cse.

Parker, William (2010). Reconstituting the depleted biome to prevent immune disorders. The *Evolution of Medicine Review*. Retrieved October 13, 2010 from http://evmedreview. com/?p=457 .

Reddy, A., Fried, B. (2007). The use of Trichuris suis and other helminth therapies to treat Crohn's disease. *Parasitology Research, 100*: 921–927.

Rook, G. (2007). The hygiene hypothesis and the increasing prevalence of chronic inflamma-tory disorders. *Transactions of the Royal Society of Tropical Medicine and Hygiene, 101:* 1072–1074.

Rook, G., Lowry, C. A. (2008). The hygiene hypothesis and psychiatric disorders. *Trends in Immunology, 29*(4): 150–158.

Schnoeller, C., Rausch, S., Pillai, S., Avagyan, A., Wittig, B. M., Loddenkemper, C., Hamann, A., Hamelmann, E., Lucius, R., Hartmann, S. (2008). A helminth immunomodulator reduces allergic and inflammatory responses by induction of IL-10-producing macrophages. *The Journal of Immunology, 180*: 4265–4272.

Summers, R. W., Elliott, D. E., Qadir, K., Urban, J. F. Jr, Thompson, R., Weinstock, J. V. (2003). Trichuris suis seems to be safe and possibly effective in the treatment of inflammatory bowel disease. *American Journal of Gastroenterology Sep;98*(9):2034–2041.

Summers, R. W., Elliott, D. E., Urban, J. F. Jr, Thompson, R., Weinstock, J. V. (2005) Trichuris suis therapy in Crohn's disease. *Gut, 54*: 87–90.

Turner, J. D., Jackson, J. A., Faulkner, H., Behnke, J., Else, K. J., Kamgno, J., Boussinesq, M., Bradley, J. E. (2008). Intensity of intestinal infection with multiple worm species is related to regulatory cytokine output and immune hyporesponsiveness. *Journal of Infectious Diseases, 197*: 1204–1212.

Walk, S.T., Blum, A.M., Ewing, S.A., Weinstock, J.V., Young, V.B. Alterations of the murine gut microbiota during infection with the parasitic helminth Heligmosomoides polygyrus. *Inflammatory Bowel Disease*, Nov;16(11):1841-9.

Warren, R. P., Margaretten, N. C., Pace, N. C., Foster, A. (1986). Immune abnormalities in patients with autism. *Journal of Autism and Developmental Disorders, 16*(2):189–197.

Weinstock, J. V., Elliott, D. E. (2009). Helminths and the IBD Hygiene Hypothesis. *Inflammatory Bowel Disease, 15*(1):128–133.

Zaccone, P., Fehervari, Z., Phillips, J. M., Dunne, D. W., Cooke, A. (2006). Parasitic worms and inflammatory diseases. *Parasite Immunology, 28*: 515–523.

Chapter 32. Homotoxicology and Beyond, by Mary Coyle

1.   Linde K, Jonas WB, Melchart D, Worku F, Wagner J, & Eitel F (1994). Critical review and meta-analysis of serial agitated dilutions in experimental toxicology. *Hum Exp Toxicol*. 481-92.

Chapter 33. Integrated Play Groups (IPG) Model, by Dr. Pamela Wolfberg

Bottema, K. (2008) *Integrated teen social groups: A qualitative analysis of peer socialization in teens with Autism Spectrum Disorder*. Unpublished position paper. University of California, Berkeley with SFSU.

California Department of Education. (1997) *Best practices for designing and delivering effective programs for individuals with Autistic Spectrum Disorders*. RiSE, Resources in Special Education, Sacramento, CA.

Fuge, G & Berry, R. (2004) *Pathways to Play! Combining Sensory Integration and Integrated Play Groups. Theme-based activities for children with Autism Spectrum and Other Sensory Processing Disorders*. Shawnee Mission, KS: Autism Asperger Publishing Company

Gonsier-Gerdin, J. (1992). *Elementary school children's perspectives on peers with disabilities in the context of Integrated Play Groups: "They're not really disabled, they're like plain kids."* (unpublished study) UC Berkeley-San Francisco State University.

Iovannone, R. Dunlop, G, Huber, H. & Kincaid, D. (2003). Effective educational practices for students with ASD. *Focus on Autism and Other Developmental Disabilities, 18* (3), 150–165.

Julius, H. & Wolfberg, P. (2009) *Integrated Play and Drama Groups for Children and Adolescents on the Autism Spectrum. Alexander von Humboldt Foundation TransCoop Program: Transatlantic Cooperation in the Humanities, Social Sciences, Law, and Economics (2009–2012)*.

Lantz, J. F., Nelson, J. M. & Loftin, R. L. (2004) Guiding Children with Autism in Play: Applying the Integrated Play Group Model in School Settings. *Exceptional Children, 37*(2), 8–14.

Mikaelan, B. (2003) *Increasing language through sibling and peer support play*. Unpublished Master Thesis, San Francisco State University, CA. National Research Council (2001) *Educating Children with Autism*. Committee on Educational Interventions for Children with Autism: Division of Behavioral and Social Sciences and Education, National Academy Press: Washington, D.C. National Autism Center (2009) *National standards project report- findings and conclusions: Addressing the need for evidence-based practice guidelines for Autism Spectrum Disorder*. Integrated Play Groups™ (IPG) model identified as "Established" practice within category of "Peer Intervention Package" based on studies reviewed; cited on p. 14, 30, & 50.

Neufeld, D. & Wolfberg, P.J. (2010) From novice to expert: Guiding children on the autism spectrum in Integrated Play Groups. In Schaefer, C. (Ed.) *Play therapy for preschool children*. Washington, D.C: American Psychological Association.

O'Connor, T. (1999). *Teacher perspectives of facilitated play in Integrated Play Groups*. Unpublished Master Thesis, San Francisco State University, CA.

Richard, V, & Goupil, G. (2005). Application des groupes de jeux integres aupres d'eleves ayant un trouble envahissant du development (Implementation of Integrated Play Groups with PDD Students). *Revue quebecoise de psychologie, 26(3), 79–103*

Vygotsky, L. (1966). Play and its role in the mental development of the child. *Soviet Psychology, 12,* 6–18 (Original work published in 1933).

Vygotsky, L. S. (1978). *Mind in society: The development of higher psychological processes*. Cambridge, MA: Harvard University Press.

Wolfberg, P. J. (1988). *Integrated play groups for children with autism and related disorders*. Unpublished master's field study, San Francisco State University.

Wolfberg, P.J. (1994). *Case illustrations of emerging social relations and symbolic activity in children with autism through supported peer play* (Doctoral   dissertation, University of California at Berkeley with San Francisco State University). *Dissertation Abstracts International,* #9505068.

Wolfberg, P. J., & Schuler, A. L. (1992). *Integrated play groups project: Final evaluation report* (Contract # HO86D90016). Washington, DC: Department of Education, OSERS.

Wolfberg, P.J. (2009). *Play and imagination in children with autism.* (second edition) New York: Teachers College Press, Columbia University.

Wolfberg, P., Turiel., E., & DeWitt, M., (2008). *Integrated Play Groups: Promoting symbolic play, social engagement and communication with peers across settings in children with autism.* Autism Speaks Treatment Grant (2008–2011).

Wolfberg, P.J. (2003) *Peer play and the autism spectrum: The art of guiding children'socialization and imagination.* Shawnee, KS: Autism Asperger Publishing Company.

Wolfberg, P.J., & Schuler, A.L. (1992). *Integrated play groups project: Final evaluation report* (Contract # HO86D90016). Washington, DC: U.S.Department of Education, OSERS.

Wolfberg, P. J. (1988). *Integrated play groups for children with autism and related disorders.* Unpublished master's field study, San Francisco State University.

Wolfberg, P. (2010).

Wolfberg, P. J., & Schuler, A. L. (1993). Integrated Play Groups: A model for promoting the social and cognitive dimensions of play in children with autism. *Journal of Autism and Developmental Disorders, 23*(3), 467–489.

Yang, T., Wolfberg, P. J., Wu, S, Hwu, P. (2003) Supporting children on the autism spectrum in peer play at home and school: Piloting the Integrated Play Groups model in Taiwan. *Autism: The International Journal of Research and Practice, 7*(4) 437–453.

Zercher, C., Hunt, P., Schuler, A. L., & Webster, J. (2001). Increasing joint attention, play and language through peer supported play. *Autism: The International Journal of Research and Practice, 5,* 374–398.

Chapter 34. Integrative Educational Care by Dr. Mary Joann Lang

1.   Humphreys A, Post T, Ellis A. (1981). *Interdisciplinary methods: A thematic approach.* Santa Monica, CA: Goodyear Publishing Company.
2.   Palmer J. (1991). Planning wheels turn curriculum around. *Educational Leadership.* 49(2);57-60.

Chapter 35. Intestine, Leaky Gut, Autism, and Probiotics, by Dr. Alessio Fasano

Fasano A. Pathological and therapeutical implications of macromolecule passage through the tight junction. *In* Tight Junctions. Boca Raton, FL: CRC Press, Inc., 2001, p. 697–722.

Fasano A. Physiological, pathological, and therapeutic implications of zonulin-mediated intestinal barrier modulation: living life on the edge of the wall. *Am J Pathol.* 173:1243–52, 2008.

White JF. Intestinal pathophysiology in Autism. *Exp Biol Med* 228:639–649, 2003.Prevalence of autism spectrum disorders - Autism and Developmental Disabilities Monitoring Network, United States, 2006. Autism and Developmental Disabilities Monitoring Network Surveillance Year 2006 Principal Investigators; Centers for Disease Control and Prevention (CDC). *MMWR Surveill Summ.* 2009; 58:1–20.

Buie T, Campbell DB, Fuchs GJ, III, et al Evaluation, Diagnosis, and Treatment of Gastrointestinal Disorders in Individuals With ASDs: A Consensus Report. *Pediatrics* 2010;125;S1–S18.

Buie T, Fuchs GJ, III, Furuta GT, Kooros K, Levy J, Lewis JD, Wershil BK, Winter H. Recommendations for Evaluation and Treatment of Common Gastrointestinal Problems in Children With ASDs. *Pediatrics* 2010;125;S19–S29

Guarner F Prebiotics, probiotics and helminths: the 'natural' solution? *Dig Dis.* 2009;27: 412–417. www.usprobiotics.org

Golnik AE, Ireland M., Complementary alternative medicine for children with autism: a physician survey. *J Autism Dev Disord.* 2009; 39: 996–1005.

Chapter 36. Intravenous Immunoglobulin (IVIG), by Dr. Michael Elice

Gupta, S, Aggarwal S., Heads, C. Dysregulated immune system in children with autism: beneficial effects of intravenous gamma globulin on autistic characteristics. J autism Dev disord 1996;26: 439–452.

Plioplys A V. Intravenous gamma globulin in children with autism. J Child Neurol 1998;13:79–82

Delgiudice-Asch G, Simon L, Schmeidler J, Cunningham-Rundles C, Hollander E. A pilot clinical triial of intravenous gamma globulin in childhood autism. *J Autism Dev Disord* 1999 199;29:157–160.

Boris M, goldblatt A, Galanko j, James J. Association of MTHFR gene variants with autism. *J Phys Surg* 2004;29:157–160.

National Institutes of Health. Intravenous immunoglobulin: prevention and treatment of disease. NIH consensus Statement 1990;8(2):1–23.

Latov N, Chaudhry V, Koski CL, Lisak RP Apatoff BR, Hahn AF, Howard AF. Use of intravenous gamma globulins in neuroimmunologic diseases. *J Allerg Clin Immunol* 2001;108:S126–132.

Comi AM, Zimmmerman AW, Frye VH, Law PA, Peeden JN. Familial Clustering of autoimmune disorders and evaluation of medical risk factors in autism. *J Child Neurol* 1999;14:388–394.

Swedo, SE. Sydenham's chorea: a model for childhood autoimmune neuropsychiatric disorders. *JAMA* 1994;272(22): 1788–1791.

Swedo SE, Rapoport JL, Cheslow DL, et al. High prevalence of obsessive-compulsive symptoms in patients with sydenham's chorea. *Am J Psychiatry*. 1989;46:335–341.

Swedo SE, Leonard HL, Garvey M, et al. Pediatric autoimmune neuropsychiatric disorders associated with streptococcal infections (PANDAS): a clinical description of the first fifty cases. Am J Psychiatry. 1998;155:264–271.

Giedd JN, Rapoport JL, Leonard HL, etal. Case study, acute basal ganglia enlargement and obsessive-compusive symptoms in an adolescent boy. J Am Acad Child Adolsc Pshychiatry. 1996,35(7):913–915

Garvey MA, Perlmutter SJ, Allen AJ, etal. A pilot study of penicillin prophylaxis for neuropsychiatric exacerbations triggered by streptococcal infections. Biol Psychiatry. 1999,45: 1564–1571

Barron KS, Sher MR, Silverman ED. Intravenous immunoglobulin therapy: magic or black magic. J Theumatol. 1992; 19:94–97

Perlmutter SJ, Leitman SF, Garvey MA etal. Therapeutic plasma exchange and intravenous immunoglobulin for obsessive-compulsive disorder and tic disorders in childhood. Lancet. 1999;50(6):429–439

Martino D, Defazio G, Giovannoni G. The PANDAS subgroup of tic disorders and childhood-onset obsessive-compulsive disorder. J Psychosom Res. 2009/Nov30;170(1):3–6

Gilbert DL, Kurlan R. PANDAS horse or zebra? Neurology. 2009 Oct 20;73(16):1252–3

Shulman ST. Pediatric autoimmune neuropsychiatric disorders associated with streptococci (PANDAS) update. Cuyrr Opin Pediatr. 2009 Feb;21(1): 127–30

Pavone P. Parano E, Rizzo R, Trifiletti RR.Autoimmune neuropsychiatric disorders associated with streptococcal infection: Sydenham chorea. PANDAS and PANDAS variants. J Child Neurol. 2006.Aug.21(8):678–689

Swedo SE, Grant PJ. Annotation: PANDAS: a model for human autoimmune disease. J child Psychol Psychiatry. 2005 Mar; 46(3): 227–34

Chapter 39. Melatonin Therapy for Sleep Disorders, by Dr. James Jan

1. JE Jan and RD Freeman. Melatonin therapy for circadian rhythm sleep disorders in children with multiple disabilities: what have we learned in the last decade? Developmental Medicine and Child Neurology. 2004, 46:776–782.
2. JE Jan, MB Wasdell, MD Weiss, RD Freeman. What is the correct dose of melatonin in sleep therapy? Biological Rhythm Research. 2007, 38:85–86.
3. JE Jan, MD Wasdell, RJ Reiter, MD Weiss, KP Johnson, A.Ivanenko, RD Freeman. Melatonin therapy of pediatric sleep disorders:recent advances,why it works,who are the candidates and how to treat. Current Pediatric Reviews.2007,3:214–324.
4. R Carr, MB Wasdell, D Hamilton, MD Weiss, RD Freeman, J Tai,WJ Rietveld, JE Jan. Long-term effectiveness outcome of melatonin therapy in children with treatment-resistant circadian rhythm sleep disorders. Journal of Pineal Research. 2007, 43:351–359.

Chapter 41. Methyl-B$_{12}$: Myth or Masterpiece, by Dr. James Neubrander

Selected References

1. Culley, D.J., Raghavan, S.V., Waly, M., Baxter, M.G., Yukhananov, R., Deth, R.C. and Crosby, G. : Nitrous oxide decreases cortical methionine synthase transiently but produces lasting memory impairment in aged rats. Anesthesia and Analgesia 105: 83-88 (2007).
2. Deth, R., Muratore, C., Benzecry, J., Power-Charnitsky, V., and Waly, M. How environmental and genetic factors combine to cause autism: A Redox/Methylation Hypothesis. Neurotoxicology (Under Review).
3. Flippo TS, Holder WD Jr. Neurologic degeneration associated with nitrous oxide anesthesia in patients with vitamin B12 deficiency. Arch Surg. 1993 Dec;128(12):1391-5.
4. Funada U, Wada M, Kawata T, Mori K, Tamai H, Kawanishi T, Kunou A, Tanaka N, Tadokoro T, Maekawa A. Changes in CD4+CD8-/CD4-CD8+ ratio and humoral immune functions in vitamin B12-deficient rats. Int J Vitam Nutr Res. 2000 Jul;70(4):167-71.
5. James SJ, Melnyk S, Fuchs G, Reid T, Jernigan S, Pavliv O, Hubanks A, Gaylor D. Efficacy of methylcobalamin and folinic acid on glutathione redox status in children with autism. Am J Clin Nutr 2009;89:425-39.
6. James SJ, Melnyk S, Jernigan S, Cleves MA, Halsted CH, Wong DH, Cutler P, Bock K, Boris M, Bradstreet JJ, Baker SM, Gaylor DW. Metabolic endophenotype and related genotypes are associated with oxidative stress in children with autism. Am J Med Genet B Neuropsychiatr Genet. 2006 Dec 5;141(8):947-56.
7. James SJ, Slikker W 3rd, Melnyk S, New E, Pogribna M, Jernigan S. Thimerosal neurotoxicity is associated with glutathione depletion: protection with glutathione precursors. Neurotoxicology. 2005 Jan;26(1):1-8.
8. James SJ, Cutler P, Melnyk S, Jernigan S, Janak L, Gaylor DW, Neubrander JA. Metabolic biomarkers of increased oxidative stress and impaired methylation capacity in children with autism. Am. J. Clinical Nutrition, Dec 2004; 80: 1611–1617.
9. Kosonen T, Pihko H. [Development regression in a child caused by vitamin B12 deficiency] Duodecim. 1994;110(6):588-91.
10. Metz J. Cobalamin deficiency and the pathogenesis of nervous system disease. Annu Rev Nutr. 1992;12:59-79.
11. Pema PJ, Horak HA, Wyatt RH. Myelopathy caused by nitrous oxide toxicity. AJNR Am J Neuroradiol. 1998 May;19(5):894-6.
12. Sharma, A., Kramer, M., Wick, P.F., Liu, D., Chari, S., Shim, S., Tan, W.-B., Ouellette, D., Nagata, M., DuRand, C., Kotb, M. and Deth, R.C.: Dopamine D4 receptor-mediated

methylation of membrane phospholipids and its implications for mental illnesses such as schizophrenia. Molecular Psychiatry 4: 235-246 (1999).

13. Waly, M, and Deth, R.C.: Glutathione and methylcobalamin-dependent methionine synthase activity in neuronal cells: Implications for neurodevelopmental and neurodegenerative disorders. (In Preparation).

14. Waly, M., Power-Charnitsky, V., Deth, R.C.: Reduced activation of phospholipid methylation by the seven-repeat variant of the D4 dopamine receptor. Eur. J. Pharmacol. (Submitted)

15. Waly, M., Banerjee, R., Choi, S.W., Mason, J., Benzecry, J., Power-Charnitsky, V.A, Deth, R.C. PI3-kinase regulates methionine synthase: Activation by IGF-1 or dopamine and inhibition by heavy metals and thimerosal Molecular Psychiatry 9: 358-370 (2004).

16. Waly M, Olteanu H, Banerjee R, Choi SW, Mason JB, Parker BS, Sukumar S, Shim S, Sharma A, Benzecry JM, Power-Charnitsky VA, Deth RC. Activation of methionine synthase by insulin-like growth factor-1 and dopamine: a target for neurodevelopmental toxins and thimerosal. Mol Psychiatry. 2004 Jan 27 [Epub ahead of print]

17. Weissbach H, Taylor R. Role of vitamin B12 in methionine synthesis. Fed Proc. 1966 Nov-Dec;25(6):1649-56.

18. Zhao W, Mosley BS, Cleves MA, Melnyk S, James SJ, Hobbs CA. Neural tube defects and maternal biomarkers of folate, homocysteine, and glutathione metabolism. Birth Defects Res A Clin Mol Teratol. 2006 Apr;76(4):230-6.

19. Zhao, R., Chen, Y., Tan, W., Waly, M., Malewicz, B., Stover, P., Rosowsky, A. and Deth, R.C.: Influence of single-carbon folate and *de novo* purine synthesis pathways on D4 dopamine receptor-mediated phospholipid methylation. J. Neurochem. 78: 788-796 (2001).

Chapter 43. Music Therapy by Leah Kmetz

1. AMTA 1999

2. Gray, Carol (2000). *The New Social Story Book*. Future Horizons Inc., Arlington, Tx.

3. Kaplan, M. (1990). *The Arts: A Social Perspective*. Rutherford, NJ:Fairleigh Dickinson University Press.

4. Merriam, Alan P. (1964). *The Anthropology of Music*. Northwestern University Press.

5. DSM-IV-TR, 2000. American Psychiatric Association.

6. Mottron, L., I. Peretz, and E. Menard (2000). *Local and Global Processing of Music in High-functioning Persons with Autism: Beyond Central Coherence?* J. Child Psychological Psychiatrist. 41. 8. 1057–1065.

Chapter 49. Parent Support, by Dr. Lauren Tobing-Puente

1. Tobing, L., & Glenwick, D. S. (2002). Relation of the Childhood Autism Rating Scale-Parent Version to diagnosis, stress, and age. *Research in Developmental Disabilities, 23*, 211–223.

2. Brobst, J.B., Clopton, J. R., & Hendrick, S.H. (2009). Parenting children with autism spectrum disorders: The couple's relationship. *Focus on Autism and Other Developmental Disabilities, 24*, 38–49.

3. Konstantareas, M. M., Homatidis, S., & Plowright, C. M. S. (1992). Assessing resources and stress in parents of severely dysfunctional children through the Clarke modification of Holroyd's Questionnaire on Resources and Stress. *Journal of Autism and Developmental Disorders, 22*, 217–234.

4. Fisman, S., & Wolf, L. (1991). The handicapped child: Psychological effects on parental, marital and sibling relationships. *Psychiatric Clinics of North America, 14,* 199–217.

5. Tobing, L. E., & Glenwick, D. S. (2006). Predictors and moderators of psychological distress in mothers of children with pervasive developmental disorders. *Journal of Family Social Work, 10,* 1–22.

6. Rodrigue, J. R., Morgan, S. B., & Geffken, G. (1990). Families of autistic children: Psychological functioning of mothers. *Journal of Clinical Child Psychology, 19,* 371–379.

7. Greenspan, S. I., & Wieder, S. (2006). *Engaging autism: Using the floortime approach to help children relate, communicate and think.* Cambridge, MA: Da Capo Press

Chapter 50. Physical Therapy, by Meghan Collins

1. Description of Physical Therapy—The World Confederation for Physical Therapy (WCPT) www.wcpt.org/description_of_physical_therapy

2. Bly, L (1983). The Components of Normal Development During the First Year of Life. Neuro-Developmental Treatment Association, Inc.

3. Schmidt, R.A. (1988). *Motor Control and Learning: A Behavioral Emphasis.* 2nd ed. Champaign, IL: Human Kinetics.

4. Campbell, SK Physical Therapy for Children Second Edition. WB Saunders, 2000 Cohen S *Targeting Autism: What we Know, Don't Know, and Can do to Help Young Children with Autism and Related Disorders.* California: University of California Press. 1998

Chapter 51. Psychotropic Medications and Their Cautious Discontinuation by Dr. Georgia A. Davis

Buie, Timothy, MD et al. Evaluation, Diagnosis and Treatment of Gastrointestinal Disorders in Individuals with ASDs: A Consensus Report. Pediatrics, Vol. 125, Supplement January 2010, pp. S1-S18

Crinnion, Walter J, ND. Toxic Effects of the Easily Avoidable Phthalates and Parabens. Alternative Medicine Review, Vol., 15, No. 3, Sept. 2010.

Dworkin, Jonathan and Shah, Ishita M. Opinion: Exit from Dormancy in Microbial Organisms. Nature Reviews Microbiology 8, 890-896 (December 2010)

Jones, David S., MD, Editor in Chief. Textbook of Functional Medicine. Gig Harbor, WA, 2006.

Lord, Richard S., Bralley, J. Alexander. Laboratory Evaluations of Integrative and Functional Medicine, Metametrix Institute, 2008.

McCandless, Jaquelyn, MD, Children With Starving Brains. Bramble Books, 2007.

McDonald, RL, McLean, MJ. Anticonvulsant drugs: mechanisms of action. Adv. Neurol. 1986:44:713-36.

Pangborn, Jon, PhD and Sidney MacDonald Baker, MD. Autism: Effective Biomedical Treatments. Autism Research Institute. Sept. 2005 Edition.

Papolos, Demetri, MD and Janice Papolos. The Bipolar Child. Broadway Books, Third Edition, 2006.

Zhang, J. and Wheeler, J. Mercury and Autism,: A Review. Education and Training in Autism and Developmental Disabilities, 2010 45(1) 107-115..

Stoll, Andrew L, MD. The Omega-3 Connection. Simon & Schuster. N.Y. 2001.

Weinberger, J, MD, W.J/ Nicklas, PhD and S. Berl, MD. Role of the differential effects on the active uptake of putative neurotransmitters. Neurology, February 1, 1976. Vol. 26, No. 2, pg. 162

Chapter 53. Sensory-Based Antecedent Interventions, by Dr. Ginny Van Rie and Dr. L. Juane Heflin

Alberto, P. A., & Troutman, A. C. (2009). *Applied behavior analysis for teachers* (8th ed.). Upper Saddle River, NJ: Pearson Merrill Prentice–Hall.

Ben-Sasson, A., Cermak, S. A., Orsmond, G. I., Tager-Flusberg, H., Carter, A. S., Kadlec, M. B., & Dunn, W. (2007). Extreme sensory modulation behaviors in toddlers with autism spectrum disorders. *The American Journal of Occupational Therapy, 61,* 584–592.

Banda, D., & Kubina Jr., R. (2006). The effects of a high-probability request sequencing technique in enhancing transition behaviors. *Education & Treatment of Children, 29,* 507–516.

Crane, L., Goddard, L., & Pring, L. (2009). Sensory processing in adults with autism spectrum disorders. *Autism: The International Journal of Research & Practice, 13,* 215–228.

Ermer, J., & Dunn, W. (1998). The sensory profile: a discriminate analysis of children with and without disabilities. *American Journal of Occupational Therapy, 52,* 283–289.

Dunn, W. (1997). The impact of sensory processing abilities on the daily lives of young children and their families: A conceptual model. *Infants and Young Children, 9(4),* 23–35.

Dunn, W. (1999). *Sensory profile.* San Antonio, TX: Pearson.

Dunn, W. (2001). The sensations of everyday life: Empirical, theoretical, and pragmatic considerations, 2001 Eleanor Clarke Slagle lecture. *American Journal of Occupational Therapy, 55,* 608–620.

Harrison, J., & Hare, D. J. (2004). Brief report: Assessment of sensory abnormalities in people with autistic spectrum disorders. *Journal of Autism and Developmental Disabilities, 34,* 727–730.

Heflin, L. J., & Alaimo, D. F. (2007). *Students with autism spectrum disorders: Effective instructional practices.* Upper Saddle River, NJ: Pearson Merrill Prentice Hall.

Hess, K., Morrier, M., Heflin, L., & Ivey, M. (2008). Autism Treatment Survey: Services received by children with autism spectrum disorders in public school classrooms. *Journal of Autism & Developmental Disorders, 38,* 961–971.

Leuba, C. (1955). Toward some integration of learning theories: The concept of optimal stimulation. *Psychological Reports, 1,* 27–32.

Keeling, K., Myles, B., Gagnon, E., & Simpson, R. (2003). Using the power card strategy to teach sportsmanship skills to a child with autism. *Focus on Autism & Other Developmental Disabilities, 18,* 103.

McIntosh, D. N., Miller, L. J., Shyu, V., & Dunn, W. (1999). Overview of the Short Sensory Profile (SSP). In W. Dunn, *Sensory Profile: User's Manual* (59–73). San Antonio, TX: Pearson.

Myles, B. S. Cook, K. T., Miller, N. E., Rinner, L. & Robbins, L. A. (2000). *Asperger syndrome and sensory issues: Practical solutions for making sense of the world.* Shawnee, KS: AAPC.

Napolitano, D., Tessing, J., McAdam, D., Dunleavy, I., & Cifuni, N. (2006). The influence of idiosyncratic antecedent variables on problem behavior displayed by a person with PDD. *Journal of Developmental & Physical Disabilities, 18,* 295–305.

National Autism Center. (2009a). *National standards report: The national standards project addressing the need for evidence-based practice guidelines for autism spectrum disorders.* Randolph, MA: Author.

National Autism Center. (2009b). *Evidence-based practice and autism in the schools: A guide to providing appropriate interventions to students with autism spectrum disorders.* Randolph, MA: Author.

Parker, R. I., & Vannest, K. J. (in press). Pairwise data overlap for single case research. *School Psychology Review.*

Reinhartsen, D., Garfinkle, A., & Wolery, M. (2002). Engagement with toys in two-year-old children with autism: Teacher selection versus child choice. *Journal of the Association for Persons with Severe Handicaps, 27*, 175–87.

Rogers, S. J., Hepburn, S., & Wehner, E. (2003). Parent reports of sensory symptoms in toddlers with autism and those with other developmental disorders. *Journal of Autism and Developmental Disorders, 33,* 631–642.

Schilling, D., & Schwartz, I. (2004). Alternative seating for young children with autism spectrum disorder: Effects on classroom behavior. *Journal of Autism & Developmental Disorders, 34,* 423–432.

Sweeney, H., & LeBlanc, J. (1995). Effects of task size on work-related and aberrant behaviors of youths with autism and mental retardation. *Research in Developmental Disabilities, 16,* 97–115.

Taber, T., Seltzer, A., Heflin, L., & Alberto, P. (1999). Use of self-operated auditory prompts to decrease off-task behavior for a student with autism and moderate mental retardation. *Focus on Autism and Other Developmental Disabilities, 14*, 159–66, 90.

Tomcheck, S. D., & Dunn, W. (2007). Sensory processing in children with and without autism: A comparative study using the Short Sensory Profile. *The American Journal of Occupational Therapy, 61,* 190–200.

Van Rie, G. L., & Heflin, L. J. (2009). The effect of sensory activities on correct responding for children with autism spectrum disorders. *Research in Autism Spectrum Disorders, 3,* 783–796.

Yack, E., Aquilla, P., & Sutton, S. (2002). *Building bridges through sensory integration* (2nd ed.). Las Vegas, NV: Sensory Solutions.

Zentall, S. S., & Zentall, T. R. (1983). Optimal stimulation: A model of disordered activity and performance in normal and deviant children. *Psychological Bulletin, 94*, 446–471.

Chapter 57. Speech-Language Therapy, by Lavinia Pereira and Michelle Solomon

Buschbacher, Pamelazita W., and Fox, Lise (2003). Understanding and Intervening with the Challenging Behavior of Young Children with Autism Spectrum Disorder. *Language, Speech, and Hearing Services in Schools, 34,* 217–227.Bibby, P., Eikeseth, S., Martin, N., Mudford, O., & Reeves, D. (2001). Progress and Outcomes for Children With Autism Receiving Parent-Managed Intensive Interventions. *Research in Developmental Disabilities,* 22, 425–447. Hegde, M.N., (1999). *PocketGuide to Assessment in Speech-Language Pathology.* San Diego, Singular Publishing Group, Inc.

Kashinath, Shubha; Woods, Juliann.; and Goldstein, Howard. (2006). Enhancing Generalized Teaching Strategy Use in Daily Routines by Parents of Children with Autism. *Journal of Speech, Language and Hearing Research*, 49, 466–485.

Kaufman, Nancy, and Tamara Kasper. "Shaping Verbal Language for Children on the Spectrum of Autism Who Also Exhibit Apraxia of Speech. Apraxia-KIDS." www.apraxia-kids.org.

Peppe, Susan; McCann, Joanne, Gibboa, Fiona; O'Hare, Anne; Rutherford, Marion. (2007) Receptive and Expressive Prosodic Ability in Children With High-Functioning Autism. *Journal of Speech, Language and Hearing Research*, 50, 1015–1028.

Prelock, Patricia PhD. "Treatment Efficacy Summary." www.asha.org.

Ruddell.R.B. (2002).*Teaching Children to Read and Write: Becoming an Effective Literacy Teacher.* Boston: Allyn & Bacon.

Schlosser, Ralf, W., and Wendt, Oliver. (2008). Effects of Augmentative and Alternative Communication Intervention on Speech Production in Children With Autism: A Systematic Review. *American Journal of Speech-Language Pathology*, 17, 221–230.

Schwartz, Heatherann and Drager, Kathryn, D.R. (2008). Training and Knowledge in Autism Among Speech-Language Pathologists: A Survey. *Language, Speech and Hearing Services in Schools*, 39, 66–77.

Siegel, Bryna. (1996). *The World of the Autistic Child*. New York, Oxford University Press, Inc.

Sweeney-Kerwin, E., Zecchin-Tirri, G., Carbone, V.J.; Janeckey, M.; Murrary, D. & McCarthy, K. (2005). Improving the Speech Production of Children with Autism. *Proceedings of the 31st Annual International Convention Association for Behavior Analysis*. Atlanta, Georgia.

Chapter 59. Part b. AAC: Augmentative and Alternative Communication by Patti Murphy

Mirenda, P. & Iacono, T. (2009). Autism Spectrum Disorders and AAC. Paul H. Brookes Publishing Co.

Gardener, R. & Gardener, B. (1969). Teaching sign language to a chimpanzee. Science, 165, 664-672

Premack, D. & Premack, A., (1974). Teaching visual language to apes and language-deficient persons. In R. Schiefelbusch & L.L. Lloyd (Eds.) Language perspectives—Acquisition, Retardation and intervention (pp. 347-376) Baltimore: University Park Press.

Rumbaugh, D. (1977). Language learning in the chimpanzee: The LANA Project. New York: Academic Press.

Savage-Rumbaugh, S., Rumbaugh, D. & Boysen, S. (1978). Symbolic communication between two chimpanzees. (Pan troglodytes). Science, 201, 641-644.

Millar, D.C. (2009). Effects of AAC on the natural speech development of individuals with autism spectrum disorders. In Mirenda, P. & Iacono, T. (Eds.) Autism Spectrum Disorders and AAC (pp. 171-192). Paul H. Brookes Publishing Co.

Mesibov, G. B., Adams, L. W., & Klinger, L. G. (1997). Autism: Understanding the disorder. New York: Plenum Press.

Light, J., Roberts, B., DiMarco, R., & Greiner, N. (1998). Augmentative and alternative communication to support receptive and expressive communication for people with autism. Journal of Communication Disorders, 31, 153-180.

Peeters, C. & Gillberg, C. (1999). Autism: Medical and educational aspects. London: Whurr Silverman, F.H. (1980). Communication for the Speechless (3rd ed.). Needham Heights, MA: Allyn & Bacon.

Berry, J.O. (1987). Strategies for involving parents in programs for young children using augmentative and alternative communication. Augmentative and Alternative Communication, 3: 90-93.

Daniels, M. (1994). The effect of sign on hearing children's language. Communication Education, 43: 291-98.

Cafiero, J. (2007). Challenging our belief system regarding people with autism and AAC: Making the least harmful assumptions, Closing the Gap 26(1)

Cafiero, J. (2004). AAC supports for engaging students with autism spectrum disorders (ASD) in group instruction, Closing the Gap, 23(4),

Behavioral supports for individuals with autism, Instructional video, Retrieved September 28, 2010 from http://www.dynavoxtech.com/training/toolkit/details.aspx?id=390

Scripting: Expanding communication abilities, Instructional video, Retrieved September 28, 2010 from http://www.dynavoxtech.com/training/toolkit/details.aspx?id=253

Visual supports for students with autism: Implementing AAC in classrooms, Retrieved http://www.voiceforliving.com/2010/11/visual-supports-for-students-with-autism

The National Professional Development Center on Autism Spectrum Disorders—Evidence-Based Practice: Social Narratives, Retrieved November 30, 2010 from http://autismpdc.fpg. unc.edu/content/social-narratives

Chapter 62. Transcranial Magnetic Stimulation by Joshua M. Baruth, et al.

American Psychiatric Association. (2000). Diagnostic and statistical manual of mental disorders (DSM-IV TR) (4th ed.). Washington, DC: American Psychiatric Association. (text revised).

Barker, A.T., Jalinous, R., Freeston, I.L. (1985). Non-invasive magnetic stimulation of the human motor cortex. *Lancet*, 1,1106-1107.

Baruth, J.M., Casanova, M., El-Baz, A., Horrell, T., Mathai, G., Sears, L., Sokhadze, E. (2010a). Low-Frequency Repetitive Transcranial Magnetic Stimulation (rTMS) Modulates Evoked-Gamma Oscillations in Autism Spectrum Disorder (ASD). *Journal of Neurotherapy*, 14, 179-194.

Baruth, J.M., Casanova, M., Sears, L., Sokhadze, E. (2010b). Early-Stage Visual Processing Abnormalities in Autism Spectrum Disorder (ASD). *Translational Neuroscience,* 1, 177-187.

Belmonte, M.K., and Yurgelun-Todd, D.A. (2003). Functional anatomy of impaired selective attention and compensatory processing in autism. Cognitive Brain Research, 17, 651-664.

Bodfish, J.W., Symons, F.J., and Lewis, M.H. (1999). Repetitive Behavior Scale. Western Carolina Center Research Reports.

Brown, C., Gruber, T., Boucher, J., Rippon, G., Brock, J. (2005). Gamma abnormalities during perception of illusory figures in autism. *Cortex*, 41, 364-76.

Casanova, M. F., Buxhoeveden, D. P., Switala, A. E., & Roy, E. (2002a). Minicolumnar pathology in autism. *Neurology*, 58, 428–432.

Casanova, M. F., Buxhoeveden, D. P., Switala, A. E., & Roy, E. (2002b). Neuronal density and architecture (gray level index) in the brains of autistic patients. *Journal of Child Neurology*, 17, 515–521.

Casanova, M.F., Buxhoeveden, D., Gomez, J. (2003). Disruption in the inhibitory architecture of the cell minicolumn: implications for autism. *Neuroscientist*, 9(6): 496-507.

Casanova, M. F., van Kooten, I., Switala, A. E., van England, H., Heinsen, H., Steinbuch, H. W. M., et al. (2006a). Abnormalities of cortical minicolumnar organization in the prefrontal lobes of autistic patients. *Clinical Neuroscience Research*, 6, 127–133.

Casanova, M. F., van Kooten, I., van Engeland, H., Heinsen, H., Steinbursch, H. W. M., Hof, P. R., et al. (2006b). Minicolumnar abnormalities in autism. *Acta Neuropathologica*, 112, 287–303.

Casanova, M.F. (2007). The neuropathology of autism. *Brain Pathology*, 17, 422-33.

Charman T. (2008). Autism spectrum disorders. *Psychiatry*, 7, 331-334.

Douglas, R. J., & Martin, K. A. C. (2004). Neuronal circuits of the neocortex. *Annual Review of Neuroscience*, 27, 419–451.

Faraday M: Effects on the production of electricity from magnetism (1831), in Michael Faraday. Edited by Williams LP. New York, Basic Books, 1965, p 531.

George and Belmaker (2007) *Transcrainial Magenetic Stimulation in Clinical Psychiatry*. Arlington, VA: American Psychiatric Publishing, Inc.

George, M.S., Wassermann, E.M., Williams, W.A., Callahan, A., Ketter, T.A., Basser, P., Hallett, M., Post, R.M. (1995). Daily repetitive transcranial magnetic stimulation (rTMS) improves mood in depression. *Neuroreport*, 6, 1853-6.

Gillberg, C., Billstedt, E. (2000). Autism and Asperger syndrome: coexistence with other clinical disorders. *Acta Psychiatrica Scandinavica*,102, 321-30.

Hoffman, R. E., & Cavus, I. (2002). Slow transcranial magnetic stimulation, long-term depotentiation, and brain hyperexcitability disorders. *American Journal of Psychiatry*, 159, 1093–1102.

Maeda, F., Keenan, J.P., Tormos, J.M., Topka, H., Pascual-Leone, A. (2000). Modulation of corticospinal excitability by repetitive transcranial magnetic stimulation. *Clinical Neurophysiology*, 111, 800-805.

Mountcastle, V.B. (2003). Introduction.Computation in cortical columns. *Cerebral Cortex*, 13, 2–4.

Mountcastle, V. B. (1997). The columnar organization of the neocortex. *Brain*, 120, 701–722.

Pascual-Leone, A., Valls-Sole, J., Wasserman, E.M., et al. (1994). Responses to rapid-rate transcranial magnetic stimulation of the human cortex. *Brain*, 117, 847-858.

Pascual-Leone, A., Walsh, V., Rothwell, J. (2000). Transcranial magnetic stimulation in cognitive neuroscience--virtual lesion, chronometry, and functional connectivity. *Current Opinion in Neurobiology*, 10, 232-7.

Quintana, H. (2005). Transcranial magnetic stimulation in persons younger than the age of 18. *The Journal of ECT*, 21:88-95.

Rippon, G., Brock, J., Brown, C., & Boucher, J. (2007). Disordered connectivity in the autistic brain: Challenges for the 'new psychophysiology'. *International Journal of Psychophysiology*, 63, 164–172.

Rubenstein, J.L.R., Merzenich, M.M. (2003). Model of autism: increased ratio of excitation/inhibition in key neural systems. *Genes, Brain, and Behavior*, 2, 255–267.

Sokhadze, E., Baruth, J., Tasman, A., Sears, L., Mathai, G., El-Baz, A., Casanova, M. (2009a). Event-related potential study of novelty processing abnormalities in autism. *Applied Psychophysiology and Biofeedback*, 34, 37-51.

Sokhadze, E., El-Baz, A., Baruth, J., Mathai, G., Sears, L., Casanova, M. (2009b). Effects of low frequency repetitive transcranial magnetic stimulation (rTMS) on gamma frequency oscillations and event-related potentials during processing of illusory figures in autism. *Journal of Autism and Developmental Disorders*, 39, 619-34.

Sokhadze, E., Baruth, J., Tasman, A., Mansoor, M., Ramaswamy, R., Sears, L., Mathai, G., El-Baz, A., Casanova, M.F. (2009c). Low-Frequency Repetitive Transcranial Magnetic Stimulation (rTMS) Affects Event-Related Potential Measures of Novelty Processing in Autism. *Applied Psychophysiology and Biofeedback*, Nov 26. [Epub ahead of print]

Wassermann, E.M. (1996). Risk and safety of repetitive transcranial magnetic stimulation: report and suggested guidelines from the International Workshop on the Safety of Repetitive Transcranial Magnetic Stimulation, June 5-7. *Electroencephalography and Clinical Neurophysiology*, 108:1-16.

Whittington, M.A., Traub, R.D., Kopell, N., Ermentrout, B., Buhl, E.H. (2000). Inhibition-based rhythms: experimental and mathematical observations on network dynamics. *International Journal of Psychophysiology*, 38, 315–336.

Wu, A.D., Fregni, F., Simon, D.K., Deblieck, C., Pascual-Leone, A. (2008). Noninvasive Brain Stimulation for Parkinson's Disease and Dystonia. *Neurotherapeutics*, 5:345-61.

Chapter 63. Vision Therapy, by Dr. Jeffrey Becker

Becker, J. (2009). Vision Therapy Can Help Spectrum Children With Visual Dysfunctions. *The Autism File USA* 33, 76–81

Cohen, A. H., Lowe, S.E., Steele, G.T., Suchoff, I.B., Gottlieb, D.D., & Trevorrow, T.L. (1988). The efficacy of optometric vision therapy, *Journal Of The American Optometric Association, 59*(2), 95–105.

Holmes, J., Rice, M., Karlsson, V., Nielsen, B., Sease, J., & Shevlin, T. (2008). The best treatment determined for childhood eye problem. *Archives of Ophthalmology, 126*(10) 1336–1349. HTS Inc. (2009). 6788 S. Kings Ranch Rd., Gold Canyon, AZ 85118. NeuroSensory Centers of America. (2009). 300 Beardsley Road, Austin, TX 78746

Taub, M.B., & Russell, R. (2007). Autism spectrum disorders: A primer for the optometrist. *Review of Optometry. 144*(5). 82–91

Trachtman, J.N. (2008). Background and history of autism in relation to vision care, *Optometry, 79*(7), 391–396.

Chapter 64. The Role of the Microbiome/Biome and Cysteine Deficiency in Autism Spectrum Disorder: the Implications for Glutathione and Defensins in the Gut-Brain Connection by Dr. Jeff Bradstreet

1.   Careaga M, Van de Water J, Ashwood P. Immune dysfunction in autism: a pathway to treatment. *Neurotherapeutics.* 2010;7(3):283-92.

2.   Gupta S, Samra D, Agrawal S. Adaptive and innate immune responses in autism: rationale for therapeutic use of intravenous immunoglobulin. *J Clin Immunol.* 2010;30(Suppl 1):90-6.

3.   Li X, Chauhan A, Sheikh AM, Patil S, Chauhan V, Li XM, Ji L, Brown T, Malik M. Elevated immune response in the brain of autistic patients. *J Neuroimmunol.* 2009;207(1-2):111-6.

4.   Weizman A, Weizman R, Szekely GA, Wijsenbeek H, Livni E. Abnormal immune response to brain tissue antigen in the syndrome of autism. *Am J Psychiatry.* 1982;139(11):1462-5.

5.   Chez MG, Dowling T, Patel PB, Khanna P, Kominsky M. Elevation of tumor necrosis factor-alpha in cerebrospinal fluid of autistic children. *Pediatr Neurol.* 2007;36(6):361-5.

6.   Vargas DL, Nascimbene C, Krishnan C, Zimmerman AW, Pardo CA. Neuroglial activation and neuroinflammation in the brain of patients with autism. *Ann Neurol.* 2005;57(1):67-81. Erratum in: *Ann Neurol.* 2005;57(2):304.

7.   Bradstreet JJ, El Dahr J, Anthony A, Kartzinel JJ, Wakefield AJ. Detection of measles virus genomic RNA in cerebrospinal fluid of children with regressive autism: s report of three cases. *J Amer Physicians Surgeons.* 2004; 9(2):38-45.

8.   Bradstreet JJ, El Dahr J, Montgomery SM, Wakefield AJ. TaqMan RT-PCR detection of measles virus genomic RNA in cerebrospinal fluid in children with regressive autism. Presented at the 2004 International Meeting for Autism Research (IMFAR), Sacramento, CA.

9.   M Dubik, PA Offit. Measles virus RNA and autism revisited. *AAP Grand Rounds.* 2004;12:56-57.

10.   Sandler RH, Finegold SM, Bolte ER, Buchanan CP, Maxwell AP, Väisänen ML, Nelson MN, Wexler HM.
Short-term benefit from oral vancomycin treatment of regressive-onset autism. *J Child Neurol.* 2000;15(7):429-35.

11.   Finegold SM, Dowd SE, Gontcharova V, Liu C, Henley KE, Wolcott RD, Youn E, Summanen PH, Granpeesheh D, Dixon D, Liu M, Molitoris DR, Green JA 3rd. Pyrosequencing study of fecal microflora of autistic and control children. *Anaerobe.* 2010;16(4):444-53.

12. James SJ, Cutler P, Melnyk S, Jernigan S, Janak L, Gaylor DW, Neubrander JA. Metabolic biomarkers of increased oxidative stress and impaired methylation capacity in children with autism. *Am J Clin Nutr.* 2004;80(6):1611-7.

13. Siesjö BK, Rehncrona S, Smith D. Neuronal cell damage in the brain: possible involvement of oxidative mechanisms. *Acta Physiol Scand Suppl.* 1980;492:121-8.

14. Jenner P. Altered mitochondrial function, iron metabolism and glutathione levels in Parkinson's disease. *Acta Neurol Scand Suppl.* 1993;146:6-13.

15. Do KQ, Trabesinger AH, Kirsten-Krüger M, Lauer CJ, Dydak U, Hell D, Holsboer F, Boesiger P, Cuénod M. Schizophrenia: glutathione deficit in cerebrospinal fluid and prefrontal cortex in vivo. *Eur J Neurosci.* 2000;12(10):3721-8.

16. Dvoráková M, Sivonová M, Trebatická J, Skodácek I, Waczuliková I, Muchová J, Duracková Z. The effect of polyphenolic extract from pine bark, Pycnogenol on the level of glutathione in children suffering from attention deficit hyperactivity disorder (ADHD). *Redox Rep.* 2006;11(4):163-72.

17. Kalebic T, Kinter A, Poli G, Anderson ME, Meister A, Fauci AS. Suppression of human immunodeficiency virus expression in chronically infected monocytic cells by glutathione, glutathione ester, and N-acetylcysteine. *Proc Natl Acad Sci U S A.* 1991;88(3):986-90.

18. Iantomasi T, Marraccini P, Favilli F, Vincenzini MT, Ferretti P, Tonelli F. Glutathione metabolism in Crohn's disease. *Biochem Med Metab Biol.* 1994;53(2):87-91.

19. Oeriu S, Tigheciu M. Oxidized glutathione as a test of senescence. *Gerontologia.* 1964;49:9-17.

20. James SJ, Melnyk S, Jernigan S, Cleves MA, Halsted CH, Wong DH, Cutler P, Bock K, Boris M, Bradstreet JJ, Baker SM, Gaylor DW. Metabolic endophenotype and related genotypes are associated with oxidative stress in children with autism. *Am J Med Genet B Neuropsychiatr Genet.* 2006;141B(8):947-56.

21. Salzman NH, Hung K, Haribhai D, Chu H, Karlsson-Sjöberg J, Amir E, Teggatz P, Barman M, Hayward M, Eastwood D, Stoel M, Zhou Y, Sodergren E, Weinstock GM, Bevins CL, Williams CB, Bos NA. Enteric defensins are essential regulators of intestinal microbial ecology. *Nat Immunol.* 2010;11(1):76-83.

22. Eisenhauer PB, Harwig SS, Szklarek D, Ganz T, Selsted ME, Lehrer RI. Purification and antimicrobial properties of three defensins from rat neutrophils. *Infect Immun.* 1989;57(7):2021-7.

23. Rowan FE, Docherty NG, Coffey JC, O'Connell PR. Sulphate-reducing bacteria and hydrogen sulphide in the aetiology of ulcerative colitis. *Br J Surg.* 2009;96(2):151-8.

24. Bäckhed F, Ley RE, Sonnenburg JL, Peterson DA, Gordon JI. Host-bacterial mutualism in the human intestine. *Science.* 2005;307(5717):1915-20.

25. Shaw SY, Blanchard JF, Bernstein CN. Association between the use of antibiotics in the first year of life and pediatric inflammatory bowel disease. *Am J Gastroenterol.* 2010;105(12):2687-92.

26. Parker W. Reconstituting the depleted biome to prevent immune disorders. *The Evolution & Medicine Review.* Web. Oct 13 2010.

27. McKay DM. The beneficial helminth parasite? *Parasitology.* 2006;132(Pt 1):1-12.

28. Elliott DE, Summers RW, Weinstock JV. Helminths as governors of immune-mediated inflammation. *Int J Parasitol.* 2007;37(5):457-64.

29. Summers RW, Elliott DE, Urban JF Jr, Thompson RA, Weinstock JV. Trichuris suis therapy for active ulcerative colitis: a randomized controlled trial. *Gastroenterology.* 2005;128(4):825-32.

30. Bager P, Arnved J, Rønborg S, Wohlfahrt J, Poulsen LK, Westergaard T, Petersen HW, Kristensen B, Thamsborg S, Roepstorff A, Kapel C, Melbye M. Trichuris suis ova therapy for allergic rhinitis: a randomized, double-blind, placebo-controlled clinical trial. *J Allergy Clin Immunol*. 2010;125(1):123-30.

31. Sewell DL, Reinke EK, Hogan LH, Sandor M, Fabry Z. Immunoregulation of CNS autoimmunity by helminth and mycobacterial infections. *Immunol Lett*. 2002;82(1-2):101-10.

32. La Flamme AC, Canagasabey K, Harvie M, Bäckström BT. Schistosomiasis protects against multiple sclerosis. *Mem Inst Oswaldo Cruz*. 2004;99(5 Suppl 1):33-6.

33. Singer HS, Morris C, Gause C, Pollard M, Zimmerman AW, Pletnikov M. Prenatal exposure to antibodies from mothers of children with autism produces neurobehavioral alterations: a pregnant dam mouse model. *J Neuroimmunol*. 2009;211(1-2):39-48.

34. Garbett K, Ebert PJ, Mitchell A, Lintas C, Manzi B, Mirnics K, Persico AM. Immune transcriptome alterations in the temporal cortex of subjects with autism. *Neurobiol Dis*. 2008;30(3):303-11.

35. Garvey J. Diet in autism and associated disorders. *J Fam Health Care*. 2002;12(2): 34-8.

36. Levy SE, Hyman SL. Novel treatments for autistic spectrum disorders. *Ment Retard Dev Disabil Res Rev*. 2005;11(2):131-42.

37. Miele E, Pascarella F, Giannetti E, Quaglietta L, Baldassano RN, Staiano A. Effect of a probiotic preparation (VSL#3) on induction and maintenance of remission in children with ulcerative colitis. *Am J Gastroenterol*. 2009;104(2):437-43.

38. Huynh HQ, deBruyn J, Guan L, Diaz H, Li M, Girgis S, Turner J, Fedorak R, Madsen K. Probiotic preparation VSL#3 induces remission in children with mild to moderate acute ulcerative colitis: a pilot study. *Inflamm Bowel Dis*. 2009;15(5):760-8.

39. Tursi A, Brandimarte G, Papa A, Giglio A, Elisei W, Giorgetti GM, Forti G, Morini S, Hassan C, Pistoia MA, Modeo ME, Rodino' S, D'Amico T, Sebkova L, Sacca' N, Di Giulio E, Luzza F, Imeneo M, Larussa T, Di Rosa S, Annese V, Danese S, Gasbarrini A. Treatment of relapsing mild-to-moderate ulcerative colitis with the probiotic VSL#3 as adjunctive to a standard pharmaceutical treatment: a double-blind, randomized, placebo-controlled study. *Am J Gastroenterol*. 2010;105(10):2218-27.

40. Guandalini S. Update on the role of probiotics in the therapy of pediatric inflammatory bowel disease. *Expert Rev Clin Immunol*. 2010;6(1):47-54.

41. Ashwood P, Anthony A, Pellicer AA, Torrente F, Walker-Smith JA, Wakefield AJ. Intestinal lymphocyte populations in children with regressive autism: evidence for extensive mucosal immunopathology. *J Clin Immunol*. 2003;23(6):504-17.

42. Bradstreet JJ, Smith S, Baral M, Rossignol DA. Biomarker-guided interventions of clinically relevant conditions associated with autism spectrum disorders and attention deficit hyperactivity disorder. *Altern Med Rev*. 2010;15(1):15-32.

43. Eggesbø M, Moen B, Peddada S, Baird D, Rugtveit J, Midtvedt T, Bushel PR, Sekelja M, Rudi K. Development of gut microbiota in infants not exposed to medical interventions. *APMIS*. 2011;119(1):17-35.

44. Adlerberth I, Wold AE. Establishment of the gut microbiota in Western infants. *Acta Paediatr*. 2009;98(2):229-38.

45. Hooper LV, Midtvedt T, Gordon JI. How host-microbial interactions shape the nutrient environment of the mammalian intestine. *Annu Rev Nutr*. 2002;22:283-307.

46. Winter HS (personal communication). MassGeneral Hospital for Children, January 2011.

47. Khoruts A, Sadowsky MJ. Therapeutic transplantation of the distal gut microbiota. *Mucosal Immunol.* 2011;4(1):4-7.

48. Russell G, Kaplan J, Ferraro M, Michelow IC. Fecal bacteriotherapy for relapsing Clostridium difficile infection in a child: a proposed treatment protocol. *Pediatrics.* 2010;126(1):e239-42.

49. Floch MH. Fecal bacteriotherapy, fecal transplant, and the microbiome. *J Clin Gastroenterol.* 2010;44(8):529-30.

50. Theoharides TC, Doyle R, Francis K, Conti P, Kalogeromitros D. Novel therapeutic targets for autism. *Trends Pharmacol Sci.* 2008;29(8):375-82.

Chapter 66. Three Drugs that Could Change Autism by Meghan Thompson.

1. Unless otherwise indicated, the information has been provided by the company or appears on its website.

2. Hughes, Virginia. "First drug for autism enters final stage of testing." Simons Foundation Autism Research Initiative. 2010. 11 Feb. 2011 <https://sfari.org/news-and-commentary/open-article/-/asset_publisher/6Tog/content/first-drug-for-autism-enters-final-stage-of-testing?redirect=/news-and-commentary/all>

3. Golden, John. "Gut Reaction Drives Biotech CEO." Westchester County Business Journal 30 October 2009.

4. Hagerman, Randi, M.D. "How do the Behaviors Seen in Persons with Fragile X Relate to Those Seen in Autism?" National Fragile X Foundation. 2011. February 13, 2011 <http://www.fragilex.org/html/autism.htm>

5. "Study Aims to Develop First Medications for Fragile-X Syndrome, Leading Inherited Cause of Mental Retardation." National Institute of Mental Health. 2008. February 13, 2011 <http://www.nimh.nih.gov/science-news/2007/study-aims-to-develop-first-medications-for-fragile-x-syndrome-leading-inherited-cause-of-mental-retardation.shtml>

AUTISM ORGANIZATIONS

NATIONAL

ACT Today!
Autism Care & Treatment Today!
19019 Ventura Blvd. Suite 200
Tarzana, CA 91356
818-705-1625
Info@act-today.org

ACT Today! is a nonprofit organization whose mission is to provide funding and support to families that cannot afford the treatments their autistic children need to achieve their full potential.

Advancing Futures for Adults with Autism (AFAA)
(917) 475-5059
AFAA@autismspeaks.org
www.afaa-us.org

AFAA was created to inform adolescents and adults with autism about living options and new developments, and promote active community involvement from adults with autism.

Global Autism Collaboration
4182 Adams Avenue
San Diego, CA 92116
(619) 281-7165
www.autismwebsite.com/gac

The Global Autism Collaboration brings together the most experienced autism advocacy organizations in an effort dedicated to advancing autism research in the interest of all individuals living with autism today and their families.

The Autism Hope Alliance
752 Tamiami Trail
Port Charlotte, FL 33953
888.918.1118
info@autismhopealliance.org

Dedicated to the recovery of children and adults from autism, the Autism Hope Alliance ignites hope for families facing the diagnosis through education and funding to promote progress in the present moment.

AutismOne
1816 W. Houston Avenue
Fullerton, CA 92833
(714) 680-0792
earranga@autismone.org
www.autismone.org

AutismOne is a nonprofit, charity organization educating more than 100,000 families every year about prevention, recovery, safety, and change.

Autism Research Institute
4182 Adams Avenue
San Diego, CA 92116
(619) 281-7165
Media Contact: Matt Kabler
matt@autism.com
www.autism.com

ARI is devoted to conducting research and to disseminating the results of research on the triggers of autism and on methods of diagnosing and treating autism.

Autism Science Digest
1816 W. Houston Ave.
Fullerton, CA 92833
(714) 680-0792
Contact: Teri Arranga, Editor in Chief
tarranga@autismone.org
www.autismsciencedigest.com

Autism Science Digest is the place for doctors, researchers, and expert mothers and fathers to get together to talk about research, treatment, and recovery. *Autism Science Digest* is the first Autism Approved™ publication of the globa lautism community. Dedicated to respecting the intelligence of parents, *Autism Science Digest* continues the philosophy of founding organization, AutismOne, featuring up-to-date biomedical information written for new and seasoned readers from clinicians and researchers you trust.

Autism Society
4340 East-West Hwy, Suite 350
Bethesda, MD 20814
www.autism-society.org
(301) 657-0881, (800)-3AUTISM x 150
info@autism-society.org

The Autism Society exists to improve the lives of all affected by autism by increasing public awareness about the day-to-day issues faced by people on the spectrum, advocating for appropriate services for individuals across the lifespan, and providing the latest information regarding treatment, education, research and advocacy.

Autism Speaks
2 Park Avenue, 11th Floor
New York, NY 10016
(212) 252-8584
contactus@autismspeaks.org
www.autismspeaks.org

Autism Speaks is dedicated to funding autism research, disseminating information, and providing a voice for autistic people's needs.

Generation Rescue
19528 Ventura Blvd. #117
Tarzana, CA 91356
1 (877) 98-AUTISM
www.generationrescue.org

Generation Rescue is Jenny McCarthy's autism organization dedicated to informing and assisting families touched by autism; it provides programs and services for personalized support, and Generation Rescue volunteers are researching causes and treatment for autism.

Helping Hand
1330 W. Schatz Lane
Nixa, MO 65714
(877) NAA-AUTISM (877-622-2884)

naa@nationalautism.org
www.nationalautismassociation.org/helpinghand.php

Helping Hand is a program from the National Autism Association that provides financial assistance for autism families.

Kids Enjoy Exercise Now (KEEN)
1301 K Street, NW
Suite 600, East Tower
Washington, DC 20005
866-903-KEEN (5336) main
866-597-KEEN (5336) fax
info@keenusa.org

KEEN is a national, nonprofit volunteer-led organization that provides one-to-one recreational opportunities for children and young adults with developmental and physical disabilities at no cost to their families and caregivers. KEEN's mission is to foster the self-esteem, confidence, skills and talents of its athletes through non-competitive activities, allowing young people facing even the most significant challenges to meet their individual goals.

National Autism Association
1330 W. Schatz Lane
Nixa, MO 65714
(877) 622-2884
naa@nationalautism.org
www.nationalautism.org

NAA raises funds for autism research and support and also provides programs, such as Helping Hand, Family First, and FOUND, designed to aid specific needs for families dealing with autism.

National Autism Center
41 Pacella Park Drive
Randolph, Massachusetts 02368
Phone: (877) 313-3833
Fax: (781) 440-0401
Email: info@nationalautismcenter.org
www.nationalautismcenter.org

The National Autism Center is a nonprofit organization dedicated to serving children and adolescents with Autism Spectrum Disorders (ASD) by providing reliable information, promoting best practices, and offering comprehensive resources for families, practitioners, and communities.

Organization for Autism Research
2000 North 14th Street
Suite 710
Arlington, VA 22201

Tel: 703.243.9710
www.researchautism.org

The Organization for Autism Research (OAR) was created in December 2001—the product of the shared vision and unique life experiences of OAR's seven founders. Led by these parents and grandparents of children and adults on the autism spectrum, OAR set out to use applied science to answer questions that parents, families, individuals with autism, teachers and caregivers confront daily. No other autism organization has this singular focus.

SafeMinds
16033 Bolsa Chica St. #104-142
Huntington Beach, CA 92649
404-934-0777
www.safeminds.org

SafeMinds is an organization dedicated to research and awareness of mercury's involvement in such neurological disorders as autism, attention deficit disorder, and more.

Talk About Curing Autism (TACA)
3070 Bristol Street, Suite 340
Costa Mesa CA 92626
949-640-4401
www.tacanow.org

TACA provides medical, diet, and educational information geared toward autistic children, and the organization also has support, resources, and community events.

U.S. Autism and Asperger Association
P.O. Box 532
Draper, UT 84020-0532
(888) 9AUTISM, (801) 649-5752
information@usautism.org
www.usautism.org

USAAA provides support, education, and resources for autistic individuals and those with Asperger's Syndrome.

Unlocking Autism
P.O. Box 208
Tyrone, GA 30290
(866) 366-3361
www.unlockingautism.org

Unlocking Autism was created to find information about autism and disseminate that information to families with autistic children; the organization also raises funds for research and awareness.

ONLINE

Age of Autism
www.ageofautism.com

Age of Autism is an online blog with daily news in the latest autism research, updates, and community happenings.

Foundation for Autism Information & Research, Inc.
1300 Jefferson Rd.
Hoffman Estates, IL 60169
info@autismmedia.org

F.A.I.R. Autism Media is a non-profit foundation creating original, up-to-date and comprehensive educational media (video documentaries) to inform the medical community and the public about the latest advances in research and biomedical & behavioral therapies for autism spectrum disorders.

Schafer Autism Report
9629 Old Placerville Road
Sacramento, CA 95827
edit@doitnow.com
www.sarnet.org

Schafer Autism Report is a publication to inform the public about autism-related issues; it can be found online.

STATE LEVEL

Alabama:

Autism Society of Alabama
4217 Dolly Ridge Road,
Birmingham, AL 35243
Jennifer Robertson, 1-877-4-AUTISM, info@autism-alabama.org
www.autism-alabama.org

ASA's mission is to improve the quality of life of persons with Autism Spectrum Disorders and their families through education and advocacy.

Alaska:

Alaska Autism Resource Center
3501 Denali Street, Suite 101
Anchorage, AK 99503-4039

866-301-7372
www.alaskaarc.org

AARC's mission is to increase understanding and support for Alaskans of all ages with autism spectrum disorder via collaboration with families, schools and communities throughout the state.

Arizona:

A.C.T. Today!
1620 N. 48th Street
Phoenix, AV 85008
Phone (602)275-1107
Fax (602) 275-1108
www.azacttoday.org

The ACT Today! Arizona chapter's mission is to support Arizona families impacted by autism by increasing their access to therapy and support. Our vision is that the quality of life for all Arizona children with autism has been improved through therapy and supports.

Southwest Autism Research & Resource Center (SARRC)
Vocational & Life Skills Academy
2225 N. 16th Street
Phoenix, AZ 85006
(602) 340-8717
sarrc@autismcenter.org
www.autismcenter.org

SARRC provides research and support as well as clinical and consultation programs for a widespread group of autistic individuals and their families.

Arkansas:

HEAR Helping Educate about Autism Recovery Arkansas Autism Resource & Outreach Center
2001 Pershing Circle, Suite 300
North Little Rock, AR 72114-1841
Telephone/TDD: 800-342-2923
Telephone: 501-682-9900
Dianna D. Varady, Parent Coordinator,
Partners for Inclusive Communities, UAMS
DDVarady@uams.edu
www.arkansasautism.org

We are a parent-run organization based in Little Rock, Arkansas, whose focus is to provide information and support to empower families, educate providers, and increase community awareness about autism spectrum disorders.

California:

ACT Today!
Autism Care & Treatment Today!
19019 Ventura Blvd. Suite 200
Tarzana, CA 91356
818-705-1625
Info@act-today.org

ACT Today! is a nonprofit 501(c)(3) organization whose mission is to provide funding and support to families that cannot afford the treatments their autistic children need to achieve their full potential.

Canine Companions for Independence
P.O. Box 446
Santa Rosa, CA 95402-0446
1-866-224-3647
www.cci.org

CCI provides support dogs for assistance to those with disabilities.

Center for Autism & Related Disorders, Inc. (CARD)
19019 Ventura Blvd
Suite 300
Tarzana CA, 91356
818-345-2345
info@centerforautism.com
www.centerforautism.com

The Center for Autism and Related Disorders, Inc. (CARD) diligently maintains a reputation as one of the world's largest and most experienced organizations effectively treating children with autism, Asperger's Syndrome, PDD-NOS, and related disorders. They follow the principles of Applied Behavior Analysis (ABA), and develop individualized treatment plans for each child.

For OC Kids Neurodevelopmental Center
1915 West Orangewood, Suite 200
Orange, CA 92868
(714) 939-6409
forockids@uci.edu
www.forockids.org

For OC Kids Neurodevelopmental Center provides education as well as treatment and support for children with developmental, behavioral, and learning issues ages 0–5.

Sensory Research Center
510 N. Prospect S-308

Redondo Beach, CA 90277
(310) 698-9008
Contact: Jennifer Hoffiz, Founder
Jhoffiz@sensorycenter.com
www.sensoryresearchcenter.org

Sensory Research Center researches treatments and provides services for children with sensory processing disorders and families without the means to participate in sensory therapy.

Colorado:

The SMART Foundation
PO Box 2181
Vail, Colorado 81658
(970) 476-7702
info@thesmartfoundation.org
www.thesmartfoundation.org

The SMART Foundation works to train professionals and provide a variety of resources and research for families dealing with autism.

Connecticut:

Autism Support Network
Box 1525
Fairfield, CT 06824
(203) 404-4929
info@AutismSupportNetwork.com
www.autismsupportnetwork.com

The Autism Support Network is a support community for individuals and groups who have dealt with autism.

Stamford Education 4 Autism, Inc.
1127 High Ridge Road PMB #315
Stamford, CT 06905
(203) 329-9310
stamforde4autism@aol.com
www.stamfordeducation4autism.org

Stamford Education 4 Autism is an organization to provide awareness and emotional support for autistic children and their families.

Delaware:

Autism Delaware
924 Harmony Road, Suite 201
Newark, DE 19713
(302) 224-6020
delautism@delautism.org
www.delautism.org

Autism Delaware provides support services, resources, and information for people with autism and their families.

Florida:

The Dan Marino Foundation
P.O. Box 267640
Weston, FL 33326
954-389-4445
www.danmarinofoundation.org

Healing Every Autistic Life
226-5 Solana Rd. #211
Ponte Vedra Beach, FL 32082
(904) 285-5651
info@healautismnow.org
www.healautismnow.org

The HEAL Foundation provides support for local autistic individuals through grants for organizations, information, and events.

Georgia:

Autism Society Of Northeast Georgia
PO Box 48366
Athens GA 30604-8366
(706) 208-0066
ga-northeastgeorgia@autismsocietyofamerica.org
http://negac-autsoc.tripod.com

The Autism Society of Northeast Georgia is a chapter of the Autism Society of America that provides support, information, and meetings for autism families in Georgia.

North Georgia Autism Center
PO Box 38
Cumming, GA 30028
770-844-8624
northgaautismcen@bellsouth.net
www.northgeorgiaautismcenter.com

NGAC's mission is to promote and provide intensive home, school, and center-based behavioral therapy to children, youth and families affected by Autism Spectrum Disorders.

Hawaii:

Pacific Autism Center
670 Auahi Street, Suite A-6
Honolulu, HI 96813
808-523-8188

laura@pacificautismcenter.com
http://pacificautismcenter.com

The mission of Pacific Autism Center is to use ABA and be a foundation for those individuals (and their families) within the autism spectrum, and to also provide access to high quality researched based services that support the individual in all areas of their life.

Idaho:

Idaho Center for Autism, LLC
5353 Franklin Road
Boise, ID 83705
(208) 342-0374
Jackie Mathias, jmathias@idahocenterforautism.com
www.idahocenterforautism.com

Idaho Center for Autism, LLC, is a small group of people who love the kids and families we work with and are committed to doing our best to help them understand that ASDs are complex disorders, with no easy answers and no guarantees, but we know that the lives of kids affected by autism can improve dramatically and are committed to working with families in order to determine and administer appropriate treatment.

Illinois:

Easter Seals Headquarters
233 S. Wacker Dr., Suite 2400
Chicago, IL 60606
(800) 221-6827 or (312) 726-6200
www.easterseals.com

Easter Seals provides services and outreach for those with autism, including medical rehabilitation, employment, and recreation information.

Illinois Center for Autism
548 Ruby Lane
Fairview Heights, IL 62208
(618) 398-7500
info@illinoiscenterforautism.org
www.illinoiscenterforautism.org

The Illinois Center aims to prevent the unnecessary institutionalization of people with autism and to help people with autism achieve their highest level of independence within their home, school and community.

Indiana:

Hamilton County Autism Support Group
19215 Morrison Way

Noblesville, Indiana 46060
(317) 403-6705
Contact: Jane Grimes, President
janegrimes@hcasg.org
www.hcasg.org

Hamilton County Autism Support Group is a local support group that provides community awareness and resources for autistic individuals and families.

Iowa:

Eastern Central Iowa Autism Society
851 16th St SE
Cedar Rapids, IA 52403
319-431-9052
Sheri Grawe, Vice President: sherigrawe@aol.com
www.eciautismsociety.org

Eastern Central Iowa Autism Society strives to be an advocate for all those affected with Autism Spectrum Disorder—to advance their quality of life through biomedicine, education, community awareness, and therapies.

Kansas:

Autism Awareness Association Inc.
PO Box 780898
Wichita, KS 67278
(316) 771-7335
Email: tralanajones@autismawareassoc.org

Heartspring
8700 East 29th Street North
Wichita, KS 67218
(316) 634-8881 , (800) 835-1043
Contact: kbaker@heartspring.org
www.heartspring.org

Heartspring is a facility that supports special-needs children through a variety of clinical and support services.

Kentucky:

Kentucky Autism Training Center
College of Education and Human Development
Dean's Office
University of Louisville
Louisville, KY 40292
800-334-8635 ext. 852-4631
katc@louisville.edu
https://louisville.edu/education/kyautismtraining

The mission of the Kentucky Autism Training Center is to strengthen our state's systems of support for persons affected by autism by bridging research to practice and by providing training and resources to families and professionals.

Louisiana:

Unlocking Autism
PO Box 15388
Baton Rouge, LA 70895
866-366-3361
www.unlockingautism.org

UA's mission is constantly evolving to meet the ever-changing needs of families who are dealing with ASDs, and it includes bringing issues of autism from individual homes to the forefront of national dialogue, joining parents and professionals in one concerted effort to fight for these children who cannot lift their voices to the nation for help, and helping those on the autism spectrum reach their greatest potential in leading fulfilling and productive lives in relationships, society and employment.

Maine:

Association for Science in Autism Treatment (ASAT)
PO Box 7468
Portland, ME 04112-7468
207-253-6058
info@asatonline.org
www.asatonline.org

ASAT's mission is to disseminate accurate, scientifically sound information about autism and treatments for autism and to improve access to effective, science-based treatments for all people with autism, regardless of age, severity of condition, income or place of residence.

Maryland:

Autism Society
4340 East-West Hwy, Suite 350
Bethesda, MD 20814
www.autism-society.org

The Autism Society exists to improve the lives of all affected by autism by increasing public awareness about the day-to-day issues faced by people on the spectrum, advocating for appropriate services for individuals across the lifespan, and providing the latest information regarding treatment, education, research and advocacy.

Center for Autism and Developmental Disabilities Epidemiology (CADDE)
Department of Epidemiology

Johns Hopkins Bloomberg School of Public Health
615 N. Wolfe Street, Suite E6031
Baltimore, MD 21205
1-877-868-8014
cadde@jhsph.edu
www.jhsph.edu/cadde

The Center serves to foster communication, coordination, and collaboration among a multi-disciplinary team of researchers around the epidemiology of Autism Spectrum Disorders (ASD) and Developmental Disabilities (DD). We also strive to bring epidemiologic data and research to public health and educational practitioners, as well as to interested ASD and DD public constituencies.

Massachusetts:

Advocates for Autism of Massachusetts
217 South Street
Waltham, MA 02453
(781) 891-6270
Contact: Judy Zacek
zacek@AFAMaction.org
www.afamaction.org

AFAM is an advocacy organization dedicated to promoting rights and providing support for those with Autism and Asperger's Syndrome.

The Autism Research Foundation (TARF)
c/o Moss-Rosene Lab, W701
715 Albany Street
Boston, MA 02118
(617) 414-7012
tarf@ladders.org
www.ladders.org/pages/TARF.html

TARF is collection of researchers looking into the neurobiological effects of autism and similar disorders.

The Doug Flutie Jr. Foundation for Autism
PO Box 767
Framingham, MA 01701
(508) 270-8855
info@flutiefoundation.org
http://dougflutiejrfoundation.org/

The Doug Flutie Jr. Foundation for Autism is committed to supporting families by providing information, resources, and access to the most current autism news and events.

First Signs
P.O. Box 358
Merrimac, MA 01860

(978) 346-4380
info@firstsigns.org
www.firstsigns.org

First Signs is an organization to inform adults about the first warning signs of autism in children.

FRAXA Research Foundation
45 Pleasant St.,
Newburyport, MA 01950
(978) 462-1866
Contact: Katie Clapp, Executive Director
info@fraxa.org, mbudek@fraxa.org, kclapp@fraxa.org
www.fraxa.org

FRAXA's mission is to accelerate progress toward effective treatments and ultimately a cure for Fragile X, by directly funding the most promising research. It also supports families affected by Fragile X and raises awareness of this important but virtually unknown disease.

The Friendship Network for Children
100 Otis St. #4B
Northborough, MA 01532
(508) 393-0030
Contact: Nancy Swanberg, Executive Director
nancy@networkforchildren.org
www.networkforchildren.org

The Friendship Network for Children is dedicated to helping promote the use of creative activities, such as music and art, to reach children with communication-related disabilities, such as autism.

The Gottschall Autism Center
2 Brandt Island Road
P.O. Box 979
Mattapoisett, MA 02739
For information call:
Pam Ferro, RN, President
508-941-4791
Cheryl Gaudino, Executive Director
774-282-0293
email: info@gottschallcenter.com

The Gottschall Autism Center partners with families to provide children and adults with optimal health interventions, support services, educational enrichment and employment.

Greenlock Therapeutic Riding Center
55 Summer St.
Rehoboth, MA 02769
508-252-5814

www.greenlock.org
Laurel Welch, PT, HPCS, Intake Therapist
greenlocktrc@gmail.com

GTRC is a non-profit organization that utilizes equine-related activities for the therapy of individuals with physical, developmental, and emotional differences.

Learning and Developmental Disabilities Evaluation & Rehabilitation Services
1 Maguire Road
Lexington, MA 02421-3114
(781) 860-1700
info@ladders.org
www.ladders.org

LADDERS is a program that evaluates patients with a variety of disabilities, including autism, and provides individual and comprehensive treatment plans.

Michigan:

Michigan Autism Partnership
1601 Briarwood Circle, Suite 500
Ann Arbor, MI 48108
P 734-997-9088
office@aacenter.org
www.mapautism.org

The Michigan Autism Partnership's vision is to create a state-wide network of parents and professionals that supports and promotes intensive, developmental, play-based programming for young children with autistic spectrum disorders.

Minnesota:

Minnesota Autism Center
5710 Baker Road
Minnetonka, MN 55345
952.767.4200
info@mnautism.org
www.mnautism.org

The Minnesota Autism Center's Mission is to promote and provide intensive home, school and center-based behavioral therapy to children, youth and families affected by Autism Spectrum Disorder.

Mississippi:

TEAAM Together Enhancing Autism Awareness in Mississippi
P.O. Box 37
Mize, MS 39116

(601) 733-0090
takeaction@TEAAM.org
www.teaam.org

TEAAM is a non-profit organization dedicated to improving the lives of Mississippians with an Autism Spectrum Disorder by cultivating and enhancing family and community supports.

Missouri:

Family First
1330 W. Schatz Lane
Nixa, MO 65714
877-NAA-AUTISM (877-622-2884)
naa@nationalautism.org
www.nationalautismassociation.org/familyfirst.php

Family First is a program by the National Autism Association that provides marital support and promotes unity in autism families.

FOUND
1330 W. Schatz Lane
Nixa, MO 65714
877-NAA-AUTISM (877-622-2884)
naa@nationalautism.org
www.nationalautismassociation.org/found.php

Found is a National Autism Association program that raises funds to counter the rise of wandering-related deaths.

Touchpoint Autism Services
1101 Olivette Executive Pkwy.
St. Louis, MO 63132
314.432.6200
info@touchpointautism.org
www.touchpointautism.org

TouchPoint directly works with hundreds of children and adults with autism spectrum disorders (ASD). They also work with families, helping them learn the special skills they need to care for a family member with autism.

Nebraska:

Autism Action Partnership
14301 FNB Parkway, Suite 115
Omaha, Nebraska 68154
(402) 496-7200
info@autismaction.org
www.autismaction.org

AAP's mission is to improve the quality of life of persons on the Autism Spectrum and their families through education, advocacy and support, thereby enabling them to be an integral part of the community.

Nevada:

Autism Coalition of Nevada
1790 Vassar St
Reno, NV 89502
(775) 329-2268
acon@aconv.org
www.aconv.org

Our mission is to support legislation for screening, diagnosis and treatment clinics, and receive appropriations.

New Hampshire:

The Birchtree Center
2064 Woodbury Avenue, Suite 204
Newington, New Hampshire, 03801
603-433-4192
www.birchtreecenter.org

The Birchtree Center's mission is to improve the quality of life for children and youth with autism and their families through nurturing relationships, therapeutic programming and specialized education.

New Jersey:

The Daniel Jordan Fiddle Foundation
P.O. Box 1149
Ridgewood, New Jersey 07451-1149
(877) 444-1149
info@djfiddlefoundation.org
www.djfiddlefoundation.org

The DJ Fiddle Foundation was created to both develop and support programs for autistic individuals, as well as spread current information.

The Devereux New Jersey Comprehensive Community Resources (DNJCCR)
286 Mantua Grove Road, Bldg. #4
West Deptford, NJ 08066
(856) 599-6400

DNJCCR serves nearly 400 children, adolescents, adults, and their families with special needs. It also has a residential/educational center that serves individuals with autism spectrum disorders.

New Horizons in Autism
600 Essex Rd.
Neptune, NJ 07753
(732) 918-0850

Contact: Michele Goodman, Executive Director
goodman@nhautism.org
www.nhautism.org/default.asp

New Horizons in Autism is an organization that operates six homes, a vocational program, and after-school, voucher stipend and behavior therapy support options.

New York:

Autism United
100 West Nicholai Street
Hicksville, NY 11801
(516) 933-4050
www.autismunited.org

Autism United is a community for families and individuals with autism that supports the professional community of autism researchers.

Foundation for Educating Children with Autism (FECA)
PO Box 813
Mount Kisco, NY 10549
(914) 941-FECA (3322)
questions@FECAinc.org
www.fecainc.org

FECA is a non-profit organization that provides educational opportunities for children with autism through the development of schools, inclusion and vocational programs, consumer advocacy and community outreach.

Special Needs Activity Center for Kids NYC (SNACK NYC)
220 E 86th Street (Lower Level)
New York, NY 10028
(212) 439-9996
info@snacknyc.com
www.snacknyc.com

SNACK is a New York-based activity center where children with special needs can socialize; it has after-school and weekend programs that include a variety of creative activities.

North Carolina:

Autism Services of Mecklenburg County, Inc.
2211-A Executive Street
Charlotte, NC 28208
704-392-9220
info@asmcinc.com
www.asmcinc.com/index.php

ASMC is a private, not-for-profit organizatio offering residential and support services for residents of North Carolina with Autism, Traumatic Brain Injuries and other developmental disabilties.

Autism Society of North Carolina
505 Oberlin Road, Suite 230
Raleigh, NC 27605
1 (800) 442-2762 (NC only), (919) 743-0204
info@autismsociety-nc.org
www.autismsociety-nc.org

The Autism Society of North Carolina provides support services and resources for individuals, professionals, and families dealing with autism in North Carolina.

North Dakota:

North Dakota Autism Center
4733 Amber Valley Parkway, Suite 200
Fargo, ND 58104
701.277.8844
info@ndautismcenter.org
www.ndautismcenter.org

North Dakota Autism Center's mission is to help children affected by autism spectrum disorders to reach their full potential through excellence in care, therapy, instruction and support

Ohio:

4 Paws for Ability
253 Dayton Ave.
Xenia, Ohio 45385
(937) 374-0385
Contact: Karen Shirk
karen4paws@aol.com
www.4pawsforability.org
4 Paws provides service dogs for disabled people, and the company specializes in dogs that are specifically trained to work with autistic people.

Ohio Center for Autism and Low Incidence (OCALI)
470 Glenmont Ave
Columbus OH 43214
(614) 410-0321, (866)-886-2254
ocali@ocali.org
www.ocali.org

OCALI's mission is to support, promote, and train individuals with autism and other low-incidence disorders to live fulfilling and successful lives.

Oklahoma:

Oklahoma Family Center for Autism
3901 Northwest 63rd St.
Oklahoma City, OK
(405) 842-9995
melinda@okautism-efca.org
www.okautism.org

The OFCA provides a way for organizations operating in the state of Oklahoma to share information and help each other advance the cause of families affected by autism. The OFCA is a resource and leadership forum for group leaders in Oklahoma who have a passion to serve their communities.

Oregon:

Autism Service Dogs of America
4248 Galewood St., Lake Oswego, Oregon 97035
info@autismservicedogsofamerica.com
http://autismservicedogsofamerica.com

Autism Service Dogs of America trains service dogs for autistic children.

Northwest Autism Foundation
519 Fifteenth Street
Oregon City , OR 97045
503-557-2111
www.autismnwaf.org

The Northwest Autism Foundation is a non-profit organization whose goal is to provide education and information for free or at a nominal cost to families, caregivers and professionals of autistic children.

Pennsylvania:

Advisory Board on Autism and Related Disorders (ABOARD)
35 Wilson Street, Suite 100
Pittsburgh, PA 15223
(412) 781-4116
support@aboard.org
www.aboard.org

ABOARD is a Pennsylvania-based support society for parents and autistic children, which provides both access to support groups and to a variety of autism information.

Autism Spectrum News
16 Cascade Drive
Effort, PA 18329
(570) 629-5960

Contact: Ira Minot, Executive Director
iraminot@mhnews.org
www.mhnews-autism.org/index.html

The Autism Spectrum News is a publication from Mental Health News Education, Inc. that informs the autism community about research, autism information, and current happenings.

Rhode Island:

About Families, CEDARR Family Center
203 Concord St., Suite 335
Pawtucket, RI 02860
401-365-6855
info@aboutfamilies.org
www.aboutfamilies.org

The About Families CEDARR Center is committed to supporting families of children who have autism spectrum disorders, mental health and substance abuse difficulties, and development, physical, and medical disabilities by providing state of the art information, evaluative, diagnostic, prescriptive, and support services that build on the strengths of the child, family, and community.

Advocates in Action
PO Box 41528
Providence, RI 02940-1528
401-785-2028
www.aina-ri.org

Together we work to help people understand information more clearly, learn about rights, participate in their communities and share their unique gifts with the rest of society.

Autism Project of RI
1516 Atwood Avenue
Johnston, RI 02919
(401) 785-2666
inquiries@riautism.org
www.riautism.org

Autism Project of RI was founded by parents intended to be a resource for other parents in the Rhode Island community who have members of their families who live with ASD.

Rhode Island Technical Assitance Project at the Department of Education
RIDE Office of Special Populations
255 Westminster St.
Providence, RI 02903
401-222-6030

Faces of Hope

Sue Constable sconstable@ritap.org
www.ritap.org

RITAP provides practitioners, parents, and policy-makers the knowledge and resources necessary to increase their capacity to provide comprehensive and coordinated services to all children including those with disabilities that result in improved educational performance and enhanced life-long outcomes.

South Carolina:

Autism Advocate Foundation
PO Box 7061
Myrtle Beach, SC 29572
(843) 213-0217
www.autismadvocatefoundation.com

To provide emotional, financial and therapeutic support for individuals with Autism Spectrum Disorders throughout their lifespan, while achieving their personal goals and dreams with integrity and distinction in their least restrictive environment.

National Autism Association
PO Box 1547
Marion, SC 29571
877-622-2884
naa@nationalautism.org
www.nationalautismassociation.org

The mission of the National Autism Association is to educate and empower families affected by autism and other neurological disorders, while advocating on behalf of those who cannot fight for their own rights.

Tennessee:

The Autism Solution Center, Inc.
9282 Cordova Park Road
Cordova, TN 38018
Phone: 901-758-8288
Fax: 901-758-1806
info@autismsolutioncenter.com

The Autism Solution Center, Inc. is a non-profit organization being developed to address an unmet, ongoing need within our communities for autism therapy, support services, research and other assistance.

Faces of Hope Children's Therapy Center
301 Hancock Street
Gallatin, Tennessee 37066
(615) 206-1176

Contact: Leslie Face, Executive Director
leslie@facesofhopetn.com
www.facesofhopetn.com

Faces of Hope provides speech, occupational, and physical therapies for autistic children in Tennessee and certain areas of Kentucky.

Texas:

ATC Rehabilitation Agency – Dallas
10610 Metric Dr., Suite 101
Dallas, TX 75243
214.221.4405

ATC Rehabilitation Agency – San Antonio
10615 Perrin-Beitel, Suite 801
San Antonio, TX 78247
210.599.7733

Autism Treatment Center – Dallas
10503 Metric Dr.
Dallas, TX 75243
972.644.2076
Anna P. Hundley, CEO

The mission of the Autism Treatment Center is to assist people with autism and related disorders throughout their lives as they learn, play, work and live in the community.

Autism Treatment Center – San Antonio
16111 Nacogdoches Road
San Antonio, TX 78247
210.590.2107
Anna P. Hundley, Executive Director

Vermont:

Howard Center
208 Flynn Avenue Suite 3J
Burlington, Vermont 05401
(802) 488-6000
Contact: Todd Centybear, Executive Director
www.howardcenter.org

Howard Center provides developmental, mental health, substance abuse, and child, youth, and family services through funding, support, and community programs.

Virginia:

Autism Learning Center
7600 Leesburg Pike #410
Falls Church, VA 22043
(703) 506-1930

autismlc@aol.com
www.autismlearningcenter.org

ALC emphasizes a positive and systematic approach to teaching skills and reducing problematic behaviors, taking a creative and flexible approach and capitalizing on the resources available for each child.

Organization for Autism Research
2000 North 14th Street, Suite 710
Arlington, VA 22201
703.243.9710
info@researchautism.org
www.researchautism.org

OAR's mission is to apply practical research that examines issues and challenges that children and adults with autism and their families face everyday to the treatment of individuals living with autism.

Washington:

Families for Effective Autism Treatment (FEAT) of Washington
14434 NE 8th St., Second Floor
Bellevue, WA 98007
206.763.3373
featwa@featwa.org
www.featwa.org

FEAT's mission is to provide families with hope and guidance to help their children with autism reach their full potential.

Washington, D.C.:

Autistic Self-Advocacy Network
1025 Vermont Avenue, NW, Suite 300
Washington, DC 20005
Contact: Ari Ne'eman, Founding President
aneeman@autisticadvocacy.org
www.autisticadvocacy.org

ASAN was created to encourage autistic individuals to seek rights and promote the positive aspects of a diverse community.

West Virginia:

Autism Services Center
The Keith Albee Building
929 4th Avenue, Second Floor
Huntington, WV 25701
(304) 525-8014

ASC is a nonprofit, licensed behavioral health care agency founded in 1979 by Ruth Christ Sullivan,

Ph. D. Though specializing in autism, the agency provides comprehensive, community integrated services for individuals with all developmental disabilities, throughout their lifespan.

West Virginia Autism Training Center
Marshall University
One John Marshall Drive
Huntington, WV 25755
1-800-642-3463
www.marshall.edu/coe/atc

The mission of the Autism Training Center is to provide education, training and treatment programs for West Virginians who have Autism, Pervasive Developmental Disorder (NOS) or Asperger's Disorder and have been formally registered with the Center. This is done through appropriate education, training and support for professional personnel, family members or guardians and other important in the life of a person with autism.

Wisconsin:

Chileda Habilitation Institute
1825 Victory Street
La Crosse, WI 54601
Ruth Wiseman, President/CEO
608-782-6480 Ext. 237
www.chileda.org

Chileda is a nationally recognized and respected program for students with exceptional needs and exceptional potential. They serve children and young adults from ages 6 to 21.

Good Friend, Inc.
808 Cavalier Drive
Waukesha, WI 53186
(414) 510-0385, (262) 391-1369
Contacts: Chelsea Budde and Denise Schamens, Founders
chelsea@goodfriendinc.com, denise@goodfriendinc.com
www.goodfriendinc.com

Good Friend, Inc. was created to spread awareness and understanding from regularly-developing children for autistic children; the organization offers information, events, and workshops.

Wyoming:

Casper Autism Society
750 West 58th Street
Casper, WY 82601

307-234-5838
cgarner@tribcsp.com
http://casperautismsociety.com/

The Casper Autism Society serves as a support group for all families affected by autism and for those on the Autism Spectrum (ASD). Monthly meetings are held and a free lending library is available.

INTERNATIONAL

Autism Canada Foundation
(519) 695-5858
www.autismcanada.org

The Autism Acceptance Project
P.O. Box 23030
Toronto, Ontario Canada M5N 3A8
Contact: Estée Klar-Wolfond, Founder and Executive Director
esteewolfond@mac.com
www.taaproject.com

TAAP is a site to promote public understanding and acceptance of autistic people. This site also has an online gallery with creations completely contributed by autistic artists.

The Autism File
PO Box 144
Hampton, TW12 2FF
England
020 8979 2525
info@autismfile.com
www.autismfile.com

The Autism File is a magazine covering autism spectrum disorders, providing information about biomedical research and treatments, education and therapies, advocacy issues, perspectives of individuals on the spectrum, and more.

The Autism Trust
Brackenwood
Hill View Road
Claygate
Surrey KT10 0TU
UNITED KINGDOM
020 8979 2525
info@theautismtrust.org.uk
www.autismtrust.com

The Autism Trust provides a variety of facilities and centers that assist autistic individuals by providing resources and support in health issues, residential needs, professional information, and more.

Child Early Intervention Medical Center, FZ LLC
Dubai Health Care City Al Razi Building, Block B, Suite 2010
P.O. Box 505122 ,Dubai, UAE
Tel: +971 4 423 3667
Fax:+971 4 429 8474
Mobile: +971505512319
www.childeimc.com

Curando el Autismo
www.curandoelautismo.org

EmergenzAutismo (Italy)
www.emergenzautismo.org

MINDD Foundation
PO Box 151 Vaucluse
NSW 2030 Australia
+61 2 9337 3600
info@mindd.org
www.mindd.org

MINDD was created to inform and provide research findings on new and alternative treatments for disorders like autism, such as Chiropractic care, Chinese medicine, and holistic care.

Research Autism
Westbourne House
14-16 Westbourne Grove
London, W2 5RH020 8292 8900
UK
info@researchautism.net
www.researchautism.net

Research Autism is a UK-based charity dedicated to autism research, and is designed for anyone with an interest in autism.

Treating Autism
222 Bramhall Lane South
Bramhall, Stockport
Cheshire SK7 3AA UK
treatingautismuk@aol.com
www.treatingautism.co.uk

Treating Autism has a membership society that receives resources and newsletters, groups that meet for support, and conferences in the UK to inform about biomedical and therapeutic developments for autism.

SCHOOLS FOR PERSONS WITH AUTISM SPECTRUM DISORDERS

Alabama:

Glenwood
The Autism and Behavioral Health Center
150 Glenwood Lane
Birmingham, Alabama 35242-5700
Main Phone: (205) 969-2880

Glenwood provides treatment and education services in a least restrictive setting, through a continuum of care, with the highest respect for individuals and families served.

Arizona:

Arizona Centers for Comprehensive Education and Life-Skills (ACCEL)
10251 North 35th Ave
Phoenix, AZ 85051
(602) 995-7366
Contact: Nancy Molder, Vice President of Educational Services.
nmolder@accel.org

ACCEL is a private, non-profit special education day school providing educational, behavioral and vocational services to students, ages 3-21, with cognitive, emotional, orthopedic, and/or behavioral challenges and Autism.

Chrysalis Academy
600 E. Baseline Rd., Ste. B6
Tempe, AZ 85283
(480) 839-6000
play.aba@gmail.com
www.play-aba.com

Chrysalis Academy is a private year-round school that serves children with autism and related disorders using ABA teaching methods.

Gateway Academy
7655 E. Gelding Drive
Suite #A-3
Scottsdale, AZ 85260
(480) 998-1071
www.gatewayacademy.us/index.htm

Gateway Academy is a private Preschool - 12th Grade day school specializing in students with Asperger's Syndrome, High Functioning Autism, and PDD-nos. It incorporates special techniques into the curriculum, such as puppy therapy, equine therapy, and music therapy.

New Way Academy
1300 North 77th Street
Scottsdale, Arizona 85257
(480) 946-9112
Contact: denise@newwayacademy.org
www.newwayacademy.org

New Way Learning Academy is Arizona's only non-profit, private K-12 day school specializing in children with learning differences.

Pieceful Solutions
6101 E. Virginia St.
Mesa, AZ 85215
(480) 309-4792
piecefulsolutions@yahoo.com
www.piecefulsolutions.com

Pieceful Solutions is an non-profit organization created specifically to offer children with autism and other developmental disabilities comprehensive schooling using innovative teaching techniques. We work cooperatively with students and parents to set, plan for and achieve goals that focus on academics, social, emotional development and life skills.

Arkansas:

The Allen School
824 N. Tyler St.
Little Rock, AR 72205
(501) 664-2961
Contact: Suzy Benham, Director
www.invitingarkansas.com/charity/allen-school.
asp

Since 1958, The Allen School has enabled children birth to five, with developmental disabilities, such as cerebral palsy, autism, epilepsy, and mental retardation, to achieve their dreams, through treatment, nurturing, and education.

California:

Beacon Day School
588 N. Glassell Street
Orange, CA 92867
Dr. Mary Jo Lang
(714) 288-4200
(714) 288-4204 FAX
contactBDS@beacondayschool.com
www.beacondayschool.com

California Autism Foundation
4075 Lakeside Drive
Richmond, CA 94806
(510) 758-0433
contactcaf@calautism.org
www.calautism.org

The mission of the California Autism Foundation is to provide people with autism and other developmental disabilities the best possible opportunities for lifetime support, training and assistance in helping them reach their highest potential for independence, productivity and fulfillment.

Camphill Communities California
Soquel, California
http://www.camphillca.org

Camphill Communities California is a residential care community for adults with developmental disabilities. We're a community of about 25 people, 12 of whom have developmental disabilities. We're located near Monterey Bay, a region famous for its rich, social, cultural and recreational opportunities.

Volunteer opportunities are available at Camphill Communities California for both long and short term coworkers. Imagine a life where the qualities of patience, tolerance, flexibility and empathy are valued. Camphill offers volunteers a path of learning that nurtures personal growth and community involvement with people with special needs. We also offer opportunities for ongoing education and training. We welcome those with idealism who want to share their life with others.

The Help Group
13130 Burbank Blvd.
Sherman Oaks, CA 91401
(877) 994-3588

The Help Group is a large organization that offers education in seven day schools for preschool through high-school aged students with autism and similar disorders. The schools practice diagnostic teaching, therapies, and physical education.

New Vista School
23092 Mill Creek Drive
Laguna Hills, CA 92653
(949) 455-1270
office@newvistaschool.org
www.newvistaschool.org

New Vista School is a grade 6-12+ progressive educational center that provides a safe, structured educational environment serving the needs of students with Asperger Syndrome, high-functioning Autism, and language learning disabilities who may benefit from social and transitional skills development.

Orion Academy
350 Rheem Blvd
Moraga, CA 94556-1516
(925) 377-0789
office@orionacademy.org
www.orionacademy.org

Orion Academy provides a quality college-preparatory program for secondary students whose academic success is compromised by a neuro-cognitive disability such as Asperger's syndrome, or NLD (Non-verbal Learning Disorder).

Pacific Autism Center for Education (School and Administrative Offices)
1880 Pruneridge Ave.
Santa Clara, CA 95050
(408) 245-3400

Contact: Jack Brown, Office Manager
admin@pacificautism.org
www.pacificautism.org

PACE has a K-12 school with programs for autistic students; an adult day program; and residential homes. The school's curriculum is based on individual assessment and programs.

PACE (Early Intervention and Sunny Days Preschool)
897 Broadleaf Ln.
San Jose, CA 95128
(408) 551-0312
Contact: Gina Baldi, Early Intervention Director
ginabaldi@pacificautism.org
www.pacificautism.org/intervention.shtml

PACE's early intervention programs focus on intellectual development for children with ASD under 6 years of age through a variety of therapies and techniques.

Pioneer Day School
4764 Santa Monica Ave.
San Diego, CA 92107
(619) 758-9424
pioneeramber@sbcglobal.net
www.pioneerdayschool.org/Home.asp

Our award winning school has created a unique and innovative model to address underlying processing deficits for students with Autism Specturm Disorders (ASD) and other special needs. We also create individualized programs for privately placed students.

Pyramid Autism Center
2830 North Glassell
Orange, CA 92865
Grace Walker, Administrative Assistant
gwalker@pyramidautismcenter.com
www.pyramidautismcenter.com

The Pyramid Autism Center (PAC) is a not-for-profit organization dedicated to serving the Orange County autism community – with specific focus on children and their families. The PAC school utilizes the Pyramid Approach to Education developed by Dr. Andrew Bondy, a world-renowned leader in autism education and research.

Sophia Project
Oakland, California
http://www.sophiaproject.org

Springstone Middle School
1035 Carol Lane
Lafayette, CA 94549
(925) 962-9660
info@thespringstoneschool.org
http://thespringstoneschool.org

The Springstone School is an independent middle school that serves students with Asperger's Syndrome, Non-verbal Learning Disability and other executive function challenges. All instruction integrates pragmatic language, occupational therapy, organizational skills and life skills in the classroom and in the community.

Colorado:

Colorado Institute of Autism
P.O. Box 50254
Colorado Springs, Colorado 80949
(719) 593-7334

Colorado Institute of Autism is a newly established private organization dedicated to children on the autism spectrum. The institution will open its doors as the first school for children with autism, utilizing Applied Behavior Analysis principles, in the State of Colorado. Available services will include a school program, outreach, assessment, workshops, and service as a resource to the community.

The Joshua School
2303 E. Dartmouth Ave.
Englewood, CO 80113
(303) 758-7171
thejoshuaschool@yahoo.com
www.joshuaschool.org

The Joshua School serves children ages 2½ to 21 years. Our programming for learners often combines many research-validated methods (within ABA) into a comprehensive but highly individualized package.

Connecticut:

Connecticut Center for Child Development, Inc.
925 Bridgeport Ave.
Milford, CT 06460
(203) 882-8810
Peggy Fitzsimmons, Private School Program
info@cccdinc.org

The Connecticut Center for Child Development Inc. is a non-profit school that is dedicated to improving the lives of children with autism, Asperger's Syndrome and other pervasive developmental disorders.

Franklin Academy
106 River Road
East Haddam, CT 06423
(860) 873-2700
admission@fa-ct.org
www.fa-ct.org

Franklin Academy is a college preparatory school for grades 9 - 12, accredited by the New England Association of Schools and Colleges, specializing in serving students with Nonverbal Learning Differences (NLD or NVLD) and Asperger's Syndrome (AS).

The Glenholme School
81 Sabbaday Lane
Washington, CT 06793
(860) 868-7377
info@theglenholmeschool.org
www.theglenholmeschool.org/home.htm

The Glenholme School is a specialized boarding school that provides a therapeutic program and exceptional learning environment to address varying levels of academic, social and emotional development in boys and girls ages 10 to 18.

Greenwich Education and Prep
62 Main Street
New Canaan, CT 06840
(203) 594-9777
Contacts: Katja Krumpelbeck, Assistant Director; Kirsten DeConti Ziotas, Director
katja@greenwichedprep.com; kdeconti@greenwichedprep.com
www.greenwichedprep.com

K-12 school with specialized services including Applied Behavioral Analysis (ABA) methods that teaches current public– and private-school curricula for easy transitions.

Greenwich Education and Prep
49 River Road
Cos Cob, CT 06807
(203) 661-1609
Contacts: Victoria Newman, Executive Director; Meredith Hafer, Director; Stacy Smegal,Assistant Director
vnewman@greenwichedprep.com; meredith@greenwichedprep.com; stacy@greenwichedprep.com
www.greenwichedprep.com

K-12 school with specialized services including Applied Behavioral Analysis (ABA) methods that teaches current public– and private-school curricula for easy transitions.

Delaware:

Delaware Autism Program
Brennen School
144 Brennen Drive
Newark, DE 19713
(302) 454-2202
(302) 454-5427 FAX

Florida:

The Chase Academy
700 Reed Canal Road
South Daytona, FL 32119
(386) 690-0893
Contact: Mimi Lundell, Executive Director
mtlundell@tcaofvolusia.org
www.tcaofvolusia.org

The Chase Academy, Inc., a private non-profit corporation located in Volusia County, Florida, was established in 2006 to provide educational services specifically tailored to meet the individualized needs of students with high-functioning Autism or any of the related Autism Spectrum Disorders (ASD) and to focus these services on maximizing the students' potential for inclusion into mainstream society.

Coral Rock Academy Operated By
Gersh Educational Development
11155 SW 112th Avenue
Miami, FL 33176
631.385.3342
www.coralrockacademy.org

The Gersh Academy's primary objective is to enable students to be emotionally available to learn. They provide customized educational services to students with neurobiological disorders. Coral Rock Academy educates students grades 4-12.

Florida Autism Center of Excellence
6400 E. Chelsea St.
Tampa, FL 33610
(813) 621-FACE (3223)
www.faceprogram.org

FACE serves students ages 3 to 22 with moderate to severe autism in pre-K through 12th grade and beyond. FACE is available to families in Hillsborough, Pinellas, Pasco, Polk, Manatee and Sarasota counties.

Jacksonville School for Autism
4000 Spring Park Rd.
Jacksonville, FL 32207
(904) 732-4343
info.jsa@comcast.net

JSA is a school for children on the autism spectrum, ages 3 to 18. The school uses a variety of curriculums based on each individual child.

The Jericho School
1351 Sprinkle Drive
Jacksonville, FL 32211
(904) 744-5110
jerichos@bellsouth.net
www.thejerichoschool.org

The Jericho School serves children with autism and developmental delays using ABA and verbal behavior treatments.

Palm Beach School for Autism
1199 W. Lantana Rd. #19
Lantana, Florida 33462
(561) 533-9917
contact@pbsfa.org
www.pbsfa.org

We serve children in our preschool program ages 3-5 years of age and children in our elementary program grades kindergarten through 5th grade.

Peace by Piece Learning Center
965 Pondella Rd.
North Fort Myers, FL 33903
(239) 652-4323
info@peacebypieceinc.com
www.peacebypieceinc.com/school.html

Here our mission is to employ our extensive education and experience, in combination with Applied Behavior Analysis, to provide evidence-based and compassionate services to individuals, families, schools and organizations.

Sydney's School for Autism
St. Patrick Catholic Church
4518 South Manhattan Avenue
Tampa, FL 33611
(813) 835-4591
Contacts: Kathy Swenson, Founder; Antia Maurer, Preschool Director
autisticangels@yahoo.com, anitam@sydneyschool.com
www.sydneysschoolhouse.com

Sydney's School for Autism serves autistic children and those with similar disorders for preschool, kindergarten, and first-grade students, based on ABA teaching methods.

Victory Center for Autism and Behavioral Challenges
18900 Northeast 25th Avenue
North Miami Beach, Florida 33180
Contact: Courtney Richel, Admission
office@thevictoryschool.org
www.thevictoryschool.org

Preschool, secondary school, and after-school program that uses Applied Behavioral Analysis (ABA) methods and one-on-one teaching in the education of children with autism and related disabilities.

Georgia:

Keystone Center for Children with Autism
1675-A Hembree Road
Alpharetta, GA 30009
404-496-4673

Keystone's mission is two-fold: first, we are dedicated to the educational and social development of children with Autism Spectrum Disorders, and second, we are committed to providing support and training to families affected by autism.

The Lionheart School
180 Academy Street
Alpharetta, Georgia 30004
770-772-4555

Lionheart's mission is to provide a developmentally appropriate program for children on the autism spectrum and other disorders of relating and communicating who need a specialized learning environment, therapeutic interventions, relationship building skills and the educational tools necessary to achieve their greatest potential.

Summit Learning Center
700 Holcomb Bridge Road
Suite 400
Roswell, Georgia 30076
Contacts: Jennifer Mitchell and Shauna Courtney, Directors
jennifer@summitlearningcenter.org, shauna@summitlearningcenter.org
www.summitlearningcenter.org/index.html

The Summit Learning Center aims to provide individualized, effective, and scientifically based treatment for children with autism and related disabilities that is not otherwise available in the state of Georgia. The Summit Learning Center provides effective treatment, based on the science of Applied Behavior Analysis (ABA).

Hawaii:

Loveland Academy Hawaii
1506 Piikoi Street
Honolulu, HI 96822
contact_information@lovelandacademyhawaii.com
808-524-4243

As a service provider in Honolulu, Oahu, Hawaii for children and young adults with autism, the mission is to provide an array of state of the art, research based, child and family centered, culturally sensitive therapeutic and educational services targeting the biological, psychological, educational, social and emotional needs of children.

Pacific Autism Center
670 Auahi St., Suite A-6
Honolulu, HI 96813
(808) 523-8188
laura@pacificautismcenter.com

The mission of Pacific Autism Center is to use ABA and be a foundation for those individuals (and their families) within the autism spectrum, and to also provide access to high quality researched based services that support the individual in all areas of their life.

Illinois:

Giant Steps Illinois
2500 Cabot Dr
Lisle, IL 60532
(630) 455-5730
Contact: Bridget O'Connor, Executive Director
boconnor@atc-gsi.org

Students in our private day school receive an intensive educational and therapeutic program based on the strengths and individual needs of the child. Using various methodologies such as ABA, repetition and practice, errorless learning, forward and backward chaining, visual supports, hands-on manipulatives, sensory strategies, etc. students focus on reading and language arts, vocabulary, functional mathematics, vocational life skills and more.

Illinois Center for Autism (Children's Special Day School Program)
548 Ruby Lane
Fairview Heights, IL 62208
(618) 398-7500
info@illinoiscenterforautism.org
www.illinoiscenterforautism.org/programs/dayschool.html

ICA serves students ages 3-21 who have been diagnosed as having autism, pervasive development disorder, Aspereger's Syndrome, and/or students who exhibit compatible characteristics of autism, such as severe communications disorders, severe behavioral disorders, uneven intellectual skills, and socially inappropriate behaviors.

Soaring Eagle Academy
PO Box 63
Riverside, IL 60546
312-683-5151
contact@soaringeagleacademy.org
www.soaringeagleacademy.org

Soaring Eagle's mission is to provide a social and academic learning environment for students with special needs supporting their individual strengths and learning styles while integrating learning and interaction within a Developmental Individual-Difference Relationship (DIR®) Based Approach.

Kansas:

HeartSpring School
8700 East 29th Street North
Wichita, KS 67226
(316) 634-8730 or (800) 835-1043 (calls outside Wichita area)
admissions@heartspring.org
www.heartspring.org/school/index.php

The Heartspring School, a residential and day program, provides a warm, loving environment for children with developmental disabilities such as autism, and teams of specialists discover and develop the whole child using a multidisciplinary approach.

Rainbows United, Inc.
340 S. Broadway, Wichita, KS 67202
Phone: (316) 267-KIDS
www.rainbowsunited.org/services-child_care.php
info@rui.org

Kids' CoveSM and Kids' PointSM services include progressive plans for all children regardless of their skill levels to provide the most trusted educational opportunities for all children ages birth through 5.

Maine:

Merrymeeting Center for Child Development
2 Davenport Circle Suite 20
Bath, ME 04530
(207) 443-6200
Contact: karenz@mccdworks.org
www.mccdworks.org/index.html

Merrymeeting Center for Child Development is committed to ensuring that children with autism, Asperger's syndrome and pervasive developmental disorder (PDD) have access to education, treatment and care that is objectively and scientifically validated as effective, delivered by professionals with specific minimum methodological competencies.

Maryland:

The IvyMount School, Inc.
11614 Seven Locks Rd.
Rockville, MD 20854
(301) 469-0223
www.ivymount.org/index.cfm

Named twice by the U.S. Department of Education as a Blue Ribbon School of Excellence, Ivymount is a non-sectarian, non-public special education day school. Ivymount's integrated approach to learning includes educational programs and therapeutic services for over 200 students annually, ages 4-21.

Linwood Center
3421 Martha Bush Drive
Ellicott City, MD 21043
(410) 465-1352
admin@linwoodcenter.org
www.linwoodcenter.org

The Linwood Center serves autistic students ages 9 to 21with residential and educational programs, and uses a variety of individualized techniques.

Massachusets:

Boston Higashi School
800 North Main Street
Randolph, MA 02368
(781) 961-0800
Contact: Deborah Donovan, President

donovan@bostonhigashi.org, admissions@bostonhigashi.org
www.bostonhigashi.org/index.php

Boston Higashi School, Inc. is the international program serving children and young adults with autism. Our philosophy is based upon the world-renowned tenets of Daily Life Therapy® developed by the late Dr. Kiyo Kitahara of Tokyo, Japan.

Eagleton School
446 Monterey Road
Great Barrington, MA 01230
(413) 528-4385
www.eagletonschool.com

Eagleton School serves boys with PDD and Asperger's, teaching and providing daily therapy with a mainly holistic approach. Students' ages range from 9 to 22.

Melmark New England
461 River Road
Andover, MA 01810
(978) 654-4300
www.melmarkne.org/index.html

Melmark New England specializes in serving those students within our clinical profiles who are currently unable to attend public school. For some children served, the goal is to return the child to the public school setting after the benefits of a Melmark New England education are achieved. For children ages 4 - 8, classroom teachers follow a theme-based curriculum into which individual goals and objectives for each student are carefully embedded

New England Center for Children
33 Turnpike Road
Southborough, Massachusetts 01772
(508) 481-1015
Contact: Cathy Welch, Director of Admissions
cwelch@neec.org
www.necc.org

NEEC provides individualized teaching methods for children with autism and related disorders, and the school provides a variety of extra-curricular activities and therapies.

Riverview School
551 Route 6A East Sandwich
Cape Cod, MA 02537
(508) 888-0489

admissions@riverviewschool.org
www.riverviewschool.org

Riverview School provides middle-school to post-secondary school education for students with learning disabilities, focusing on transitions, personal growth, and wellness.

Minnesota:

Camphill Village Minnesota
Sauk Centre, Minnesota
http://www.camphillvillage-minnesota.org

Camphill Village Minnesota is a spiritually striving intentional community of approximately 45 people, including adults with disabilities. Our Village is nestled among 470 acres of gently rolling hills and sparkling lakes and waterways in the beautiful Heartland of America, about 2 hours west of the city of Minneapolis. The life, work, and celebrations of our community are based on the strong belief that every individual, regardless of ability, is an independent spiritual being. Developmental disabilities are treated not as illnesses, but as a part of the fabric of human experience, and we believe that people with these disabilities are worthy of recognition, respect, and honor. Our community has a strong agricultural component with farming, gardening, and a small goatherd. Our craft shops include a bakery, weavery, woodworking shop, card shop, hemp jewelry shop, and a food processing and cheese-making kitchen. All members of the community are cared for within the context of healthy home environments and an active village life.

The Fraser School
2400 W. 64th St
Minneapolis, MN 55423
612-861-1688
school@fraser.org
www.fraser.org

Fraser's mission is to make a meaningful and lasting difference in the lives of children, adults and families with special needs. We accomplish this by providing education, healthcare and housing services.

Lionsgate Academy
3420 Nevada Ave N.
Crystal, MN 55427
(763) 486-5359

Contact: Elaine Campbell, Administrative Coordinator
ecampbell@lionsgateacademy.org
www.lionsgateacademy.org

Lionsgate Academy provides a transition-oriented and personalized learning program focused on secondary (grades 7-12) higher-functioning students on the autism spectrum that supports their full potential.

Missouri:

Oakwood
West Plains, Missouri
For information, contact:
ottow1@peoplepc.com

Ozark Center for Autism
3006 McClelland Boulevard
Joplin, Missouri 64804
(417) 347-7600
Contact: Paula Baker, Ozark Center CEO
pfbaker@freemanhealth.com
www.freemanhealth.com/ozarkcenterforautism

Ozark Center for Autism impacts lives daily through the use of Applied Behavior Analysis. Students attend school six hours a day, five days a week to minimize loss of skill.

New Jersey:

The Allegro School
125 Ridgedale Avenue
Cedar Knolls, NJ 07927
973-267-8060
www.allegroschool.org

The Allegro School is a non-profit school that provides quality education, keeps autistic children with their families, and prepares them for community living. The school serves approximately 105 students ages 3-21.

Alpine Learning Group
777 Paramus Road
Paramus, NJ 07652
201-612-7800
Bridget A. Taylor, Executive Director
btaylor@alpinelearninggroup.org
alpinelearninggroup.org/default.asp

The Alpine Learning Group is a non-profit education and treatment program facility for leraners 3 to 21 years of age that utilizes the Applied Behavior Analysis (ABA) treatment for autism.

Bancroft Schools
425 Kings Highway East, P.O. BOX 20
Haddonfield, NJ 08033
(800) 774-5516
Contact: Theresa Tolatta, Director of Admissions
and Marketing
inquiry@bnh.org.
www.bancroft.org/ID_DD/IDDD_bancroftschool_
home.html

The Bancroft School offers early education
through secondary education for autistic students
with a variety of techniques, including ABA, community-based instruction, and incidental learning.

Bright Beginnings Learning Center
1660 Stelton Road
Piscataway, NJ 08854
(732) 339-9331
Wendy Eaton, Principal
www.mcesc.k12.nj.us/special/bright.htm

The Bright Beginnings Learning Center provides
specialized, classroom based instruction, based
on the principles of Applied Behavior Analysis
for students with autism or autistic-like behavior,
ages 3 to 12.

Celebrate the Children School
345 South Main Street
Wharton , NJ 07885
(973) 989-4033
Contact: Monica G. Osgood, Director
info@celebratethechildren.org
www.celebratethechildren.org

Celebrate the Children School uses the developmental, individual, relationship-based model to
teach autistic students ages 3 to 19 with a focus
on a positive and social educational experience.

The Children's Institute
One Sunset Avenue
Verona, NJ 07044
973-509-3050
Bruce Ettinger, Ed.D., Superintendent/ CEO
webmaster@tcischool.org
www.tcischool.org/default.aspx

TCI uses a model alternative program in which
each student's social/emotional and cognitive
learning needs are addressed in a prescriptive
Individualized Educational Plan (IEP).

Douglass Developmental Disabilities Center
151 Ryders Lane

New Brunswick, NJ 08901-8557
732-932-4500
Dr. Lara Delmolino, Ph.D., BCBA, Acting Director,
Adult Services
www.dddc.rutgers.edu

The Douglass Developmental Disabilities Center
(DDDC) was established by the Board of Governors of Rutgers, The State University of New
Jersey in 1972 to meet the needs of people with
autism spectrum disorders and their families
and continues to do so by employing ABA-based
therapies.

Garden Academy
P.O. Box 188
Maplewood, NJ 07040-0188
(973) 761-6140
info@gardenacademy.org
www.gardenacademy.org

Garden Academy will serve individuals with autism
ages 3-21. Garden Academy uses scientific, data-
based and accountable interventions to provide an
individualized education to students with autism
so that they may lead lives of the greatest possible
independence.

The Midland School
94 Readington Road
PO Box 5026
North Branch, New Jersey 08876
(908) 722-8222
info@midlandschool.org
www.midlandschool.org/index.asp

The Midland School is a nationally recognized program approved by the New Jersey Deparment of
Education that serves children with special needs.

New Beginnings
28 Dwight Place
Fairfield, NJ 07004
(973) 882-8822
www.nbnj.org

New Beginnings is dedicated to working with
children ages three to 21 diagnosed on the
autism spectrum. We use a variety of techniques
and resources aimed at helping individuals reach
their potential and live productively—increasing
social, educational and employment opportunities through integration into all aspects of community life.

Reed Academy
85 Summit Ave.
Garfield, NJ 07026
(973) 772.1188
info@reedacademy.org
www.reedacademy.org

Reed Academy is a private, not-for-profit program for individuals with autism spectrum disorders ages 3-21 using ABA techniques. In addition to an individualized full day school program, we also provide family consultation services and parent training.

Somerset Hills Learning Institute
1810 Burnt Mills Road
Bedminster, NJ 07921
(908) 719-6400
info@somerset-hills.org
www.somerset-hills.org/home.html

With our reliance on education and treatment approaches derived from the science of applied behavior analysis, some of our students will graduate to traditional education settings. Others will graduate into the workforce and independent living. None will be relegated to a bleak and inhumane future.

Stepping Stone School
45 County Road 519
Bloomsbury, NJ 08804
(908) 995-1999
Frank Jiorle, Executive Director
frankji@ptd.net
www.sstoneschool.com/page1.html

Stepping Stone School serves Children and Adolescents with Emotional Disorders,Learning Disabilities, Asperger's Syndrome, ADD,ADHD. An individualized instructional and restorative counseling program is provided as an integral part of the school experience.

Y.A.L.E. School Atlantic
(Hamilton Township, NJ)
(856) 346-0007
www.yaleschool.com/schools/atlantic

This school provides year-round, full-day educational programming to children with autism or pervasive developmental disorder not otherwise specified (PDD-NOS), ages 3-7.

Y.A.L.E. School Southeast
1004 Laurel Oak Road
Voorhees, NJ 08043
(856) 346-0007
www.yaleschool.com/schools/southeast

This school provides year-round, full-day educational programming to children with autism or pervasive developmental disorder not otherwise specified (PDD-NOS). The program provides educational services to students ages 3 to 14 years.

Y.A.L.E. School Southeast II
(856) 346-0007
www.yaleschool.com/schools/southeasttwo

This school provides year-round, full-day educational programming to children with autism or pervasive developmental disorder not otherwise specified (PDD-NOS). The program provides educational services to students ages 14 to 21 within a public Jr/Sr high school in Audubon, NJ.

New York:

Anderson Center for Autism
4885 Route 9, P.O. Box 367
Staatsburg, New York 12580
(845) 889-4034
info@ACenterforAutism.org
www.andersoncenterforautism.org

The Anderson Center for Autism is a private center with residential and educational programs for both children and adults with autism, based on ABA treatment.

Ascent: A School for Individuals with Autism
819 Grand Boulevard
Deer Park NY 11729
(631) 254-6100
Nancy Shamow, PH.D., Executive Director
NShamow@aol.com
www.ascentschool.org

Ascent is a private, non-profit school for children diagnosed with autism and atypical pervasive developmental disorders. It provides a full day, 12 month academic and behavioral treatment program to preschool and school age children ranging in age from 3 to 21 years.

Brooklyn Autism Center Academy
111 Remsen Street
Brooklyn, NY 11201
718.554.1027
info@brooklynautismcenter.org
www.brooklynautismcenter.org

The BAC is a non-profit school serving children with Autism Spectrum Disorders (ASD) in Brooklyn. Their philosophy is grounded in the Applied Behavior Analysis (ABA) model, which is the educational standard and best practice for children with autism.

For Adults

Camphill Village U.S.A.
Copake, New York
http://www.camphillvillage.org

Camphill Village is a unique therapeutic residential community in Copake, New York, where dedicated volunteers and people with developmental disabilities share a full life together. Located in rural Columbia County 100 miles north of New York City, the Village comprises 600 acres of wooded hills, gardens and pastures. Villagers (adults with disabilities), coworkers and coworkers' children live together in extended family households and work together in a variety of craft shops and work areas. Crafts include candle making, stained glass, bookbinding, weaving, and woodworking. Land work includes a biodynamic dairy farm, vegetable gardens, a Healing Plant garden and workshop, and Turtle Tree Seed biodynamic seed workshop. The Village also has a medical care center, culture and arts center, bakery, Café and Gift Shop.

The Center for Developmental Disabilities
72 South Woods Road
Woodbury NY, 11797
(516) 921-7650
vprew@centerfor.com
www.centerfor.com

The Center for Developmental Disabilities has a residential program for autistic and developmentally disabled individuals ages 5 to 21, with educational programs, access to therapy, and clinical services.

Gersh Academy (multiple locations)
358 Hoffman Lane
Hauppauge, NY 11788
254-04 Union Turnpike
Glen Oaks, NY 10004
631.385.3342
www.gershacademy.org

The Gersh Academy's primary objective is to enable students to be emotionally available to learn. They provide customized educational services to individuals with neurobiological disorders, grade 3-12.

The Gersh Experience
North Tonowanda, NY 14120
Post Secondary Program
631-385-3342
www.coralrockacademy.org./index.php/schools/the-gersh-experience

The Gersh Experience provides a customized educational program that allows students with neurobiological disorders to successfully experience college life away from the home.

The LearningSpring Elementary School
247 East 20th Street
New York, NY 10003
(212) 239-4926
Margaret Poggi, Head of School
mpoggi@learningspring.org
www.learningspring.org

The LearningSpring elementary school uses a Cooperative Learning Paradigm, where academics is integrated with mastery of social/emotional, pragmatic language, organization and sensory-motor skills.

McCarton School
350 East 82nd Street
New York, New York 10028
Phone: (212) 996-9035
info@mccartonschool.org
www.mccartonschool.org

The McCarton School provides an educational program for autistic children by using an integrated one-to-one model of therapy that is grounded in Applied Behavioral Analysis (ABA) combined with speech and language therapy, motor skills training, and peer interaction.

Millwood Learning Center
12 Schumann Road
Millwood, NY 10546
(914) 941-1991
www.devereux.org

Located in Westchester County, the Center provides year-round, full-day, intensive educational and behavioral interventions to students with autism and other pervasive developmental disorders.

New York City Center for Autism Charter School
433 E. 100 Street

New York, NY 10029
(212)-860-2580
Contact: Julie Fisher, Principal
http://schools.nyc.gov/SchoolPortals/04/M337/default.htm

This school serves grades 1 through 8 and provides special services and extra-curricular activities for children with autism.

Rebecca School
40 East 30th Street
New York, NY 10016-7374
(212) 810-4120
info@rebeccaschool.org
www.rebeccaschool.org

Therapeutic day school for children 4 to 18 that uses the Developmental Individual Difference Relationship-based (DIR) model in the education of children with PDD and autism.

Shema Kolainu-Hear Our Voices
4302 New Utrecht Ave.
Brooklyn, NY 11219
718-686-9600
info@skhov.org
www.shemakolainu.org

SK-HOV's mission is to hear the voices of the children and families they serve as they strive to achieve their full potential for independence, productivity and inclusion in the community. Shema Kolainu is dedicated to the education of children with autism spectrum disorders (ASD). Their vision is to provide the best opportunity offered anywhere for children with ASD to achieve recovery.

Summit Academy
150 Stahl Rd.
Getzville, NY 14068
Phone: 716.629.3400
Fax: 716.629.3499
www.summited.org/early.asp

For Young Adults: 18-28
Triform Camphill Community
Hudson, New York
http://www.triform.org

Triform Camphill Community is a residential therapeutic community, founded in 1979. Triform is a growing energetic community. In the past five years, we have built a residential house and a weavery-therapy building. As a youth-guidance community, Triform endeavors to accompany young adults with

special needs to adulthood, self-development, and fulfillment of their potential through education and work training. About 60 people live on 125 acres of land. The community is rich in agriculture, crafts, festivals, and arts. Triform is located in upstate New York, near the city of Hudson and the Hudson River, 2 hours from New York City, 3 hours from Boston, and 1 hour from Albany, New York State's capital as well as 10 miles from the Camphill Village in Copake, New York.

West Hills Montessori School (operated by Gersh Academy)
313 Round Swamp Road
Melville, NY 11747
631.385.3342
www.gershacademy.org

It is a private, co-educational day school that serves 100 students, ages 18 months to 12 years (Toddler through 6th grade), from both Nassau and Suffolk counties.

North Carolina:

Mariposa School for Children with Autism
The Mariposa School for Children with Autism
203 Gregson Drive
Cary, NC 27511
(919) 461-0600
Contact: Dr. Jacqueline Gottlieb, Head of Mariposa School
info@MariposaSchool.org
www.mariposaschool.org

The Mariposa School staff serves and teaches autistic children by reassessing their needs constantly and giving each child an individual teaching plan.

Ohio:

Autism Academy of Learning
219 Page Street
Toledo, Ohio 43620
(419) 865-7487
Anthony Gerke, Director of Education agerke@theautismacademy.org
www.theautismacademy.org/

The Autism Academy of Learning is structured to provide every student with Autism Spectrum Disorder an appropriate foundation in the areas of academics, behavior, daily living skills, vocational skills, and independence. Our goal is to promote a higher quality of life, and the realization of the full intellectual and social development of students with Autism Spectrum Disorder.

Haugland Learning Center
3400 Snouffer Rd.
Columbus, OH 43235
614-602-6473
hlccolumbus.com

Haugland Learning Center (HLC) serves the educational needs of over 120 children with Autism or Asperger syndrome throughout the state of Ohio, accepting students from preschool through twelfth grade (including those with behaviors) and is therefore an excellent alternative to public school. All students with an Autism or Asperger's diagnosis are eligible to receive the Autism Scholarship from the Ohio Department of Education, which can be used to pay for educational services at HLC.

Oakstone Academy
5747A Cleveland Avenue
Columbus, OH 43231
(614) 865-9643

The Oakstone Academy is a non-profit, fully inclusive, chartered school dedicated to serving children with autism and their families, and we are determined to use the principles of applied behavior analysis within the natural environment and implement the most effective empirically based strategies to promote language, social, behavioral, and academic competency in children with autism.

Summit Academy Schools
www.summitacademies.com

Oregon:

Building Bridges
3533 Southeast Milwaukie
Portland, OR 97202
(503) 235-3122
http://bridgespdx.wordpress.com
Beth Mishler, Board Certified Behavior Analyst beth@bridgespdx.com

Building Bridges is pleased to offer three behavioral classrooms for children with language and social disorders including autism spectrum disorder: primary (ages 6-8), kindergarten (ages 5-6), and preschool (ages 3-4). The curriculum includes instruction in language arts, mathematics, science, social studies, language, social skills and

graphomotor skills, and functional and play skills needed in the classroom are also taught.

The Child Development School of Oregon
12208 NW Cornell Road
Portland, OR 97229
(503) 646-9135
Therese Steward

Our mission is to provide state-of-the-art education for students with autism and related disabilities and to help all our students reach their full potential in school, in the community, and in life.

School of Autism
7714 N Portsmouth
Portland, OR 97203
503-283-9603
schoolofautism@yahoo.com
www.schoolofautism.com

The School of Autism is a place that families with children with autism can go to get therapy, support and education. Through play, sensory immersion and guidance by people who actually have been through the same process, families and children with autism can be treated AND educated in one place.

Pennsylvania:

Autistic Endeavors Learning Center
7340 Jackson Street
Philadelphia, PA, 19136
Barbara A. Butkiewicz Co-Founder/President
aelcinfo@yahoo.com
www.autisticendeavors.org
(215) 360-1569

The mission of Autistic Endeavors Learning Center is to promote independent functioning of children with Autistic Spectrum Disorders. The Center will provide an intensive instructional program using, but not limited to, methods of Applied Behavior Analysis to help children with Autism acquire effective communication and socialization skills.

For Children: Pre-K to Grade 12
Camphill Special School
Glenmoore, Pennsylvania
http://www.camphillspecialschool.org

Children, ages 5-19 years, live in an extended family with coworkers—often with their own children—and other volunteers in specially designed homes. The education program is adapted from Waldorf education focusing on experiential learning and emphasizing social, artistic and practical skills, and is supported by a variety of therapies that are available to help the child in his or her development. The community consists of approximately 90 students, 40 teachers and teacher aides, 10 therapists, 70 additional coworkers and 11 staff and is located in the same general area of southeastern Pennsylvania as Camphill Village Kimberton Hills and Camphill Soltane.

Camphill Soltane
Glenmoore, Pennsylvania
http://www.camphillsoltane.org

Camphill Soltane is a life-sharing community of 80 people, including young adults, ages 18-35, with developmental disabilities. At Soltane, we encourage self-advocacy for those with disabilities, help coworkers reach their aspirations through effective and inspiring training, and encourage teamwork in home and work areas. Soltane's mission is to build a bridge to adulthood for young people with disabilities, and our cornerstone is an attempt to actively involve every person in the process of creating community. We are located 1 hour west of Philadelphia, PA, in a semi-rural setting.

Camphill Village Kimberton Hills
Kimberton, Pennsylvania
http://www.camphillkimberton.org

Camphill Village Kimberton Hills is a 432 acre, land-based, life-sharing community located about an hour west of Philadelphia in Chester County Pennsylvania. Made up of 120 members, Kimberton Hills strives to restore vitality to our ecosystems and societal structures through Anthroposophy, the spiritual philosophy of Rudolf Steiner. Adults who have developmental disabilities live and work side by side with volunteers in family households to form a supportive community based on shared responsibilities and caring. The community features a large biodynamic CSA Garden which offers a two year apprenticeship study program, an award winning organic dairy, a café and bakery which serve the village and surrounding region, weavery and fiber arts workshops, as well as land and building maintenance programs. Kimberton Hills is known locally for its sustainable buildings and its strong cultural life of festivals, music, and art.

The Comprehensive Learning Center (CLC)
150 James Way
Southampton, PA 18966
(215) 322-7852
clcschool@clcschool.net
www.clcschool.net

The Comprehensive Learning Center's primary mission is to ensure that each of its students reaches their maximum potential through an intensive, comprehensive education and treatment program based on the scientifically validated procedures of applied behavior analysis.

Devereux Kanner/Kanner CARES
390 East Boot Road
West Chester, PA 19380
610-431-8100
www.devereux.org/site/
PageServer?pagename=kan_cares

Devereux Childhood Autism Research and Education Services (CARES) is a state of the science center-based, day education program for young children with autism using contemporary strategies and methodologies consistent with Applied Behavior Analysis (ABA).

The Melmark School
2600 Wayland Road
Berwyn, Pennsylvania 19312
(610) 325-4969
admissions@melmark.org
www.melmark.org

The Melmark School offers day and residential special education services to children and adolescents ages 5 to 21 with learning difficulties and/or challenging behaviors secondary to a diagnosis of Autism Spectrum Disorder; Acquired Brain Injury; Mental Retardation, mild to profound; Cerebral Palsy; and/or Neurological Disorders.

TALK Institute and School
(formerly Magnolia)
395 Bishop Hollow Road
Newtown Square, PA 19073
610.356.5566
www.talkinc.org/about.html
New Students
phone 610.356.5566
Email mikeabramson@comcast.net
Media Inquiries
phone 610.356.5566
Email melkot@aol.com

The Vista School
1249 Cocoa Avenue
Hershey, PA 17033
(717) 835-0310
Kristen Yurich, Clinical Director kyurich@
thevistaschool.org

Vista serves children with ASD ranging in age from pre-kindergarten to secondary school age from Berks, Cumberland, Dauphin, Franklin, Juniata, Lancaster, Lebanon, and Perry Counties, who are functioning on the moderate to severe end of the autism spectrum, who often display severe delays in communication skills, engage in higher rates of problematic or challenging behaviors, require assistance for activities of daily living, have little or limited ability to appropriately occupy their leisure time, and need one-on-one instruction for learning new skills.

Tennessee:

The King's Daughters' School for Autism
900 Trotwood Avenue
Columbia, Tennessee 38401
(931) 388-3810

The mission of The King's Daughters' School is to serve the educational and training needs of children and adults with developmental disabilities. The school strives to provide a high-quality program of personal development in a wholesome residential atmosphere aimed at allowing each person to reach his or her fullest potential as an independent and productive citizen.

Texas:

Autism Treatment Center – Dallas
10503 Metric Drive
Dallas, Texas 75243
(972) 644-2076
www.atcoftexas.org

The mission of the Autism Treatment Center is to assist people with autism and related disorders throughout their lives as they learn, play, work and live in the community.

Capitol School of Austin
2011 West Koenig Lane
Austin, Texas 78756
(512) 467-7006

The mission of Capitol School of Austin is to provide an enriched learning environment where children with speech, language, and learning differences can reach their full potential and develop skills necessary to succeed in future educational settings.

Focus On The Future Training Center
3405 Custer Rd. Suite 100
Plano, TX 75023
(972) 599-1400
Contact: Brenda M. Batts, Director
focussped@yahoo.com
www.focussped.com/index.html

Focus on the Future Training Center is a highly regarded Pre-K to Grade 12 private school for children with autism and other mental disabilities. They offer some of the best autism early intervention and other individualized curriculum featuring Speech Therapy, Occupational Therapy, and Music Therapy.

The Monarch School
1231 Wirt Rd.
Houston, TX 77055
(713) 479-0800
Contact: Sharon Duval
sduval@monarchschool.org
www.monarchschool.org
Developmental Individuarl Difference / FloorTime based program.

Newfound School
2206 Heads Lane, Suite 110
Carrollton, TX 75006
(214) 390-1749
www.newfoundschool.com

Newfound School is a small private school for grades PreK - 12 for children with learning and/ or behavior challenges. It is designed to provide meaningful instruction and learning in a caring, nurturing atmosphere. Students are provided life-long learning strategies for academics, behavior, and social skills.

The Westview School
1900 Kersten Drive
Houston, TX 77043
713.973.1900
Jane G. Stewart, Director
www.westviewschool.org

The Westview School is a private, non-profit school which was founded in 1981 to provide a structured, nurturing, and stimulating learning environment for children with learning differences which prevent them from being successful in regular programs.

Utah:

The Carmen B. Pingree Center for Children with Autism
780 South Guardsman
UT 84108
(801) 581-0194
Contact: Pete Nicholas, Director
petern@vmh.com
www.carmenbpingree.com

The Pingree Center is a preschool and kindergarten program for children with autism that uses a unique 5-step approach for a discrete trial format method of teaching.

Spectrum Academy
575 Cutler Drive
North Salt Lake, UT 84054
(801) 936-0318
http://spectrumcharter.org/

The Spectrum Academy is the premier charter school in Utah that tailors learning environment and curriculum to accommodate the unique needs of children with Asperger's Syndrome and other high-functioning Autism Spectrum Disorders. Our mission encompasses all children, and we are pleased to be free and offer enrollment open to the public.

Vermont:

Heartbeet
Hardwick, Vermont
http://www.heartbeet.org

Howard Center
208 Flynn Avenue Suite 3J
Burlington, Vermont 05401
(802) 488-6000
debs@howardcenter.org
www.howardcenter.org

The Autism Spectrum Program (ASP) at Howard Center provides intensive, specialized instructional and behavioral treatment and support services year-round to individuals with Autism Spectrum Disorders, ages 2-21 years. Services are provided in home, school, and community settings and target the teaching and shaping of essential communication, social, adaptive behavior, daily living, and functional learning skills. Multiple treatment methodologies under the principles of Applied Behavior Analysis are utilized.

INSPIRE for Autism
77 Dylan Rd.
Brattleboro, VT 05301
802-251-7301
info@inspireforautism.org
http://inspire4autism.com/

I.N.S.P.I.R.E. for Autism, Inc. will strive to maximize the potential for adolescents and young adults with Autism Spectrum Disorders to lead satisfying, self-sustaining lives in connection with their communities.

Virginia:

Alternative Paths Training School--Alexandria
5632 Mt. Vernon Memorial Highway
Alexandria, VA 22309
(703) 766-8708
Renee Loebs, Curriculum Specialist
rloebs@aptschool.org
www.aptschool.org

ATPS's mission is to provide students with the knowledge and practical skills essential for their successful integration into the community Locations in Alexandria and Fredericksburg.

Blue Ridge Autism Center
312 Whitwell Drive
Roanoke, VA 24019
540-366-7399
BRAC.1@juno.com
www.blueridgeautismcenter.com

BRAC is committed to providing resources and training to families and professionals throughout the Roanoke Valley and surrounding areas.

Dominion School for Autism
4205 Ravenswood Rd.
Richmond, VA 23222
804-355-1011
wendy.brown@dominionautism.org
www.dominionautism.org

The mission and educational philosophy of The Dominion School is to provide children with autism an individualized, ABA-based educational program in a loving and supportive atmosphere.

Spiritos School
400 Coalfield Road
Midlothian, Virginia 23113
(804) 897-7440
Janet@spiritosschool.com

www.spiritosschool.com

Our mission is to create a wealth of individualized instructional and treatment experiences that provide continual educational programming in an atmosphere of love and acceptance for children with autism and developmental delay.

The Aurora School
420 Wildman St.
Leesburg, VA 20176
540-751-1414
Courtney Deal, Program Director
cdeal@aurora-school.org

At Aurora, we believe that education works best for students and families when valid research findings from the fields of education and psychology, behavior analysis in particular, are constantly applied in the classroom, so teaching practices at the school are derived primarily from applied behavior analysis (ABA).

The Faison School
1701 Byrd Avenue
Richmond, VA 23230
804-612-1947
Dr. Kathy Mathews, Director of Education
kathy@kmaba.com
www.thefaisonschool.org

The Faison School for Autism/ACV is dedicated to giving each child the best chance he or she has to improve their life's journey by employing a three-pronged approach of empirically-driven treatment, research, and training to best serve our students. Our philosophy is a holistic one, focusing on the child, their family, and all those who touch and enrich their lives.

Virginia Institute for Autism
1414 Westwood Road
Charlottesville, VA 22901-5149
(434) 923-8252
information@viaschool.org
www.viaschool.org

VIA is dedicated to providing comprehensive, outcome-based education to people with autism; supporting families coping with the challenges that come with autism; and developing and supporting primary research, advocacy and training in the education of people with autism.

Washington:

DIR®/Floortime™ Summer Camp

20310 19th Ave NE
Shoreline, WA 98155
(206) 367-5853
Contact: Rosemary White, OTR/L, DIR® Faculty
pedptot@comcast.net

Various Locations:

Lovaas Institute
Various Locations
(856) 616-9442 (East Clinical Treatment Headquarters)
(310) 410-4450 (West Clinical Treatment Headquarters)
info@lovaas.com
www.lovaas.com

Intensive Applied Behavioral Analysis (ABA) Program that uses the Lovaas Method for autistic children ages 2 to 8 (children over the age of 5 qualify for consultative services, but not clinic-based services).

May Institute (Headquarters)
41 Pacella Park Drive
Randolph, MA 02368
(781) 440-0400
info@mayinstitute.org
www.mayinstitute.org

May Institute is one of the largest providers of private schools specifically serving children with autism. Our four May Centers for Child Development offer full-day, year-round educational services to children and adolescents with autism spectrum disorders (ASD) and other developmental disabilities. Schools are located in Massachusetts and California.

CANADA:

Autism Society Canada
PO Box 65
Orangeville
ON, L9W 2ZS
Canada
1-866-874-3334
info@autismsocietycanada.ca
www.autismsocietycanada.ca

Autism Society Canada's mission is to work with our many partners to address the national priorities facing the Autism community.

Camphill Communities Ontario

Angus, Ontario, Canada

http://www.camphill.on.ca

Camphill Communities Ontario, a life sharing endeavor serving people with developmental disabilities, has two locations: Camphill Nottawasaga is a rural community with adults and made up of several homes and workshops including woodwork, pottery, forestry and a vegetable garden. Our work is to care for each other, our homes, our gardens and our land. We share this work, each one according to his wishes and capabilities. The aim is to build a vital community life that offers each person the conditions for healing growth and renewal. Camphill Sophia Creek is developing residential workshop opportunities in an urban environment in the downtown core of Barrie, which is 1 hour north of Toronto.

The Cascadia Society

North Vancouver, British Columbia, Canada

http://www.cascadiasociety.org

The Cascadia Society is a life-sharing community that includes adults with special needs. Cultural, artistic and therapeutic experiences are provided through residential home care and day activities within the urban setting of Vancouver's North Shore. The Cascadia Society is dedicated to bringing healing to human beings and to the earth. Their primary task is to allow the potential in each person to unfold and to be in harmonious relationship with the environment.

The Ita Wegman Association of BC

Duncan, British Columbia, Canada

http://www.glenorafarm.com

The Ita Wegman Association of operates Glenora Farm, a rural, agriculturally based community for adults with special needs. The community operates a biodynamic farm. At Glenora Farm, those who are in need of special care, and those who provide it, relate to each other as companions, rather than as professionals and clients. In the way they live together, care for the land and in the things they make, they uphold the ideals of Camphill, in which each contributes what he or she is able to, and receives in turn what he or she needs.

St. Marcellinus School

730 Courtneypark Dr W

Mississauga, ON L5W 1L9, Canada

(905) 564-6614

Contact: Lynda Arsenault, Admissions

lynda.arsenault@dpcdsb.org

www.dpcdsb.org/MARCL

RECOMMENDED
READING

Bailey, Sally, *Wings to Fly: Bringing Theatre Arts to Students with Special Needs* (Woodbine House, 1993) and *Barrier-Free Drama*

Barbera, Mary Lynch, and Tracy Rasmussen. *The Verbal Behavior Approach: How to Teach Children with Autism and Related Disorders*. Jessica Kingsley Publishers, 2007.

Bluestone, Judith. *The Fabric of Autism: Weaving the Threads into a Cogent Theory*. The HANDLE Institute, 2004.

Bock, Kenneth, and Cameron Stauth. *Healing the New Childhood Epidemics: Autism, ADHD, Asthma, and Allergies: The Groundbreaking Program for the 4-A Disorders*. Ballantine Books, 2008.

Buckley, Julie A. *Healing Our Autistic Children: A Medical Plan*. Palgrave Macmillan 2010.

Casanova, Manuel F. Brain and *Brain, Behavior and Evolution* magazines, *Recent Developments in Autism Research* (Nova Biomedical Books, 2005), *Asperger's Disorder* (Medical Psychiatry Series) [Informa Healthcare, 2008], *Neocortical Modularity And The Cell Minicolumn* (Nova Biomedical Books, 2005)

Chauhan, Abha, Ved Chauhan, and Ted Brown, editors. *Autism: Oxidative Stress, Inflammation, and Immune Abnormalities*. CRC Press, 2009.

Chinitz, Judith Hope, *We Band of Mothers:Autism, My Son, and the Specific Carbohydrate Diet* (Autism Research Institute, 2007)

Davis, Dorinne S., *Every Day A Miracle: Success Stories through Sound Therapy*. Kalco Publishing LLC (October 6, 2004)

Davis, Dorinne. *Sound Bodies through Sound Therapy*. Kalco Publishing LLC, 2004.

Delaine, Susan K. *The Autism Cookbook: 101 Gluten-Free and Dairy-Free Recipes*. Skyhorse Publishing, 2010.

Fine, Aubrey, and Nya M. Fine, editors. *Therapeutic Recreation for Exceptional Children : Let Me In, I Want to Play*. Delta Society, 1996.

Fine and Eisen. *Afternoons with Puppy*. Purdue University Press 2008.

Fine, Aubrey. *The Handbook on Animal Assisted Therapy: Theoretical Foundations and Guidelines for Practice*. Academic Press, 1999.

Gabriels, R. "Art therapy with children who have autism and their families." *Handbook of art therapy*. Ed. C. Malchiodi. Guilford Press, 2003.

Goldberg, Michael J., with Elyse Goldberg. *The Myth of Autism: How a Misunderstood Epidemic Is Destroying Our Children*. Skyhorse Publishing, 2011.

Gottschall, Elaine G. *Breaking the Vicious Cycle: Intestinal Health Through Diet*. Kirkton Press, 1994.

Grandin, Temple and Catherine Johnson. *Animals in Translation Using the Mysteries of Autism to Decode Animal Behavior*. Houghton Mifflin Harcourt, 2005.

Greenspan, Stabley and Wieder, Serena. *Engaging Autism: Using the Floortime Approach to Help Children Relate, Communicate, and Think*. Da Capo Press, 2006.

Greenspan, Stanley, with Jacob Greenspan. *Overcoming ADHD: Helping Your Child Become Calm, Engaged, and Focused—Without a Pill*. Da Capo Lifelong Books, 2009.

Grinspoon, Lester, *Marihuana Reconsidered* (Harvard University press 1971, 1977, and American archives press classic edition, 1994) and *Marijuana, the Forbidden Medicine* (Yale University press, 1993, 1997)

Heflin, Juane, *Spectrum Disorders: Effective Instructional Practices* (Prentice Hall,2006)

Henley, D. R. *Exceptional children, exceptional art: Teaching art to special needs*. Worcester, MA: Davis Publications,1992.

Herskowitz, Valerie. *Autism & Computers: Maximizing Independence Through Technology*. AuthorHouse, 2009.

Heflin, L. Juane. *Students with Autism Spectrum Disorders: Effective Instructional Practices,* Prentice Hall, 2007.

Hogenboom, Marga. *Living with Genetic Syndromes Associated with Intellectual Disability*. Jessica Kingsley Publishers, 2001.

Jepson, Bryan Jepson. *Changing the Course of Autism: A Scientific Approach for Parents and Physicians*. Sentient Publications, 2007.

Kaufman, Barry Neil. *Son Rise: The Miracle Continues*. H J Kramer, 1994.

Kawar, Frick and Frick. *Astronaut Training: A Sound Activated Vestibular-Visual Protocol for Moving, Looking & Listening*. Vital Sounds LLC, 2006.

Kirby, David. *Evidence of Harm: Mercury in Vaccines and the Autism Epidemic: A Medical Controversy*. St. Martin's Press, 2005.

Lansky, Amy L. *Impossible Cure: The Promise of Homeopathy*. R.L. Ranch Press, 2003.

Lewis, Lisa. *Special Diets For Special Kids I & II*. Future Horizons, 2001.

Levinson, B. M. *Pet-oriented Child Psychotherapy*. Springfield, IL: Charles C. Thomas. 1969.

Lyons, Tony. *1,001 Tips for the Parents of Autistic Girls: Everything You Need to Know About Diagnosis, Doctors, Schools, Taxes, Vacations, Babysitters, Treatment, Food, and More*. Skyhorse Publishing, 2010.

Marohn, Stephanie. *The Natural Medicine Guide to Autism*. Hampton Roads Pub Co, 2002.

Martin, Nicole. *Art as an Early Intervention Tool for Children with Autism*. Jessica Kingsley Publishers, 2009.

Matthews, Julie. *Nourishing Hope for Autism: Nutrition Intervention for Healing Our Children, 3rd ed*. Healthful Living Media, 2008.

Maurice, Catherine. *Let Me Hear Your Voice: A Family's Triumph over Autism*. Ballantine Books, 1994.

McCandless, Jaquelyn. *Children with Starving Brains: A Medical Treatment Guide for Autism Spectrum Disorder, 4th ed*. Bramble Books, 2009.

McCarthy, Jenny and Jerry Kartzinel. *Healing and Preventing Autism: A Complete Guide*. Penguin, 2009.

McCarthy, Jenny. *Louder Than Words: A Mother's Journey in Healing Autism*. Penguin, 2007.

McCarthy, Jenny. *Mother Warriors*. Penguin, 2008.

Mehl-Madrona, Lewis, *Coyote Medicine* (Touchstone, 1998), *Coyote Healing* (Bear & Company, 2003) *Coyote Wisdom* (Bear & Company, 2005) *Narrative Medicine* (Bear & Company, 2007) and *Healing the Mind through the Power of Story: The Promise of Narrative Psychiatry* (Bear & Company (June 15, 2010)).

Noble, J. "Art as an instrument for creating social reciprocity: Social skills group for children with autism." *Group process made visible: Group art therapy*. Ed. S. Riley. Brunner-Routledge, 2001.

Pereira, Lavinia, and Solomon Michelle, *First Sound Series* by Trafford Publishing

Prizant, Barry, Amy Wetherby, Emily Rubin, Amy Laurent and P. Rydell. *The SCERTS Model: A Comprehensive Educational Approach for Children with Autism Spectrum Disorders*. Baltimore, MD: Paul H. Brookes Publishing, 2006.

Rimland, Bernard. *Infantile Autism: The Syndrome and Its Implication for a Neural Theory of Behavior.* Prentice Hall,1964.

Rimland, Bernard, Jon Pangborn, Sidney Baker. *Autism: Effective Biomedical Treatments (Have We Done Everything We Can For This Child? Individuality In An Epidemic)*. Autism Research Institute, 2005.

Rimland, Bernard, Jon Pangborn, Sidney Baker. *2007 Supplement - Autism: Effective Biomedical Treatments (Have We Done Everything We Can for This Child? Individuality In An Epidemic)*. Autism Research Institute, 2007.

Robbins, Jim. *A Symphony in the Brain: The Evolution of the New Brain Wave Biofeedback.* Grove Press, 2008.

Rogers, Sally J. and Geraldine Dawson. *Early Start Denver Model For Young Children With Autism: Promoting Language, Learning, And Engagement*. Guilford Press, 2009.

Seroussi, Karyn. *Unraveling the Mystery of Autism and Pervasive Developmental Disorders*. Simon & Schuster, 2000.

Seroussi, Karyn and Lisa Lewis. *The Encyclopedia of Dietary Interventions for the Treatment of Autism and Related Disorders*. Sarpsborg Press, 2008.

Sicile-Kira, Chantal. *Autism Spectrum Disorders: The Complete Guide to Understanding Autism, Asperger's Syndrome, Pervasive Developmental Disorder, and Other ASDs*. Penguin, 2004.

Sicile-Kira, Chantal. *Adolescents on the Autism Spectrum: A Parent's Guide to the Cognitive, Social, Physical, and Transition Needs of Teenagers with Autism Spectrum Disorders*. Penguin, 2006.

Sicile-Kira, Chantal. *Autism Life Skills: From Communication and Safety to Self-Esteem and More - 10 Essential Abilities Every Child Needs and Deserves to Learn*. Penguin, 2008.

Silva, Louisa. *Helping your Child with Autism: A Home Program from Chinese Medicine*. Guan Yin Press, 2010.

Silver, R. A. *Developing cognitive and creative skills through art: Programs for children with communication disorders or learning disabilities* (3rd ed. revised). New York: Albin Press 1989.

Siri, Kenneth, *1001 Tips for Parents of Autistic Boys*. Skyhorse Publishing, 2010.

Stagliano, Kim. *All I Can Handle: I'm No Mother Teresa: A Life Raising Three Daughters with Autism*. Skyhorse Publishing, 2010.

Theoharides, Theoharis C., *Pharmacology* (Essentials of Basic Science) (Little Brown and Company, 1992) *Essentials of Pharmacology* (Essentials of Basic Science) (Lippincott Williams & Wilkins, 1996)

Wiseman, Nancy D. *The First Year: Autism Spectrum Disorders: An Essential Guide for the Newly Diagnosed Child*. Da Capo Lifelong Books, 2009.

Wolfberg, Pamela J. *Play and Imagination in Children with Autism, 2nd ed*. Autism Asperger Publishing Company, 2009.

Woodward, Bob and Marga Hogenboom. *Autism: A Holistic Approach*. Floris Books, 2001.

Yasko, Amy. *Autism: Pathways to Recovery*. Neurological Research Institute, 2009.

Yasko, Amy. *Genetic Bypass: Using Nutrition to Bypass Genetic Mutations*. Neurological Research Institute, 2005.

Index

Adaptive Behavior, 17, 37, 202-204, 207, 324
Aggression, 29, 66, 68, 71, 78, 90, 95, 140, 143-144, 151, 168-170, 190, 222, 229-230, 313, 341, 372, 382
Allergic, 4, 151
conditions, 420
diseases, 118
disorders, 7, 215
reaction(s), 3-4, 8-9, 24, 26, 151, 284, 286, 308-309
response, 8
rhinitis, 7
sensitivity, 174
skin reaction, 52
symptomatology, 7-8
symptoms, 3, 7-9, 11
triggers, 4
Allergies, 2-5, 7-8, 11, 58, 207, 269-270, 286, 309, 311-312, 350
dairy, 69 See also Dairy
food, 8, 118, 128, 147, 270, 286 See also Food Intolerance
respiratory, 421
symptoms of, 8
treatment of, 3
Allergy, 5, 8, 151, 175
attack, 186
desensitization, 2-3
food, 3, 7-8, 69 See also Food Intolerance
groups, 271
injections, 4
non-IgE food allergy, 7
reactions, 3
shots, 3
symptoms (of), 2-4, 6, 421
test(s)(ing), 3-5, 7-8, 151
Androgen(s), 140-143
elevated levels, 140-145
production, 141
-related conditions, 145
Animal-Assisted Activities (AAA), 15
Interventions (AAI), 13, 15-16
Therapy (AAT), 12, 15, 17
Anti-androgen medication, 143-144 See also Medication
therapy, 144-145
Antibiotics, xii-xiv, 29, 67-68, 124, 173, 221, 281, 420, 422-423
decreasing use of, 284
exposure to, 29
oral, 97, 100
prophylactic, 219, 221
treatments with, 34
Antiepileptic,
adverse effects of, 24
drugs, 24-26
medication, 23-24, 26
Treatments, 23-24
Antifungal(s), 31 -32, 67-70, 173, 272, 281
drug, 31, 34
effect, 32
medication, 32, 271
properties, 31
regiments, 32
therapy, 211
treatment, 28, 32
Antihistamines, 3, 7

Anthroposophy, 77-78, 85
Applied Behavior Analysis (ABA), xvi-xvii, 35-41, 56, 88, 90-95, 134, 159, 207, 241-244, 246, 327-328, 348, 358, 360-361, 382, 401
Journal of, 87, 92, 158
therapies, 39, 399
Applied Verbal Behavior (AVB), 40
Aquatic Therapy, 42-43, 47
University, 47
Arranga, Teri, 435
Art Therapy, 56-59, 83
art therapist, 56-59
Augmentative and Alternative Communication (AAC), 353, 357, 363, 369-373, 375-377, 383
AutismTrack, 379, 381-382
Bailey, Sally, 129
Baruth, Joshua , 402
Beacon Day School, 202-203
Becker, Dr. Jeffrey, 412
Beckman Oral Motor, 348, 353
Berkley, Alison, 72, 327-328, 333-334
Berard Auditory Integration Training, 61, 340
Betts, Dr. Donna, 56
Betz, Dr. Alison, 92
Biofilm Protocol, 66, 68, 313
Biological Therapies, 28
Biome Depletion Theory, The, 175
Bleecker, Tim, 152
Bolles, Mary, 335
Bradstreet, Dr. James, 417
Brain Inflammation, 192, 419, 421, 423-424
Brockett, Dr. Sally, 61, 64
Camphill Communities, The, 76-77, 85
Cannabis, 229-234
Center for Autism and Related Disorders (CARD), 35, 40-41, 86-87, 90-91, 147
eLearning, 86-88, 90-91
Cellular Reprogramming Therapy, 188
Chapple, Dr. Charles, 101
Chelation, 97-99, 211, 289-290
agents, 189
Cherry, Cathy Purple , 48
Chinitz, Judith, 121, 171
Chiropractic Therapy, 101
Clark, Jenifer, 241
Collins, Meghan, 305
Computer-Based Intervention (CBI), 363-365, 367
Coppin, Rachel, 363, 383
Core Muscle Weakness, 306
Coyle, Mary 191
Craniosacral Therapy, 101-102
Critical Thinking, 330
Crohn's Disease, 165, 167-169, 226, 420-421
Curative Education, 77, 81
Dairy, 68, 115, 118-120, 126, 147, 214, 250, 271
allergies, 69 See also Allergies
foods, 147
-free diet, 282 See also Diet
intolerance, 67
products, 147, 212-213, 271

Dance/Movement Therapy (DMT), 109-113, 389
Davis, Dorinne, 339
Davis, Dr. Georgia A., 308
Davis Model of Sound Intervention, 339, 341, 345, 347
Dawson, Dr. Geraldine, 133
Denver Model, 134
Detoxification, 114, 187-189, 284, 286-289, 309, 435
detox 192
detoxifiers, 289
detoxify, 252, 286
detoxing, 347
reaction, 71
Development(al)
ladder, 152-153, 157
milestones, 153, 254, 306, 320-321, 338, 350
models, 241, 246
motor, 104, 202, 305
perceptual motor, 111
sensorimotor, 112
Diet(s), 2, 26-27, 30, 34, 67, 83, 114-116, 118-122, 124-128, 147, 151, 168, 171, 189-190, 211, 254-256, 271, 280-283, 285, 313, 381, 422, 424, 432
Body Ecology Diet, 115
dairy-free, 282 See also Dairy
dietetic measures, 121
elimination(s), 27, 272, 309
GF/CF, 115, 147, 224, 281-282
gluten-free, 58, 114-115, 128
ketogenic, 26-27, 255-256
liquid, 314
low carbohydrate, 26, 127, 255
low-oxalate, 30, 115
restricted(ive), 115, 168
restrictions, 58, 350
sensory, 205, 293
Specific Carbohydrate Diet, 69, 115, 121-122, 124-127, 171, 281, 424
therapeutic, 149-150
yeast-free, 31
Dietary
changes, 27, 424
formulation, 9
infractions, 313-314
interventions, xvii, 34, 83, 114-115, 120-121, 149, 167, 207
modulation, 124
options, 211
requirements, 119
restriction, 124, 128, 224
sugar, 31
supplement(s), 10, 148, 212, 216, 281-283, 285
supports, 81
treatment, 26, 122
Digestive 126-127, 214
deficiencies, 432
difficulties, 28
discomforts, 285
disorders, 177, 179
disturbances, 81, 83
enzyme(s), 69, 146, 148, 150-151, 281, 283, 285, 288 See also Enzyme

functioning, 176
issues, 122
juices, 71
problems, 68, 148, 179
process(es), 83, 125, 147, 179, 283
sensitivities, 151
support, 146
symptoms, 28
system(s), 122, 125, 151, 172, 280
tract, 28, 150, 283
Discrete Trial Training (DTT), 37, 40, 95
Drama Therapy, 129-132, 389
Drugs, xi, xvi, 11, 32, 147, 188, 215-216, 225, 229-230, 232-233, 254, 281, 289, 392, 430
anti-allergic, 9
antiepileptic, 24-26 See also Antiepileptic
antifungal, 31
antipsychotic, 228-229
Cellceutix KM-391, 430-431,
Curemark, LLC CM-AT, 430, 432
hypnotic, 236
long-term effects of, 229
pharmaceutical, 230
psychotropic, 169
Seaside Therapeutics STX 209, 430, 433-434
steroid, 3, 9, 26, 226, 254, 418
Early Intervention Program, 92-94, 294
Early Start Denver Model (ESDM), 133-138
Elice, Dr. Michael, 217
Emerge and See, 72, 327
EnListen, 343
Enzymes
digestive, 69, 146, 148, 150-151, 281, 283, 285, 288 See also Digestive
Enzymatic System, 194
Equine-Assisted Therapy, 15-16
Fasano, Dr. Alessio, 210
Fast ForWord, 345, 365
Fine, Dr. Aubrey H., 12
Floortime, 72, 152-153, 156-157, 291, 327-328, 348
Food Intolerance, 7, 118, 147, 151
feeding disorders, 87, 158-159, 162
food allergy, 3, 7-8, 69 See also Allergy
food selectivity, 158,
selective eating behavior, 159
Friedman, Amanda, 72, 327-328, 331
Frye, Dr. Richard E., 23, 253
Functional Communication Training (FCT), 38
Gastrointestinal (GI)
abnormalities, 254-255
ailments, 165
cause, 169
complaint(s), 163, 165
diagnosis(es), 169-170
disease, 163-164, 168, 170
disorders, 26, 226, 280-281
disturbances, 280

dysfunction, 68
evaluation, 170, 281, 285
function, 144
inflammation, 418
issues, 67-69, 97, 284, 286
pain, 285
pathology, 165-166, 435-436
problem(s), 3, 144-145, 163-165, 280-281, 284
side-effects, 24
stress, 192
symptoms, 11, 25, 163-164, 166, 168, 211, 281
system, xx, 151, 254, 280, 435
tract, xvii, xx, 67, 71, 166, 172, 188, 211, 280, 284
treatments, 211
ulceration, 26
Geier, David A., 139
Geier, Dr. Mark R., 139-140
Gemmotherapy, 188
Gluten, 68, 71, 114-117, 120, 147, 211, 224, 313-314, 350, 424 See also Diet
-free diet, 58, 147, 281, 350
Goldberg, Dr. Michael, 268
Gonzalez, Kristin Selby, 149
Granpeesheh, Dr. Doreen, 35-36, 86-87
Greenspan, Jake, 152
Griffin, Cindy, 190
Grinspoon, Dr. Lester, 228
Gut-Brain Connection, 280, 417, 419
Gut Inflammation, 123, 225-226, 422
Handhold Adaptive, 379, 381-382
Hanen Approach, The, 352
Heflin, Dr. L. Juane, 323
Helminthic Therapy, 171, 421
helminths, 173-175, 420-421
Herskowitz, Valerie, 363-364
Hippotherapy, 16, 388
Hogenboom, Dr. Marga, 76
Holistic Approach to Neurodevelopment and Learning Efficiency, The (HANDLE), 178-183
Homeopathy, 2, 184-187, 190-191
homeopathic remedies
Houston Homeopathy Method, 184-185, 188, 190
Sequential, 184-185, 187-188, 190-191
Homeostasis, 122, 187
Homotoxicology, 188, 191-196
Horse(s), 15-16, 19-21, 83, 375, 387-389 See also Equine-Assisted Therapy and Therapeutic Horseback Riding
Houston, Dr. Devin, 146,
Human BioAcoustics, 346
Hygiene Hypothesis, 173-174, 176
Hynes, Laura, 315
Immune, 270
aberrations, 418
abnormalities, 30, 171
activation, 418
activity, 420
allergic response, 8
balance, 423

barrier function, 284
benefit, 225
biasing, 420
boosting nutrients, 287
cells, 8, 171
cytokines, 174
defenses, 122
deficiencies, 286
disorder(s), 7, 174, 177
dysfunction, 2-3, 192, 254, 282
dysfunctional state, 271
dysregulation, 68, 268, 418, 421, 423, 435-436
effects, 280
enhancer, 225
environments, 424
function(ing), 2-3, 172-173, 195, 226, 275, 286, 419
inflammatory cells, 211
inflammatory condition, 66
issues, 284
mechanisms, 3
mediated diseases, 420
mediated disorder(s), 269
panel, 270
parameters, 224
pathways, 174
problems, xiii, xvii, xx, 2, 269, 286-287
process, 270
programming, 420
reactions, 5
related, 286
response(s), 30, 123, 283-284, 287, 289, 418, 424
signaling, 172
status, 224
stressed, 269
stimulation, 174
system(s), xiv, 3, 9, 29-30, 34, 67-68, 122-123, 151, 171-174, 176, 183, 187-188, 220, 224, 226, 254, 269-272, 275-277, 280, 283, 286-287, 308, 421-422, 435
Immunotherapy, 2-7
subcutaneous (SCIT), 3
sublingual (SLIT), 3-5
Individualized Education Program (IEP), 59, 203
Ingels, Dr. Darin, 2
Integrated Play Groups, 198
Integrative(Integrated)
Educational
care, 202
model, 203-204
Interactive Metronome, 346
iPrompts, 363, 379, 380
Jan, Dr. James, 235
Jarrow, Markus, 291
Kaufman, Nancy R., 359
Kaufman Speech to Language Protocol (K-SLP), 359, 361-362
Kmetz, Leah, 257
Kodak, Dr. Tiffany, 92
Krigsman, Dr. Arthur, 163, 166
Lang, Dr. Mary Joann, 202
Lanham, Lindyl, 184-185, 190
Leaky Gut, 210-212, 284, 288
LeFeber, Mariah Meyer, 109
Lovaas Therapy, 39
Low Dose Naltrexone (LDN), 224-227
Low Muscle Tone, 179, 299, 306, 338, 360

Martin, Nicole, 56
Mast Cell Activation, 7-9, 11
Idiopathic mast cell activation disorder, 7
non-clonal mast cell activation syndrome, 7
Mastocytosis, 7-8, 11
McCandless, Dr. Jaquelyn, 224
Medication(s)
anti-androgen, 143-144
See also Anti-androgen
antiepileptic, 23 See also Antiepileptic
antifungal, 32, 271 See also Antifungal
discontinuation, 36, 308
discontinuing, 310-311, 313
non-antiepileptic, 23
psychotropic, 60, 308, 312-313
Medicinal Marijuana, 228
marijuana, 229-234
Mehl-Madrona, Dr. Lewis, 28, 387
Melatonin, 235-240, 285, 312
Therapy, 235-240
Mentalization Enhanced Remediation Integrated Treatment (MERIT), 241-244, 247
Methyl-B12, 249-252
Microbiome, 211-212, 417-424
Medicinal Marijuana
Moraine, Paula, 76
Movement-Based Activities, 331-333
Munroe-Meyer Institute, 92-94, 158-159
Murphy, Patti, 363, 369
Music Therapy, 257-261, 389, 393
Najdowski, Dr. Adel C., 87
Natural Environment Training (NET), 37, 39-40
Neubrander, Dr. James, 248
Neurofeedback, 262-267
Neuroimmune Dysfunction, 268-269
Newman, Larry, 279
Nutrigenomics, 273-274
Nuyens, Carolyn, 178
Occupational Therapy, 17, 159, 203, 291-292, 294, 335
Oligotherapy, 188
Oral-Motor Therapy, 352
Othmer Ph.D., Siegfried, 262
Othmer, Susan F., 262
Parasite Therapy, 171, 176-177, 211
Pediatric Feeding Disorder Program, 93
Pereira, Lavinia, 348
Pet Therapy, 15 See also Animal-Assisted Therapy, Animal-Assisted Intervention, Equine-Assisted Intervention, Therapeutic Horseback Riding
Physical Therapy, xvii, 42, 305-307, 340, 412
Piazza, Dr. Cathleen, 158
Picture Exchange Communication System (PECS), 40, 260, 353-354, 357, 370
Pivotal Response Training (PRT), 37, 39-40, 134

Probiotics, 31, 67, 69, 71, 124-125, 210, 212-213, 215-216, 281, 284-285, 309, 313-314, 421, 422, 424
Proloquo2Go, 363, 383-386
PROMPT (Prompts for Restructuring Oral Muscular Phonetic Targets) Treatment, 134, 348, 352
Puente, Ph.D. Lauren Tobing, 300
Rogers, Dr. Sally, 133
Salzman, Andrea, 42
Samonas Method, The, 344
Schneider, Dr. Harry, 394
Sensory
gym, 72, 293-294, 327, 329
integration therapy, xvii, 65, 205, 293, 297
Sensory-Based Antecedent Interventions, 323
Sensory Learning Program, The, 335-338
Sentence Developer, 366
Sequential Therapy, 187, 190
Siri, Ken, x, xviii, 66
Sleep
disorders, 68, 235-236, 238
disturbances, 3, 71, 176, 236-237
regulation, 235
Social Therapy, 77
Solomon, Michelle, 348
Sound-Based Therapies, 339-341, 343, 346-347
Speech-Language
Therapy, 348, 350, 376
Pathologist, 90, 158-159, 348-358, 360, 369, 376-377, 383
Spotlight Program, The, 131
Sulfation, 283, 287-288
Suliteanu, Marlene, 178
Sykes, Lisa, 139
TalkTools Therapy, 352, 360
Tarbox, Jonathan, 35
Technological-Based Interventions, 363
Tedesco, Robert C., 379
Theoharides, Dr. Theoharis, 6
Therapeutic (Horseback) Riding, 15-16, 19-21, 83 See also Animal-Assisted Intervention, Animal-Assisted Therapy, Equine-Assisted Therapy, Pet Therapy
Thompson, Meghan, 430
Tomatis Method, The, 342-343
Transcranial Direct-Current Stimulation (tDCS), 395, 398-399, 401
Transcraniel Magnetic Stimulation, 402, 404
TSO, 175-177, 421, 424
Van Rie, Ginny, 323
Vaz, Dr. Petula, 158
Verbal Behavior Analysis (VBA), 40
Vision Therapy, 65, 335, 412, 414, 416
Vismara, Dr. Laurie, 133, 137
Wolfberg, Dr. Pamela, 198-199
Yasko, Dr. Amy, 273